Social Behaviour

Genes, Ecology and Evolution

Humans live in large and extensive societies and spend much of their time interacting socially. Likewise, most other animals also interact socially. Social behaviour is a source of constant fascination to biologists and psychologists of many disciplines; from behavioural ecology to comparative biology and sociobiology. The two major approaches used to study social behaviour involve either the mechanism of behaviour – where it has come from and how it has evolved – or the function of the behaviour studied. Featuring guest contributions from leaders in the field, this book presents both theoretical foundations and recent advances to give a truly multidiscplinary overview of social behaviour for advanced undergraduate and graduate students. Topics include aggression, communication, group living, sexual behaviour and cooperative breeding. With examples ranging from bacteria to social mammals including humans, a variety of research tools are used, including candidate gene approaches, quantitative genetics, neuroendocrine studies, cost–benefit and phylogenetic analyses and evolutionary game theory.

Tamás Székely is an evolutionary biologist with a main research interest in breeding system evolution. Most of his work uses birds as model organisms, studied mostly through field work but also with the use of mathematical modelling and phylogenetic analyses to dissect behaviour. He has co-edited four books, including one on sex, size and gender roles. He is Professor of Biodiversity at the University of Bath, and was recently awarded a research fellowship by the Leverhulme Trust. He has also been a visiting fellow at Harvard University.

Allen J. Moore is an evolutionary biologist whose research interests include quantitative genetic studies of behaviour and morphology, the development of behaviour, theoretical investigations of evolution and behavioural ecology. He is Professor of Evolutionary Genetics at the University of Exeter, as well as head of school and director of the university's Centre for Ecology and Conservation. He is a former secretary of the Society for the Study of Evolution, and is currently editor-in-chief of the *Journal of Evolutionary Biology*.

Jan Komdeur has a strong reputation in experimental evolutionary ecology. He established the Seychelles warbler as a model system, and his many long-standing international collaborations with leading biologists connect aspects of behavioural ecology, population genetics and theoretical modelling. He has published many papers in international journals, serves on several editorial boards, and has received a number of prestigious international awards and grants. He is Professor of Avian Evolutionary Ecology at the University of Groningen and Director of the Top Master's programme in evolutionary ecology.

Social Behaviour

Genes, Ecology and Evolution

Edited by

Tamás Székely
University of Bath

Allen J. Moore
University of Exeter

Jan Komdeur
University of Groningen

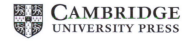
CAMBRIDGE
UNIVERSITY PRESS

CAMBRIDGE UNIVERSITY PRESS
Cambridge, New York, Melbourne, Madrid, Cape Town, Singapore,
São Paulo, Delhi, Dubai, Tokyo, Mexico City

Cambridge University Press
The Edinburgh Building, Cambridge CB2 8RU, UK

Published in the United States of America by
Cambridge University Press, New York

www.cambridge.org
Information on this title: www.cambridge.org/9780521883177

First published 2010

Printed in the United Kingdom at the University Press, Cambridge

A catalogue record for this publication is available from the British Library

Library of Congress Cataloguing in Publication data
Social behaviour : genes, ecology and evolution / [edited by] Tamás Székely, Allen J. Moore, Jan Komdeur.
p. ; cm.
Includes bibliographical references and index.
ISBN 978-0-521-88317-7 (hardback) – ISBN 978-0-521-70962-0 (pbk.)
1. Sociobiology. 2. Social interaction. 3. Behavior evolution.
4. Behavior genetics. I. Székely, T. (Tamás) II. Moore, Allen J. (Allen Jonathan) III. Komdeur, J. IV. Title.
[DNLM: 1. Social Behavior. 2. Ecology. 3. Evolution. 4. Genetics, Behavioral. HM 1106]
HM628.S63 2010
304.5–dc22   2010027383

ISBN 978-0-521-88317-7 Hardback
ISBN 978-0-521-70962-0 Paperback

Contents

Contributors

Elizabeth Adkins-Regan
Department of Psychology, Cornell University, Ithaca,
New York, USA

Suzanne H. Alonzo
Department of Ecology and Evolutionary Biology,
Yale University, New Haven, Connecticut, USA

Leanna M. Birge
Department of Biology, University of Maryland,
College Park, Maryland, USA

Tim Birkhead
Department of Animal and Plant Sciences,
University of Sheffield, UK

Bronwyn H. Bleakley
School of Biosciences, University of Exeter, UK

Daniel T. Blumstein
Department of Ecology and Evolutionary Biology,
University of California Los Angeles, California, USA

Russell Bonduriansky
School of Biological, Earth and Environmental Sciences,
University of New South Wales, Sydney, Australia

Andrew Cockburn
Evolutionary Ecology Group, School of Botany and
Zoology, Australian National University, Canberra,
Australia

Nicholas B. Davies
Department of Zoology, University of Cambridge, UK

Timothy J. DeVoogd
Department of Psychology, Cornell University, Ithaca, New York, USA

Niels J. Dingemanse
Animal Ecology Group, University of Groningen, the Netherlands

Marion L. East
Institute for Zoo and Wildlife Research, Berlin, Germany

Jan Ekman
Department of Ecology and Evolution, Uppsala University, Sweden

Kevin R. Foster
Center for Systems Biology, Harvard University, Cambridge, Massachusetts, USA

Robert P. Freckleton
Department of Animal and Plant Science, University of Sheffield, UK

Raghavendra Gadagkar
Centre for Ecological Sciences, Indian Institute of Science, Bangalore, India

Louise Gallagher
Department of Psychiatry, University of Dublin, Trinity College, Dublin, Ireland

Andy Gardner
Department of Zoology, University of Oxford, UK

David Haig
Museum of Comparative Zoology, Harvard University, Cambridge, Massachusetts, USA

Mark E. Hauber
School of Biological Sciences, University of Auckland, New Zealand

Heribert Hofer
Institute for Zoo and Wildlife Research, Berlin, Germany

Bert Hölldobler
School of Life Sciences, Arizona State University, Tempe, Arizona, USA

Alasdair I. Houston
School of Biological Sciences, University of Bristol, UK

Sarah B. Hrdy
Department of Anthropology, University of California Davis, California, USA

Robert Huber
Biological Sciences, Bowling Green State University, Ohio, USA

Laurent Keller
Department of Ecology and Evolution, University of Lausanne, Switzerland

Jan Komdeur
Animal Ecology Group, University of Groningen, the Netherlands

Jens Krause
Faculty of Biological Sciences, University of Leeds, UK

Edward A. Kravitz
Department of Neurobiology, Harvard Medical School, Boston, Massachusetts, USA

Joel D. Levine
Department of Biology, University of Toronto at Mississauga, Ontario, Canada

Ruth Mace
Department of Anthropology, University College London, UK

Lisa McGraw
Yerkes National Primate Research Center, Emory University School of Medicine, Atlanta, Georgia, USA

John M. McNamara
Department of Mathematics, University of Bristol, UK

Manfred Milinski
Max Planck Institute for Evolutionary Biology, Plön, Germany

Allen J. Moore
School of Biosciences, University of Exeter, UK

Jordan M. Moore
Department of Psychology, Cornell University, Ithaca, New York, USA

Ronald Noë
Ethologie des Primates, Université Louis-Pasteur, Strasbourg, France

Mark Pagel
School of Biological Sciences, University of Reading, UK

Geoff A. Parker
School of Biological Sciences, University of Liverpool, UK

Marion Petrie
Evolutionary Biology Group, Institute of Neuroscience, Newcastle University, UK

Tommaso Pizzari
Department of Zoology, University of Oxford, UK

David C. Queller
Department of Ecology and Evolutionary Biology, Rice University, Houston, Texas, USA

Paul B. Rainey
New Zealand Institute for Advanced Study, Biosciences, Massey University, Auckland, New Zealand

Denis Réale
Département des sciences biologiques, Université du Québec à Montréal, Canada

Michael G. Ritchie
School of Biology, University of St Andrews, UK

Gene E. Robinson
Department of Entomology, University of Illinois at Urbana-Champaign, Illinois, USA

Graeme Ruxton
Division of Environmental & Evolutionary Biology, University of Glasgow, UK

Ben C. Sheldon
Department of Zoology, University of Oxford, UK

Paul W. Sherman
Department of Neurobiology and Behavior, Cornell University, Ithaca, NY, USA

Laura K. Sirot
Department of Molecular Biology and Genetics, Cornell University, Ithaca, New York, USA

David Skuse
Behaviour and Brain Sciences Unit, Institute of Child Health, London, UK

Marla B. Sokolowski
Department of Biology, University of Toronto at Mississauga, Ontario, Canada

Tamás Székely
Department of Biology and Biochemistry, University of Bath, UK

Michael Taborsky
Department of Behavioural Ecology, University of Bern, Switzerland

Robert Trivers
Department of Anthropology, Rutgers University, New Brunswick, New Jersey, USA

Franz J. Weissing
Centre for Ecological and Evolutionary Studies, University of Groningen, the Netherlands

Tom Wenseleers
Zoological Institute, Catholic University of Leuven, Belgium

Gerald S. Wilkinson
Department of Biology, University of Maryland,
College Park, Maryland, USA

Edward O. Wilson
Museum of Comparative Zoology, Harvard University,
Cambridge, Massachusetts, USA

Jason B. Wolf
Faculty of Life Sciences, University of Manchester, UK

Mariana F. Wolfner
Department of Molecular Biology and Genetics, Cornell
University, Ithaca, New York, USA

Alex Wong
Department of Biology, University of Ottawa, Ontario,
Canada

Larry J. Young
Yerkes National Primate Research Center, Emory
University School of Medicine, Atlanta, Georgia, USA

Amotz Zahavi
Department of Zoology, Tel Aviv University, Israel

Marlene Zuk
Department of Biology, University of California,
Riverside, California, USA

Introduction
The uphill climb of sociobiology: towards a new synthesis

Tamás Székely, Allen J. Moore and Jan Komdeur

Social behaviour garners broad interest: biologists, social scientists, psychologists and economists all incorporate a consideration of social behaviour in their studies. This breadth of interest is unsurprising, as the vast majority of animals (and all that reproduce sexually) live partly (or fully) in social environments. As Robert Trivers (1985) succinctly put it, 'Everybody has a social life.' Some of this interest undoubtedly emerges because members of our own species (*Homo sapiens*) live in extensive societies and spend much time interacting with each other. Yet you do not have to be human for social behaviour to have a strong influence on biological processes. The significance of social behaviour is easy to see: if you isolate an ant, a fish or a bird from its peers in a sort of Kaspar Hauser setup, within a short time many of its 'normal' behaviours will change and be impaired. Social behaviour, heuristically defined as activities among members of the same species that have fitness consequences for both the focal individual and other individuals in the group, is thus ubiquitous.

The perplexing causes and far-reaching implications of social behaviour make it a rich subject to help understand evolution (Gardner & Foster 2008). The understanding of social evolution is challenging, given that social behaviour is often costly. Furthermore, unlike many traits that are passively selected by the environment, in the context of social behaviour the animals create selection for themselves by interacting with each other. This added complexity requires

more complex models and clever experiments to disentangle cause and effect. Although the study of social behaviour goes back thousands of years (Dugatkin 1997), it is this complexity arising from interactions that fascinates evolutionary biologists.

Our enthusiasm for social behaviour led us to discuss the various ways we can study and understand social behaviour among animals. In 2006 the three of us drafted an outline of an ambitious book, and contacted Cambridge University Press with the outline. Our main motivation was the lack of a comprehensive volume that would cover both proximate and ultimate aspects of social behaviour, and go beyond taxon-specific treatises on some of the workhorses of social evolution (e.g. social insects, birds and mammals). Social behaviour has come a long way since the pioneering papers of Hamilton (1964) and Maynard Smith and Price (1973), and the landmark syntheses of Wilson (1975) and Trivers (1985). Given the stimulus of these papers and books, researchers investigated social behaviour with renewed vigour. Furthermore, the subsequent decades have applied new tools and new perspectives, and have gained new insights: advances in molecular genetics, neurobiology, mathematical theories of social behaviour and phylogenetic methods fundamentally changed the way we study animal behaviour, and what we know about social traits. We thought that to further advance sociobiology would require a comprehensive book which provides an overview of theoretical foundations and recent advances, and looks at implications beyond evolutionary biology.

E. O. Wilson (1975) defined sociobiology as a 'systematic study of the biological basis of all social behavior'. Sociobiology was created by population biologists and zoologists, and indeed Wilson wrote his tome as a true synthesis with the aim of pulling together theory and empirical data for (primarily) vertebrate social behaviour, having covered insect behaviour in an earlier book (Wilson 1971). For this reason, most scholars consider sociobiology sitting conveniently within the broad field of population biology. The agenda we set in this book, however, is broader and explicitly embraces genetics, developmental biology and physiology. We take Wilson's definition literally, and argue that investigation of any trait that has a bearing on social behaviour should justly be called *sociobiology*. Therefore, a developmental biologist who studies limb development may be labelled as a sociobiologist, if his/her objective is to understand how limb development and locomotion contributes to social traits – for instance, group foraging. Therefore, we view sociobiology as any aspect of evolutionary biology research that targets social traits.

Sociobiology is in the midst of a major paradigm shift. Early ethologists such as Konrad Lorenz, Niko Tinbergen, Karl von Frisch and their students provided a scientific basis of social behaviour by investigating group and family life, fighting, communication, display behaviours and mating. This ethological paradigm later split into studies of mechanisms (neuroethology, behavioural genetics) and function (behavioural ecology, sociobiology), as predicted by E. O. Wilson (1975). The two distinct approaches are now moving back towards each other. On the one hand, behavioural ecologists have begun to realise that functions cannot be fully understood without an appreciation of underlying mechanisms. For example, where traditionally behavioural ecologists studied how parents influence their offspring through nest attendance and feeding, modern researchers might investigate the same problem by considering the constituents of the egg in which the embryo developed, the architecture of the nest and how it influences physiological processes, and basic biochemical processes such as the role of antioxidants in offspring and parent fitness. Furthermore, there is an increasing interest in how these factors might interact and intersect.

On the other hand, geneticists, developmental behavioural biologists and neuroscientists are beginning to acknowledge that many of the genetic/genomic/neural processes may not make sense unless they are placed into an ecological context. There is a recognition that we need to understand the selective processes to which animals are subject in their natural environment. The most exciting studies of proximate influences on behaviour examine the interactions between the genome, development and the environment. We believe that investigating behaviour from this integrative perspective will lead our understanding of *eco-evo-devo*: the interplay between ecology, evolution, genes and development.

We have three major objectives with this book. Our first is to provide an overview of proximate and ultimate approaches to social behaviour. Social behaviour is all too often branded as a field dominated by behavioural ecologists, evolutionary psychologists and theoretical evolutionary biologists. We believe this perception is mistaken, because what makes social behaviour exciting is its fundamentally multidimensional nature. By contrasting examples from both mechanism and function, we anticipate that novel syntheses will emerge. For this reason, we have selected contributors who investigate organisms ranging from bacteria to humans, and who use a variety of research tools including a candidate gene approach, quantitative genetics, neuroendocrine studies, ecological studies of cost–benefit analyses, evolutionary game theory and phylogenetic analyses.

Our second objective is to produce an accessible overview of key topics in social behaviour for all students of behaviour, both academic and non-academic. Social behaviour appeals to a broad audience in diverse biological fields and beyond biology: for instance, clinical scientists, psychiatrists and philosophers of science may find some chapters useful. Although the target audience for each chapter is undoubtedly the research field in which the authors work, we asked contributors to make their review broad. We hope that the book's accessible style will elicit cross-fertilisation between varied disciplines.

Finally, we also hope to inspire the new generation of students and young scientists. To fulfil this goal, we invited 21 guests to explain why they are interested in social behaviour. These guest profiles are short personal accounts from some of the most influential researchers in the field of social behaviour. Scientists are notorious for avoiding public attention; indeed, a major part of the scientific tradition is to remain objective, impersonal and neutral. However, this often hides extraordinary personalities, and conceals the persistence that drives many of us to study what we believe is interesting or important. The reader may find common themes among the elite of behaviour researchers. Those who have successfully altered how we view behaviour were often driven by pure curiosity. In an age where 'accountability' is increasingly used to mean 'applied' in research, it is refreshing to see that the main motivation for many researchers is a love of their subject, the organisms they study, or both.

When we embarked on this project, we were also hoping to establish common principles (or even a unifying theory) of social behaviour. We quickly realised, however, that our ambition could be only partially fulfilled (see Chapter 21). First, the field has expanded enormously since 1975, and each topic for which we envisaged one chapter would be more realistically covered by a whole book, or a set of books. Second, we had hoped to cover both proximate and ultimate aspects of social behaviour by soliciting contributors to tackle both. By and large we failed on the latter point, because in spite of promising (but often limited) interactions between researchers working on mechanistic *or* ultimate aspects of social behaviour, the field of social behaviour has remained divided due to the different scientific traditions and funding agencies. An alternative subtitle for our book could have been 'towards a new synthesis', because a synthesis, if achievable, is not yet complete.

We anticipate that the primary audience of this book will be graduate students, teachers, university lecturers and researchers. We envisage that the book will be suitable for graduate (or advanced undergraduate) discussions, and lecture courses in animal behaviour, behavioural ecology, evolutionary biology and psychology. The book is divided into three major parts: theoretical foundations (Part I), key themes (Part II) and implications (Part III). Chapters in Part I deal with modelling social behaviour from four perspectives (evolutionary genetics, game theory, phylogenetic inference and population genetics), and one chapter overviews how neuroendocrinologists investigate social traits. In Part II we selected some of the key themes in social-behaviour research (e.g. aggression, communication, group living, sexual behaviour, parental care and family life), and also invited contributions to dissect three pinnacles of social evolution: microorganisms, mammals and humans. Social insects are discussed in Chapter 6, and in profiles by Raghavendra Gadagkar, Bert Hölldobler, Laurent Keller, Gene Robinson and Edward O. Wilson. The main purpose of Part III is to look beyond these specific themes, and to investigate how sociobiology can be enriched by, and in turn can enrich, personality research, social cognition, population ecology, speciation and biodiversity conservation.

Having discussed various arrangements for the guest profiles, we decided to put these contributions in alphabetical order by name. We strongly recommend reading all of them: they are a testament to the diversity of approaches and personal philosophies that pervade some of the best research programmes. Most profiles are relevant to several chapters, and one chapter is often relevant to several profiles. The following chapters and profiles have the most obvious overlap: Chapter 1 (profiles by Keller, Queller, Robinson), 2 (Keller, Ritchie, Robinson), 3 (Haig, Robinson, Sherman), 4 (Haig, Milinski, Parker, Taborsky), 5 (Cockburn, Davies, Gadagkar, Hölldobler), 6 (Gadagkar, Queller, Taborsky, Trivers, Wilson, Zahavi), 7 (Gadagkar, Hölldobler, Hrdy), 8 (Hölldobler, Ritchie, Trivers, Zahavi), 9 (Milinski, Rainey, Sherman), 10 (Birkhead, Cockburn, Davies, Parker, Petrie), 11 (Birkhead, Davies, Parker, Petrie), 12 (Cockburn, Sherman, Taborsky, Zahavi), 13 (Queller, Rainey, Zahavi), 14 (Hrdy, Noë, Trivers), 15 (Hrdy, Noë, Wilson), 16 (Milinski, Noë, Petrie), 17 (Hrdy, Milinski, Trivers), 18 (Haig, Parker, Rainey), 19 (Birkhead, Keller, Queller, Ritchie), 20 (Cockburn, Milinski, Wilson).

This was an ambitious project, and we appreciate the enthusiasm expressed by our colleagues for such a book. A number of people supported the project right from its conception, in particular Amotz Zahavi, David Haig, Geoff Parker, Gene Robinson, Kevin Foster, Marla Sokolowski and Tim Birkhead, and we appreciate their continued encouragement. We further gratefully acknowledge the advice and comments of the following colleagues on book chapters and on profiles: Elizabeth Adkins-Regan, Suzanne H. Alonzo, Olaf Bininda-Edmonds, Bronwyn H. Bleakley, Russell Bonduriansky, Carlos A. Botero, Martha Brians, Charles R. Brown, Carel J. ten Cate, Andrew Cockburn, Patrizia D'Ettorre, Sasha Dall, Martin Daly, Anne Danielson-Francois, René van Dijk, Veronica Doerr, Jan Ekman, Gabriel Garcia-Pena, Patricia Adair Gowaty, Wolfgang Goymann, Kristine L. Grayson, Jim Groombridge, Elizabeth A. D. Hammock, Freya Harrison, Ben J. Hatchwell, Rebecca Kamila Hayward, Richard James, Laurent Keller, Bart Kempenaers, Min-Ho Kim, Clemens Küpper, Joel Levine, Erez Lieberman, Peter R. Long, Donna L. Maney, Manfred Milinski, Patricia J. Moore, Philip L. Munday, Ronald Noë, Ákos Pogány, Geoff Parker, John L. Quinn, Mike Ritchie, Stephan J. Schoech, Catherine E. Selbo, Andy Sih, Kevin M. Sinusas, Rhonda R. Snook, Nancy G. Solomon, Colleen Cassady St Clair, Áron Székely, Tamás Székely Jr, Gavin H. Thomas, Nina Wedell, Jonathan Wright and Gergely Zachar. Martin Griffiths, Abigail Jones, Hugh Brazier and Rachel Eley at Cambridge University Press provided unfailingly cheerful advice and help. The illustrations were kindly redrawn by Dick Visser, Groningen University. The stunning cover photo was provided by Alex Badyaev.

TS is grateful to Harvard University, in particular to David Haig, Brian Farrell and Jonathan Losos; this book was started whilst he held a Hrdy Visiting Fellowship at Harvard University. TS was also supported by the Leverhulme Trust (ID200660763) and NERC (NE/C004167/1). AJM acknowledges the importance and influence of endless discussions with his collaborators, particularly Butch Brodie and Trish Moore, in addition to his coauthors on Chapter 2, Bronwyn Bleakley and Jason Wolf. An invitation from Butch Brodie to teach a summer course at Mountain Lake Biological Station (University of Virginia) on the evolution of social behaviour was invigorating and stimulated a re-reading of Wilson's books, as well as helpful discussions with Butch and Joel McGlothlin. AJM was supported by NERC (NE/B503709/2 and NE/D011337/1). JK acknowledges the importance and influence of discussions with his collaborators, particularly Joost Tinbergen, Christiaan Both, Niels Dingemanse, Franjo Weissing, Ido Pen, Michael Magrath, David Richardson, Jan Ekman, Terry Burke and Ben Hatchwell. JK was supported by grants from the Netherlands Organisation for Scientific Research (NWO–VICI/ 865-03-003, NWO–ALW/809-34-005 and 810-67-022,) and the Netherlands Foundation for the Advancement of Tropical Research (WOTRO/84-519). All three of us were funded by GEBACO (FP6/2002–2006, no. 28696) and INCORE (FP6–2005-NEST-Path, no. 043318). We also thank the authors, who met the deadlines we set and rose to the challenge of producing both readable and interesting chapters that stimulate thought and debate. All authors responded with good cheer and support, for which we are grateful.

Finally, we owe much gratitude to our parents, wives and children, who taught us first-hand the benefits, the significance (and sometimes the costs) of social environment.

References

Dugatkin, L. A. (1997) *Cooperation Among Animals*. New York, NY: Oxford University Press.

Gardner, A. & Foster, K. R. (2008) The evolution and ecology of cooperation: history and concepts. In: *Ecology of Social Evolution*, ed. J. Korb & J. Heinze. Berlin: Springer, pp. 1–36.

Hamilton, W. D. (1964) The genetical evolution of social behaviour, I & II. *Journal of Theoretical Biology*, **7**, 1–52.

Maynard Smith, J. & Price, G. R. (1973) The logic of animal conflict. *Nature*, **246**, 15–18.

Trivers, R. (1985) *Social Evolution*. Menlo Park, CA: Benjamin/Cummings.

Wilson, E. O. (1971) *The Insect Societies*. Cambridge, MA: Harvard University Press.

Wilson, E. O. (1975) *Sociobiology: the New Synthesis*. Cambridge, MA: Harvard University Press.

Undiminished passion

Tim Birkhead

My career in sperm competition has been a roller-coaster ride, energised by a number of particularly special moments. One occurred while I was studying guillemots *Uria aalge* on a group of uninhabited islands off the coast of Labrador in the early 1980s. Surrounded by sea-ice, magical auroras, humpback whales *Megaptera novaeangliae* and thousands of promiscuous birds, this was a wonderful study site. Plotting the results from my notebook at the end of one day, I became aware of what at that time seemed like a remarkable emerging pattern: extra-pair copulations were occurring exactly at the time in a female's cycle when they were most likely to result in fertilisation. It was one of those extraordinary moments when it was clear that everything was going to work out. Not only would this be (at that time) one of the most detailed studies of extra-pair behaviour in birds, it would also suggest that extra-pair copulations were adaptive (Birkhead *et al.* 1985). DNA fingerprinting was still a few years in the future, so it would be a while before we knew how this pattern would impact on fitness, but the behaviour was clear, and at the time my results seemed tremendously exciting. Importantly, they also raised many new questions. My obsession with seabirds, islands and sex, however, had started long before I went to the Arctic.

Like many of my generation of behavioural ecologists, I was a fanatical naturalist as child, encouraged by my father, a keen birdwatcher, and my mother, an accomplished artist. I was indulged – as a teenager I kept birds in my bedroom, whose walls (and carpet, inadvertently) I painted in my own designs. My mother fostered my enthusiasm and my father instilled in me two traits that today might seem old-fashioned: a strong work ethic and always to do my best. We lived in northern rural England, outside Leeds, and with a freedom almost unknown today I spent many days bird-watching alone or with friends. My life revolved around natural history: I raised young magpies *Pica pica*, rooks *Corvus frugilegus*, tawny owls *Strix aluco* and starlings *Sturnus vulgaris*. I collected insects and was the proud owner of an aviary of foreign birds. When I was 12 during a family holiday in north Wales I was taken by my father to Bardsey Island for the day. It was almost surreal in its perfection: thrift-covered cliffs, an azure sea and cerulean skies full of choughs *Pyrrhocorax pyrrhocorax*. As we walked across the island towards the end of the day we saw a young man sitting with a telescope and a notebook studying birds, and my father casually said to me, 'You could do something like that' – little realising how prophetic his comment was.

At school I was uninterested in (and therefore pretty useless at) everything except biology and art, frustrated at being imprisoned when I could have been outdoors. Maths, physics and chemistry were difficult because they were too abstract: I liked art and biology precisely because you could see them. I was

Social Behaviour: Genes, Ecology and Evolution, ed. Tamás Székely, Allen J. Moore and Jan Komdeur. Published by Cambridge University Press. © Cambridge University Press 2010.

encouraged and inspired by one or two extraordinary teachers – the combination of not finding all school-work easy, together with seeing how valuable good teaching could be, later made me aspire to be an effective teacher myself.

At about 17 I started to 'study' the grey heron *Ardea cinerea*, a species, like the peregrine *Falco peregrinus* and other raptors, whose numbers had been reduced by toxic chemicals. I knew I wanted to study herons, but with no guidance, I had no real idea of what to do. My 'studies' consisted of watching the birds at a daytime winter roost near Farnley Park, a beautiful estate where 150 years previously J. M. W. Turner had painted landscapes, herons and other birds. I spent entire winter days huddled in the under-growth watching these majestic birds, elated by the occasional flurry of raised plumes as birds disputed the best roost location. If nothing else, my heron-watching honed my observational skills and powers of endurance.

I went to Newcastle University to read zoology in 1969 and loved it. My most inspiring teacher there was Robin Baker, who told us about the then unpub-lished work of Geoff Parker and Bob Trivers on sperm competition and sexual selection. Hearing about this and seeing the logic of individual selection for the first time was an extraordinary moment. I was inspired, and decided there and then that I would pursue the study of sperm competition in birds.

During one university vacation I worked on a rela-tive's farm in Cornwall. Knowing of my interest in herons, he told me that an old school friend of his, Ian Prestt, was investigating the effect of pesticides on herons and other birds at Monks Wood Experimental Station. A letter secured me an invitation to experi-ence this research first hand, and before I knew it I had the keys of a Land Rover and was allowed to study the herons' social behaviour on my own. It was exhilarating. I felt I was doing something construct-ive, and it was great to be able to come back each day and enthuse about what I had seen. At Monks Wood I met John Parslow, who later offered me a vacation job looking at guillemots on Skomer Island, Wales.

John was also interested in the effects of toxic chemi-cals on seabirds, and found an excuse for me to go to Skomer.

Before that, I attended the Edward Grey Institute student conference in Oxford in the spring of 1972. David Lack was director of the EGI, and he asked the gathered group of students if anyone was interested in undertaking a DPhil. He preferred to walk rather than sit, so my 'interview' took place walking up and down outside St Hugh's College in light rain. I babbled on about my interest in individual selection, social behaviour and sperm competition, and Lack, who didn't say much, merely commented that he knew more about ecology than behaviour. By the time I returned to Newcastle I had an offer. With no further discussion, Lack presumed that I would study guil-lemots on Skomer, since that was what I was going to do for John Parslow as soon as I graduated. With hind-sight, I realise that Parslow and Lack had colluded – luckily for me.

The guillemot was a fortuitous choice. Although I was interested in sperm competition I had no idea when I started my DPhil. that the guillemot, despite being socially monogamous, was sexually rather promis-cuous. The observations I made were promising, but I soon realised that without a large number of individu-ally marked birds in close proximity, guillemots would take me only so far in sperm competition. On moving to Sheffield in 1976 I started what would become a 10-year study of magpies to look at mate-guarding and extra-pair behaviour. But I was still in love with sea-birds, and I spent the next seven summers in various parts of the Canadian Arctic. Labrador, however, was the tipping point. The colonies there provided exactly the opportunity I needed to follow the behaviour of individually recognisable guillemots. As all the pieces started to fit together, I made the decision in the spring of 1983 that from then on sperm competition would be the main focus of my research.

Social behaviour was only part of the story. A true understanding of sperm competition also required a proper understanding of the mechanistic aspects of reproduction: how sperm were utilised, where and

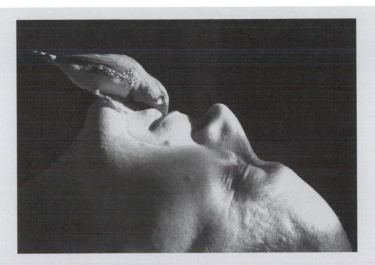

Tim Birkhead and zebra finch. Photo: Francesca Birkhead.

when fertilisation occurred, and so on. Capitalising on avicultural skills acquired as a teenager, I made the zebra finch *Taeniopygia guttata* one of the two model species I would study (Birkhead 1996).

The second was a serendipitous choice – the fowl *Gallus gallus*. In the late 1980s I was invited to a meeting at the University of Stockholm's field station at Tovetorp in southern Sweden. During a tour of the facilities we were shown enclosures containing lynx *Lynx lynx*, moose *Alces alces* and other macho large mammals, all of which were being studied by rather macho research students. Suddenly a group of feral fowl (a primitive domestic fowl very similar to the red jungle fowl) scuttled past us and a male forced a copulation almost at our feet. Taken aback, I asked my host which of the various research students was studying these birds. Slightly incredulous, he said 'no one' – they were simply 'decoration'. I was intrigued, and a year or two later Tom Pizzari (see Chapter 10) was there as my PhD student studying their behaviour. I had mentioned to Tom that if he could persuade the cockerels to copulate with a stuffed female we might be able to obtain natural ejaculates, as I had done with zebra finches, and thereby gain new insights into both their copulation behaviour and the mechanics of sperm competition. It seems surprising that after decades of poultry research, no one knew how many sperm a male transferred during copulation. Despite his best efforts, Tom was unable to persuade the males to perform with his stuffed female. I went out to Sweden and one afternoon, as we watched the birds together, Tom was called away to the phone. In his absence I caught a live female (they were habituated and extremely docile) and, placing her feet between my fingers, crawled on my belly, with her rear end facing away from me, towards a cockerel. Slightly incredulous at his good fortune, the male mounted and inseminated the female. I let her go and tried another female. It worked again. I knew then that we were on the threshold of something exciting. Tom returned from his phone call, and I said to him, 'Watch this.' Once again the birds performed. Within a matter of hours we had devised a way of collecting ejaculates from the female, allowing us to measure ejaculate size and opening up a rich new avenue of research (Pizzari & Birkhead 2000, Pizzari *et al.* 2003).

What has guided my research? (1) First and foremost, a ceaseless intellectual curiosity about the natural world. The freedom I had as a youth to spend countless hours watching birds and other animals honed my field skills, fuelled my fascination for biology and gave me a strong sense of what I call biological intuition. That is, recognising what is biologically meaningful, what is likely to work and what isn't. (2) Enthusiasm. I'm not sure where enthusiasm comes from, but my zeal was fostered and encouraged by my parents, and it has continued to provide the drive and tenacity that research requires. (3) Excellent teachers and wonderful colleagues. The Edward Grey Institute provided a particularly stimulating, challenging and instructive environment when I was a DPhil. student. Subsequently I have been extraordinarily fortunate to have had a succession of outstandingly able research students and other colleagues to keep me on my toes. (4) Open-mindedness. By this I mean reading and interacting widely (not just within behavioural ecology), and embracing broad horizons. There is no better way of generating new ideas than looking beyond the boundaries of one's own discipline (Birkhead 2008).

Finally, the best thing of all about being a behavioural ecologist is that one's enthusiasm for the natural world actually increases over time. The more we discover, the more we discover that there is still more to discover. Even after 40 years in the business, my passion for birds and for biology in general is even greater than when I started.

References

Birkhead, T. R. (1996) Mechanisms of sperm competition in birds. *American Scientist*, **84**, 254–262.

Birkhead, T. R. (2008) *The Wisdom of Birds: an Illustrated History of Ornithology.* London: Bloomsbury.

Birkhead, T. R., Johnson, S. D. & Nettleship, D. N. (1985) Extra-pair matings and mate guarding in the common murre *Uria aalge. Animal Behaviour*, **33**, 608–619.

Pizzari, T. & Birkhead, T. R. (2000) Female fowl eject sperm of subdominant males. *Nature*, **405**, 787–789.

Pizzari, T., Cornwallis, C. K., Lovlie, H., Jakobsson, S. & Birkhead, T. R. (2003) Sophisticated sperm allocation in male fowl. *Nature*, **426**, 70–74.

PART I

Foundations

Foundations

Nature–nurture interactions

Marla B. Sokolowski and Joel D. Levine

Overview

Inheritance is associated with a paradox: it roars with the survival of the species, while at the same time it whispers a fragile message that is constantly modified even among kin. The genes, the environmental context and the traits that arise from their interaction are interrelated. A complexity that characterises this three-way relationship has been attributed to the nature–nurture dichotomy. Traditionally, *nature* is understood to mean *the genes*, whereas *nurture* denotes *the environment*. So, for example, people may debate why one pumpkin is superior to another – was it the quality of the soil or other growth conditions in the pumpkin patch, or was it the specific combination of alleles in that pumpkin's genome?

In recent years, there has been a long-overdue paradigm shift from a limited focus on the nature–nurture dichotomy to a more expansive view that includes gene by environment (G × E) interactions and even gene-environment (G ↔ E) interdependencies, as defined and discussed in this chapter (Rutter 2007). A mechanistic basis for the concept of interdependency arose from advances in molecular biology and genomics which show that DNA is not only inherited but is also environmentally responsive. The latter argument is supported by findings that individuals with dissimilarities in their DNA (DNA polymorphisms) are differentially affected by the same environment. Different environments through development and adulthood can affect individuals with one genetic variant but not another. Individuals, by virtue of their genetic variants, may prefer certain environments, and, in turn, the experiences they acquire in a chosen environment affect the expression of their genes. And finally, the DNA of individuals with the same genetic variants is differentially modified by experience, and this modification is inherited. Studies of gene-environment interdependencies in social behaviour are tremendously challenging. The environmental term is necessarily multifaceted and laced with abiotic and biotic factors that vary in time and space. However, the developing union between this conceptual framework and the new tools in genetics, molecular biology, genomics, animal tracking and imaging greatly facilitates these studies.

In this chapter we address the paradigm shift from (a) nature–nurture to (b) G × E and onwards to (c) G ↔ E interdependencies, with an emphasis on social behaviour. We first approach this shift from a historical perspective, and then move on to discuss experimental designs, behavioural plasticity,

Social Behaviour: Genes, Ecology and Evolution, ed. Tamás Székely, Allen J. Moore and Jan Komdeur. Published by Cambridge University Press. © Cambridge University Press 2010.

norms of reaction, development and epigenetics from both mechanistic (proximate) and evolutionary (ultimate) perspectives. We do not cover quantitative genetic approaches to G–E interactions and correlations, as they have been described elsewhere (Falconer & Mackay 1996; see also Chapter 2). Rather, we present a rationale for moving from the statistical analysis of these relationships to an understanding of how genes and genomes interact and respond to environmental variation

The term *social behaviour* is used broadly here for scenarios where organisms interact with one another, as for instance in courtship and mating, social foraging, parenting, aggression, defence, social learning, rhythmicity, play and communication. This view of social behaviour differs from the term *eusocial* used in studies of the highly social insects, honey bees, ants and termites (Wilson 1971). By contrast, the term *eusocial* is used specifically to describe a society that has a reproductive division of labour (with or without sterile castes), overlapping generations and cooperative care of young (Wilson 1971). This chapter is not a literature review, but it includes examples from social and eusocial animals, as both offer important insight into nature–nurture interdependencies. Although many of the examples used here come from model genetic organisms, the available resources (genetic tools, genome sequences, high-throughput behavioural analyses, sophisticated monitoring of animals in nature) are rapidly expanding. Thus, we are poised to expand our research from quantitative genetic analysis to investigations of how specific genes, genomes and environments affect behaviour.

1.1 Introduction: a historical overview of the nature–nurture dichotomy

The nature–nurture dichotomy is rooted in the centuries-old questions about the origins of individual differences (for review see Logan & Johnston 2007). It concerns the importance of innate or inborn characteristics versus those obtained by experience. In other reincarnations the nature–nurture dichotomy has been called instinct–learning, innate–acquired or gene–environment. In present day terminology, the nature–nurture dichotomy is comparable to gene–environment determinism.

Ever since the late nineteenth century, Darwin's evolutionary theory has provided a context for biologists and psychologists to think about the evolution of behavioural traits – see *The Descent of Man* (Darwin 1871) and *The Expression of the Emotions* (Darwin 1872). Because of this focus on natural selection, Darwin's work emphasised the importance of behaviours that were heritable. Darwin and his contemporaries did not think of nature and nurture as being disconnected, rather they viewed instinctive and learned behaviours as lying on a continuum. Near the end of the nineteenth century, Galton thought that nature was what an organism brought into the world whereas nurture reflected how the organism was influenced after birth. However, in the first half of the twentieth century a wedge was firmly driven between instinct and learning. As the theory of evolution became the unifying theory in the biological sciences, biologists focused primarily on heritable behavioural variation. As a result, by the 1920s, 'nature' rested primarily in the domain of biologists and 'nurture' in the domain of psychologists.

Niko Tinbergen and Konrad Lorenz, prominent European zoologists in the 1950s, developed the field of ethology and argued that most behaviours were instinctive; they focused on evolutionary explanations for behaviour (Tinbergen 1951, Lorenz 1981). Ethologists studied the stereotyped behaviour of animals in their natural settings. Although they recognised a role for learning in an individual's behavioural responses, Tinbergen and Lorenz emphasised a view of behaviour as fully developed without environmental input, with stimuli in the environment merely acting to trigger the full behavioural pattern (Kruuk 2003, Burkhardt 2005).

The ethologists imparted valuable lessons central to modern-day studies of behaviour. These include the ethogram (i.e. a strict description of all behaviours performed by the organism), the value of observing animals in their natural setting, and the dangers of teleological and anthropomorphic thinking. However, some of the ethologists' research depended on deprivation experiments, and as a result they defined behaviour as instinctive by exclusion (for a criticism of deprivation experiments see Lehrman 1953, 1970). In their experiments, the organism was deprived of all stimuli during development prior to measuring its subsequent behaviour. If the behaviour pattern was performed in full after the deprivation experiment, then the behaviour was said to be instinctive. For example, if a bird reared in total isolation could wholly perform its courtship song, ethologists would argue that song was instinctive ('genetic' in today's terminology). Deprivation experiments, however, only manipulate the environment. They do not assess whether genes influence behaviour, as is implied by the term *nurture*. To assess genetic differences, the genes need to be manipulated.

Meanwhile, the psychologists of the time, Skinner and Watson in America and MacDougall in the UK, studied learning and asserted that most behaviours are acquired through nurture (Kruuk 2003, Burkhardt 2005). Although they designed experiments that were in the range of the organism's abilities, the behavioural tasks often differed dramatically from those performed by the organism in its natural setting. Their experimental designs were thought to limit any 'natural' predispositions brought to the experiment by the animal so that the experimental results would not be confounded. Since learning, by definition, requires environmental input, the experiments designed by these psychologists were used mainly to study 'nurture'. The intricacies of learning were studied within one inbred rat *Rattus norvegicus* strain, thereby limiting genetic contributions to variation in learning. Thus the psychologists of the time manipulated environmental, not genetic factors. They also believed that animals are born with a blank slate and that experiences write on this slate, thereby shaping the individual throughout development. In conclusion, during

this time period, the disciplines of biology and psychology themselves were firmly rooted in a nature–nurture dichotomy.

By the last quarter of the twentieth century it was generally accepted that both nature and nurture contribute to behavioural variation (Sokolowski & Wahlsten 2001). The nature–nurture controversy had evolved into questions of how much of the variation is inherited (*heritability*) and how much is due to the environment (*plasticity*). Plasticity refers to the modifiability of behaviour via the environment; while, in general, heritability denotes the ability of a trait to be inherited. The quantitative genetic definition of heritability is not really akin to the English word *inherited* because some traits are inherited but have zero heritability. For example, having one nose in humans is inherited but its heritability is zero because variation in the number of noses in humans is not found. The term *heritability* is used by quantitative geneticists to assess how much of the phenotypic variation in a trait arises from genetic variation. It is especially useful in predicting responses to selection.

There are a number of ways to measure heritability using quantitative genetics (Falconer & Mackay 1996). One is broad-sense heritability, which partitions sources of variation into 'genetic' and 'environmental' components, imposing an additive model and ignoring G × E interactions (Sokolowski & Wahlsten 2001):

$$V_p = V_g + V_e \tag{1.1}$$

where V_p is the variation in phenotype, V_g variation due to genes, and V_e variation due to the environment. The broad-sense heritability ($= V_g/V_p$) changes according to the environment. Quantitative genetic measures of heritability can be substantially more sophisticated than broad-sense heritability; narrow-sense heritability removes non-additive and environmental sources of variation (Falconer & Mackay 1996). However, it is worth pointing out that heritability does not contain information about the specific genes that contribute to variation in a trait or how they interact with the environment.

Wahlsten and Gottlieb (1997) state that 'Environment regulates the actions of genes, and genes, via changes in the nervous system, influence the sensitivity of an organism to changes in the environment. The two causes are not separable developmentally.' Partitioning behavioural variation into a genetic and an environmental component reveals little about natural variation in the development and functioning of behaviours. Just as phenotypes do not arise from nature or nurture, an explanation of nature and nurture is also inadequate. Simply put, genetic factors do not act independently of the environment, and the social environment cannot act independently of the genome. As development progresses there is a constant interchange between genes and environment. Investigations of the interactions and interdependencies between genes and the environment are critical for developing a deep understanding of both the proximate and ultimate contributions to individual differences in behaviour.

More than 40 years ago, Donald Hebb, a well-known psychologist, was asked the question, 'What is more important to human personality, nature or nurture?' His now famous reply can be paraphrased as 'What is more important to a rectangle, the length or the width?' (Meaney 2001). This inspired response really says it all. For too many years, the over-simplistic nature–nurture dichotomy has shrouded the important and complex interactions between genes, environment and development, and has limited our ability to investigate gene–environment interdependencies. Moving on is long overdue.

1.2 Gene-by-environment interactions

Here we use the term *genetic* to denote variation in genes, in the DNA specifically. Briefly, a gene is a long stretch of DNA which can have variation in its sequence of bases (e.g. ATCGGG vs. ATCGCG). This difference in DNA sequence can have consequences for the RNA that gets transcribed from the DNA and the protein that gets translated from the RNA. The DNA variation may be in the coding region, whose information is used to make the protein, or in the regulatory region, which indicates where and when the protein should get expressed. What then is required to conclude that there is a genetic contribution to differences in behaviour? Deprivation and common garden-variety experiments (Fig. 1.1) do not suffice.

They generally do not assess genetic contributions to differences in behaviour because they only involve environmental manipulations. Also, repeated measures of behaviour in an individual over time, or measures of behaviour in genetic clones (where all individuals in a group are genetically identical at all loci) do not address the question of genetic contributions to behavioural variation. Genes do not strictly determine, control or cause behaviour. 'Genetic determinism' describes direct mapping of a gene onto a trait. According to this model, when the allele for a behavioural trait is present, then the organism will always exhibit the trait. Thus, deterministic thinking ignores environmental input into the behavioural variation as well as gene-by-environment interactions. It now appears that, rather than determining behavioural traits, genes may influence the probability that behavioural traits will be expressed in a given environment. Genetic determinism *rarely, if ever*, applies to behavioural traits, either in individuals or in populations.

Recent technological advances enable us to measure G × E interactions both from a statistical perspective and also at the levels of the gene and the genome. G × E interactions predominate in the animal and the human literature (Rutter 2007). In this respect phrases like 'genetic *control* of a trait', 'genes *determine* behaviour' and 'genetic *basis* of trait differences' mislead the reader into thinking that genes dictate behaviour. Although it might garner more attention to say 'a gene for this behaviour, a gene for that behaviour', it is nevertheless incorrect because genes always influence individual *differences* in behaviour.

Even in the case when a major gene influence on behaviour has been identified (Falconer & Mackay 1996), the environment still affects the expression of behavioural differences. Take for example the *foraging* gene in the fruit fly *Drosophila melanogaster*, whose rover allele, for^R, increases the probability of a larva moving more within and between food patches and eating less compared to the sitter allele, for^s (Sokolowski 1980, Kaun *et al.* 2007). The allelic variants of the *foraging* gene encode a cGMP-dependent protein kinase (PKG) (Osborne *et al.* 1997), and differentially affect many hundreds of downstream genes (Kent *et al.* 2009). The *foraging* gene also plays

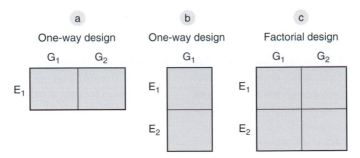

Figure 1.1 Experimental designs involving two environments (E_1 and E_2) and two groups of organisms of the same species with different genotypes (G_1 and G_2). There is significant genetic variation between groups (organisms in G_1 and G_2) but no genetic variation within each group (organisms within G_1 or within G_2). (a) Testing the behaviour of two different groups of genotypes in the same environment (common garden experiment). (b) Testing the behaviour of genetically identical individuals in different environments. (c) This factorial design can detect genotype × environment interactions if they are present.

a role in plastic responses to environmental change. Interestingly, a genetic predisposition to behave as a rover or a sitter does not constrain plasticity in these behaviours. For example, when rovers are food-deprived they behave like sitters and the PKG enzyme activity level decreases (Kaun *et al.* 2007). Moreover these data demonstrate that the relationship between nature and nurture is non-additive.

Indeed, there is a common misunderstanding about the relationship between heritability and plasticity. The misconception is that when a trait is 'more genetic' it will have a narrower range of responses to changes in the environment, and when a trait is 'less genetic' (more environmental) it will have a wider range of phenotypic possibilities. In other words, environmental influences are thought to cause greater variability than genetic ones. This misguided view is found in some of the human literature with regard to traits such as IQ, sexual orientation and psychiatric disorders (Sokolowski & Wahlsten 2001), and often G × E interactions and G ↔ E interdependencies are ignored in this view.

1.2.1 Gene-by-environment interactions: analysis of variance

Gene-by-environment interactions can be statistically quantified using a number of experimental designs. For purposes of illustration, below we discuss the quantification of G × E interactions using a two-way ANOVA in a comparison of inbred strains. This approach can be used to measure G × E interaction at the level of allelic variation in a gene or at the genomic level, which takes into account most of the genes in the organism. The experimental design requirements are briefly discussed below.

In the laboratory, G × E interactions are measured in genetically different organisms in well-defined environments. For example, collections of inbred strains, groups of individuals that differ in a set of known alleles or at the level of the entire genome, can be used for these studies. Ideally, studies of G × E interactions should be done on genetically different clones in well-defined environments but alas, nature rarely provides us with the best research material. Thus the aim becomes to maximise the between-group genetic variation while minimising the within-group variation for the behaviour of interest. This can most easily be accomplished using genetic model organisms (i.e. organisms with a long history of genetic analysis such as *Drosophila melanogaster, Caenorhabditis elegans, Mus musculus*). It is notably more difficult for organisms used by behavioural ecologists. Fitzpatrick *et al.* (2005) proposed a candidate gene approach that incorporates information garnered from previous studies of genetic model organisms into the study of specific candidate genes in ecological model organisms.

Measuring a specific behaviour in groups of genetically distinct organisms (as defined above) in one environment gives us a rough estimate of genetic contributions to behavioural differences (Fig. 1.1a). Measuring the same behaviour in one group of genetically identical organisms across environments gives us a measure of plasticity, the modifiability of the behaviour (Fig. 1.1b). When there are at least two distinct groups of organisms whose behaviour is measured in at least two environmental contexts, it becomes possible to estimate G × E interactions if they are present (Fig. 1.1c). G × E interactions cannot be measured if data have not been collected for any of the four experimental design 'cells'. So, for example, having information on two cells only – such as the learning-ability scores of one group with low socio-economic status and another group with high socio-economic status – tells us nothing about how genes, environment or G × E interactions contribute to learning within or between these two groups (Sokolowski & Wahlsten 2001).

Here we discuss how a simple two-way analysis of variance (ANOVA) can be used to measure the significance of genetic, environmental and G × E contributions to variation in a behavioural trait. More complex models of G × E interactions and G–E covariance are discussed elsewhere (Falconer & Mackay 1996). The simplest design would measure two genetically different groups across two environments (Fig. 1.2). G × E interaction is indicated by a significant two-way interaction in the ANOVA. From a behavioural perspective, a significant G × E interaction means that the genotypes (or groups) each respond differently to the different environments.

1.2.2 Gene-by-environment interactions: implications and limitations

Studies of inbred strains of mice *Mus musculus* show that it is not always possible to predict the strength and significance of G, E or G × E interactions even when all possible conditions are controlled between laboratories (Crabb *et al.* 1999, Wahlsten *et al.* 2003, 2006). Data were collected from eight strains of mice on five behavioural tests done in three labs. Ethanol preference and water escape learning showed comparable

results in all labs. Data for open field activity and for cocaine activation showed that five of the eight strains were similar in the three labs. In anxiety tests, mice in Edmonton scored higher than those in Portland. These differences could not be attributed to differences in rearing, shipping, ageing and testing of the mice as all these factors were carefully controlled. These results are informative, as they speak to how G × E interaction influences the lack of reproducibility of experiments from one study to another and for some traits in some strains. The results show that genes can be incredibly sensitive to tiny differences in the environment that cannot be controlled experimentally. Additionally, some genotypes and behaviours are more sensitive to these environmental differences than others.

G × E interactions are also studied from the perspective of allelic variation in a single gene. A functional polymorphism in the promoter region of the serotonin transporter (5-HTT) gene moderates the effect of stressful life experiences. When exposed to stressful life events, people with one or two copies of the short allele of the 5-HTT promoter polymorphism show more depression than those homozygous for the long allele (Caspi *et al.* 2003).

Finally, G × E interaction is measured at the genomic level using the balanced square experimental design described above. RNA microarrays can be performed on species whose DNA has been sequenced or where a set of expressed sequence tag (EST) clones exist (National Center for Biotechnology Information 2004). For example, rover and sitter *D. melanogaster*, which have different *foraging* alleles, can be fed or food-deprived before RNA from their heads is extracted and compared using microarray analysis. ANOVA performed on this genome-wide dataset reveals individual genes and pathways where G × E interactions are significant (Kent *et al.* 2009). This approach can provide insight into the pathways that act downstream of the allelic variants of the gene under study.

The concept of 'norms of reaction' was developed to illustrate the phenotypic response, in this case behaviour (B) of a single genotype across a range of

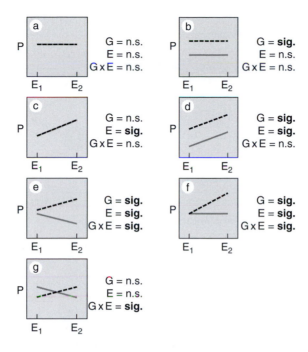

Figure 1.2 Gene-by-environment interactions. As in Figure 1.1, two groups, G_1 and G_2, which differ genetically, have their behaviour tested in two different environments (E_1 and E_2). (a) shows no gene (G) environment or G × E interaction because the lines are horizontal and G_1 and G_2 do not differ from each other (the dashed line is directly on top of the solid line). (b) shows a significant G but no E or G × E because the lines are horizontal but the levels of behavioural response differ between the groups. (c) shows a significant effect of E because the lines are not horizontal; there is plasticity in the response of the strains across the two environments. Since G_1 and G_2 respond the same to the two environments, there is no G or G × E effect. (d) shows a significant effect of G and E because the lines are not horizontal, and the levels of behavioural response differ between the two groups. Since the slope of the response is the same in both groups, there is no significant G × E interaction. (e) and (f) both show significant G, E and G × E where the groups differ in their response to the environment. (g) shows significant G × E, but G and E are not statistically significant because the patterns are symmetrical in this drawing.

environments. When the norms of reaction are compared for many genotypes the relationships can be readily observed (Fig. 1.3). The additive model called the *reaction range* (G + E) predicts parallel curves where there is no G × E interaction (Fig. 1.3a). The model best supported by the behavioural literature is the *norm of reaction* model, in which knowledge of how a genotype or group performs in one environment does not allow you to predict how it will perform in another environment (Fig. 1.3b). The concept of G × E interaction has more recently been extended to G ↔ E interdependencies.

1.3 The interdependence of genes and the environment

Individuals do not passively experience their environment. Environments are chosen and modified on the basis of an individual's behavioural tendencies, for example the propensity to take risks or to be social (see Chapter 16). Such propensities can be influenced by genes. Because of the variability in the ways organisms interact with their environments, certain environmental influences may significantly affect some individuals but not others (Meaney 2001).

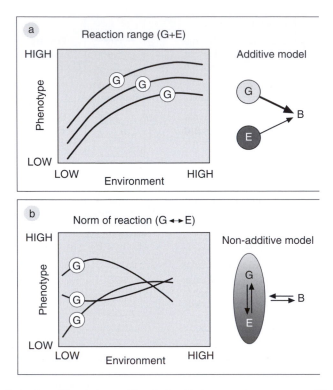

Figure 1.3 Two models of behaviour (B) and the possible relationship between three genotypes (G_1, G_2, G_3) and the environment in a gradient from low to high. (a) The reaction range predicts the shapes of the curves for all genotypes. It predicts that the causal effects of genes and environment are additive. (b) The norm of reaction predicts that the shape of the curves arise from gene-by-environment interactions which enable reversals of rank orders in different environments. For any one genotype, knowledge of the level of phenotype in one environment does not predict its level in another environment. Genotype and environment are interdependent. After Sokolowski and Wahlsten (2001).

What do we mean by G ↔ E interdependence? As is traditionally thought, the environment influences the genes, but the idea of interdependence also incorporates the newer idea that the effects of the environment may result from an indirect consequence of the animal's genotype. For example, animals with certain genotypes may have an increased probability of choosing a particular habitat, and this habitat choice can have consequences for the animals' subsequent pattern of gene expression. Indeed there may be long-term consequences for the frequency of the alleles that facilitated a specific habitat preference. More specifically, individuals with alleles that predispose them to take risks are therefore more likely to encounter risky situations.

This can result in reward or punishment which affects the subsequent gene expression and behaviour of the risk takers, and which also has long-term fitness consequences. G ↔ E interdependencies are most common in the case of social interactions, because the social environment produces large effects on individual behaviour with consequences that can, say, through stress, alter an individual's gene expression. Thus, social behaviour is a special case of G ↔ E interdependence because conspecifics represent an environmental factor that can then change the organisms' gene expression and subsequent behaviours (see also Chapter 2). As is the case with habitat selection and risk taking, organisms can choose social situations. From this perspective, social context can be considered to be an environmental factor.

1.4 Different kinds of environments

The previous sections illustrate that G × E interactions capture – more or less – the relationship between a phenotype and its genetic substrate. The emphasis on G × E interaction is an analytical advance over G + E. The interaction term recognises that the response of a genotype may vary across environments in a complex manner. This analysis is further refined by considering what is meant by 'environment'.

As described above, the term *environment* can refer to abiotic factors (temperature, humidity) and biotic factors (density of individuals, social groupings, parenting). Increasingly, the social environment is considered an important influence on an individual's gene expression and behaviour (see Chapters 10, 11 and 18). As discussed below, an individual's experience of social interactions may affect reproductive success. This establishes an interesting feedback loop whereby the group influences individual group members in a manner that tweaks the population of genes and alleles across generations. This idea is not new: a relationship between social life and the genetic landscape was articulated by the ecologist W. C. Allee in the early part of the 19th century. Allee suggested that life in groups is adaptive – within limits. He linked his own observations on the phylogeny of social life to Sewall Wright's quantitative theories of population genetics (Allee 1958). Recently, Allen Moore and colleagues (Moore *et al*. 1997, Wolf *et al*. 1998; Chapter 2) have reintroduced the idea that there is something special about the social environment. They proposed a theory of *indirect genetic effects* (IGE). Broadly put, this theory states that social experience shapes phenotypic variability and thereby influences the frequency of alleles in a population. According to this view, an individual's phenotype is a function of genotype, physical environment and social environment. The quantitative statement of the theory is remarkable because it is written in terms of how an individual is affected by his or her social experience

and because, in principle, the effects of genotype and at least two types of environment (physical and social) may be quantified. Partitioning the environmental variable into physical and social parts is an essential feature of the theory.

Several studies have demonstrated indirect genetic effects. For example, in their studies on display traits in wild caught *Drosophila serrata*, Blows and colleagues have shown that individual flies, males and females, adjust the expression of pheromonal signals in accord with their social environment (Petfield *et al*. 2005; see also Wolf *et al*. 1999, 2002, 2003, Wolf 2000). Moreover, Krupp *et al*. (2008) have demonstrated that the composition of a social group influences patterns of gene expression and pheromonal signalling as well as levels of mating in *D. melanogaster*. Consistent with the theoretical ideas noted in the previous paragraph, this study demonstrates that the frequency of copulation increases with increasing genotypic diversity among males in a social group (Krupp *et al*. 2008). In a related study, Kent *et al*. (2008) found significant G × S (S is the social environment) interactions for nearly all of the chemical signals found on the surface of male *D. melanogaster*. In some cases the G × S interaction factor accounted for more variability than others in the model (Kent *et al*. 2008). Kent *et al*. also show quantitatively that male flies exert indirect genetic effects on other males. In these experiments, individual pheromonal displays are predicted by the genotypic composition of a social group. This demonstration of social effects on individual behaviours is especially salient because studies that take molecular and cellular approaches to understanding a phenotype tend to be framed around individual subjects (e.g. how does the individual smell or learn or court or eat?). In this respect, the theory of indirect genetic effects may provide a bridge between quantitative genetics and molecular genetics, as demonstrated by the studies of Krupp *et al*. and Kent *et al*.; it is all the more noteworthy that this bridge depends on the important role of the social environment.

Although not usually studied within the theoretical framework associated with IGE and quantitative genetics, an influence of the social environment on individual development defines another important class of effects. Eusocial insects, such as the honey bee *Apis mellifera*, are known to maintain a highly structured social environment, but even for eusocial insects there is some plasticity associated with the division of labour in the hive (Robinson 2004, Robinson *et al.* 2005). This is evident based on developmental, molecular, and behavioural criteria. Indeed, the social role of a honey bee within the hive is a complex trait that may be determined in part by social density. Ordinarily, nurses become foragers when they are about three weeks old. A marker for this new job is the onset of a functional circadian clock mechanism in the brain. Prior to assuming the role of a forager, clock genes, such as *period*, are expressed but not in a pattern that is consistent with a timing function. Once the transition from nurse to forager occurs, levels of *period* transcription oscillate throughout the day, a signature feature of circadian clock function. However, when caste ratios within the hive are manipulated to leave mostly young nurses with a shortage of foragers, some of the nurses undergo a precocious development of circadian function and make an early transition to become foragers (Bloch *et al.* 2001, Bloch & Robinson 2001). These remarkable studies show that a change in the social environment induces precocious changes in gene expression in some individuals. The interaction between social environment and gene expression can alter development and social role even within the rigid context of a beehive.

In general, studies within the framework of indirect genetic effects and in eusocial insects support the idea that the social environment plays an important role in shaping the relationship between phenotype and genotype. We have described examples related to courtship and foraging behaviours. The example from the bees points towards the theme of development. From a biological standpoint many adult behavioural phenotypes require developmental forerunners (Ganguly-Fitzgerald *et al.* 2006), just as the nurse–forager transition requires that all the components needed for a functional circadian clock are ready. In the next section, we address the role of development per se.

1.5 Development

Previous sections have emphasised ideas and methods from quantitative genetics as a framework for understanding the relationship between phenotype and genotype. Early development is a time when interactions between the environment and genotype may be critical for establishing the mature individual in terms of physiology and behaviour. Although, in statistical terms, an emphasis on development is not consistent with the analytic framework we have been presenting (development is not independent of genes and environment), it is noteworthy because of its special role in many behavioural phenotypes.

The timing of environmental input is critical for the development and performance of individual differences in behaviour. In some cases sensitive periods have been reported for normal behavioural development. A 'sensitive period' is a time in the development of an organism when it shows a heightened sensitivity to particular environmental stimuli. The organism's development is altered due to its experiences during the sensitive period. If the organism does not get the appropriate stimuli during the sensitive period, its development, behaviour and health may be compromised later in life (Hensch 2005).

Research on both humans and rhesus monkeys *Macaca mulatta* shows persuasive evidence for specific G × E interactions framed by a sensitive period in development. In general, the short-allele polymorphism in the promoter region of the serotonin transporter gene is associated with poor neuronal function in infancy and poor control of aggression in the juvenile and adolescent stages of development when monkeys are reared in infancy with peers but no mothers. Monkeys with the short allele raised during this period of development with their mothers and their peers did not exhibit these deficiencies. And finally, monkeys with the long allele are normal for all of these factors regardless of their early social rearing (Suomi 2006).

Like genes, environmental factors can affect the development and/or functioning of behaviour. The gene's product may be required during development, for example, to construct a nervous system that facilitates the later performance of a behaviour pattern. Alternatively, the gene's product may only be required to function during the performance of the behaviour pattern. Another possibility is that the gene's product may be involved in both developmental and functional aspects of the behavioural phenotype. This can be assessed using genetic tools, such as transgenics, to express or turn off gene expression at different times during development and adulthood. Molecular techniques can be applied to resolve details of genetic contributions to behaviour.

The importance of development, of maternal and other social input and of certain sensory stimuli during sensitive periods of development is well established for a diverse array of animals including insects, rodents and primates. The ease with which we might slip into the language of 'nature–nurture' dichotomies may be partly due to the powerful influence of the maternal nurturing that is thought to be so important for human development. It is therefore noteworthy that recent developments in the study of mothering suggest that there are mechanisms of inheritance that may not arise from variation in the DNA sequence which we now discuss.

1.6 Epigenetic changes as an interface between nature and nurture

A new level of complexity in the evaluation of inheritance has appeared within the last decade. Epigenetics introduces a wrinkle into the relationship between phenotype and genotype because this source of inheritance does not depend directly on DNA sequence. Instead, epigenetics emphasises the relationship between phenotype and environment; this mechanism feeds back to regulate gene expression without altering the genotype. This view is especially compelling because one of the best examples of an epigenetic effect relates to a paradigm of social behaviour, the maternal influence on stress response.

Bird (2007) defines epigenetic events as 'the structural adaptation of chromosomal regions so as to

register, signal, or perpetuate altered activity states.' In a seminal review, he goes on to write that 'epigenetic processes are buffers of genetic variation, pending a change of state that leads an identical combination of genes to produce a different developmental outcome.' This definition includes the use of the term in developmental biology as well as in behavioural studies, and it declares that an epigenetic event is a response.

Szyf, Meaney and colleagues have characterised an epigenetic mechanism for determining stress responses in rats. They call it *maternal programming* (Weaver *et al.* 2004, 2005, Szyf *et al.* 2005). The response to stress is mediated by glucocorticoid receptors in the hippocampus. Levels of glucocorticoid receptors are affected by licking and grooming provided by mothers during the first week of life. Offspring of mothers that lick and groom at high levels produce higher number of copies of glucocorticoid receptor mRNA, while offspring that receive less licking and grooming make fewer copies. In addition, the offspring of mothers with higher levels of licking and grooming show increased hippocampal receptor sensitivity, increased sensitivity to steroid feedback, decreased hypothalamic levels of corticotrophin releasing factor, and decreased startle responses compared to offspring that received less maternal stimulation. In general, individuals that received higher maternal stimulation were less reactive to stressful stimuli, based on a variety of behavioural, neural and neuroendocrine measures.

Two critical observations call attention to this work. First, the expression of the glucocorticoid receptor is influenced by patterns of DNA methylation within the gene that encodes the receptor. DNA methylation is a type of chemical modification of the DNA that does not change the original DNA sequence. In this case the promoter of the glucocorticoid receptor is methylated (a methyl group is added), resulting in a decrease in the expression of this gene. These patterns are established by the level of licking and grooming received by the pup. The patterns are maintained into later stages of life, and they can be manipulated to alter responses to stressful stimuli based on experience. Thus the changes in gene activity in response to stress are controlled by patterns of methylation that define an epigenetic response to mothering. Second, the stress response-related effects of maternal licking and grooming are passed on to female offspring. The female offspring treat their offspring according to how they themselves were reared (with high or low levels of licking and grooming). Szyf *et al.* (2005) describe evidence that the transmission of this maternal behaviour across generations is related to methylation of the oestrogen receptor gene passed from mother to daughter.

Although there are not yet many examples of robust epigenetic effects on behaviour, the example of maternal behaviour in rats implies a level of complexity that is greater than G × E interactions. If such epigenetic effects prove to be common, then the inheritance of a phenotype must account for several tiers of plasticity both within the genome and 'around' it.

1.7 Conclusions and future directions

The relationship between phenotype and genotype is an ongoing matter of study. Traditionally, behavioural studies have oscillated between the ideas that behaviour may be determined more by the genes than the environment or vice versa. However, this 'nature–nurture' dichotomy has proved false. Statistical approaches associated with quantitative genetics have shown that including interaction terms between genotype and environment (G × E) is more realistic than a restricted additive view (G + E).

The concepts associated with G × E interactions have been expanding. One such expansion has to do with the interdependence of genes and the environment. Moreover, the environment itself may be partitioned into abiotic and biotic factors. A compelling example of this approach is illustrated by the theory of indirect genetic effects (IGE). This theory quantifies the influence of genotype, physical environment and social environment on an individual's phenotype. While calling attention to the importance of the social milieu, IGE provides a conceptual bridge between quantitative effects and the analysis of how specific genes contribute to an individual's

phenotype; it implies that a molecular substrate for social experience can be described experimentally, and such examples are beginning to appear (Krupp *et al.* 2008, Kent *et al.* 2008).

Although developmental processes lie outside current quantitative frameworks, recent studies in monkeys and humans have suggested the profound importance of sensitive periods for social function and the development of behavioural responses in general. It is tempting to link developmental input to a role for epigenetic mechanisms that may underlie the inheritance of behavioural phenotypes. Studies on maternal care in rodents have shown that licking and grooming provided by a mother to her offspring within the first week after birth influences stress responses in the offspring once they mature. In addition, some qualities of the maternal behaviour style (high licking and grooming versus low) are transmitted from mother to daughter. These effects of maternal 'programming' are associated with methylation of DNA sequences that in turn affect the transcription of steroid receptors in the brain. Such epigenetic effects may represent a new level of analysis that mediates the relationship between genes and behaviour.

Throughout this chapter we have endeavoured to emphasise the importance of social context and social experience as an environmental stimulus that affects gene expression in individuals and, thus, phenotypic variability within a population. We emphasise new approaches and technologies that advance our understanding of the relationships between genes and environment and how they affect behaviour. These newer approaches expand our knowledge from quantitative genetic analyses to include an understanding of the molecular genetic mechanisms underlying behavioural variation. In the past, these quantitative genetic analyses were the only good approach to questions of gene–environment relationships, because we had little to no knowledge of the genes and genomes of most animals. However, in just a few years we will be able to obtain the complete DNA sequence of any animal's genome for well under $1000! And knowledge of these sequences will enable us to measure changes in the expression of all genes in the genomes of any species with different social behaviours and in ecologically relevant environments. For example, we will be able to test hypotheses about suites of genes and pathways that are up- or downregulated in response to a social situation, and ask why. These findings could then be compared between individuals, populations and species to further frame our evolutionary hypotheses.

This integration requires interdisciplinary approaches and dialogue between those of us in different subfields. Initially, we may have to make simplifying assumptions about social groups in order to investigate molecular mechanisms that underlie social influences on perception, physiology and behaviour. We may have to relax ideas about examining social interactions at all life-history stages in ecological contexts. Once some of the mechanisms underlying the gene–environment relationships in social behaviour are understood then follow-up experiments can be done to include more complex social manipulations in ecologically relevant contexts. The examples we have presented in this chapter focus attention on genes and genomes. As more details become available, the critical tissues and developmental stages will become known. In this way, we will be able to carry the questions we have been asking from the level of genes and environment to fill in other levels. For example, neural, endocrine, muscular and metabolic systems may all be important contributors to variation in social behaviour and may have evolved in interesting ways – yet to be determined. Finally, technologies associated with high-throughput molecular methods and approaches from systems biology are advancing with great rapidity. It is likely that industrial-scale analyses (the –omics) of questions about social life and G × E interactions will be possible for many organisms in the near future. Exciting times are ahead.

Acknowledgements

We thank Dr Craig Riedl for advice and comments on the writing of this chapter, as well as two anonymous reviewers who provided valuable comments that improved the manuscript. Christie DesRoches helped with the preparation of the figures. JDL and MBS are supported by the Natural Science and Engineering Council of Canada and the Canada Research Chairs Programme.

Suggested readings

Krupp J. J., Kent, C., Billeter, J.-C. *et al.* (2008) Social experience modifies pheromone expression and mating behaviour in male *Drosophila melanogaster. Current Biology*, **18**, 1373–1383.

Rutter, M. (2007) Gene–environment interdependence. *Developmental Science*, **10**, 12–18.

Sokolowski, M. B. & Wahlsten, D. (2001) Gene–environment interaction and complex behavior. In *Methods in Genomic Neuroscience*, ed. S. O. Moldin. Boca Raton, FL: CRC Press, pp. 3–27.

Suomi, S. J. (2006) Risk, resilience, and gene × environment interactions in rhesus monkeys. *Annals of the New York Academy of Sciences*, **1094**, 83–104.

Szyf, M., Weaver, I. C., Champagne, F. A., Diorio, J. & Meaney, M. J. (2005) Maternal programming of steroid receptor expression and phenotype through DNA methylation in the rat. *Frontiers in Neuroendocrinology*, **26**, 139–162.

References

Allee, W. C. (1958) *The Social Life of Animals*. Boston, MA: Beacon Press.

Bird, A. (2007) Perceptions of epigenetics. *Nature*, **447**, 396–398.

Bloch, G. & Robinson, G. E. (2001) Reversal of honeybee behavioral rhythms. *Nature*, **410**, 1048.

Burkhardt, R. W. (2005) *Patterns of Behavior: Konrad Lorenz, Niko Tinbergen, and the Founding of Ethology*. Chicago, IL: University of Chicago Press.

Caspi, A., Sugden, K., Moffitt, T. E. *et al.* (2003) Influence of life stress on depression: moderation by a polymorphism in the 5-HTT gene. *Science*, **301**, 386–389.

Crabbe, J. C., Wahlsten, D. & Dudek, B. C. (1999) Genetics of mouse behavior: interactions with laboratory environment. *Science*, **284**, 1670–1672.

Darwin, C. (1871) *The Descent of Man, and Selection in Relation to Sex*. London: John Murray.

Darwin, C. (1872/1965) *The Expression of the Emotions in Man and Animals*. Chicago, IL: University of Chicago Press.

Falconer, D. S. & Mackay, T. F. C. (1996) *Introduction to Quantitative Genetics*, 4th edn. Harlow: Longman.

Fitzpatrick, M. J., Ben Shahar, Y., Smid, H. M. *et al.* (2005) Candidate genes for behavioural ecology. *Trends in Ecology and Evolution*, **20**, 96–104.

Ganguly-Fitzgerald, I., Donlea, J. & Shaw, P. J. (2006) Waking experience affects sleep need in *Drosophila*. *Science,* **313**, 1775–1781.

Hensch, T. K. (2005) Critical period plasticity in local cortical circuits. *Nature Reviews Neuroscience*, **6**, 877–888.

Kaun, K. R., Riedl, C. A. L., Chakaborty-Chatterjee, M. *et al.* (2007) Natural polymorphism in a cGMP-dependent protein kinase affects food intake and absorption in *Drosophila*. *Journal of Experimental Biology*, **210**, 3547–3558.

Kent, C., Azanchi, R., Smith B., Formosa, A. & Levine J. D. (2008) Social context influences chemical communication in *D. melanogaster* males. *Current Biology*, **18**, 1384–1389.

Kent, C. F., Daskalchuk, T., Cook, L., Sokolowski, M. B. & Greenspan, R. J. (2009) The Drosophila foraging gene mediates adult plasticity and gene–environment interactions in behaviour, metabolites, and gene expression in response to food deprivation. *PLoS Genetics*, **5** (8): e1000609.

Krupp J. J., Kent, C., Billeter, J.-C., So, A.-K. *et al.* (2008) Social experience modifies pheromone expression and mating behaviour in male *Drosophila melanogaster*. *Current Biology*, **18**, 1373–1383.

Kruuk, H. (2003) *Niko's Nature: A Life of Niko Tinbergen and his Science of Animal Behaviour.* Oxford: Oxford University Press.

Lehrman, D. S. (1953) A critique of Konrad Lorenz's theory of instinctive behavior. *Quarterly Review of Biology*, **28**, 337–363.

Lehrman, D. S. (1970) Semantic and conceptual issues in the nature–nurture problem. In: *Development and Evolution of Behavior*, ed. L. R. Aronson, E. Tobach, D. S. Lehrman & J. S. Rosenblatt. San Francisco, CA: W. H. Freeman, pp. 17–50.

Logan, C. A. & Johnston, T. D. (2007) Synthesis and separation in the history of 'nature' and 'nurture'. *Developmental Psychobiology*, **49**, 758–769.

Lorenz, K. Z. (1981) *The Foundations of Ethology.* Berlin: Springer-Verlag.

Meaney, M. J. (2001) Nature, nurture, and the disunity of knowledge. *Annals of the New York Academy of Sciences*, **935**, 50–61.

Moore, A. J., Brodie, E. D. & Wolf, J. B. (1997) Interacting phenotypes and the evolutionary process: I. Direct and indirect genetic effects of social interactions. *Evolution*, **51**, 1352–1362.

National Center for Biotechnology Information (2004) ESTs: gene discovery made easier. Science Primer. www.ncbi. nlm.nih.gov/About/primer/est.html (accessed 26 October 2009).

Osborne, K., Robichon, A., Burgess, E. *et al.* (1997) Natural behaviour polymorphism due to a cGMP-dependent protein kinase of *Drosophila*. *Science,* **277**, 834–836.

Petfield, D., Chenoweth, S. F., Rundle, H. D. & Blows, M. W. (2005) Genetic variance in female condition predicts indirect genetic variance in male sexual display traits. *Proceedings of the National Academy of Sciences of the USA*, **102**, 6045–6050.

Robinson, G. E. (2004) Beyond nature and nurture. *Science*, **304**, 397–399.

Robinson, G. E., Grozinger, C. M. & Whitfield, C. W. (2005) Sociogenomics: social life in molecular terms. *Nature Reviews Genetics*, **6**, 257–270.

Rutter, M. (2007) Gene-environment interdependence. *Developmental Science*, **10**, 12–18.

Sokolowski, M. B. (1980) Foraging strategies of *Drosophila melanogaster*: a chromosomal analysis. *Behaviour Genetics*, **10**, 291–302.

Sokolowski, M. B. & Wahlsten, D. (2001) Gene–environment interaction and complex behavior. In: *Methods in Genomic Neuroscience*, ed. S. O. Moldin. Boca Raton, FL: CRC Press, pp. 3–27.

Suomi, S. J. (2006) Risk, resilience, and gene × environment interactions in rhesus monkeys. *Annals of the New York Academy of Sciences*, **1094**, 83–104.

Szyf, M., Weaver, I. C., Champagne, F. A., Diorio, J. & Meaney, M. J. (2005) Maternal programming of steroid receptor expression and phenotype through DNA methylation in the rat. *Frontiers in Neuroendocrinology*, **26**, 139–162.

Tinbergen, N. (1951) *The Study of Instinct.* Oxford: Oxford University Press.

Toma, D. P., Bloch, G., Moore, D. & Robinson, G. E. (2000) Changes in *period* mRNA levels in the brain and division of labor in honeybee colonies. *Proceedings of the National Academy of Sciences of the USA*, **97**, 6914–6919.

Wahlsten, D. & Gottlieb, G. (1997) The invalid separation of effects of nature and nurture: lessons from animal experimentation. In: *Intelligence, Heredity and Environment*, ed. R. J. Sternberg & E. Grigorenko. New York: Cambridge University Press, pp. 163–192.

Wahlsten, D., Metten, P., Phillips, T. J. *et al.* (2003) Different data from different labs: lessons from studies of gene-environment interaction. *Journal of Neurobiology*, **54**, 283–311.

Wahlsten, D., Bachmanov, A., Finn, D. A. & Crabbe, J. C. (2006) Stability of inbred mouse strain differences in behavior and brain size between laboratories and across decades. *Proceedings of the National Academy of Sciences of the USA*, **103**, 16364–16369.

Wang, Y., Jorda, M., Jones, P. L. *et al.* (2007) Functional CpG methylation system in a social insect. *Science*, **314**, 645–647.

Weaver, I. C., Cervoni, N., Champagne, F. A. *et al.* (2004) Epigenetic programming by maternal behavior. *Nature Neuroscience*, **7**, 847–854.

Weaver, I. C., Champagne, F. A., Brown, S. E. *et al.* (2005) Reversal of maternal programming of stress responses in adult offspring through methyl supplementation: altering epigenetic marking later in life. *Journal of Neuroscience*, **25**, 11045–11054.

Wilson, E. O. (1971) *The Insect Societies*. Cambridge, MA: Harvard University Press.

Wolf, J. B. (2000) Gene interactions from maternal effects. *Evolution*, **54**, 1882–1898.

Wolf, J. B. (2003) Genetic architecture and evolutionary constraint when the environment contains genes. *Proceedings of the National Academy of Sciences of the USA*, **100**, 4655–4660.

Wolf, J. B., Brodie, E. D., Cheverud, J. M., Moore, A. J. & Wade, M. J. (1998) Evolutionary consequences of indirect genetic effects. *Trends in Ecology and Evolution*, **13**, 64–69.

Wolf, J. B., Brodie, E. D. & Moore, A. J. (1999) Interacting phenotypes and the evolutionary process II. Selection resulting from social interactions. *American Naturalist*, **153**, 254–266.

Wolf, J. B., Vaughn, T. T., Pletscher, L. S. & Cheverud, J. M. (2002) Contribution of maternal effects QTL to genetic architecture of early growth in mice. *Heredity*, **89**, 300–310.

Social evolution, sexual intrigue and serendipity

Andrew Cockburn

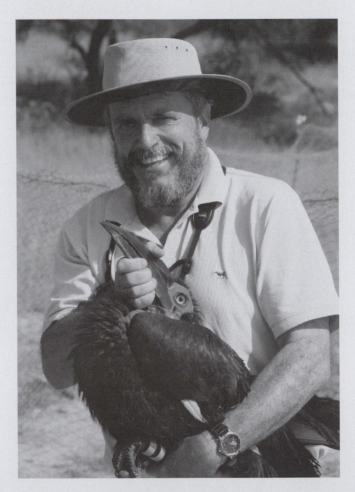

Ground hornbills *Bucorvus leadbeateri* breed cooperatively, and their chicks rely on the group for food for longer than any other social species except our own. Photo: Morne DuPlessis.

Social Behaviour: Genes, Ecology and Evolution, ed. Tamás Székely, Allen J. Moore and Jan Komdeur. Published by Cambridge University Press. © Cambridge University Press 2010.

Like many aspects of science, my interest in social evolution came about at least in part by accident. My early training was in population and community ecology, on plants and rodents living rather asocial lives. Although I had read much of Peter Klopfer's 1973 book *Behavioral Aspects of Ecology*, my own evolutionary interests were primarily focused on life-history evolution. The first turning point came when Mike Cullen, formerly from Oxford but recently appointed to a chair in the Monash Zoology Department where I was studying for my doctorate, popped into the office I shared with Dick Braithwaite, another aficionado of rodent population biology, and dropped off what I am fairly sure was the first copy in Australia of the landmark 1978 textbook by Krebs and Davies. This book, with its excitement and clarity of thought, should remain compulsory reading for everybody, despite its subsequent eclipse by later editions.

There is no doubt that the next greatest influence was the classic book and series of articles produced in the early 1980s by Tim Clutton-Brock, Steve Albon and Fiona Guinness on the ecology of red deer *Cervus elaphus* (Clutton-Brock *et al.* 1983). Their focus on lifetime estimates of fitness in free-living animals seemed to me to be the work I would like to do. I also felt that I had found the perfect study animal. The commonest marsupials in nearby forests were antechinuses, small shrew-like animals with strange sex lives. Unlike deer, they lived their rather miserable lives with drama and panache at a pace that meant I could potentially track them over many generations. Females become sexually receptive for a week or so at the same time each year, after which every single male in the population dies abruptly, before their young are born. The non-overlapping generations of males seemed to me to throw a variety of theoretical questions into sharp relief, and despite the disadvantages of crawling round leech-infested rainforest in the middle of the night, we were able to tease apart a number of questions that had otherwise proved intractable (Lee & Cockburn 1985). For example,

the hypothesis that natal dispersal by young males occurs because of competition with older males cannot apply if the older males do not live to see their young (Cockburn *et al.* 1985).

Antechinuses also introduced to me the wonderful world of social evolution. When we started working on these strange little animals it was believed that the males exhausted themselves chasing females through the forest, but we soon showed that this was untrue. Instead, male *Antechinus agilis* aggregated in nest cavities high in trees, which females visited to seek matings (Lazenby-Cohen & Cockburn 1988). The demise of the males came about because they fed off their bodies optimistically awaiting the visits of females. This realisation led me steadily towards an interest in grouping behaviour, and ultimately to switch my primary attention to the evolution of cooperative breeding, a long-standing issue of critical importance in social evolution. Returning from the field with a combination of leech-induced anaemia and weather-induced flu to hear a graduate student who was studying cooperative superb fairy-wrens *Malurus cyaneus* boast of his success in negotiating a staff discount on croissants at the local café also precipitated the switch.

When I was at least a decade younger than is currently the case, I had the opportunity to show one of the chief architects of the behavioural ecology synthesis around my field site. He seemed bemused by the whole operation and, somewhat awestruck, asked me at the end of the morning whether I knew anyone else my age who still did field work. My apparently dogged persistence in continuing to love spending time in the field preadapted me to the study of cooperative breeding in birds, for here was a field replete with long-term studies of exquisite detail, where the chief practitioners were not really interested in talking to 'newcomers' until they had 10 years of obsessive field work under their belt.

Over the last two decades I have been involved in an inexorable attack on the view of the world that had emerged among these practitioners – that philopatry was driven by constraints on dispersal, and that kinship was the primary stimulus for helping behaviour (Cockburn 1998; see also Chapter 12). Why are my own emphases on mating competition and phylogenetic effects on cooperative breeding distinct from those of my colleagues? Again I put it down to happenstance. Avian cooperative breeding is as easy to study from my university as anywhere in the world, with perhaps 20 common species in the immediate neighbourhood of my university. We started with two of the most charismatic: white-winged choughs *Corcorax melanoramphos* and superb fairy-wrens, and have worked on both for more than 20 years, amply qualifying for membership of the long-term study club. However, by choosing two study species at the same time, we committed ourselves to a fundamentally different path of discovery to our predecessors. Instead of bravely proceeding on the assumption that we could extrapolate glibly from one species to all the others, we found that every year the two species appeared to have less and less in common. Increasingly, it seemed that none of the generalisations applied, and if there was generalisation to replace them, it is that the social and mating systems of Australian birds are profoundly complex and idiosyncratic (Cockburn 2004). I suspect it will take me another two decades to sort this out, as I suspect that at the moment we do not know a lot more than Byron, who many years ago wrote:

What men call gallantry, and gods adultery,
Is much more common where the climate's sultry

Against this background, what advice or principles can I offer a beginning researcher? First, never ignore natural history. For almost any question, there will be an organism particularly well-suited to exploring the nuances of theory. Second, and a related point, animals do not read textbooks, and they do some very weird things. Resist the temptation to force your observations into the straitjacket of theory. Third, stay attuned to the opportunities of technological advances from other fields. I first heard about DNA fingerprinting, the technique that has most changed the study of social behaviour, through a chance conversation at a conference. Finally, when things are going wrong, remember the big picture. I still struggle to think of better ways to have fun than studying the social lives of animals.

References

Clutton-Brock, T. H., Guinness, F. E. & Albon, S. D. (1983) *Red Deer: Behavior and Ecology of Two Sexes*. Edinburgh: Edinburgh University Press.

Cockburn, A. (1998) Evolution of helping behavior in cooperatively breeding birds. *Annual Review of Ecology and Systematics*, **29**, 141–177.

Cockburn, A. (2004) Mating systems and sexual conflict. In: *Ecology and Evolution of Cooperative Breeding in Birds*, ed. W. D. Koenig and J. L. Dickinson. Cambridge: Cambridge University Press, pp. 81–101.

Cockburn, A., Scott, M. P. & Scotts, D. J. (1985) Inbreeding avoidance and male-biased natal dispersal in *Antechinus* spp. (Marsupialia: Dasyuridae). *Animal Behaviour*, **33**, 908–915

Klopfer, P. H. (1973) *Behavioral Aspects of Ecology*, 2nd edn. Englewood Cliffs, NJ: Prentice-Hall.

Krebs, J. R. & Davies, N. B., eds. (1978) *Behavioural Ecology: an Evolutionary Approach*. Oxford: Blackwell.

Lazenby-Cohen, K. A. & Cockburn, A. (1988) Lek promiscuity in a semelparous mammal, *Antechinus stuartii* (Marsupialia: Dasyuridae)? *Behavioral Ecology and Sociobiology*, **22**, 195–202.

Lee, A. K. & Cockburn, A. (1985) *Evolutionary Ecology of Marsupials*. Cambridge: Cambridge University Press.

2

The quantitative genetics of social behaviour

Bronwyn H. Bleakley, Jason B. Wolf and Allen J. Moore

Overview

How and when social behaviour evolves has long been a focus of study within evolutionary biology, yielding the entire subfield of sociobiology and behavioural ecology. Although social behaviours may be explored in the same way as any other type of phenotype, the genetics underlying social behaviours differ from traits that do not vary depending on the social environment in which they are expressed. Social behaviour is best described as an *interacting phenotype*: a phenotype that depends at least in part on interactions with social partners for its expression. Models of indirect genetic effects provide a quantitative genetic framework for understanding the sources of variation underlying interacting phenotypes. They also suggest a genetic mechanism for inheriting traits that are expressed among rather than within individual animals, and identify selection arising from the interactions (termed *social selection*).

This chapter will first introduce the concepts of interacting phenotypes, indirect genetic effects, and social selection. We build a quantitative genetic model for interacting phenotypes and discuss how the evolution of such traits differs from non-interacting traits. We then explore the parameters of the model in more depth. We subsequently summarise existing empirical studies of indirect genetic effects, discuss the implications for the evolution of behavioural traits through social selection, and discuss transitions between quantitative genetic and molecular genetic approaches to studying behavioural evolution. Finally, we highlight potential future avenues of research.

A change improving competitive ability is always favored (unless checked by selection in another context). Each successive improvement sets a new standard which the next can profitably surpass. This is due to the fact that conspecific rivals are an environmental contingency that can itself evolve.

Mary Jane West-Eberhard (1979, p. 228)

2.1 Introduction

Animals often spend a significant portion of their lives engaged in interactions with conspecifics (Allee 1927), and engage in helping, aggression, competition, mating and cooperation, to name but a few possible exchanges. As a result, many behaviours, if not the majority, have a social facet, and even those behaviours

Social Behaviour: Genes, Ecology and Evolution, ed. Tamás Székely, Allen J. Moore and Jan Komdeur. Published by Cambridge University Press. © Cambridge University Press 2010.

that are not inherently 'social' can often be expressed in or influenced by social contexts (e.g. foraging in a group, anti-predator behaviour). Not surprisingly, then, social behaviour has held a pre-eminent place in evolutionary studies of behaviour. However, the interest in social behaviour goes beyond simple popularity. Evolution of social behaviour is complicated by the need to consider groups or multiple individuals and their behaviour simultaneously. Initially researchers focused on the problem of understanding how selection acts on social behaviour. While it is the population that evolves, natural selection generally operates on individuals. Understanding how selection acts on social behaviour remains one of the predominant problems in behavioural ecology, and is the focus of many of the chapters in this book. But selection alone does not result in evolution. As Darwin noted in *The Origin of Species* (1859), for natural selection to occur, individuals must vary in traits relevant to survival and reproduction. Since Fisher (1918) we have known that this variation must reflect genetic influences; selection occurs when this variation influences survival or reproduction. A complete understanding of the evolution of social behaviour therefore requires us to identify the sources of genetic variation as well as the fitness consequences of this variation. Identifying the sources of genetic variation among individuals is the fundamental goal of evolutionary quantitative genetics, and in this chapter we describe a quantitative genetic approach to understanding how social behaviour evolves.

As West-Eberhard (1979, 1983, 1984) observes, selection may arise from competitive interactions within social contexts, and is pervasive because of the ubiquity of interactions among conspecifics. She identifies this as *social selection*, which can be defined as 'differential success in social competition, whatever the resource at stake' (West-Eberhard 1983), and which results from any interaction between conspecifics that influences the fitness of the participants. Hamilton (1964) defined the fitness consequences of four categories of social behaviour: cooperation, selfishness, altruism and spite. Competition for mates (which falls within the selfish category) is an especially salient source of variation among individuals

(Darwin 1871), and as a result, sexual selection is the best-characterised source of social selection. Kin selection is another specific form of social selection generated by interactions among relatives (Hamilton 1964). Social selection differs from natural selection (or ecological selection) because an individual's fitness is determined in part by influences of social partners on that individual's phenotype (Wolf *et al.* 1999a). Selection operating on individuals may therefore be partitioned into natural and social selection (Queller 1992a, 1992b, Frank 1997).

Social selection is only one half of the evolutionary equation because, for there to be phenotypic evolution (i.e. changes in mean phenotypes across generations), the changes in phenotype distributions within a generation resulting from selection must be translated into cross-generation changes. It is the genetic variation underlying traits that determines how within-generational changes in phenotype distributions result in cross-generational changes; therefore, to evolve, social behaviour must have a genetic component. In this chapter we show that the evolution of behaviour expressed in (or affected by) social interactions is fundamentally the *same* as that for any other traits. That is, there are genetic and environmental influences on social behaviour, and genetic variation underlying phenotypic variation in a social trait allows it to evolve. We simultaneously argue that the genetics of such traits are *different* from most other sorts of traits (e.g. morphological or physiological). Consequently, understanding the evolution of behaviour influenced by the social environment requires a very different theoretical and empirical approach (Box 2.1). Social behaviour is the product of an interaction, and therefore becomes a composite trait that cannot be attributed solely to a single individual (Fuller & Hahn 1976, Meffert 1995, Hahn & Schanz 1996). This is not a newly recognised problem; in one of the first studies to apply quantitative genetics to behaviour in an evolutionary context, Manning (1961, p. 84) wrote 'There is perhaps little reality in the heritability of a character which involves the interaction between two individuals' (but went ahead and calculated a realised heritability anyway). Fuller and Hahn (1976) and, in a follow-up, Hahn and

Schanz (1996) noted some of the special problems of studying genetics of social behaviour, including the fact that social behaviour involves, by definition, the interaction of two or more individuals. In addition, they noted that the unit observed is a group, and that the behavioural output of a group is hard to attribute to the genetic or experimental history of only one member of the group.

Box 2.1 Extended and interacting phenotypes

Extended phenotype includes abiotic

Interacting phenotype interactions among conspecifics, need not be related

Maternal/paternal/kin effects interactions among relatives

Targets of social selection

In this figure we try to capture some of the ways that researchers have dealt with the unusual nature of behaviour as a phenotype, and how these approaches overlap or subsume each other. At the simplest level, relatives interact and models of maternal, paternal and kin effects capture how these interactions influence a focal phenotype and its evolution (Lynch 1987, Kirkpatrick & Lande 1989, Cheverud & Moore 1994). Unrelated individuals interacting have been captured by interacting-phenotype models (Moore *et al.* 1997, Wolf & Moore 2010). Most general of all are the verbal models of the extended phenotype, which include interactions both within and between species (Dawkins 1982). The first two approaches include formal mathematical modelling; the extended phenotype is not yet captured mathematically.

Many of the studies described in this chapter refer specifically to 'extended' rather than 'interacting' phenotypes. Furthermore, interacting phenotypes are also described in the context of maternal, sib-social or indirect genetic effects. Here we briefly describe how these concepts may be integrated. The figure above depicts the overlap among extended phenotypes, interacting phenotypes and maternal/paternal/kin effects. *Extended phenotypes* have classically been used to describe extensions of phenotype outside an individual such as gall formation (Stone & Cook 1998), spider webs and beaver dams (Dawkins 1982). An obvious extension of extended phenotype is the influence of an individual on the phenotype of its social partners. *Interacting phenotypes* describe interactions among conspecifics; however, those conspecifics need not be kin. *Maternal and paternal effects*, which can be expanded to include any class of relative and therefore 'kin effects' (Lynch 1987), describe a special case of interacting phenotypes (Moore *et al.* 1997). Extended phenotypes, interacting phenotypes and maternal/paternal/kin effects are all underlain by indirect genetic effects to the extent that variation in the effector trait (the trait in one partner that influences the expression of a trait in another partner) is influenced by genetic variation.

Box 2.1 Continued

The category to which a trait or an effect is assigned will depend on the perspective applied. For example, gall formation by larval insects growing in their plant hosts is likely induced by larval secretions; however, gall formation is often described as an extended phenotype because the gall is external to a larva but is the result of larval characteristics. Gall formation may be categorised as an interacting phenotype because gall characteristics reflect the influence of social partners: galls that house multiple larvae are morphologically different from those that house single larvae. In addition, gall formation may be described in terms of maternal effects, as oviposition behaviour of the mother determines how many larvae develop within a gall (influences on gall formation are reviewed in Stone & Cook 1998). Phenotypic variation in galls is likely influenced by genetic variation in individuals (e.g. for amount or potency of secretions), siblings within the gall (e.g. for secretions they contribute or competition among individuals) and mothers (for oviposition behaviour). Indirect genetic effects in this system comprise genetic variation in social partners and mothers that influence the formation of galls. Galls are a target of selection, as they confer varying degrees of protection to the larvae they house (Weis *et al.* 1992) as well as nutrition (Weis *et al.* 1988), and it follows intuitively that a larva developing alone in a gall will experience selection differently than one developing in a gall housing multiple larvae. Social selection will therefore act on gall characteristics if social partners or parents influence gall formation.

Models of evolution and empirical studies require an explicit description of the phenotype of interest. How do we account for the nature of interactions in descriptions of phenotypes? There have been a number of approaches to describing behavioural phenotypes expressed in social interactions, but the only approach that incorporates inheritance when the individuals are not related is that of *interacting phenotypes* (Moore *et al.* 1997). Related to models of maternal effects, where the environment provided by relatives is genetically influenced (Lynch 1987, Kirkpatrick & Lande 1989, Cheverud & Moore 1994), interacting-phenotype models allow us to reconcile how genetic variation influences traits expressed in social interactions (Moore *et al.* 1997). This allows us to consider the complete evolution of traits expressed in social environments because the evolution of both the trait and the social environment can be considered simultaneously. Where optimality and game theory suggest a predicted outcome of evolution, interacting-phenotype models describe the direction and rate of evolution towards an optimum. Models of interacting phenotypes define which traits should be measured, and how we should measure these traits if we are interested in evolution. Interacting-phenotype models are related, conceptually, to the model of extended phenotypes proposed by Dawkins (1982). However, where extended phenotype and the more recently proposed niche construction (Odling-Smee *et al.* 2003) paradigms consider interacting phenotypes, they ignore the consequences of genetic variation and covariation on the behaviour of either interactant.

It is clear that considering genetic influences on social behaviour requires something of a different approach. There is likely to be more than one solution. Fuller and Hahn (1976) and Hahn and Schanz (1996) advocated treating pairs of animals as the unit to measure, and combining different identified genotypes. While this works, it generally requires inbred strains, constraining its applicability to many studies of behaviour. Moore *et al.* (1997) coined the term 'interacting phenotype' to capture the essence of the difference in phenotypes expressed during and influenced by interactions. Traits other than social behaviour can have a phenotypic expression contingent on an interaction (for example, body mass of an offspring may be contingent on parental feeding behaviour or sibling competition: Lock *et al.* 2004); however, all social behaviours are interacting phenotypes. This approach is more general, explicitly evolutionary, and can be applied more widely to any organism where quantitative genetic studies are possible (including plants: Mutic & Wolf 2007). Here we briefly review the theoretical underpinnings of quantitative genetics of social behaviour from an interacting-phenotype perspective, and provide empirical examples showing the consequences of the contingent nature of social traits.

2.2 Evolution and behaviour

Adaptive evolution proceeds by selection acting on a trait to cause changes in the distribution of the trait, which then persists in the next generation in proportion to the degree to which variation underlying the trait is heritable. This type of inheritance is often described in terms of heritability, the degree to which phenotypic variation in a trait can be explained by additive genetic variation (Falconer & Mackay 1996, Roff 1997, Lynch & Walsh 1998). Inheritance is then a key component of evolution but is largely neglected in most evolutionary studies of behaviour, which often focus on selection. We must therefore ask whether we can reconcile genetics and behaviour. One of Tinbergen's (1953) lasting legacies was to promote the idea that behaviour does not differ from any other morphology, and can therefore be studied like any other type of trait. As such, behaviour should reflect an evolutionary history, develop and be affected by genetic as well as both internal and external environmental influences, and have adaptive value. In apparent conflict with this view is the underlying premise of much of behavioural ecology that there is remarkable phenotypic plasticity of behaviour. Most behaviour is not 'fixed', and can change on timescales of minutes, hours, days, weeks and years, not just generations. Bateson (2004) makes these points succinctly: animals make choices, change their environment, modify their behaviour to match current conditions, and expose themselves to novel conditions. Much of this

results in behaviour as an agent of evolutionary change, causing selection on the organism. But behaviour is, nonetheless, widely thought to evolve differently than morphology. Behaviour is considered to be especially sensitive to environmental inputs (West-Eberhard 2003, Bateson 2004). Moreover, the evolution of behaviour is thought to 'lead' the evolution of morphology (Bateson 2004); that is, behaviour may be more likely to be the first trait that changes in the face of selection, or to be the trait that results in selection. Can we reconcile these views with that of genetics, where traits are reduced to the input of genes and environment?

Behaviour influencing selection presents few significant challenges for modern biologists. After all, sexual selection is primarily behaviour (Darwin 1871), as is kin selection (Hamilton 1964). But herein lies the problem – if behaviour can evolve, then does that mean the environment (and therefore the agent of selection itself) is evolving as well? As West-Eberhard (1979, 1983, 1984) and Lande (1981) showed, the answer can be yes, and this can lead to unusual evolutionary outcomes such as runaway evolution. So behaviour may present unique properties as a phenotype because it can both cause evolution (by being the agent of selection) and evolve itself – i.e. behaviour can be an evolving environment. This is because behaviours expressed in a social context involve an interaction and so depend, at least in part, on the social environment. Selection that occurs in the context of intraspecific interactions is termed social selection because the fitness benefits and costs accrued by individuals depend at least partially on the interactions those individuals have with their social environment. The phenotypic value of an interacting trait expressed by any individual reflects the influence of the social environment, therefore an individual's fitness also reflects the influence of the social environment. It is intuitive to categorise sexual selection as a subset of social selection because an individual's fitness will depend in part on the phenotype of its mate (see Chapter 10; West-Eberhard 1979, 1983, 1984).

Behaviour is somewhat different from other phenotypes because we must consider the influence of social environments when defining many behavioural phenotypes. For simplicity, we will refer to any trait that is influenced by social environment as a *social behaviour*. Using this definition, social behaviour is a wide category, including obvious traits such as aggression and social dominance, courtship, communication, parental care, cooperation, social foraging, copying, learning and others. Although most people think of the obvious candidates with social behaviour (cooperation, conflict), many if not most behaviours can be influenced by social context (e.g. activity levels of *Drosophila*: Higgins *et al.* 2005). This does not diminish the value of social behaviour, but instead enhances the richness of the field. Social behaviour is ubiquitous. Therefore, we need to model influences on behaviour within a context that allows the social environment to be included.

2.3 Behavioural genetics and social behaviour

2.3.1 Concepts

One of the most common approaches to understanding inheritance of phenotypes is through quantitative genetics. However, the application of quantitative genetics to behaviour was, is and remains controversial. There has been no resolution of the nature–nurture controversy (see Chapter 1; West-Eberhard 2003). But why should this be? Quantitative genetic approaches are designed to determine the relative importance of various factors that influence the expression of any trait that varies among individuals that we can observe and measure. At the simplest level we are interested in knowing how heritable factors that can be passed from one generation to the next (additive or direct genetic effects) influence variation in trait expression within a population. We are most often interested primarily in additive genetic effects because they are the stuff of evolution; it is primarily the additive genetic effects that make offspring resemble their parents and, therefore, it is the additive effects that translate changes within a generation into cross-generation changes. That is, while selection within a generation determines the distribution of a trait, evolution only occurs if this change in distribution is translated into a permanent shift in the next generation. It is for this reason that quantitative genetics rapidly branched out from its evolutionary

roots into an applied field as humans used artificial selection to permanently change animal and plant populations to better match the whims of the human architects of selection.

Quantitative genetics was invented by Fisher (1918) and developed over the ensuing 80-plus years into a fully mature field of study in evolutionary biology (Falconer & McKay 1996, Roff 1997, Lynch & Walsh 1998). The study of the quantitative genetics of a trait is relatively straightforward, and the underlying principles have changed little since Fisher, although there has been considerable development of methods and expansion of ideas. Sources of variation are statistically partitioned among individuals, using breeding studies (Falconer & McKay 1996, Roff 1997, Lynch & Walsh 1998) or pedigrees (Kruuk 2004), and used to distinguish heritable effects from those that reflect non-additive genetic effects, and random or specific environmental influences. Manipulated breeding designs or pedigrees provide information about relatedness (or relationships) among individuals and the ability to quantify the trait of interest, as well as sufficient sample sizes to produce reasonably robust estimates of quantitative genetic parameters. The statistical partitioning of variation into genetic and environmental variances therefore allows us to estimate parameters such as heritability (h^2), evolvability (typically the coefficient of additive genetic variation, CV_A) and genetic correlations (r_A), which allow us to make evolutionary predictions and inferences (Lynch & Walsh 1998).

Quantitative genetics of social behaviour is the same as quantitative genetics of any other trait, but with social behaviour there are additional considerations. As we suggest above, social behaviour is contingent on the biotic (social) environment, an environment that can itself evolve. We need to take this contingency into consideration when we describe genetic influences on social behaviour. To do this we will very briefly review quantitative genetic models of inheritance. We briefly introduce these models here to illustrate the differences between social and non-social traits. The relevant models and their development are presented in Wolf and Moore (2010).

2.3.2 Basic quantitative genetic theory

We can use linear equations to model the quantitative genetics of any trait. These linear equations are really nothing more than mathematical representations or statements of the factors that contribute to variation in trait expression. In the simplest case, the value of some trait that we measure for an individual (denoted z, where z represents the 'phenotypic value' of a trait) reflects both genotypic (g) and environmental (e) influences:

$$z = g + e \qquad (2.1)$$

We can partition the genetic influences (g) further, separating genetic effects into additive (a, the predictable effects of alleles, independent of all other genetic influences), dominance (d, the effect attributable to the interaction of alleles at a locus) and epistatic (i, the effects of genetic interactions between loci) effects:

$$z = a + d + i + e \qquad (2.2)$$

Equation 2.2 allows us to partition the effects on trait expression into any categories that we wish to understand. This might include partitioning the environmental effects into those attributable to particular causative factors (e.g. the environmental influence of temperature), or might include contingent influences, such as the interaction between the genetic and environmental effects (genotype-by-environment interactions, denoted G × E: see Chapter 1).

These linear equations describe the contributions of various factors to the expression of a trait we measure, but what we are really interested in is how variation among individuals reflects variation in these underlying effects. Using basic covariance mathematics and a few simplifying assumptions (such as no genotype-environment covariance, i.e. individuals are randomly distributed with respect to environment; no genotype-environment interactions; and all non-additive genetic influences are combined with the random environmental influences), we can express the phenotypic variance as:

$$Z = G + E \qquad (2.3)$$

where Z is the phenotypic variance (variance of z), G is the additive genetic variance (or variance of a) and E is the environmental variance (or variance of e, including all non-additive genetic and environmental influences). With our assumptions we can partition the variances in the same way we partitioned individual influences.

This basic quantitative genetic model has been used and expanded upon for the past 90 years since first devised by Fisher (1918), and has a rich history in evolutionary studies. It allows us to partition influences on traits and quantify the relative importance of different genetic and environmental influences. However, it clearly does not capture the socially contingent nature of some behavioural traits. For this we need an expanded model.

2.4 A model of interacting phenotypes

2.4.1 Indirect genetic effects

Our early theoretical work focused on developing this basic model to allow us to understand the importance of other individuals on the expression of a behavioural phenotype (Moore *et al.* 1997, 1998). Although our interest in this problem was stimulated originally by a consideration of the evolution of social dominance (as noted by numerous authors, social dominance has little meaning outside of an interaction, but this does not negate genetic influences on an individual's dominance; Fuller & Hahn 1976, Hahn & Schanz 1996, Moore *et al.* 2002), we clearly saw that many other traits fell into this category. Our approach was stimulated by 'maternal effects' models (e.g. Kirkpatrick & Lande 1989; see also Cheverud & Moore 1994), where the phenotypes of offspring are contingent on the environment provided by their parents. In these maternal-effects models, variation in the environment provided by mothers can be attributed to traits expressed by those mothers, and because these parental traits can reflect heritable variation, the maternally provided environment can be heritable (Kirkpatrick & Lande 1989, Cheverud & Moore 1994). These models capture what is known by all parents: children are influenced both by genetics and by the environment provided by their parents. But variation in the environment provided by parents may reflect genetic differences among parents. The extension beyond the parent–offspring relationship is simple: phenotypes of individuals may reflect additive genetic influences, the environment provided by another individual, and other environmental influences. Of course variation in the environment provided by other individuals may, as in the maternal-effects models, be influenced by genetic differences among those individuals.

To incorporate the environment provided by other individuals we simply take our model for trait expression (equations 2.1 and 2.2) and divide the environment into 'random' (e_n) and social (e_s) components, where the latter is the environment provided by other (conspecific) individuals:

$$z = a + e_n + e_s \qquad (2.4)$$

Because the social environment is composed of traits (i.e. features) of other individuals, we can replace the social environment term (e_s) in equation 2.4 with a term that reflects the influence that some trait (trait j) has in one individual on the expression of a trait (trait i) measured in the first individual (our *focal individual*):

$$z_i = a_i + e_i + \psi_{ij} z_j' \qquad (2.5)$$

where a_i is the additive genetic influences on trait i, e_i is the non-social environmental influences on the trait (including, for simplicity, the non-additive genetic influences), and $\psi_{ij} z_j'$ is social environmental effect, which in this case is the effect of trait j expressed in one individual on the expression of trait i in the focal individual. This last term has two parts: ψ_{ij} is the *interaction effect coefficient* and scales the strength of this effect (i.e. the influence that trait j expressed in one individual has on the expression of trait i in the focal individual) while z_j' is simply the value of trait j expressed in an individual that our focal individual interacts with (specifically, it is termed the *effector trait*). Trait i might be influenced by the same trait (also $j = i$) or a different trait ($j \neq i$) in the social partner. We use a prime to indicate that z_j' is the phenotype of a different individual. We discuss the interaction effect coefficient further below, but note that when $\psi_{ij} = 0$ (that is, the trait is not

at all contingent on the social environment) we return to the original model of quantitative genetics given in equation 2.1.

Although we have modelled the trait j as an environmental influence on the expression of trait i, this trait can also be influenced by genetics and evolve. Therefore, we can also decompose trait j into genetic and environmental influences:

$$z_j = a_j + e_j \qquad (2.6)$$

Substituting equation 2.6 into equation 2.5, we get:

$$z_i = a_i + e_i + \psi_{ij} \left(a_j' + e_j' \right) \qquad (2.7)$$

which illustrates how the trait of our focal individual is influenced both by genes expressed in itself (a_i) and by genes expressed in the interacting individual (a_j). Genes expressed in another individual that influence the trait of the focal individual are called *indirect genetic effects* (Riska *et al.* 1985, Moore *et al.* 1997), to contrast with the 'direct' additive genetic effects expressed within the individual and passed across generations as defined by Fisher (1918). Maternal genetic effects (sometimes simply referred to as maternal effects) are therefore a special case of indirect genetic effects.

We can develop this model into equations for evolutionary change (Moore *et al.* 1997), or consider how interactions and indirect genetic effects (IGEs) influence selection (Wolf *et al.* 1999a). For example, developing equation 2.7 into the simplest model for evolutionary change in the mean of trait i ($\Delta \bar{z}_i$) arising from the genetic aspects of interacting phenotypes among unrelated individuals, we get:

$$\Delta \bar{z}_i = \left[G_{ii} \beta_i + G_{ij} \beta_j \right] + \psi_{ij} \left[G_{jj} \beta_j + G_{ij} \beta_i \right] \qquad (2.8)$$

where G_{ii} is the additive genetic variance of trait i, G_{ij} is the genetic covariance between traits i and j, G_{jj} is the genetic variance of trait j, β_i is selection on trait i (β_i is a selection gradient that gives the linear relationship between z_i and fitness), and β_j is selection on trait j (Moore *et al.* 1997, 1998; see also Wolf & Moore 2010 for a discussion of this same model).

This model of interacting phenotypes has six major consequences for or changes from the standard model of quantitative genetics (Wolf & Moore 2010). First, and most obvious, social effects on trait expression provide the opportunity for indirect genetic effects (see equation 2.7). Second, social effects can result in genetically based genotype–environment covariances, where a genotype may experience a predictable social environment because of genetic associations between interacting individuals (for the details of how genotype–environment covariances may emerge see Wolf et al. 1999a, Wolf & Moore 2010). This is important because one of the fundamental assumptions of quantitative genetics is no genotype–environment association (as opposed to genotype–environment interaction (G × E), which is readily accommodated in quantitative genetic models). This point may be especially prevalent in behaviour, where individuals seek out other, specific, individuals or social environments with which to interact. The third major consequence of social effects is that they can alter the genotype–phenotype relationship (Moore et al. 1997, Wolf et al. 1998). We develop this further below. Fourth, social effects can produce an association (covariance) between the traits expressed in interacting individuals because the trait(s) of one individual alter the traits expressed by the interacting partner (see Wolf et al. 1999a, Wolf 2003 for more in-depth mathematical development). This covariance can affect quantitative genetic studies by changing the resemblance of relatives, leading to an over- or underestimate of the genetic variance underlying a trait (Wolf 2003, Bijma & Wade 2008). In practical terms, partitioning the variance attributable to social effects (some methods are discussed below) will allow more accurate measurements of the genetic variance underlying the traits of interest. The fifth major consequence of social effects is that they can generate social selection on traits, where social interactions lead to components of selection acting on traits (Wolf et al. 1999a). Social selection occurs when an individual's fitness is influenced by interactions with conspecifics and a covariance between traits expressed in interacting individuals (as in the fourth major consequence above; see Wolf et al. 1999a). The sixth major consequence of social effects is that they can lead to altered

trait evolution due to the evolution of the (mean) social environment. This has a number of implications, including evolution of traits even in the absence of direct genetic effects, and differences in trait values between populations can be due, at least partly, to differences in the average social environments in those populations (Moore et al. 1997, Agrawal et al. 2001a).

Consideration of IGEs also resolves some controversies over social evolution (Bijma & Wade 2008). Recently, Bijma et al. (2007a, 2007b) considered how IGEs and group selection interact using offspring performance models of IGEs (see Cheverud & Moore 1994 for a description of the difference between trait-based and offspring performance models in the context of maternal effects). Bijma and Wade (2008) further develop offspring performance models of IGEs and show how a consideration of IGEs allows a fuller understanding of the similarities and differences between kin selection and multilevel selection. They further show that while the evolution of social traits by kin selection depends on relatedness, multi-level selection can result in the evolution of social traits when interacting individuals are not related and populations are not structured along kin lines. We leave the mathematical development and support for all these points to the papers we have referenced, and especially Wolf and Moore (2010), which reviews and develops the mathematical models in great detail. In this chapter we focus on the empirical investigations into interacting phenotypes and indirect genetic effects. First, however, we explore the interaction effect coefficient, ψ, further.

2.4.2 The interaction effect coefficient, ψ

The constant that scales the strength of the influence of the effector trait on the focal trait is called the *interaction effect coefficient* and is symbolised by ψ (Moore et al. 1997). This coefficient is conceptually homologous to m, the maternal effect coefficient in maternal-effects models, which measures the relative influence of a mother's phenotype on the phenotype of her offspring (Kirkpatrick & Lande 1989). As m is calculated by taking the partial regression of the offspring's phenotype on the phenotype of the mother, holding genetic sources of variation constant (Kirkpatrick & Lande 1989), so is ψ measured by taking the partial regression of the phenotype of the focal individual on the phenotype of the social partner, also holding genetic sources of variation constant (Moore *et al.* 1997).

The coefficient ψ is typically represented as a single value, but in reality a matrix summarises the different effect of coefficients for a set of traits (each can be viewed as a path coefficient; see Moore *et al.* 1997 for diagram). Each value of ψ gives the effect of one trait on the expression of another trait, such as:

$$\begin{bmatrix} \psi_{ii} & \psi_{ji} \\ \psi_{ij} & \psi_{jj} \end{bmatrix}$$

where ψ_{ij} denotes the influence of trait j in the social partner on the expression of trait i in the focal individual. There are two things to note about this matrix: first, entries along the diagonal give the reciprocal effects that a trait has on its own expression and, second, the matrix is not symmetric, meaning that entries on the off diagonal with opposite subscripts are not the same. This latter point is important because it means that, for example, the effect of trait i on trait j does not have to be the same as the effect of trait j on trait i (i.e. ψ_{ij} does not have to equal ψ_{ji}). If the trait values are standardised (mean = 0, standard deviation = 1), then ψ will range from –1 to 1, providing an intuitive scale for measuring the relative influence of social partners on our focal individuals (Moore *et al.* 1997).

This interaction effect coefficient is probably best understood using an example. Consider the expression of trait i (for example grooming) in a focal individual (z_i). This trait might be influenced by the expression of two traits in a social partner: grooming (z_i') and aggression (z_j'), where the prime indicates the trait in the social partner. Substituting these into equation 2.5 from above, the amount of grooming (trait value z_i) we expect to see in our focal individual is then described by the linear equation:

$$z_i = a_i + \psi_{ii} z_i' + \psi_{ij} z_j' + e_i \tag{2.9}$$

In heuristic terms, this equation simply describes that the amount of allogrooming an individual performs

will reflect its own genes, the amount of allogrooming performed by its social partner and the aggressiveness of its social partner (both of which are influenced by the social partner's own genes), and other environmental influences. Different combinations of traits may be described by coefficients of interaction that differ in sign and magnitude. In our example, if allogrooming functions as an appeasement, it may increase as partner aggression increases, meaning that the social effect of aggression on allogrooming is positive (i.e. $\psi_{ij} > 0$). Alternatively, if allogrooming is only possible when social partners are not behaving in an aggressive manner, then ψ_{ij} (grooming in our focal individual influenced by aggression in the partner) will be negative. It is reasonable to predict that aggression and grooming in the social partner might affect grooming in our focal individual to different degrees, potentially even in different directions. Although the example above describes a unidirectional interaction, in reality social partners are likely to affect each other: if the expression of allogrooming in the social partner is influenced by that same trait in the focal individual (we assume in this example that $\psi_{ii} \neq 0$), the expression of allogrooming will involve reciprocal effects. Furthermore, the aggression of the focal individual will influence the expression of allogrooming in the social partner, so there will be complex reciprocal effects in the expression of allogrooming.

2.4.3 The importance of ψ

The magnitude of ψ determines the degree that evolutionary outcomes deviate from those predicted under standard quantitative genetic models of evolution. For example, for moderate values of ψ for a single trait influenced by the same trait in the social partner (e.g. $\psi_{ii} = 0.60$) rates of evolution increase about threefold compared to evolution occurring in the absence of an interaction (because of the reciprocal effects). Large values of ψ for any two traits may alter the rate, magnitude and (depending on the sign) direction of evolution. Those interactions where the trait in the focal individual is influenced by the same trait in the social partner (e.g. grooming in the social partner influences grooming in the focal individual), however, are expected to generate the greatest change because the interactions are reciprocal between the partners (Moore *et al.* 1997). Therefore, small changes in the average genetic contribution to trait expression can be exaggerated by the interaction of individuals caused by this feedback loop between them. In practical terms, the diagonal of a ψ matrix therefore becomes the most important component of the matrix for making predictions about how interacting traits are likely to evolve.

The coefficient ψ has typically been modelled as a population constant (Moore *et al.* 1997). However, intuitively we might expect ψ to vary among individuals or among social partners of different genotypes (Wolf *et al.* 1999a). Specifically, social effects may not be additive or constant in all cases, making the value of ψ context-dependent (Agrawal *et al.* 2001a). Quantification of ψ is important for understanding patterns of evolution in interacting traits because the strength of ψ will directly affect the magnitude of the response to selection and the rate of evolution (Wolf *et al.* 1998). In addition, if ψ itself is to evolve, variation in ψ must be present.

The degree to which individuals respond to their social environment may vary among individuals and among populations, as individuals are differentially responsive in many species and in many contexts (e.g. Komers 1997). A hypothetical example may help to illustrate this phenomenon. Suppose three inbred strains of mice exhibit different degrees of allogrooming (what we will call trait *g*), which we will characterise as Low, Medium and High. If individuals respond to their social environment, in this case the specific amount of grooming performed by their social partners, then regressing focal behaviour (z_g) on the behaviour of the social partner (z'_g) produces a relationship such as that pictured in Figure 2.1a. We quantify ψ for the Low strain by pairing focal individuals from the Low strain with social groups each comprised entirely of one of the other strains and measure allogrooming in both the focal individual and its social partners. If ψ is large and positive, we would generate a regression much like that pictured in Figure 2.1b. If we then repeated the experiment using the other strains as the focal strain, we might find variation in ψ such that although individuals from all strains increase their allogrooming as their social group does, they differ in the degree to which they increase (Fig. 2.1c). If

we selected for individuals exhibiting more allogrooming, we would also predict an increase in allogrooming in the social group because how much allogrooming an individual performs results not only from its own genes (whether it comes from the Low or High strain, for example) but also from the group with which it is paired. The converse is also true: selecting groups that exhibit more grooming will also lead to increases in grooming by individuals. The degree to which the group responds to selection on the individual (or vice versa) will be a direct function of the magnitude of ψ (Moore *et al.* 1997, Agrawal *et al.* 2001a).

Additionally, individuals may exhibit non-additive responses to a given social group, with their responses differing not only in magnitude but potentially in direction as well (Wolf 2000a). The presence of such non-additive interactions further complicates our predictions about how selection acting at one level will manifest at other levels (Brodie 2000). In the previous example, selection acting on an individual can lead to evolution in the social group because variation in individual behaviour actually represents, at least in part, genetic variation in social partners. But if combinations of social partners from other strains yield differences in observed behaviour, the response of the group to selection acting on a focal member cannot be predicted without specific knowledge of the individuals involved (Brodie 2000). If ψ is additive, then any individual from any of the three strains will groom less when paired with a social group from the Low strain and more when paired with a social group from the High strain. If focal individuals from different strains respond differently to a particular social group, however, ψ is non-additive. Continuing with our mouse example, imagine we have two Low and two Medium grooming strains. Each strain will serve as both a focal strain (LowFocal strain and MediumFocal strain respectively), and as social partners (LowPartner strain and MediumPartner strain) for each other. If LowFocal mice groom more with social partners from the LowPartner strain than with partners from the MediumPartner strain, while MediumFocal mice groom more when paired with the MediumPartner strain than with the LowPartner strain, ψ is non-additive (Figure 2.1d). In other words, predicting the outcome of the interaction requires specific

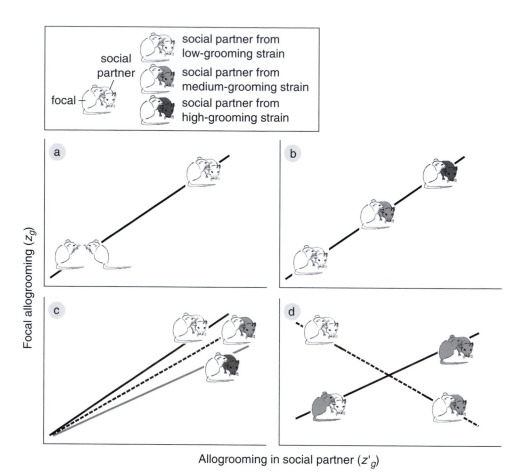

Figure 2.1 Hypothetical measurements of the interaction effect coefficient (ψ) for grooming behaviour in inbred strains of mice obtained from regressing the phenotype of the focal individual (z_g) on the phenotype of the social partner/s (z'_g). (a) Shows a large positive value for ψ where the slope of the regression line gives ψ. (b) Describes ψ measured in a focal strain paired with social partners from multiple other inbred strains. (c) Demonstrates variability in ψ such that although all focal strains increase their grooming behaviour as that of their social partners increases, they do so at different rates with different strains of partners. (d) Depicts non-additivity of ψ resulting from G × G epistatic interactions where different focal strains respond differently to the same phenotype of a social partner (i.e. LowFocal mice decrease their grooming when paired with a MediumPartner mouse while MediumFocal mice increase their grooming with MediumPartner mice).

information about the phenotype and genotype of both interactants. Thus, selecting for individuals that exhibit more allogrooming will actually generate different evolutionary results in the social group depending on the specific combination of focal and group strains that is utilised. Although we can infer such non-additive ψ for behaviour ranging from competition (e.g. Lewontin & Matsuo 1963) to mating behaviour (reviewed in Wolf 2000b), only two direct measurements of ψ have been made, both of which found evidence for non-additivity of ψ: predator inspection in guppies *Poecilia reticulata*, with the time a female spends schooling with her social partners depending on both her strain and the strain of her social group (Bleakley & Brodie 2009); and chemical signalling in *Drosophila melanogaster*, with the influence of a social group on a male's chemical profile depending on both his and the group's strain (Kent *et al.* 2008).

2.4.4 The measurement of ψ

To date, direct measures of the magnitude of ψ, other than measures of the maternal effect coefficient m, are rare, primarily because controlling the genetic component of the social environment is difficult. Maternal effects studies often control the genetic component of the environment through breeding design (such as half-sib analysis) and cross-fostering, and even then there are few direct measures of the influence of individual maternal traits on specific offspring traits (but see Agrawal *et al.* 2001b, Kölliker & Richner 2001). Interactions among unrelated individuals can be explored using methods analogous to cross-fostering in breeding designs that control for family identity but require large sample sizes. The use of inbred or isogenic strains of animals provides a means of controlling both the direct effects of genes on behaviour in the focal individual and the indirect effects of genes carried in social partners (see also Fuller & Hahn 1976, Hahn & Schanz 1996). In addition to being genetically distinct, inbred lines used for studies of IGEs must also be behaviourally distinct, thus allowing us to control the genetic component of the social environment while varying the social environment an individual experiences by changing the strain from which an individual's social group is drawn (Moore *et al.* 1997). Pairing an inbred focal individual with an inbred social group therefore allows the direct quantification of the influence of the genetic component of the social environment on the behaviour of a focal individual. Finally, inbred lines allow us to replicate the combination of genotypes over many groups (Fuller & Hahn 1976, Hahn & Schanz 1996).

Direct measurements of ψ allow us to address broader evolutionary questions. For simplicity, all existing models and empirical tests of IGEs assume that the strength of ψ is constant within a population. However, the models also predict that ψ should vary and evolve if it is an individual trait with a genetic basis, and must evolve for interacting phenotypes to also evolve (Moore *et al.* 1997, Agrawal *et al.* 2001a). Measurements of ψ completed for two different focal strains of guppies and for wild-type and mutant *Drosophila* varied both as a result of the focal strain and the strain with which the individual was paired (Kent *et al.* 2008, Bleakley & Brodie 2009). In these studies, differences in ψ, measured for two focal strains with respect to the same social group and non-additive interactions between strains suggest that genetic variation in ψ may exist, providing a substrate on which selection may act to drive the evolution of interacting phenotypes.

2.5 Experimental studies of indirect genetic effects

Classic quantitative genetic studies have developed numerous approaches to partition the relative influences of all aspects of the genetic and environmental variation, including genetic variation contained in the social environment. Fuller and Hahn (1976) and Hahn and Schanz (1996) review the classic methods for studying genetics of social behaviour, including *homogenous sets*, *standard tester* and *panel of tester* designs. These are particularly powerful ways to control for experience effects and are well suited to studies of inbred lines (their research involves laboratory mice *Mus musculus*). While these are important approaches, for many evolutionary geneticists inbred lines are not available. Nevertheless, the cautions and lessons of this research should be considered.

Indirect genetic effects and an interacting-phenotype approach can have applications to many problems in evolutionary biology. Moore *et al.* (1998) applied the concept to sexual selection in general, and Wolf *et al.* (1997, 1999b) and Miller and Moore (2007) considered how IGEs (particularly maternal effects) might relate to and influence sexual selection and mate choice. Moore and Pizzari (2005) developed an IGE model for sexual conflict. As West-Eberhard (1984) has discussed, communication influences (competitive) interactions, and D'Ettorre and Moore (2008) consider how indirect genetic effects and social selection might influence the evolution of cues and signals during social communication. Mating is clearly a behaviour that in dioecious organisms requires an interaction, and that goes beyond the initial behavioural interactions. Simmons and Moore (2008) consider how IGEs might influence traits of sperm as a result of sperm competition. The aforementioned papers illustrate the studies that need to be done and the diversity of approaches that can be adopted in genetic studies of interacting phenotypes.

2.5.1 Breeding designs

Given that the theory is relatively new, studies of social behaviour as interacting phenotypes, with measures of indirect genetic effects and ψ, are in their infancy. Nevertheless, the work that has been done has shown that it is important to consider effects of interactions and indirect genetic effects on social behaviour. Most of these studies adapt classical quantitative genetic approaches and use controlled breeding studies in the laboratory. For example, patterns of heritable variation in morphology (e.g. body size at pupation) of *D. melanogaster* strongly depend on whether individuals were reared with full siblings, half-siblings or unrelated individuals (Wolf 2003). Similarly, genetically based differences in rearing conditions (the social environment experienced by the pupae) created by variation in patterns of relatedness influence worker mass, caste ratio and sex ratio in acorn ants *Temnothorax curvispinosus* (Linksvayer 2006). Acorn ants live and breed in small colonies housed entirely within acorns, making them amenable to laboratory manipulations. Seven treatments, including combinations of removing the queen, mixing the workers and mixing the larvae, were utilised to tease apart the relative influences of maternal effects (the presence of the mother), indirect genetic effects ('sib-social effects' of being reared by siblings) and direct genetic effects (Fig. 2.2), and to identify the presence of genetic variation for all three effects. Although not as important as direct genetic effects, both maternal and sib-social effects influence worker mass, caste ratios and sex ratios (Linksvayer 2006). It should be noted that while both these studies measured morphological and life-history characters, these characters directly reflect the endpoint of behaviour present in the rearing environments, such as dominance and competitive interactions in the *Drosophila* and feeding and larval care behaviour in the ants.

Quantitative genetic breeding designs can create known levels of relatedness among individuals who have their phenotype measured. One of the most common and powerful of these is the paternal full-sib/half-sib study, where each male (sire) is mated to multiple females (dams), and multiple offspring are measured from each family. Petfield *et al.* (2005) used a half-sib breeding study to show that IGEs arising from females influenced the cuticular hydrocarbon phenotypes of males in *D. serrata*. These cuticular hydrocarbons are important sexual signals and influence female mate choice; males apparently assess female condition during interactions and alter their signal accordingly. House *et al.* (2008) used a half-sib study of males and females to identify IGEs that may be involved in re-mating behaviour of the burying beetle *Nicrophorus vespilloides*. Where controlled breeding is not possible, it may be possible to use pedigree information and the 'animal model' to measure quantitative genetic parameters (Kruuk 2004). Wilson *et al.* (2009) recently used this approach to measure the direct and indirect genetic contributions, and the correlations between them, to agonistic behaviour in deer mice *Peromyscus maniculatus*.

Experiments utilising breeding designs have been more commonly used in quantifying the presence and strength of maternal and paternal effects for a broad range of physiological and life-history traits (reviewed in Bernardo 1996, Mousseau & Fox 1998). For example, paternal effects from male accessory-gland products in crickets *Gryllus bimaculatus* have significant consequences for offspring viability (Garcia-Gonzalez & Simmons 2005), and immune function in offspring is often the result of maternal antibody transmission (Grindstaff *et al.* 2003). Offspring survival and development reflect aspects of maternal care in a wide range of species (e.g. *Parus major*, Kölliker *et al.* 2000; *Nicrophorus pustulatus*, Rauter & Moore 2002; *Poecilia reticulata*, Reznick *et al.* 1996), and offspring behaviour often reflects maternal and paternal effects (*Mus musculus*, Isles *et al.* 2004; *Poecilia reticulata*, Evans *et al.* 2004).

Studies that partition the relative influences that genetic variation and environmental variation have on phenotypes may identify suites of interactions,

Treatment	Remove queen	Mix worker	Mix larvae	Diagram of three colonies per treatment
L	X	X	–	
Q	–	X	X	
W	X	–	X	
WL	X	–	–	
QL	–	X	–	
QW	–	–	X	
QWL	–	–	–	

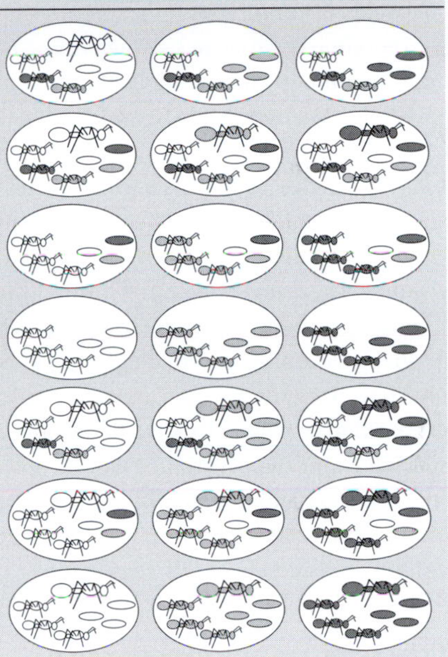

Figure 2.2 The experimental conditions utilised by Linksvayer (2006) to isolate direct, maternal and indirect genetic effects associated with rearing conditions provided by siblings, by removing the queen (Q), mixing the workers (W) or mixing the larvae (L) in acorn ant *Temnothorax curvispinosus* colonies. Three experimental manipulations were used to create seven possible treatments. X indicates which manipulations were used in each treatment. The figure depicts three colonies for each treatment and shading is used to indicate the colony of origin for the queen, workers and larvae. Treatments L, Q and W vary only in shading for larvae, workers or queens respectively to indicate the source of among-colony variance for each treatment. The last row (QWL) is an unmanipulated control, and therefore the queen, workers and larvae are all the same shade.

often from different sources. Longevity of female dung beetles *Onthophagus taurus*, and consequently the number of broods reared over the course of a lifetime, are significantly affected by the male with which the female mates (Kotiaho *et al.* 2003). Development, specifically brood mass, reflects maternal effects resulting from differences in provisioning of eggs. However, maternal provisioning depends on the male a female was mated with, with the greatest brood masses resulting from differential provisioning (females provision more) after mating with males with large horns and body sizes. The interaction between parental provisioning and offspring solicitation, and family conflicts in general, are fertile ground for studies of IGE. The consequences of family interactions for evolution

have been extensively modelled (Wolf & Brodie 1998, Kölliker 2005, Kölliker *et al.* 2005). There are only a few empirical studies, however (Kölliker 2005). Most clear-cut are those in insects using cross-fostering designs. Offspring condition and survival in burrowing bugs *Sehirus cinctus* depend on maternal genes for provisioning behaviour (Agrawal *et al.* 2001b). However, offspring also genetically vary in their ability to solicit food from the mother. Recall from above that one consequence of IGEs is that social effects (in this case offspring soliciting mom, and mom feeding offspring) can generate covariance between the traits expressed in interacting individuals (Wolf 2003, Bijma & Wade 2008). As a result of genetic variation underlying offspring solicitation and maternal provisioning in these bugs, final levels of provisioning reflect an interaction between maternal effects and IGEs, and a genetic covariance between feeding behaviour and solicitation emerges. The same covariance between offspring solicitation and parental provisioning is observed in the burying beetle *Nicrophorus vespilloides* (Lock *et al.* 2004). However, the sign of the covariance is positive in burying beetles (individuals with high levels of provisioning have high levels of begging in their offspring) while it is negative in burrowing bugs (high-provisioning families have low-begging offspring). The sign of this covariance reflects the relative strength of selection on provisioning or solicitation: where maternal behaviour is highly selected the covariance will be negative, whereas when offspring behaviour is under stronger selection the covariance will be positive (Kölliker *et al.* 2005). Thus the quantitative genetic model of Kölliker *et al.* (2005) based on IGEs helps us to understand the resolution of family conflicts.

2.5.2 Artificial selection and experimental evolution

Indirect genetic effects may be characterised with lines that have been artificially selected for differences in behaviour or bottlenecked to encourage inbreeding, thus increasing genetic differences among strains and reducing genetic variance in the social environment. Male house flies *Musca domestica* compensate for female mating thresholds that change as a result of bottlenecking by altering their courtship behaviour (Meffert 1995, Aragaki & Meffert 1998). This result was demonstrated quantitatively using combinations of selection lines to observe interactions between the genotype of a male and the genotype of his potential mate, termed genotype × genotype epistasis or G × G (developed more fully below; see also Wade 1998, Wolf & Brodie 1998, Wolf 2000b). G × G interactions are analogous to G × E interactions, but rather than the same genome generating a different phenotype in response to different environments, when G × G interactions occur, the expressed phenotype reflects an interaction between the genotype of the focal individual and the genotype of the social partner (Wade 1998, Wolf & Brodie 1998, Wolf 2000b). Meffert (1995) found two large principal

components (PC) describing male courtship in house flies. Four sets of selection lines were created, high (+) and low (−) expression of each PC, and males were then allowed to court females in all four possible combinations (+male paired with +female, +male paired with −female, etc.). Male behaviour often reflected the selection line from which his social partner was derived. For example, −males increased the intensity of their displays when paired with +females (Aragaki & Meffert 1998, Meffert & Regan 2002).

Similarly, IGEs reflecting interactions between male and female genotype have been identified for a number of aspects of sperm competition and male contributions to seminal fluid. Female *D. melanogaster* lay eggs at a faster rate after mating with males derived from a short-generation selection line than when mated to males from a long-generation selection line in response to heritable differences in the constituents of seminal fluid (reviewed in Clark & Begun 1998). Replicated experimental evolution lines of *D. pseudoobscura* were established with selection imposed by different operational sex ratios (OSR) during mating interactions within each line (1:1, 3:1, 6:1 male-to-female ratio). This generated different levels of social competition among males. After 50 generations, courtship behaviour evolved differently in the lines. While mean courtship rates and mating durations did not differ among the lines, the shape of the phenotypic covariance matrix changed, suggesting rapid non-linear evolution due to indirect genetic effects arising from different social interactions (Bacigalupe *et al.* 2008).

Selection lines have also been utilised to explore the evolution of social dominance, but in a qualitatively different way. In the cockroach *Nauphoeta cinerea* stable linear dominance hierarchies are formed, dominance status influences mating success, and males exhibit a heritable badge of status based on a pheromone blend (reviewed in Moore *et al.* 2002). Allowing only the most dominant or most subordinate males to breed, using within-family selection, created dominant and subordinate lines. As a result, selection was not operating directly on any specific trait of a male, such as body size, but rather on the predictable outcome of a set of interactions. No changes in levels of agonistic behaviour were identified for hierarchies within either the high or low lines after seven generations of selection (i.e. males from the dominant line were not consistently more aggressive). Pairing males from both selection lines, however, demonstrated the response to selection, with males from the dominant line predictably dominant over males from the subordinate lines. A male's dominance status directly reflected the selection line from which his social partner was drawn, and dominance evolved under the two selection regimes (Moore *et al.* 2002).

2.5.3 Inbred lines and G × G

Perhaps the most straightforward means of detecting indirect genetic effects is to look for interactions between different genomes (G × G). Meffert (1995) pursued this approach with selection lines, but a more straightforward and perhaps more common method is to use inbred lines. For example, male and female genotypes interact in inbred lines of *D. melanogaster* to determine sperm precedence in multiply mated females, significantly influencing both the fitness of the males and the resultant distribution of offspring phenotypes in the subsequent generation (Clark & Begun 1998, Clark *et al.* 1999). The influences of indirect genetic effects have been identified for several categories of behaviour in *Drosophila*. Higgins *et al.* (2005) utilised inbred lines originating from natural populations of *D. melanogaster* to create social groups. Groups consisted of five males and five females, all of the same genotype, and were replicated with multiple groups from each possible genotype. All individuals were scored for a suite of behaviours that in total represents a composite of general activity levels for groups of interacting flies. They identified significant effects of genotype – direct genetic effects explaining 14% of variation in observed behaviour – for total activity levels, as well as the relative proportion of time a given genotype performed particular behaviours. Indirect genetic effects explained a comparable amount of variation in group behaviour (19%).

Danielson-François *et al.* (2009) examined the relative influence of IGEs on competitive ability in wax moths, also using inbred lines. Larval lesser wax moths *Achroia grisella* infest honeycombs of the western honey bee *Apis mellifera*, eating the honeycomb and other organic material within the hive. Competition within the honeycomb can be extreme, with individuals carving out tunnels that are vigorously defended against other individuals, sometimes resulting in the death of a competitor. Inbred lines were created from natural populations and sets of larvae were obtained from three different lines (summarised here as lines A, B and C). Fifteen larvae from line B were then reared with fifteen larvae from either line A or line C, replicated five to nine times, and weighed at eclosion. The genetic identity of the competitors had a significant influence on the competitive ability of larvae from line A, with larvae attaining much larger body masses when pitted against line A than line C. In fact, individuals from line B were better able to compete against individuals from line A than against individuals from their own line (Fig. 2.3; Danielson-François *et al.* 2009).

Inbred lines are infrequently used to explore maternal effects, with three notable behavioural exceptions. Cowley *et al.* (1989) explored prenatal maternal effects imposed by differences in the uterine environment using two inbred strains of mice *Mus musculus* and their F_1 hybrid. Reciprocal embryo transfer between all three strains was performed and body weight and tail length were monitored through maturation. Although the impact of uterine genotype on the growth of the progeny was typically less than the direct genetic effects of progeny genotype, the genotype of the surrogate mother was nevertheless very important in determining offspring phenotype in virtually all stages of development. Additionally, interactions between surrogate-maternal and progeny genotype significantly influenced progeny phenotype at many points during development. The importance of maternal effects on offspring phenotype varied through time (Cowley *et al.* 1989), consistent with other studies that often find the strength of maternal effects declining through offspring development (reviewed in Messina 1998). Maternal effects that can be extrapolated to maternal behaviour are found in inbred litters of mice fostered by mothers of their own or a different strain (Hager & Johnstone 2003). As in the studies of insect parental care discussed above, and in other studies of parent–offspring interactions, there is a strong maternal genetic effect (*Sehirus cinctus*, Kölliker *et al.* 2005). Maternal genotype strongly

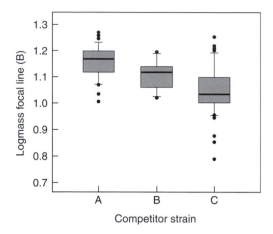

Figure 2.3 The outcome of competition of larvae from one inbred line of wax moth *Achroia grisella* when paired with larvae from the same or each of two additional inbred lines. Competitive ability is significantly influenced by the genetic identity of the larvae's competitors. Redrawn after Danielson-François *et al.* (2009).

influences the level of provisioning a litter receives, and an interaction between offspring and maternal genotype is also important, with offspring receiving more resources from foster mothers from the same strain as their biological mother. This result may reflect strain-specific differences in soliciting food, with young better able to solicit from mothers of their own strain, or kin discrimination by the mothers (Hager & Johnstone 2003). Finally, using isogenic lines of *D. melanogaster* (lines that are completely homozygous across most or all of the genome), Ruiz-Dubreuil and del Solar (1993) found that maternal effects impact gregarious oviposition behaviour, although they are not as influential as additive genetic effects or dominance effects.

2.5.4 Measuring ψ

The most precise quantitative measures of ψ are obtained from regressing the phenotype of the focal individuals on the phenotypes of their social partners (Moore *et al.* 1997, Chenoweth & Blows 2006). If both the focal individuals and their social partners come from inbred strains, controlling the variance in phenotype resulting from both direct and indirect genetic

effects respectively, the slope of the regression is equal to ψ. The coefficient ψ could be estimated in this way with outcrossed individuals, using breeding design to control for direct and indirect genetic effects, but would require very large sample sizes. As with any regression, the greater the number of social-partner genotypes present, the more accurate and precise the measurement of ψ (Moore *et al.* 1997, Chenoweth & Blows 2006). In addition, more combinations of focal and partner genotypes allow us to identify possible interaction effects, which indicate different magnitudes or even different signs of ψ for different combinations of social partners. A multiple regression including all the relevant behaviours is used to construct the ψ matrix (Moore *et al.* 1997). However, a critical issue in this approach is the need to control for shared or common environmental effects among interactants. For example, if one is interested in the influence of aggression expressed in one individual on the expression of aggression in another individual, it is important to rule out the possibility that shared environmental effects modulate the aggression of both individuals simultaneously. This is best done by controlling environmental effects where possible (e.g. temperature, rearing group) and randomly grouping individuals.

The influences of IGEs on guppy anti-predator behaviour have been explored in this manner. Inbred lines of guppies are both genetically and behaviourally distinct and respond to their specific social environment (Bleakley *et al.* 2006, 2007, 2008). Female guppies from each of two inbred focal strains were paired with social groups comprised of one of four other strains and assayed for anti-predator and social behaviour in the presence of a model predator. Multiple regression was used to explore the influence of each behaviour in the social group on each behaviour in the focal female (in other words, to quantify ψ). Influences of both direct and indirect genetic effects were observed, as well as interactions between strains. In general, the factor that best explained variance in focal female behaviour was the same behaviour performed by the social group with which she was paired. In all cases where this was true, greater levels of expression of a behaviour in the social group led to increases in the behaviour in the focal individual, generating a strong positive relationship between the behaviour performed by the social group and the behaviour performed by the focal female. Measurements of ψ associated with these homologous pairs of traits (ψ_{11} or ψ_{22}, etc.) for guppy anti-predator behaviour ranged from zero to 1 (the maximum), but were usually greater than 0.5 (Bleakley & Brodie 2009). For example:

$$\begin{array}{c} & z'_{prox} \quad z'_{insp} \\ \begin{array}{c} z_{prox} \\ z_{insp} \end{array} & \begin{bmatrix} 0.80 & -0.22 \\ 0 & 0.85 \end{bmatrix} \end{array}$$

where z_{prox} refers to proximity to the predator model and z_{insp} refers to predator inspections. Recall that the prime indicates the phenotypic value of the social partner. Such large values of ψ for homologous traits suggest that the evolution of guppy anti-predator behaviour could be significantly greater in rate or magnitude compared to the evolution of non-interacting phenotypes (Moore et al. 1997). In addition, squaring the individual path coefficients provides a lower estimate for the proportion of variance explained by indirect genetic effects (sensu Price 1998). At least 25% of the variance in guppy behaviour in this experiment can be attributed to indirect genetic effects.

One other study to date has measured ψ. Joel Levine's laboratory used the genetic tools of D. melanogaster along with a clever experimental design to measure the effect of the social environment on indirect genetic effects influencing chemical signals. Many behavioural interactions are mediated by chemical signalling, including mating interactions in D. melanogaster. Kent et al. (2008) manipulated both the physical environment and the social environment and compared the effects of each on male cuticular hydrocarbon (odour) signals. Males interacted in groups of 40 consisting of all wild-type males, all (clock) mutant males, or 32 wild-type and 8 mutant flies. Large direct genetic effects exist, with a male's own genotype a significant influence on his chemical signalling profile. However, the genotype of the social group also explains a significant proportion of the observed variation and, importantly, interactions between genotypes were identified as influencing the production of

all but one cuticular hydrocarbon. Altogether, social environment accounted for at least 33% of observed variation in male signalling. Along with identifying influences of direct and indirect genetic effects, Kent et al. (2008) measured ψ. Within homogenous groups, ψ was greater than zero for virtually all cuticular hydrocarbons. Non-additivity of ψ was observed in the heterogenous groups, where the influence of mutants on wild-type males generated strongly positive values of ψ, while influences of the wild-type males on mutants were negative or not significantly different from zero.

2.6 Molecular genetics, genomics and interacting phenotypes

So far we have reviewed studies that begin with an examination of the phenotype (behaviour) of interest and then find the sources of variation, such as environmental, direct or indirect genetic effects, on this phenotype. An alternative to this 'top-down' methodology is to start with genes – i.e. to adopt a 'bottom-up' approach (Boake et al. 2002). Social interactions have been demonstrated to modulate gene expression in a number of systems including male song and female mating behaviour in zebra finches Taeniopygia guttata, dominance status in cichlids Astatotilapia (Haplochromis) burtoni, mate choice in swordtails Xiphophorus nigrensis, and aggressive behaviour in D. melanogaster (Winberg et al. 1997, Jarvis et al. 1998, Burmeister et al. 2005, Cummings et al. 2008, L. Wang et al. 2008, Woolley & Doupe 2008). Additionally, patterns of gene expression, including G × G interactions, may be used to explain species-level differences in behaviour (Linksvayer 2007).

The studies measuring ψ in guppy anti-predator behaviour and chemical signalling in D. melanogaster suggest that indirect genetic effects are often large and positive. Combined with studies utilising recombinant lines of Arabidopsis or Drosophila, the above studies suggest a means of integrating an indirect genetic-effects approach with molecular genetics and genomics by straddling the top-down and bottom-up approaches. For example, Mutic and Wolf (2007) identified 15 quantitative trait loci (QTL: stretches of

DNA statistically associated with the measured trait) that directly influenced size, development and fitness phenotypes in *Arabidopsis thaliana*. Of those 15 QTL, 13 also influenced the expression of traits in neighbouring plants, demonstrating significant indirect genetic effects and suggesting that indirect genetic effects may be a necessary consequence of direct genetic effects in some systems. Consistent with the guppy and *Drosophila* studies, the direct and indirect effects were almost always of the same sign (meaning that neighbours generally had positive effects on each other), suggesting that selection on any given trait could generate strong positive feedback across neighbours, potentially accelerating or magnifying evolutionary change. The IGEs identified in this study suggest that facilitation among neighbouring plants may be the consequence of direct genetic effects within a plant extending beyond that individual to influence its neighbours, for example through changes in soil chemistry. Similarly, J. Wang *et al.* (2008) found that gene expression for chemical communication in fire ants *Solenopsis invicta* is more influenced by the genotype of colony mates than by an individual's own genotype, even though variation for the trait is associated with a single Mendelian factor. This example is also illustrative of the feedback between components of the social environment and social selection, as the particular colony expression of this chemical-communication trait regulates the number of queens present and influences the behaviour of individual workers, thus shaping the selective pressures acting within and on the colony. Finally, Krupp *et al.* (2008) found that the genetic composition of the group with which a male interacts significantly affects the transcription of clock genes in both the head and oenocytes, altering the pattern of pheromone accumulation on the cuticle and therefore the mating behaviour of the focal male in *D. melanogaster*.

2.7 Conclusions and future directions

Studies of behaviour have long recognised that animals respond to the environment provided by their social partners with changes in their behaviour (Allee 1927,

Tinbergen 1953), and questions about how, when and with whom an animal interacts and the consequences of those interactions form the basis of behavioural ecology, the study of social behaviour from a functional perspective. In the preceding pages we have highlighted a number of behaviours that are best categorised as interacting phenotypes, including competitive ability, group activity, anti-predator behaviour and mating behaviour, to name but a few. Impacts of indirect genetic effects (IGEs) on all types of phenotypes appear to be widespread. Maternal effects have been found in almost every taxon imaginable, influencing life-history, physiological and behavioural traits, and they are often equivalent in magnitude to additive genetic effects on offspring phenotype (reviewed in Mousseau & Fox 1998). IGEs have been found in a slowly growing number of taxa, and also for a variety of life-history and behavioural traits. When the strength of IGEs has been quantified, they are often found to be as important as, if not more important than, additive genetic effects on phenotypes.

Studies of social behaviour often implicitly, if not explicitly, include information about the phenotype and genotype of social partners, and such studies could thus be informed by explicit consideration of IGEs. Many studies have demonstrated the dependence of mating behaviour (e.g. preferences) on the genotype of the potential mate, and often an interaction between the genotypes of the male and female (reviewed in Tregenza & Wedell 2000, Kempenaers 2007). Sexual conflict explicitly contains interactions between the genotype of one partner for a coercive trait and the genotype in the other partner for susceptibility, which is predicted to lead to antagonistic coevolution between male and female genomes within the same species (reviewed in Chapman *et al.* 2003). For example, *D. melanogaster* males produce accessory-gland proteins that are transferred during mating and manipulate female behaviour. A female's post-mating behaviour thus reflects, at least in part, the genes of her mate and therefore IGEs (Simmons & Moore 2008). The outcome of agonistic interactions often depends on genes carried in the partner for body size, ornamentation or expressed levels of aggression. Nelson (2005) provides a comprehensive review of the genetics, endocrine mechanisms and social influences on aggression, all of which implicitly incorporate genes carried in the social partner. Cannibalism, as a specialised form of aggression, is also best characterised as an interacting phenotype reflecting both the genes in one partner for traits that facilitate cannibalism, such as the likelihood of aggression and body size or other specialised morphology (e.g. dentition), and genes in the other social partner that influence susceptibility to cannibalism (see Elgar & Crespi 1992 for a review of mechanisms and manifestations of cannibalism). Although the formulation of the model presented above refers to a single social partner, many animals interact in larger groups. Population structure can be added to the model (Agrawal et al. 2001a), but for most purposes the mean phenotype of the group can be used in place of a single social partner (Moore et al. 1997). An unexplored facet of these models is the degree to which the composition of a social network might structure IGEs in a population. Finally, because the presence of indirect genetic effects allows selection to operate at multiple levels of organisation, IGEs may contribute to the organisation and evolution of social networks, such as those formed by social insects (Fewell 2003).

To illustrate how information about IGEs might be incorporated into studies of social behaviour, we will develop one final example involving a conservation application of behaviour. Conservation of threatened and endangered species frequently requires explicit understanding of both animal behaviour and evolutionary genetics (reviewed in Chapter 20; Caro 1998, Gosling & Sutherland 2000, Frankham et al. 2002). Conservation efforts rely on establishing successful interactions among individuals in zoos or in at-risk populations – interactions predicated on animal phenotypes that are best described as interacting phenotypes such as mating, aggression and parent–offspring relations (see Chapters 7, 10 and 11). Understanding IGEs should influence how zoo or threatened populations are managed to best facilitate recruitment of new members, breeding and appropriate parental behaviour, as well as to minimise aggression.

The importance of considering interacting phenotypes in conservation efforts is highlighted by the importance of the Allee effect in conservation biology (Stephens & Sutherland 1999). The Allee effect describes situations whereby individuals benefit from, or even require, the presence of conspecifics to forage efficiently, locate mates or express effective anti-predator behaviour. For example, Glanville fritillaries *Melitaea cinxia*, an endangered butterfly, experience decreased mating success in small populations. This is compounded by the effect of neighbours on emigration: these butterflies emigrate more frequently from small populations than from large populations (Kuussaari et al. 1998). The specific mechanism by which social environment influences migration patterns for Glanville fritillaries remains unknown, but could plausibly include group patterns of chemical signalling, such as those demonstrated by Kent et al. (2008) and J. Wang et al. (2008), or gene expression contingent on the specifics of social interaction such as that found in zebra finches and cichlids (Jarvis et al. 1998, Burmeister et al. 2005). Accounting for the role the social environment plays in facilitating mating could improve captive breeding or breeding/release programmes. Explicit understanding of interacting phenotypes influencing behaviour within a group adds to our understanding of population structure, facilitating our ability to successfully manage populations for which population structure is critical.

We suggest that adopting the interacting-phenotype perspective and acknowledging the social environment as unique – it is a genetically influenced environment and can also evolve – will go some way towards furthering our understanding of how traits expressed or influenced by social interactions might evolve. Yet despite the probable ubiquity and influence of indirect genetic effects on behavioural traits, there are only a few studies aimed at understanding the proximate and evolutionary consequences for IGEs. Explorations of the genetic architecture underlying interacting phenotypes must take into account the potential impacts of IGEs. Predictions from models suggest that IGEs may be especially important in influencing population structure, an important facet of conservation efforts. Our understanding of how interacting phenotypes evolve would greatly benefit from studies aimed at teasing apart the genetics, including genes carried in social partners, of social interactions.

Acknowledgements

We thank Butch Brodie III, John Hunt, Clement Kent, Joel Levine, Joel McGlothlin and Trish Moore for discussions. Two anonymous reviewers improved the manuscript with their comments. Our work is supported by NERC (AJM and JBW) and NSF (BHB).

Suggested readings

Theoretical studies

Bijma, P. & Wade, M. J. (2008) The joint effects of kin, multilevel selection and indirect genetic effects on response to genetic selection. *Journal of Evolutionary Biology*, **21**, 1175–1188.

Cheverud, J. M. & Moore, A. J. (1994) Quantitative genetics and the role of the environment provided by relatives in behavioral evolution. In: *Quantitative Genetic Studies of Behavioral Evolution*, ed. C. R. B. Boake. Chicago, IL: University of Chicago Press, pp. 67–100.

Wolf, J. B. & Moore, A. J. (2010) Interacting phenotypes and indirect genetic effects: a genetic perspective on the evolution of social behavior. In: *Evolutionary Behavioral Ecology*, ed. D. F. Westneat & C. W. Fox. Oxford & New York: Oxford University Press, pp. 225–245.

Empirical studies

Hunt, J. & Simmons, L. (2001) Status-dependent selection in the dimorphic beetle *Onthophagus taurus*. *Proceedings of the Royal Society B*, **268**, 2409–2414.

Kent, C., Azanchi, R., Smith, B., Formosa, A. & Levine, J. D. (2008) Social context influences chemical communication in *D. melanogaster* males. *Current Biology*, **18**, 1384–1389.

Linksvayer, T. A. (2006) Direct, maternal, and sibsocial genetic effects on individual and colony traits in an ant. *Evolution*, **60**, 2552–2561.

References

Agrawal, A. F., Brodie, E. D. & Wade, M. J. (2001a) On indirect genetic effects in structured populations. *American Naturalist*, **158**, 308–323.

Agrawal, A. F., Brodie, E. D. & Brown, J. (2001b) Parent–offspring coadaptation and the dual genetic control of maternal care. *Science*, **292**, 1710–1712.

Allee, W. C. (1927) Animal aggregations. *Quarterly Review of Biology*, **II**, 367–398.

Aragaki, D. L. R. & Meffert, L. M. (1998) A test of how well the repeatability of courtship predicts its heritability. *Animal Behaviour*, **55**, 1141–1150.

Bacigalupe, L. D., Crudginton, H. S., Slate, J., Moore, A. J. & Snook, R. R. (2008) Sexual selection and interacting phenotypes in experimental evolution: a study of *Drosophila pseudoobscura* mating behavior. *Evolution*, **62**, 1804–1812.

Bateson, P. (2004) The active role of behavior in evolution. *Biology and Philosophy*, **19**, 283–298.

Bernardo, J. (1996) Maternal effects in animal ecology. *American Zoologist*, **36**, 83–105.

Bijma, P. & Wade, M. J. (2008) The joint effects of kin, multilevel selection and indirect genetic effects on response to genetic selection. *Journal of Evolutionary Biology*, **21**, 1175–1188.

Bijma, P., Muir, W. M. & Arendonk, J. A. M. V. (2007a) Multilevel selection 1: Quantitative genetics of inheritance and response to selection. *Genetics*, **175**, 277–288.

Bijma, P., Muir, W. M., Ellen, E. D., Wolf, J. B. & Arendonk, J. A. M. V. (2007b) Multilevel selection 2: Estimating the genetic parameters determining inheritance and response to selection. *Genetics*, **175**, 289–299.

Bleakley, B. H. & Brodie, E. D. (2009) Indirect genetic effects influence antipredator behavior in guppies: estimates of the coefficient of interaction psi and the inheritance of reciprocity. *Evolution*, **63**, 1796–1806.

Bleakley, B. H., Martell, C. M. & Brodie, E. D. (2006) Variation in anti-predator behavior among five strains of inbred guppies, *Poecilia reticulata*. *Behavior Genetics*, **36**, 783–791.

Bleakley, B. H., Parker, D. J. & Brodie, E. D. (2007) Nonadditive effects of group membership can lead to additive group phenotypes for anti-predator behaviour of guppies, *Poecilia reticulata*. *Journal of Evolutionary Biology*, **20**, 1375–1384.

Bleakley, B. H., Eklund, A. C. & Brodie, E. D. (2008) Are designer guppies inbred? Microsatellite variation in five strains of ornamental guppies. *Poecilia reticulata*, used for behavior research. *Zebrafish*, **5**, 39–48.

Boake, C. R. B., Arnold, S. J., Breden, F. *et al.* (2002) Genetic tools for studying adaptation and the evolution of behavior. *American Naturalist*, **160**, S143–159.

Brodie, E. D. (2000) Why evolutionary genetics does not always add up. In: *Epistasis and the Evolutionary Process*, ed. J. B. Wolf, E. D. Brodie & M. J. Wade. New York: Oxford University Press, pp. 3–19.

Burmeister, S. S., Jarvis, E. D. & Fernald, R. D. (2005) Rapid behavioral and genomic responses to social opportunity. *PLoS Biology*, **3** (11), e363.

Caro, T., ed. (1998) *Behavioral Ecology and Conservation Biology*. New York, NY: Oxford University Press.

Chapman, T., Arnqvist, G., Bangham, J. & Rowe, L. (2003) Sexual conflict. *Trends in Ecology and Evolution*, **18**, 41–47.

Chenoweth, S. F. & Blows, M. W. (2006) Dissecting the complex genetic basis of mate choice. *Nature Reviews Genetics*, **7**, 681–692.

Cheverud, J. M. & Moore, A. J. (1994) Quantitative genetics and the role of the environment provided by relatives in behavioral evolution. In: *Quantitative Genetic Studies of Behavioral Evolution*, ed. C. R. B. Boake. Chicago, IL: University of Chicago Press, pp. 67–100.

Clark, A. G. & Begun, D. J. (1998) Female genotypes affect sperm displacement in *Drosophila*. *Genetics*, **149**, 1487–1493.

Clark, A. G., Begun, D. J. & Prout, T. (1999) Female × male interactions in *Drosophila* sperm competition. *Science*, **283**, 217–220.

Cowley, D. E., Pomp, D., Atchley, W. R., Eisen, E. J. & Hawkins-Brown, D. (1989) The impact of maternal uterine genotype on postnatal growth and adult body size in mice. *Genetics*, **122**, 193–203.

Cummings, M. E., Larkins-Ford, J., Reilly, C. R. L. *et al.* (2008) Sexual and social stimuli elicit rapid and contrasting genomic responses. *Proceedings of the Royal Society B*, **275**, 393–402.

Danielson-François, A., Zhou, Y. & Greenfield, M. D. (2009) Indirect genetic effects and the lek paradox: inter-genotypic competition may strengthen genotype × environment interactions and conserve genetic variance. *Genetica*, **136**, 27–36.

Darwin, C. (1859) *On the Origin of Species by Means of Natural Selection*. London: John Murray.

Darwin, C. (1871) *The Descent of Man, and Selection in Relation to Sex*. London: John Murray.

Dawkins, R. (1982) *The Extended Phenotype: the Gene as the Unit of Selection*. San Francisco: Freeman Press.

D'Ettorre, P. & Moore, A. J. (2008) Chemical communication and the coordination of social interactions in insects. In: *Sociobiology of Communication: an Interdisciplinary Perspective*, ed. P. D'Ettorre & D. P. Hughes. Oxford & New York: Oxford University Press, pp. 81–96.

Elgar, M. A. & Crespi, B., eds. (1992) *Cannibalism, Ecology and Evolution Among Diverse Taxa*. Oxford: Oxford University Press.

Evans, J. P., Kelley, J. L., Bisazza, A., Finazzo, E. & Pilastro, A. (2004) Sire attractiveness influences offspring performance in guppies. *Proceedings of the Royal Society B*, **271**, 2035–2042.

Falconer, D. S. & Mackay, T. F. C. (1996) *Introduction to Quantitative Genetics*, 4th edn. Harlow: Longman.

Fewell, J. H. (2003) Social insect networks. *Science*, **301**, 1867–1870.

Fisher, R. A. (1918) The correlation between relatives on the supposition of Mendelian inheritance. *Transactions of the Royal Society of Edinburgh*, **52**, 399–433.

Frank, S. A. (1997) Fisher's fundamental theorem, kin selection, and causal analysis. *Evolution*, **51**, 1712–1729.

Frankham, R., Ballou, J. D. & Briscoe, D. A. (2002) *Introduction to Conservation Genetics*. Cambridge: Cambridge University Press.

Fuller, J. L. & Hahn, M. E. (1976) Issues in the genetics of social behavior. *Behavior Genetics*, **6**, 391–406.

Garcia-Gonzalez, F. & Simmons, L. W. (2005) The evolution of polyandry: intrinsic sire effects contribute to embryo viability. *Journal of Evolutionary Biology*, **18**, 1097–1103.

Gosling, L. M. & Sutherland, W. J. (2000) *Behaviour and Conservation*. Cambridge: Cambridge University Press.

Grindstaff, J. L., Brodie, E. D. & Ketterson, E. D. (2003) Immune function across generations: integrating mechanism and evolutionary process in maternal antibody transmission. *Proceedings of the Royal Society B*, **270**, 2309–2319.

Hager, R. & Johnstone, R. A. (2003) The genetic basis of family conflict resolution in mice. *Nature*, **421**, 533–535.

Hahn, M. E. & Schanz, N. (1996) Issues in the genetics of social behavior: revisited. *Behavior Genetics*, **26**, 463–470.

Hamilton, W. D. (1964) The genetical theory of social behavior I. *Journal of Theoretical Biology*, **7**, 1–16.

Higgins, L. A., Jones, J. M. & Wayne, M. L. (2005) Quantitative genetics of natural variation of behavior in *Drosophila melanogaster*: the possible role of social environment on creating persistent patterns of group activity. *Evolution*, **59**, 1529–1539.

House, C. M., Evans, G. M. V., Smiseth, P. T. *et al.* (2008) The evolution of repeated mating in the burying beetle, *Nicrophorus vespilloides*. *Evolution*, **62**, 2004–2014.

Isles, A. R., Humby, T., Walters, E. & Wilkinson, L. S. (2004) Common genetic effects on variation in impulsivity and activity in mice. *Journal of Neuroscience*, **24**, 6733–6740.

Jarvis, E. D., Scharff, C., Grossman, M. R., Ramos, J. A. & Nottebohm, F. (1998) For whom the bird sings: context-dependent gene expression. *Neuron*, **21**, 775–88.

Kempenaers, B. (2007) Mate choice and genetic quality: a review of the heterozygosity theory. *Advances in the Study of Behavior*, **37**, 189–278.

Kent, C., Azanchi, R., Smith, B., Formosa, A. & Levine, J. D. (2008) Social context influences chemical communication in *D. melanogaster* males. *Current Biology*, **18**, 1384–1389.

Kirkpatrick, M. & Lande, R. (1989) The evolution of maternal characters. *Evolution*, **43**, 485–503.

Kölliker, M. (2005) Ontogeny in the family. *Behavior Genetics*, **35**, 7–18.

Kölliker, M. & Richner, H. (2001) Parent-offspring conflict and the genetics of offspring solicitation and parental response. *Animal Behaviour*, **62**, 395–407.

Kölliker, M., Brinkhof, M. W. G., Heeb, P., Fitze, P. S. & Richner, H. (2000) The quantitative genetic basis of offspring solicitation and parental response in a passerine bird with biparental care. *Proceedings of the Royal Society B*, **267**, 2127–2132.

Kölliker, M., Brodie, E. D. & Moore, A. J. (2005) The coadaptation of parental supply and offspring demand. *American Naturalist*, **166**, 506–516.

Komers, P. E. (1997) Behavioural plasticity in variable environments. *Canadian Journal of Zoology-Revue Canadienne De Zoologie*, **75**, 161–169.

Kotiaho, J. S., Simmons, L. W., Hunt, J. & Tomkins, J. L. (2003) Males influence maternal effects that promote sexual selection: a quantitative genetic experiment with dung beetles *Onthophagus taurus*. *American Naturalist*, **161**, 852–859.

Krupp, J. J., Kent, C., Billeter, J.-C. *et al.* (2008) Social experience modifies pheromone expression and mating behavior in male *Drosophila melanogaster*. *Current Biology*, **18**, 1373–1383.

Kruuk, L. E. B. (2004) Estimating genetic parameters in natural populations using the 'animal model'. *Philosophical Transactions of the Royal Society B*, **359**, 873–890.

Kuussaari, M., Saccheri, I., Camara, M. & Hanski, I. (1998) Allee effect and population dynamics in the Glanville fritillary butterfly. *Oikos*, **82**, 384–392.

Lande, R. (1981) Models of speciation by sexual selection on polygenic traits. *Proceedings of the National Academy of Sciences of the USA*, **78**, 3721–3725.

Lewontin, R. & Matsuo, Y. (1963) Interaction of genotypes determining the viability in *Drosophila busckii*. *Proceedings of the National Academy of Sciences of the USA*, **49**, 270–278.

Linksvayer, T. A. (2006) Direct, maternal, and sibsocial genetic effects on individual and colony traits in an ant. *Evolution*, **60**, 2552–2561.

Linksvayer, T. A. (2007) Ant species differences determined by epistasis between brood and worker genomes. *PLoS ONE*, **2** (10), e994.

Lock, J. E., Smiseth, P. T. & Moore, A. J. (2004) Selection, inheritance and the evolution of parent-offspring interactions. *American Naturalist*, **164**, 13–24.

Lynch, M. (1987) Evolution of intrafamilial interactions. *Proceedings of the National Academy of Sciences of the USA*, **84**, 8501–8511.

Lynch, M. & Walsh, B. (1998) *Genetics and Analysis of Quantitative Traits*. Sunderland, MA: Sinauer Associates.

Manning, A. (1961) The effects of artificial selection for mating speed in *Drosophila melanogaster*. *Animal Behaviour*, **9**, 82–92.

Meffert, L. M. (1995) Bottleneck effects on genetic variance for courtship repertoire. *Genetics*, **139**, 365–374.

Meffert, L. M. & Regan, J. L. (2002) A test of speciation via sexual selection on female preferences. *Animal Behaviour*, **64**, 955–965.

Messina, F. J. (1998) Maternal influences on larval competition in insects. In: *Maternal Effects as Adaptations*, ed. T. A. Mousseau & C. W. Fox. New York, NY: Oxford University Press, pp. 227–243.

Miller, C. W. & Moore, A. J. (2007) A potential resolution to the lek paradox through indirect genetic effects. *Proceedings of the Royal Society B*, **274**, 1279–1286.

Moore, A. J. & Pizzari, T. (2005) Quantitative genetic models of sexual conflict based on interacting phenotypes. *American Naturalist*, **165**, S88–97.

Moore, A. J., Brodie, E. D. & Wolf, J. B. (1997) Interacting phenotypes and the evolutionary process. I. Direct and indirect genetic effects of social interactions. *Evolution*, **51**, 1352–1362.

Moore, A. J., Wolf, J. B. & Brodie, E. D. (1998) The influence of direct and indirect genetic effects on the evolution of behavior: social and sexual selection meet maternal effects. In: *Maternal Effects as Adaptations*, ed. T. A. Mousseau & C. W. Fox. New York, NY: Oxford University Press, pp. 23–41.

Moore, A. J., Haynes, K. F., Preziosi, R. F. & Moore, P. J. (2002) The evolution of interacting phenotypes: genetics and evolution of social dominance. *American Naturalist*, **160**, S186–197.

Mousseau, T. A. & Fox, C. W., eds. (1998) *Maternal Effects as Adaptations*. New York, NY: Oxford University Press.

Mutic, J. J. & Wolf, J. B. (2007) Indirect genetic effects from ecological interactions in *Arabidopsis thaliana*. *Molecular Ecology*, **16**, 2371–2381.

Nelson, R. J., ed. (2005) *Biology of Aggression*. New York, NY: Oxford University Press.

Odling-Smee, F. J., Laland, K. N. & Feldman, M. W. (2003) *Niche Construction: the Neglected Process in Evolution*. Princeton, NJ: Princeton University Press.

Petfield, D., Chenoweth, S. F., Rundle, H. D. & Blows, M. W. (2005) Genetic variance in female condition predicts indirect genetic variance in male sexual display traits. *Proceedings of the National Academy of Sciences of the USA*, **102**, 6045-6050.

Price, T. (1998) Maternal and paternal effects in birds: effects on offspring fitness. In: *Maternal Effects as Adaptations*, ed. T. A. Mousseau & C. W. Fox. New York, NY: Oxford University Press, pp. 202-226.

Queller, D. C. (1992a) A general model for kin selection. *Evolution*, **46**, 376-380.

Queller, D. C. (1992b) Quantitative genetics, inclusive fitness, and group selection. *American Naturalist*, **139**, 540-558.

Rauter, C. M. & Moore, A. J. (2002) Evolutionary importance of parental care performance, food resources, and direct and indirect genetic effects in a burying beetle. *Journal of Evolutionary Biology*, **15**, 407-417.

Reznick, D., Callahan, H. & Llauredo, R. (1996) Maternal effects on offspring quality in poeciliid fishes. *American Zoologist*, **36**, 147-156.

Riska, B., Rutledge, J. J. & Atchley, W. R. (1985) Covariance between direct and maternal genetic effects in mice, with a model of persistent environmental influences. *Genetical Research*, **45**, 287-297.

Roff, D. A. (1997) *Evolutionary Quantitative Genetics*. New York, NY; London: Chapman & Hall.

Ruiz-Dubreuil, D. G. & del Solar, E. (1993) A diallele analysis of gregarious oviposition in *Drosophila melanogaster*. *Heredity*, **70**, 281-284.

Simmons, L. W. & Moore, A. J. (2008) Evolutionary quantitative genetics of sperm. In: *Sperm Biology: an Evolutionary Perspective*, ed. T. R. Birkhead, D. J. Hosken & S. Pitnick. London: Academic Press, pp. 405-434.

Stephens, P. A. & Sutherland, W. J. (1999) Consequences of the Allee effect for behaviour, ecology and conservation. *Trends in Ecology and Evolution*, **14**, 401-405.

Stone, G. N. & Cook, J. M. (1998) The structure of cynipid oak galls: patterns in the evolution of an extended phenotype. *Proceedings of the Royal Society B*, **265**, 979-988.

Tinbergen, N. (1953) *Social Behaviour in Animals, with Special Reference to Vertebrates*. London: Wiley.

Tregenza, T. & Wedell, N. (2000) Genetic compatability, mate choice and patterns of parantage: Invited review. *Molecular Ecology*, **9**, 1013-1027.

Wade, M. J. (1998) The evolutionary genetics of maternal effects. In: *Maternal Effects as Adaptations*, ed. T. A. Mousseau & C. W. Fox. New York, NY: Oxford University Press, pp. 5-21.

Wang, J., Ross, K. G. & Keller, L. (2008) Genome-wide expression patterns and the genetic architecture of a fundamental social trait. *PLoS Genetics*, **4** (7), e1000127.

Wang, L., Dankert, H., Perona, P. & Anderson, D. J. (2008) A common genetic target for environmental and heritable influences on aggressiveness in *Drosophila*. *Proceedings of the National Academy of Sciences of the USA*, **105**, 5657-5663.

Weis, A. E., Walton, R. & Crego, C. L. (1988) Reactive plant tissue sites and the population biology of gall makers. *Annual Review of Entomology*, **33**, 467-486.

Weis, A. E., Abrahamson, W. G. & Andersen, M. C. (1992) Variable selection on *Eurosta's* gall size, I. The extent and nature of variation in phenotypic selection. *Evolution*, **46**, 1674-1697.

West-Eberhard, M. J. (1979) Sexual selection, social competition, and evolution. *Proceedings of the American Philosophical Society*, **123**, 222-234.

West-Eberhard, M. J. (1983) Sexual selection, social competition, and speciation. *Quarterly Review of Biology*, **58**, 155-183.

West-Eberhard, M. J. (1984) Sexual selection, competitive communication, and species-specific signals in insects. In: *Insect Communication*, ed. T. Lewis. London: Academic Press, pp. 283-324.

West-Eberhard, M. J. (2003) Gaps and inconsistencies in modern evolutionary thought. In: *Developmental Plasticity and Evolution*. Oxford: Oxford University Press, pp. 3-20.

Wilson, A. J., Gelin, U., Perron, M.-C. & Réale, D. (2009) Indirect genetic effects and the evolution of aggression in a vertebrate system. *Proceedings of the Royal Society of London B*, **276**, 533-541.

Winberg, S., Winberg, Y. & Fernald, R. D. (1997) Effect of social rank on brain monoaminergic activity in a cichlid fish. *Brain, Behavior and Evolution*, **49**, 230-236.

Wolf, J. B. (2000a) Indirect genetic effects and gene interactions. In: *Epistasis and the Evolutionary Process*, ed. J. B. Wolf, E. D. Brodie & M. J. Wade. New York: Oxford University Press, pp. 158-176.

Wolf, J. B. (2000b) Gene interactions from maternal effects. *Evolution*, **54**, 1882-1898.

Wolf, J. B. (2003) Genetic architecture and evolutionary constraint when the environment contains genes. *Proceedings of the National Academy of Sciences of the USA*, **100**, 4655-4660.

Wolf, J. B. & Brodie, E. D. (1998) The coadaptation of parental and offspring characters. *Evolution*, **52**, 299-308.

Wolf, J. B. & Moore, A. J. (2010) Interacting phenotypes and indirect genetic effects: a genetic perspective on the evolution of social behavior. In: *Evolutionary Behavioral Ecology*, ed. D. F. Westneat & C. W. Fox. Oxford & New York: Oxford University Press, pp. 225-245.

Wolf, J. B., Moore, A. J. & Brodie, E. D. (1997) The evolution of indicator traits for parental quality: the role of maternal and paternal effects. *American Naturalist*, **150**, 639–649.

Wolf, J. B., Brodie, E. D., Cheverud, J. M., Moore, A. J. & Wade, M. J. (1998) Evolutionary consequences of indirect genetic effects. *Trends in Ecology and Evolution*, **13**, 64–69.

Wolf, J. B., Brodie, E. D. & Moore, A. J. (1999a) Interacting phenotypes and the evolutionary process. II. Selection resulting from social interactions. *American Naturalist*, **153**, 254–266.

Wolf, J. B., Brodie, E. D. & Moore, A. J. (1999b) The role of maternal and paternal effects in the evolution of parental quality by sexual selection. *Journal of Evolutionary Biology*, **12**, 1157–1167.

Woolley, S. C. & Doupe, A. J. (2008) Social context-induced song variation affects female behavior and gene expression. *PLoS Biology*, **6** (3), e62.

Mating systems: integrating sexual conflict and ecology

Nicholas B. Davies

When I began as a research student in 1973, the key to understanding mating systems was thought to be through a study of ecology. My bible was David Lack's recent book (1968), which showed how variation in bird mating systems could be linked to differences in the type, abundance and dispersion of resources, such as food and nest sites. Lack concluded that most bird species were monogamous because a male and female each maximised their reproductive success if they cooperated to rear a brood together. Two quotes from Lack's book convey the prevailing view of that time: a comparative approach was needed rather than experiments because 'no one has yet found how to make a monogamous species polygynous' (p. 8); 'given that the marvellous adaptations of the brood parasites are a product of natural selection, it is ... hard to concede that this same powerful force is likewise responsible for the dull, conventional habits of the monogamous song birds which raise their own young' (p. 97).

Two changes heralded a revolution during the next decade. The first was a new idea, namely the recognition of sexual conflict in mating and parental care (Trivers 1972, Parker 1979). The second was a new technique, namely DNA profiles for assigning parentage with precision. A new idea and a new technique was an inspiring combination for a fresh look at bird mating systems. So, in 1980, I began a long-term study in the Cambridge University Botanic Garden of a little brown bird, the dunnock *Prunella modularis*, to see how sexual conflict and ecology interacted to influence its variable mating system. My research agenda was simple: to mark individuals, watch them closely and relate their behaviour to their reproductive payoffs.

It soon became clear that social conflicts arose through reproductive conflicts of interest. Furthermore, it was these conflicts which generated the various mating systems. A male dunnock had greatest reproductive success with polygyny, and promoted this by attempting to expand his territory to encompass a second female. However, dominant females tried to drive subordinate females away because polygyny reduced their success through the costs of shared male care. A female had greatest success with polyandry, where sharing matings between two unrelated males led to help from both with chick feeding. However, dominant males tried to drive subordinate males away because the benefits of another male's help did not compensate him for the costs of paternity loss. Sometimes the conflicts produced a 'stalemate', in which two males shared two females (polygynandry). Here, neither female could evict the other and so claim both males for herself, while the dominant male was unable to evict the subordinate male to claim both females. Monogamy occurred where

Social Behaviour: Genes, Ecology and Evolution, ed. Tamás Székely, Allen J. Moore and Jan Komdeur. Published by Cambridge University Press. © Cambridge University Press 2010.

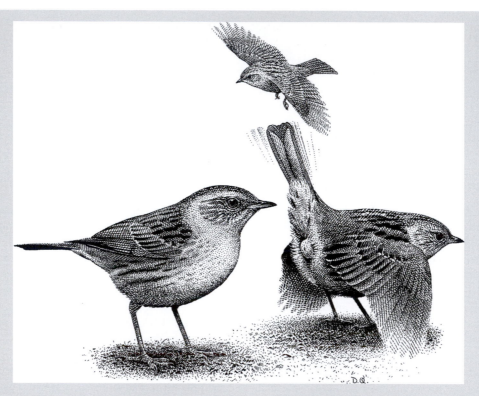

A female dunnock soliciting to the beta male; the alpha male is about to fly in and interrupt. Drawing by David Quinn, from Davies (1992).

neither partner could gain a second mate (Davies & Houston 1986, Davies 1992).

The key question now became: under what circumstances will particular individuals gain their preferred outcomes despite the conflicting preferences of others? This depended partly on differences in competitive ability; for example, older males were more likely to be polygynous. Ecological factors were also important; for example, denser vegetation increased the chance that a female could escape mate guarding by the dominant male and so give a mating share to a subordinate male.

To see whether changes in the ecological stage led to changes in the form of sexual conflict, we turned to a congener of the dunnock, the alpine accentor

P. collaris, which breeds on high mountain tops. Our studies in the French Pyrenees (1950–2410 m) showed that alpine accentors bred in larger polygynandrous groups, with 2–4 unrelated males sharing 2–4 females in a large range, 30 times the size of a dunnock territory. On the mountain tops, invertebrate prey were scarcer and more patchily distributed in space and time than at lower elevations. The alpine accentor's large ranges were necessary because the best places to feed varied widely depending on snow, wind and sunshine. The causes of sexual conflict were the same as in dunnocks; females gained increased male help with chick feeding by sharing matings among several males, whereas dominant males did best by attempting to monopolise matings (Davies *et al*. 1995, Hartley *et al*. 1995, Nakamura 1998a, 1998b). However, the social conflicts differed in form: alpine accentors in a polygynandrous group often all fed together, so there was more intense scramble competition for mates. Males competed for paternity with even higher rates of copulation than dunnocks. Females competed for male attention by developing bright red cloacas, reminiscent of the sexual swellings of female primates which live in multi-male groups (Nakamura 1990), by extraordinarily high rates of copulation solicitation (Davies *et al*. 1996), and by singing to attract males away from other females in the group (Langmore *et al*. 1996).

The most direct test of whether these social differences were caused by ecological differences was by experiment. Could we manipulate dunnocks into adopting alpine accentor-like social behaviour? At regular feeding sites, where we provided food daily, dunnocks defended small exclusive territories. However, at variable feeding sites, where more food was allocated each day, but to one of several randomly chosen adjacent sites (to simulate the more patchy food on mountain tops), dunnocks adopted larger, overlapping ranges, more typical of alpine accentors, with 2–5 males overlapping 2–4 females (Davies & Hartley 1996). Unfortunately, we were unable to follow the consequences for mating because in spring the dunnocks turned to natural food supplies. However, in another experiment we removed females to intensify female competition for males. This also induced a change to alpine accentor-like behaviour, with an increase in female calling, and occasional song, to attract males away from other fertile females (Langmore & Davies 1997).

David Lack would have been astonished at the variation in mating systems generated by sexual conflict. However, progress in understanding the influence of ecology requires better analyses of scarce resources. Owens and Bennett (1997) have proposed a promising way forward by recognising that different factors might explain variation

at different taxonomic levels: within populations, variation arises through sexual conflict; between populations and closely related species, ecological differences are important; between higher taxonomic levels, variation is linked to differences in life histories. Exploring these three sources of variation is a challenge for the future.

References

Davies, N. B. (1992) *Dunnock Behaviour and Social Evolution*. Oxford: University Press.

Davies, N. B. & Hartley, I. R. (1996) Food patchiness, territory overlap and social systems: an experiment with dunnocks *Prunella modularis*. *Journal of Animal Ecology*, **65**, 837–846.

Davies, N. B. & Houston, A. I. (1986) Reproductive success of dunnocks *Prunella modularis* in a variable mating system. II. Conflicts of interest among breeding adults. *Journal of Animal Ecology*, **55**, 139–154.

Davies, N. B., Hartley, I. R., Hatchwell, B. J. *et al*. (1995) The polygynandrous mating system of the alpine accentor, *Prunella collaris*. I. Ecological causes and reproductive conflicts. *Animal Behaviour*, **49**, 769–788.

Davies, N. B., Hartley, I. R., Hatchwell, B. J. & Langmore, N. E. (1996) Female control of copulations to maximize male help: a comparison of polygynandrous alpine accentors, *Prunella collaris*, and dunnocks, *P. modularis*. *Animal Behaviour*, **51**, 27–47.

Hartley, I. R., Davies, N. B., Hatchwell, B. J. *et al*. (1995) The polygynandrous mating system of the alpine accentor, *Prunella collaris*. II. Multiple paternity and parental effort. *Animal Behaviour*, **49**, 789–803.

Lack, D. (1968) *Ecological Adaptations for Breeding in Birds*. London: Methuen.

Langmore, N. E. & Davies, N. B. (1997) Female dunnocks use vocalizations to compete for males. *Animal Behaviour*, **53**, 881–890.

Langmore, N. E., Davies, N. B., Hatchwell, B. J. & Hartley, I. R. (1996) Female song attracts males in the alpine accentor, *Prunella collaris*. *Proceedings of the Royal Society B*, **263**, 141–146.

Nakamura, M. (1990) Cloacal protuberance and copulatory behaviour of the alpine accentor (*Prunella collaris*). *Auk*, **107**, 284–295.

Nakamura, M. (1998a) Multiple mating and cooperative breeding in polygynandrous alpine accentors. I. Competition among females. *Animal Behaviour*, **55**, 259–275.

Nakamura, M. (1998b) Multiple mating and cooperative breeding in polygynandrous alpine accentors. II. Male mating tactics. *Animal Behaviour*, **55**, 277–289.

Owens, I. P. F. & Bennett, P. M. (1997) Variation in mating systems among birds: ecological basis revealed by hierarchical comparative analysis. *Proceedings of the Royal Society B*, **264**, 1103–1110.

Parker, G. A. (1979) Sexual selection and sexual conflict. In: *Sexual Selection and Reproductive Competition in Insects*, ed. M. S. Blum & N. A. Blum. New York, NY: Academic Press, pp. 123–166.

Trivers, R. L. (1972). Parental investment and sexual selection. In: *Sexual Selection and the Descent of Man, 1871–1971*, ed. B. Campbell. Chicago, IL: Aldine, pp. 136–179.

3

Social behaviour and bird song from a neural and endocrine perspective

Elizabeth Adkins-Regan, Timothy J. DeVoogd and Jordan M. Moore

Overview

Tinbergen (1963) proposed that in order to understand behaviour it is necessary to discover not only its adaptive function and phylogenetic history (now often referred to as ultimate causation) but also its development and physiology (proximate causation). In recent years there has been increasing appreciation of the importance of pursuing these four aims not only separately but also in an integrated manner that allows them to inform each other. Hormonal and neural mechanisms are best understood in an ecological and evolutionary context. An appreciation of how they work is essential both for understanding the ecology and evolution of behaviour, and for linking genes to behaviour.

This chapter will discuss hormonal and neural bases of social behaviour, emphasising basic principles, recent trends and questions for the future, with a more extended discussion of bird song as a prime example of a social behaviour that has inspired a substantial body of integrative research. Special attention will be given to learned song and the songbird neural song system that underlies the learning, production and perception of song. As a neural system that is anatomically well defined, dedicated to an important category of social behaviour, and hormonally influenced, the song system is uniquely valuable for elucidating general principles of the mechanisms of social behaviour.

3.1 Introduction to peripheral hormones and social behaviour

It is well established that mating behaviour is often causally related to circulating levels of sex steroid hormones produced by the gonads. These same hormones can be involved in many other social behaviours serving to promote reproductive success, such as territorial aggression and singing by birds (Adkins-Regan 2005, Nelson 2005). A substantial literature reports correlated increases in certain forms of social behaviour and in circulating sex-hormone levels at the onset of reproductive adulthood and at the onset of each breeding season in free-living animals. Both social behaviour and sex-hormone levels often differ between the sexes, and experimental manipulations of hormones show that some of these correlations reflect a causal influence of sex hormones on social behaviour. Most common are manipulations of testosterone in males. Similarly, correlations between prolactin (a peptide hormone) and parental behaviour have been reported, although experimental support for a causal role in parental behaviour is limited to a small number of species (Rosenblatt & Snowdon 1996). These are important findings, especially when backed up by manipulation experiments. (Correlation is never evidence of causation, a principle that applies just as much to hormones and behaviour as to any other scientific domain.) They have been over-generalised and over-simplified, however, so as to equate testosterone with male social behaviour, oestradiol with female behaviour, and prolactin with parental behaviour. These generalisations go well beyond, or even contradict, current knowledge. Additional principles have emerged from the literature that help establish the limits of generality. In the following sections, some of these limits will be clarified.

3.1.1 Maleness is not testosterone and femaleness is not oestradiol

There are no sex-specific steroid or other hormones in most (perhaps all) vertebrates. For example, both sexes produce both androgens and oestrogens. The equating of testosterone with male behaviour and oestradiol with female behaviour has its origins in research with species (mainly mammals but also some other vertebrates) in which reproductively active males have higher circulating levels of testosterone than females, and females have higher circulating levels of oestradiol.

Many vertebrates (including some mammals) do not fit this pattern, however. Females of some species have testosterone levels that are similar to or higher than those of males – for example, many lizards and turtles (Norris 2007). Males of some species have oestradiol levels similar to or higher than those of females – for example, zebra finches *Taeniopygia guttata* (Adkins-Regan *et al.* 1990).

Even when males have lower oestradiol levels, experiments may reveal that conversion of testosterone to oestradiol (aromatisation) in brain regions such as the preoptic area that contain the aromatase

(oestrogen synthase) enzyme are an essential part of the neuroendocrine pathway leading to male behaviour. For example, all of the male-specific courtship and mating behaviours of zebra finches, including singing, require oestrogenic metabolites of testosterone (Harding *et al.* 1983), and in Japanese quail *Coturnix japonica* both an interest in females and copulatory mounting require brain aromatisation of circulating testosterone (Balthazart *et al.* 1997). In both species, androgens that are potent stimulators of avian masculine morphological characters such as vasa deferentia or quail foam glands, but that cannot be aromatised, fail to stimulate all of the masculine social behaviours that are critical for reproductive success.

When female testosterone levels are equal to or higher than those of males, it is important to find out what this testosterone is doing for the females' behaviour, and to understand the ultimate causes of the marked species differences in whether and by how much the sexes differ in testosterone levels (Ketterson *et al.* 2005). Equating testosterone with aggressiveness suggests the hypothesis that there is greater female–female competition in species with high female testosterone, but if that equation is an over-simplification, the hypothesis could be incorrect.

3.1.2 Are individual, sex and species differences related to circulating hormones?

If individual males differ markedly in courtship vigour or frequency, are they sure to have different testosterone levels? Individual differences are the raw material for evolutionary change, and it is crucial to discover the mechanistic bases of individual differences in social behaviour. Understanding the mechanisms responsible for the evolution of sex and species differences in behaviour is equally important, and there is always the possibility that similar mechanisms could produce all three kinds of differences (individual, sex and species) in social behaviour.

With respect to individual differences, more often than not, male hormone levels do not differ in the expected way (i.e. more vigorously courting males do not necessarily have higher testosterone levels), especially if care is taken to measure baseline hormone levels rather than levels caused by recent social interactions. Nor can the repeatability of those baseline levels be safely assumed. Instead, what is striking is the enormous range of circulating hormone levels that are compatible with active breeding behaviour in free-living animals (Kempenaers *et al.* 2008). In addition, experiments reveal that hormone–behaviour relationships more often resemble a threshold step-function than the kind of monotonically increasing dose–response curve that would result in positive hormone–behaviour correlations (Adkins-Regan 2005).

Some of the most notable cases in which circulating hormone levels do predict individual differences in social behaviour are found in species with alternative phenotypes, usually male morphs (Brantley *et al.* 1993, Knapp 2004). Such findings from bimodally distributed categories of males cannot be assumed to generalise to the kind of continuous variation seen in most species, but they are interesting on their own terms, providing exceptional opportunities for research integrating proximate causation (what mechanisms make the phenotypes behave differently?) with ultimate causation (why did one sex evolve into two or more different phenotypes?). A notable example that will tie into the chapter's emphasis on learned song and the song system is that both sexes of the white-throated sparrow *Zonotrichia albicollis* occur as two morphs, white-striped and tan-striped. When compared with tan-striped birds of the same sex, white-striped birds are more aggressive, sing more, have higher testosterone levels (males only), and have larger song-system nuclei (DeVoogd *et al.* 1995, Spinney *et al.* 2006). White-striped males do not sing more *because* they have higher testosterone, however (Maney *et al.* 2009).

In some species with sex differences in social behaviour, experimental sex reversal of hormone levels produces behavioural sex reversal. For example, female canaries *Serinus canaria* and a number of other female songbirds (oscine passerines) that do not normally sing begin to sing the elaborate songs typical of males when given testosterone (reviewed in Balthazart & Adkins-Regan 2002). Here activational effects of sex hormones (those occurring in adulthood that are reversible) appear to be a key mechanistic basis for the expression of the normal sex differences (e.g. lack of singing by female canaries).

Sometimes, however, such hormone treatments do not produce behavioural sex reversal. An alternative type of hormonal basis is early organisation, in which sex steroid hormones produced by the embryonic, fetal or neonatal gonads permanently establish the future sex of the behavioural phenotype through actions on the developing brain during a limited critical period. Hormonal organisation has been conclusively established as a major route to adult sex differences in social behaviour in a number of species of mammals, and in Japanese quail and chickens *Gallus gallus domesticus* (Balthazart & Adkins-Regan 2002, Wallen & Baum 2002). Activational effects of adult hormones then allow the expression of what has been organised earlier, and there will be no expression if the behavioural capacity was omitted earlier in life. The general principle for mammals is that exposure to high (male-typical) sex steroids early in development causes masculinisation and/or defeminisation of behaviour, producing a male-typical behavioural phenotype, regardless of the genetic sex of the animal, whereas their absence will produce a female-typical behavioural phenotype. Japanese quail and chicken organisation occurs according to the opposite principle from mammals. Exposure to high (female-typical) levels of sex steroids (especially high oestrogen-to-androgen ratios) as embryos causes behavioural demasculinisation, sending the individuals down the path to a female-typical behavioural phenotype, whereas lower levels and ratios send them down the path to a male-typical phenotype.

Hormonal organisation not only accounts for the development of sex differences in social behaviour in some animals, but also suggests additional hypotheses for individual differences (Crews 1998, Ball & Balthazart 2008). For example, perhaps male quail that crow less frequently were exposed to a little more oestrogen as embryos. Such hypotheses are difficult to test, however. Thus far, there are few cases where evidence has firmly established an organisational hormone source for individual differences.

It has been proposed that maternal steroids present in vertebrate egg yolks might have long-term (possibly organisational) effects on fitness mediated by later consequences for adult social behaviour such as competitive aggression (Schwabl 1993). Experiments designed to test this hypothesis are still rare, and the assumption that embryonic exposure to testosterone will necessarily produce a more male-like phenotype is questionable in light of what is known about avian sexual differentiation (Balthazart & Adkins-Regan 2002, Carere & Balthazart 2007).

Hormonal organisation has also been hypothesised to contribute to species differences in social behaviour. One particularly well-known example is the proposal that the greater aggressiveness and genital masculinisation of female spotted hyenas *Crocuta crocuta* compared to other hyenas are due to greater neonatal androgen exposure (Frank *et al.* 1991). This hypothesis is no longer well supported, however (Chapter 14; Forger 2001, Goymann *et al.* 2001). Among other problems, blocking neonatal androgen exposure with drugs does not cause females to lack masculinised genitalia.

Thus a role for circulating hormones in social behaviour variation has been best established for sex differences. One major difficulty in looking to hormonal organisation of behaviour and brains as a source of ideas for a developmental mechanism producing individual and species differences is that sexual differentiation of social behaviour is poorly understood except in mammals, a few lizards and galliform birds.

3.1.3 Could hormonal targets in the brain be a source of individual, sex and species differences?

In hormone–behaviour relationships, much of the action is on the receiving end of hormones, at the target organs (Fig. 3.1). The brain regions that have been most closely associated with social behaviour (the social behaviour network: Newman 2002, Goodson 2005) contain receptors or other mechanisms for hormones to alter the structure and activity of neurons. A hormone-sensitive behaviour could increase even if circulating hormone level had not changed, because

of an increase in hormone receptors or metabolising enzymes such as aromatase. A hormone-sensitive behaviour could be maintained throughout the year even when hormone levels are low if the receiving mechanisms are upregulated to become more sensitive. Sexes could differ behaviourally not because of dimorphic circulating hormone levels, but because of dimorphism in the brain targets, including dimorphism in numbers of steroid receptors. For example, singing is oestrogen-dependent in zebra finches, and males have the same circulating oestradiol levels as females, but only males sing.

Similarly, in the evolution of species differences, changes in circulating hormone levels are not the only way for selection to change hormone-dependent behaviour such as male courtship and aggression, and may not even be a particularly common way (Hau 2007). Species in the same family can differ in hormone receptor distributions in the brain. Neuroendocrine mechanisms such as steroid receptors and steroidogenic enzymes are gene products and thus important bridges to the genetic basis of social behaviour (Zera *et al.* 2007). As more is discovered about the molecular cascades at the receiving end of hormones, it will be possible to identify some of the genes involved and see how they vary in form or expression to produce individual, sex and species differences in social behaviour (see Chapters 11 and 17).

3.1.4 Neurohormones are key mechanisms for social behaviour

The brain is a neuroendocrine organ in addition to its other functions. The production of oestrogens in the brain is but one of many cases that have been discovered in which hormones or hormone-like molecules are produced and act centrally to regulate behaviour. Peptides of the oxytocin family (including oxytocin, vasopressin, vasotocin, mesotocin and isotocin) are either produced within specific hypothalamic nuclei (the paraventricular and supraoptic nuclei in mammals and birds), and released from the posterior pituitary to enter the circulation, or produced in other brain regions (for example, the bed

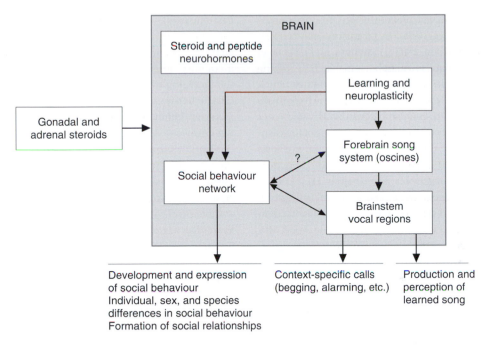

Figure 3.1 Key hormonal and neural mechanisms for vertebrate social behaviour. Steroids influencing social behaviour can come either from the peripheral circulation (gonads and adrenals), or from steroid synthesis within the brain itself. Peptides of the oxytocin family that influence social behaviour are produced within the brain. The six nodes of the social behaviour network contain both steroid and peptide mechanisms. In oscine passerine birds, the forebrain neural song system underlies the production and perception of learned song. Relationships between this system and the social behaviour network are not yet well understood. Learning and neural plasticity are essential properties of both systems.

nucleus of the stria terminalis) and released within the brain to influence behaviour. Several of the key nodes of the social behaviour network express these peptides or their receptors (Newman 2002, Goodson 2005). Depending on the animals, peptides of the latter type cannot be assumed to pass through the blood–brain barrier. The circulating levels of peptides from the posterior pituitary are not necessarily the relevant molecules for social behaviour, and direct brain manipulations of peptides and their receptors, rather than systemic treatments, may be required to test causal hypotheses. Such experiments have confirmed that oxytocin-family peptides are regulators of vocal and aggressive behaviour across vertebrates, and of affiliative and parental behaviour in several mammals (Carter *et al.* 1995, Goodson & Bass 2001, Lim & Young 2006). Because these peptides and their receptors are gene products, such research provides

exceptional opportunities for linking social behaviour to the genome in order to understand the mechanistic basis of evolutionary changes in social behaviour. Two examples will serve to show the potential of neuropeptide research for illuminating evolutionary diversity.

One body of work seeks to understand whether the vasotocinergic system is responsible for species differences among birds in sociality (Goodson & Wang 2006, Goodson *et al.* 2006). Using multiple species of estrildid finches ranging from highly gregarious to territorial, it was found that (a) the gregarious species have more vasotocinergic neurons in the medial bed nucleus of the stria terminalis, and those neurons respond more to same-sex stimuli, and (b) the gregarious species have more vasotocin receptors in the medial septum and portions of the lateral septum. The lateral septum had been identified earlier as an area where vasotocin infusions produce opposite effects on aggression in gregarious and territorial birds (Goodson 2005). Vasotocin has also been shown to regulate social behaviours such as singing and aggression in an array of other vertebrates, which bodes well for the species generality of the hypothesis (Maney *et al*. 1997, Goodson & Bass 2001).

The other body of work has targeted one of the vasopressin receptor subtypes, the V1a receptor, as a basis for the evolution of species differences in the mating system in *Microtus* voles (see Chapter 11). Males of the socially monogamous prairie vole *M. ochrogaster* have more V1a receptors in the ventral pallidum than males of promiscuous congeners. Male mice *Mus musculus* and meadow voles *Microtus pennsylvanicus* (both promiscuous species) that are genetically engineered to have prairie-vole levels of V1a receptor expression in the ventral pallidum prefer to spend time with familiar rather than novel females following vasopressin administration or cohabitation, the preference shown by male prairie voles but not by controls of the two promiscuous species (Young *et al*. 1999, Lim *et al*. 2004). The breakthrough in these experiments is the use of a direct experimental manipulation of gene expression to test a comparative hypothesis about the neuroendocrine basis for the evolution of a species difference in social behaviour. In addition, marked individual differences in the numbers of V1a receptors have been found in the brains of wild prairie voles that could be a source of individual differences in monogamous tendencies (Phelps & Young 2003, Ophir *et al*. 2008).

These findings about brain peptide pathways and social behaviour are providing new hypotheses for the mechanistic bases of within- and between-species diversity. It is important to find out whether they generalise to other mammals and non-mammalian systems.

3.1.5 Mechanisms differ for the formation and maintenance of social relationships

Social relationships such as dominance and parental care of offspring have an initial formative stage (see Chapters 7, 11 and 14), when the individuals first encounter each other and establish the relationship, and a subsequent maintenance stage, characterised by some degree of stability and predictability (dominance) along with adjustment to the changing needs of the other party (parenting). Classic bodies of research on both dominance and maternal behaviour have established that circulating hormones are mainly involved, if at all, during the initial formative stage, and that once formed, the relationships continue regardless of changes in hormonal status (Adkins-Regan 2005). This principle appears to apply to invertebrate dominance and parental care as well, even though the relevant hormones are chemically different (Trumbo 1996). Similarly, male birds that undergo a precipitous drop in testosterone at the onset of the incubation stage of the breeding cycle nonetheless retain their territories and mates.

In the case of parental behaviour, the essential experimental manipulations (prolactin administration and suppression) required to confirm a causal role in the onset of the behaviour have been done in very few species (Buntin 1996, Mann & Bridges 2001). Prolactin elevations occur during the parental-care breeding stage in a number of birds, mammals and teleost fishes, but as always experimental manipulations will be necessary to find out whether there is any causal relationship.

3.2 Learned song and the song system

The preceding sections presented a number of principles covering the ways in which social behaviour and endocrinology (or neuroendocrinology) may be coupled – or may not. Song in songbirds is a paradigmatic example where extensive research has both related endocrinology and neurobiology to the behaviour, and elucidated the functions and development of the behaviour. Because of the variety of insights that have come from study of this system, we will review it in more depth than some of the other social behaviours that have been described. We will explore proximate causes of song, but place them in the context of ultimate causes.

Songbirds learn their vocalisations and use them in social interactions (Thorpe 1958). Typically, males sing during the reproductive season to attract mates, to define territories, and as a component of agonistic displays with other males. A variety of influences come together to affect song acquisition and expression. Learning involves choice of a model at a time that is right in terms of brain development, model availability, and appropriate patterns of circulating steroids. Song production involves correct timing – it must be produced during the correct season, at the right time of day, and coordinated with other aspects of social behaviour such as territory ownership or stage of reproduction. Song perception is equally important – both males and females must be able to recognise conspecifics from song, and furthermore often can judge aspects of male quality from song and even recognise and respond appropriately to individual males on the basis of their songs. Finally, a quality that makes this system both intensely exciting and challenging is interspecies variation in the content and usage of song. Examples of each of these observations are presented below.

3.2.1 Song is learned – at the right time, from the right source

Songbirds acquire song through a multistage process. During an early sensitive period, song is internalised if an acceptable model is available (Nelson 1998). Songs heard during this period of auditory learning will later be produced by the bird; songs heard before or after this period typically will not be produced. Individuals in many species then exhibit a phase of subsong in which brief, low-volume, highly variable sounds are produced (Marler *et al.* 1988). In species in which only males normally sing, a phase of plastic song follows, in which the males practise recognisable models. As the birds become sexually mature, these vocalisations crystallise into full song, in which males produce a discrete set of sounds in a highly stereotyped way in territorial defence or the courtship process (Marler 1956, Kroodsma 1996). Whereas this pattern characterises song acquisition in many of the songbird species in which it has been

studied (reviewed by Marler & Nelson 1993, Marler 1997), bird species can vary substantially from it. Brown thrashers *Toxostoma rufum*, mockingbirds *Mimus polyglottos* and European starlings *Sturnus vulgaris*, for example, continue to alter and augment their songs throughout life (open-ended learners). In zebra finches, the species most commonly studied in the lab, juveniles learn most of the elements of their song from their fathers. Males in other species may acquire parts of their song from several different adult males. This learning pattern, however, is not universal. Juvenile brown-headed cowbirds *Molothrus ater* are shaped by adult females to produce some of their song elements (Miller *et al.* 2008). European sedge warblers *Acrocephalus schoenobaenus* will improvise an elaborate song if external models are not available (Leitner *et al.* 2002).

Much of what is known of the factors that initiate or terminate song learning comes from experiments in zebra finches. Initiation of learning is associated with attaining a level of brain development at which brain areas involved in song acquisition can communicate with auditory association areas. The end of the sensitive period appears to be tied to androgen level – raising circulating levels of steroids can cause the acquisition period to terminate abnormally early, leading to an abnormally simple song. The sensitive period is prolonged for a time if juveniles are isolated from song (Eales 1987, Jones *et al.* 1996). Perhaps links between experience and the close of the sensitive period can explain how initial song learning in individuals that hatch late can occur when the birds are a year old for some species that sing and reproduce seasonally (Kroodsma & Pickert 1980).

3.2.2 Adult song is coordinated across seasons and time of day, and with mating status

Songbirds from temperate zones breed seasonally, and singing activity usually peaks during these periods. Some species of open-ended learners maintain stereotyped song patterns during each breeding season but readily augment them in between. Species differ widely in the details of song expression – in some, song is prominent while forming a territory and attracting a mate, but then decreases dramatically. In others, it continues to be expressed throughout reproduction. However, within a species, the coordination of song with mating and reproduction is striking. How is the production of a complex learned motor behaviour timed so precisely? How is this iconic social behaviour linked to the appropriate social situation? The proximate answer to such questions comes from having a constrained brain system used for song production that is linked to sensory association areas and to the endocrine system.

The major brain nuclei that control song production (Fig. 3.2) consist of caudal projections from the HVC (a brain nucleus analogous to the premotor cortex: Reiner *et al.* 2004) through the robust nucleus of the arcopallium (RA) and the hypoglossal nucleus to the muscles used for vocalising. HVC also projects to area X, a striatal region thought to be important in motor song learning that ultimately feeds back to the caudal nuclei (reviewed by DeVoogd & Lauay 2001).

Nottebohm (1981) first observed neural changes in these regions associated with seasonal plasticity in singing: HVC, RA and area X of males are nearly twice as large during spring as they are during autumn, and the time at which these nuclei begin to expand coincides with the onset of renewed song rehearsal. More detailed anatomical analyses showed that the changes in volumes accompanied changes in the length of dendrites and of synapses (DeVoogd *et al.* 1985, Hill & DeVoogd 1991). In the HVC, additional neurogenesis and/or neuronal survival contribute to the spring increase in volume (Kirn *et al.* 1991, Tramontin & Brenowitz 1999). Although large seasonal shifts in anatomy occur in many temperate-zone species, they are not universal. They are not found in wild canaries (Leitner *et al.* 2001) or in black-capped chickadees (Smulders *et al.* 2006). Thus the consequences of massive gain and loss of synaptic networks must be more complex than simply linking song to reproduction.

Since song is learned from auditory models, neural connections must exist between brain regions involved in perception and in production. Experiments measuring expression of immediate early genes (IEGs) have been central to starting to

understand these relations (reviewed by DeVoogd & Lauay 2001). Neuronal activity often leads to synthesis of new proteins that might be used to replace transmitter molecules, or to restructure the synapses that contributed to the activation. Immediate early genes create proteins that coordinate this transcription. Staining for IEG mRNA or protein, then, gives an image of the neurons that have recently been active. Producing song is associated with expression of IEGs in all the major nuclei of the motor song system, both in the lab and in the wild (reviewed by DeVoogd & Lauay 2001). In dramatic contrast, merely hearing a song is not associated with activation of any of these nuclei, but rather with activation of a variety of regions not previously associated with song processing: subdivisions L1 and L3 of field L (analogous to the primary auditory cortex), zones adjacent to HVC and RA, as well as caudomedial nidopallium (NCM) and caudomedial mesopallium (CMM), areas believed analogous to auditory association cortex (Figure 3.2). NCM and CMM are reciprocally connected with field L, with auditory nuclei elsewhere in the brain, as well as with nuclei of the motor song system, thus forming a link between audition and singing (reviewed by DeVoogd & Lauay 2001).

The NCM is especially responsive to song content (reviewed by Theunissen & Shaevitz 2006). Different sorts of syllables evoke distinct patterns of IEG activation in canary NCM (Ribeiro *et al.* 1998). Playing more attractive songs to female starlings causes greater activation in NCM than less attractive songs (Gentner *et al.* 2001). More IEG expression is induced in NCM in female white-crowned sparrows *Zonotrichia leucophrys* hearing songs of their natal dialect than songs of another dialect (Maney *et al.* 2003), and in zebra finches that are hearing the song with which they were tutored versus other songs (Terpstra *et al.* 2004). Expression of IEGs and physiological activity in NCM of adult male zebra finches presented with tutor song are positively correlated with the number of syllables these birds accurately copied from that song (Bolhuis *et al.* 2000, 2001, Terpstra 2004, Phan *et al.* 2006).

The NCM is also sensitive to recent experience. Repeated presentation of a song results in a decrement of the IEG activation that it evokes in NCM (Mello *et al.*

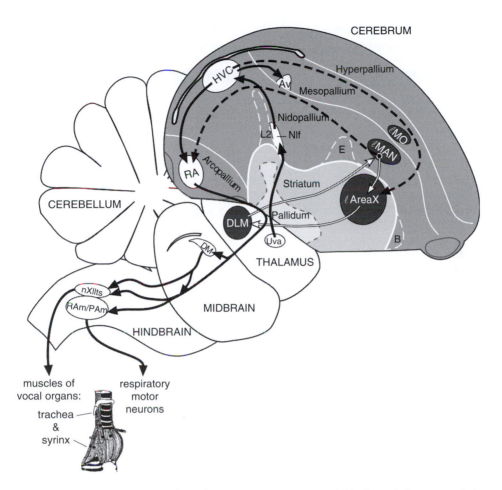

Figure 3.2 Brain (top) and singing apparatus (syrinx) of a songbird. Areas such as field L (L2 and adjacent areas), the caudo-medial area of the nidopallium (NCM) and the caudomedial area of the mesopallium (CMM) respond to hearing songs. The nearby high vocal centre (HVC) projects to the robust nucleus of the arcopallium (RA), which in turn stimulates hindbrain nuclei that control the muscles used for singing (nXIIts – the tracheosyringeal portion of the hypoglossal nucleus) and breathing (retroambigualis and parambigualis – RAm/PAm). Song acquisition or production are modulated by inputs from several other regions, including area X in the striatum, the medial nucleus of the dorsal lateral thalamus (DLM), the lateral magnocellular nucleus of the anterior nidopallium (lMAN) and an adjacent medial area (mMAN, not shown), as well as the nuclei interface (NIf) and Uva. From Wilbrecht & Kirn (2004).

1995). This decrement only occurs if the context of presentation is also kept fixed (Kruse *et al.* 2004), suggesting that the NCM is involved in perceiving context as well as song. Neuronal firing in the NCM increases when the bird hears conspecific song (Stripling *et al.* 1997). This response habituates (to 60–70% of its initial level) with repeated presentation of that specific song (Chew *et al.* 1996, Stripling *et al.* 1997). Varied song presentations followed by IEG measures demonstrated that birds simultaneously adapt to a variety of conspecific songs, and retain the decreased response for at least 24 hours (Chew *et al.* 1996). Vicario and colleagues have found decrements in electrophysiological responses to particular songs up to 40 hours after exposure (Phan *et al.* 2006). Intriguingly, both the IEG and the physiological responses (and their adaptation) do not differ between adult male and female zebra finches (Chew *et al.* 1996, Terleph *et al.* 2007). These results suggest that the NCM is the brain region that forms memories of songs, and functions in individual recognition on the basis of song in both sexes (see also Sockman *et al.* 2002).

Thus, the motor song system is activated to produce stereotyped vocalisations. These are perceived by auditory association areas, in which the amount of activity that is induced is related to the nature of the original learning, to the content that is being heard and to recent and current context. Whereas these observations provide a framework for thinking about the use of song as a social signal, they do not explain changes across seasons and across phases of reproduction. These attributes appear to be regulated by gonadal steroids and other hormones acting on the production and perception regions.

3.2.3 Gonadal steroids coordinate song and social behaviours with reproduction

Changes in gonadal steroids often affect male song. Adult male chaffinches *Fringilla coelebs* cease singing in winter or following castration, but will resume doing so if injected with testosterone (T) (Poulsen 1951, Thorpe 1958). Similarly, castrated adult male zebra finches decrease their song rate, but will return to their normal frequency if administered T implants (Pröve 1974, Arnold 1975). In some species females are also sensitive to such manipulations. Female white-crowned sparrows and canaries, both of which can sing but do so infrequently, increase their song rate and enhance their repertoire size in response to T in adulthood (Leonard 1939, Kern & King 1972, Nottebohm 1980), as do non-singing female chaffinches (Thorpe 1958). Even female zebra finches will acquire song if treated with exogenous steroids early in development (Gurney & Konishi 1980, Gurney 1981). In species that sing seasonally, endogenous changes in steroid level seem to modulate singing in similar ways.

Steroid manipulations that cause onset of song or increase its frequency also increase the size of song-system brain nuclei and cause neuronal dendrites to grow and add synapses (reviewed in DeVoogd & Lauay 2001). Increasing day length in spring stimulates gonadal production of steroids and alters melatonin production, both of which may then induce elaboration of the motor nuclei for song production (Gahr & Kosar 1996, Whitfield-Rucker & Cassone 1996, Bentley *et al.* 1999). Such a scenario could lead to singing that is coordinated with activation of the reproductive system.

3.2.4 Sex differences in singing are based in song-system dimorphism

Brain regions involved in producing song are usually much larger in males than in females (reviewed by Brenowitz 1997). Some of the earliest studies on mechanisms controlling bird song demonstrated that sex differences in song are often mediated by gonadal steroids acting on neurons within the song system (reviewed in Balthazart & Adkins-Regan 2002). Early autoradiographic analyses showed that cells within HVC and the lateral magnocellular nucleus of the nidopallium (lMAN) of zebra finches accumulate T or its metabolites, and that males, in addition to possessing larger song nuclei than females, also contain a higher proportion of androgen-accumulating cells in these regions (Arnold *et al.* 1976, Arnold & Saltiel 1979). These results suggested both that intrinsic properties of the song system regulate its responsiveness to these hormones and, further, that gonadal steroids alone might masculinise the song circuit. Indeed, treatment with exogenous steroids near the time of hatching significantly enlarges the volumes of HVC and RA in female zebra finches and increases the number of neurons they contain (Gurney & Konishi 1980). Discerning the precise roles of androgens and oestrogens in the ontogeny of the song system has been difficult, however, because there are multiple sources of steroids (including the brain as well as the gonads), multiple steroid metabolites, some with multiple receptor types, and the actions of each are widespread. Organisational effects of gonadal sex steroids have been largely ruled out as the source of the song-system dimorphism, because genetic males with ovaries develop a male neural song system and sing, and genetic females with testes develop a female song system and do not sing (Wade 1999). Furthermore, while it is clear that steroids are synthesised in the brain, it can be difficult to determine the sites of synthesis, transport and use within the song system. Additionally, the treatments that masculinised female song circuitry used much higher levels of steroids than normally would impact the brains of males (Adkins-Regan *et al.* 1990). Therefore, the contributions of T and oestradiol to the sexual differentiation of the neural song circuit remain unclear (Arnold 1997). Comparative studies can help to resolve some of the ambiguity. In particular, they can elucidate general relationships between naturally occurring variation in endocrine, neuroanatomical and behavioural attributes, and these findings can then be used to formulate more directed hypotheses.

If androgens and oestrogens truly function to masculinise the song circuit, and if the neural mechanisms controlling song acquisition are conserved across species and sexes, then interspecific variation in sex patterns of song ought to covary with differences in neuroendocrinology. As mentioned above, sexual dimorphisms in hormone sensitivity of the song system were first detected in zebra finches. Males have both more densely concentrated and a greater overall number of androgen-accumulating cells in HVC and lMAN than females (Arnold & Saltiel 1979). Consistent with the hypothesis that these differences are related to their distinct singing abilities, Brenowitz and Arnold (1985) found no differences in either of these traits between sexes in the duetting bay wren *Thryothorus nigricapillus*. Interestingly, neither canaries nor rufous-and-white wrens *T. rufalbus* show a dimorphism in the percentage of androgen-target cells in HVC and lMAN despite the fact that females of these species have smaller repertoires and sing less frequently than males (Bottjer & Maier 1991, Brenowitz & Arnold 1992). Females of these species do have fewer total cells of this type than males, however, because these nuclei are smaller in females. The size of this dimorphism parallels the extent of their behavioural differences. Female canaries sing drastically simpler songs than males, and have only

approximately 25% the number of T-target cells, whereas female rufous-and-white wrens acquire a repertoire half the size of males and possess about 40% the number of T-target cells compared to males (Brenowitz & Arnold 1992, Brenowitz 1997).

Brenowitz and Arnold (1992) highlighted one scenario that could account for the pattern of sexual dimorphisms in hormone receptivity seen in these four species. The basic ability to sing may be related to the proportion of androgen-accumulating cells (and thereby sensitivity to circulating steroids), whereas variation in more subtle features of song could be associated with the overall number of such neurons (perhaps related to acuity in controlling vocalisation muscles). In other words, a bird must have a certain minimum percentage of androgen-target cells in HVC, lMAN, and potentially other song nuclei in order to possess the capacity to sing. Female zebra finches, unlike the other three species, presumably fail to meet this criterion. Provided that this condition is met, the overall number of cells that concentrate T or its metabolites may then influence more subtle features of song, such as repertoire size and production rate (Brenowitz & Arnold 1992, Brenowitz 1997). Available experimental data are consistent with this idea. Female canaries increase their song rate, develop a larger repertoire, and grow a larger HVC when exposed to exogenous T (Nottebohm 1980).

These studies do not discriminate between cells that accumulate T per se and those that concentrate its metabolites, and, as a consequence, they may mask the true patterns of androgenic and oestrogenic receptivity. However, studies that localised the sites of oestrogen action argue against this possibility. First, songbirds appear to be unique among avian taxa in that they contain oestrogen receptors (ERs), both ERα and ERβ subtypes, in the NCM, an area implicated in song perception, and ERα in the HVC. In contrast to the prevalence of androgen receptors (ARs) throughout the song system, the HVC is the only song control nucleus that contains ERs. Autoradiographic analyses revealed low incidences of this cell type in the HVC of juvenile female and adult male zebra finches (~5% and ~4%, respectively), restricted to the ventromedial portion of the nucleus (Nordeen *et al.* 1987). This lack of oestrogen-accumulating cells in zebra finches is seemingly characteristic of estrildid finches, but contrasts with other oscines and underscores how studying neuroendocrinology substantially in a single species may obscure more general patterns. In contrast to zebra finches, approximately 45% of HVC neurons in male canaries contain ERs, and these cells are located uniformly throughout the nucleus. Most cells express either ERs or ARs, but few possess both. Female canaries possess a density of ERα-immunolabelled cells equivalent to that of males but, as with androgen-target cells, they have fewer overall because they have a smaller HVC. Likewise, male and female bay wrens and rufous-and-white wrens also have equal proportions of HVC neurons that accumulate oestradiol or its metabolites. In each of these species, then, males and females have the same proportions of cells that accumulate oestrogen or that express ERα, regardless of whether the sexes also differ in their singing abilities. Thus, the degree of dimorphism in song production appears more closely related to anatomical dimorphisms than to sex differences in steroid receptivity (steroid distribution reviewed by DeVoogd & Lauay 2001, Wade & Arnold 2004).

3.2.5 Song perception goes with song production

Females of many species sing little if at all, but song often has major effects on females. For example, female pied flycatchers *Ficedula hypoleuca* and European starlings are attracted to nest-boxes that broadcast male song, whereas they pay less attention to silent nest-boxes (Eriksson & Wallin 1986, Mountjoy & Lemon 1991). Females react differently to songs that differ in content (Ratcliffe & Otter 1996, Nowicki *et al.* 2002, Riebel 2003). Females respond differently to songs of their mates or fathers than to the songs of other males (Miller 1979a, 1979b, Riebel *et al.* 2002), suggesting that they can remember individual identities. Female zebra finches readily choose to move towards normal song over the impoverished song produced by males reared in isolation (Lauay *et al.* 2004), and prefer to mate with males who sing full songs over isolate songs (Williams *et al.* 1993).

Females of several species choose males with more complex songs as mates or for extra-pair copulations (Catchpole 1987, Eens *et al.* 1991, Bensch & Hasselquist 1992, Hasselquist *et al.* 1996). Adult females can make precise discriminations of conspecific song (Miller 1979a, 1979b, Wiley *et al.* 1991, Cynx & Nottebohm 1992, Williams *et al.* 1993). They prefer familiar to unfamiliar songs (King *et al.* 2003, Hernandez & MacDougall-Shackleton 2004). Female song sparrows *Melospiza melodia* give more copulation solicitation displays to songs containing many learned elements than to equally complex songs with more improvised elements (Nowicki *et al.* 2002). These studies indicate that females readily identify conspecific song, but importantly, adult females can make sophisticated judgements about the nature of the song. Such findings underscore the social uses of song – it is a social communication signal to which conspecifics attend closely. Variation in the quality and content of the signal affects the responses of the hearers. Acuity of perception is as important as control of production. Indeed, elaboration of song is only meaningful to the extent that it can be perceived by receivers. Sexual selection has driven evolution of singing abilities, by modifying the brain regions responsible for perception as well as production.

To fully understand song learning, it is necessary to understand how songbirds perceive and respond to it. Such ventures have become more feasible with the recent identification of novel brain regions that selectively upregulate IEG transcription in response to hearing conspecific song (reviewed by DeVoogd & Lauay 2001). As indicated above, NCM and CMM, in particular, respond more strongly to conspecific songs than to songs of other species or noise. At a time when so little is known about how birds perceive songs, comparative studies could be of great use in identifying potential functions of these areas and how they differ between species that use song in different ways.

In females, CMM is important in processing song. Adult female zebra finches trained in a two-choice operant paradigm choose to play back their tutor song over an unfamiliar song (Riebel 2000). Tutor song induces greater IEG activation than novel song in CMM, but not in NCM (Terpstra *et al*. 2006). Also, physiological activity of CMM neurons in adult female European starlings is selective for learned songs (Gentner & Margoliash 2003). Neurons in CMM also respond to songs experienced in associative learning tasks (Gentner *et al*. 2004).

Relatively little is known of the development of perceptual acuity in females. We have found that formation of synapses in NCM is affected by social experience during development. Female zebra finches raised without hearing song do not select normal song over isolate (abnormally simple) song as adults (Lauay *et al*. 2004), and have fewer dendritic spine synapses in NCM than do normally reared females (Lauay *et al*. 2005). It is not clear whether they have an early sensitive period for learning about song, or whether they could learn to make such judgements about song at any time.

3.2.6 Huge (understudied) variation in the forms of learning and production

Phylogenetic comparative study (see Chapter 5) is a powerful means by which to relate social behaviours to song, and song to neuroendocrinology and neurobiology. Aspects of song are learned in every species within the oscine suborder of Passeriformes in which this has been studied. Across the more than 4000 species of this suborder, interspecific variation has been observed in nearly every measurable aspect of song. Species differ in the amount they can learn, the accuracy and precision with which they reproduce tutor songs, the types of sounds they attempt to copy, the time of life during which memorisation and vocal modification occurs, and the social interactions necessary and/or sufficient to produce normal learning. Indeed, such extensive behavioural diversity as that typifying song development is seldom found within such recently evolved lineages (Catchpole & Slater 1995). The vast majority of research on song and the song system to date has used zebra finches, and most of the remaining studies have used canaries and starlings. What is more, some of the behaviours and learning mechanisms of the more popular subject species are not

representative of most other songbirds. However, intriguing data from other species suggest that more systematic comparative study may yield powerful insights into the relations between such social qualities as mating pattern, group size and duration of association, and song content and usage, as well as the neural and endocrine factors that regulate song. Many reviews are available that survey primary findings in the song system. The following sections will highlight research in some less frequently studied species, especially research that has used an explicitly comparative perspective.

3.2.7 Individual and species differences in brain space allocated to song predict song complexity

Intraspecific studies

Why do some males within a species sing more elaborate songs than others (e.g. Bensch & Hasselquist 1992), or why do some include more notes that are especially salient to females (e.g. Vallet & Kreutzer 1995) than do other males? At a proximate level, some males can learn more song components than others. Song complexity is typically measured as the number of unique syllables or song types constituting an individual's repertoire (but see Kroodsma 1996), and it can vary substantially both within and across species. Most efforts to identify neural correlates of these differences have focused on single species and, overall, have produced ostensibly contrasting results. In canaries, a male's song complexity is correlated with the volume of both the HVC and the robust nucleus of the arcopallium (RA; Nottebohm *et al*. 1981). This first report linking the complexity of a learned behaviour to the amount of neural substrate specifically devoted to performing it inspired several additional studies that sought to replicate the findings in different species.

In an early experiment on allopatric populations of marsh wrens *Cistothorus palustris*, Canady *et al*. (1984) found that males from western North America both sing significantly more song types and possess significantly larger HVCs than males living in the east. Moreover, HVC volumes are positively related to song repertoires within both populations. Syllable repertoires are also correlated with HVC volume (relative to that of telencephalon) in European sedge warblers and in zebra finches (Airey *et al.* 2000a, Airey & DeVoogd 2000). Experiments in red-winged blackbirds *Agelaius phoeniceus*, rufous-sided towhees *Pipilo erythrophthalmus*, European starlings and brown-headed cowbirds have not found this association (Brenowitz *et al.* 1991, Bernard *et al.* 1996, Kirn *et al.* 1989, Hamilton *et al.* 1998). Still other experiments have reported intermediate associations. For example, Ward *et al.* (1998) did not find an association between HVC volume and syllable repertoire size in zebra finches, but did find a significant relation between HVC neuron number and the number of sounds in the song that had been accurately copied. Finally, this topic was revisited in canaries (Leitner & Catchpole 2004). While the authors did not replicate the original finding of Nottebohm *et al.* (1981), they did find a significant positive relation between HVC volume and the proportion of sexy syllables (Vallet & Kreutzer 1995, Vallet *et al.* 1998) within a bird's repertoire. These latter results highlight two important caveats to the general correlations. First, song-nucleus volumes provide only a gross measure of circuit complexity and may be influenced by multiple factors. Second, the songs of different species have undergone distinct selection pressures, and features other than repertoire have been accentuated to varying degrees in different species (discussed below). Such differences are not accounted for in these types of broad comparisons.

What, then, is to be made of these incongruent results? This was the focus of a recent meta-analysis that synthesised data from most of the studies listed above (Garamszegi & Eens 2004). This approach identified strong positive relationships between HVC and RA volumes and measures of song complexity. Moreover, the authors attributed the preponderance of non-significant relationships to small sample sizes and type II errors, suggesting that insufficient statistical power led to the erroneous failure to reject the null hypothesis. Thus, a general relationship between

the volume of song nuclei HVC and RA and song complexity exists within species.

Interspecific studies

One of the fascinating features that distinguish songbird species is their varying capacity to learn multiple song components. Some, like the chipping sparrow *Spizella passerina* and several warblers within the genus *Locustella*, learn only a single syllable that they sing repetitiously thereafter (Borror 1959, Thorpe 1957). Others can sing multiple syllables and organise them into distinct song types, as does the song sparrow (Borror 1965). A few species, such as the brown thrasher and common nightingale *Luscinia megarhynchos*, can acquire staggering repertoires consisting of hundreds to thousands of unique syllables (Kroodsma & Parker 1977, Hultsch & Todt 1981). This remarkable interspecific variation is accompanied by consistent differences in the song system. In a wide phylogeny of 41 species spanning eight families, evolutionary changes in the relative volume of HVC were positively correlated with changes in song type repertoire (DeVoogd *et al.* 1993). Interestingly, positive relationships were also evident between genera and between families, suggesting that residual HVC volume and song complexity have been linked throughout the evolution of the oscine clade.

We have observed the same pattern of associations in a more focused comparative analysis of eight European reed-warbler species from the two closely related genera *Acrocephalus* and *Locustella* (family Sylviidae; Székely *et al.* 1996). More recently, similar analyses on 36 further species drawn from 14 families also indicated a positive correlation between syllable repertoire and relative HVC volume (Moore *et al.* 2004). Song was not related to the relative volumes of RA, lMAN, or area X. Moreover, there was no relationship between song complexity and the volume of the mesopallium, a telencephalic region whose volume is positively correlated with feeding-innovation rate in several groups of birds (Lefebvre *et al.* 1997, 1998). This last result highlights the modularity of the song system – associations between singing behaviours and neural attributes are very specific.

The wide-ranging diversity of bird song begs for more comparisons. Whereas studies like those cited above can help to identify general relationships between brains and behaviour, they also encounter comparability problems that warrant consideration (Kroodsma 1996). The songs of different species are rarely, if ever, directly comparable. As one example, the spectrotemporal structures of song components vary drastically, and it is next to impossible to identify equivalent units across all birds. Compounding this problem, different classification criteria and terminology are often used to quantify repertoires of different species, and different species selectively accentuate different features. Secondly, even when distinct syllable or song types can be easily discriminated, they almost certainly differ in their difficulty of memorisation and/or production. Yet broad interspecific comparisons like those listed above treat all elements as if they are equivalent. Finally, syllable or song-type repertoires are frequently measured to indicate song complexity because they are highly variable and easily quantified, but birds certainly attend to features of their song other than repertoire, and species likely differ in this respect as well. As a consequence, the specific functions of song nuclei may have diverged, to some extent, across lineages. In spite of these many limiting factors, a significant correlation between HVC volume and song complexity is detectable and apparently well conserved across the oscine suborder.

In summary, comparative studies on the song system can provide valuable insights into general relationships between song learning and its associated anatomy. Researchers generally agree that interspecific comparisons ought to be interpreted within an evolutionary context (Chapter 5). Ideally, studies that incorporate many diverse species can be accompanied by others that focus on fewer, more closely related species in order to minimise the influence of comparability problems. Whether made across wide phylogenies, or restricted to more closely related species, these analyses can provide insights into the neurobiological processes that mediate divergent behaviours and direct the testing of more specific hypotheses.

3.2.8 Constraints and costs of a plastic system

The sections above review evidence that species and individuals within species vary in the amount of song they learn. They use song in multiple social contexts. Hearers vary in their responses to song, depending on context, season and, of course, species. At its most elementary level, song indicates the existence of a conspecific. However, data reviewed above demonstrate that it is often used for so much more – commonly as an agonistic signal between males and an affiliative signal towards females. The ability to sing appropriately is essential to reproduction. In species in which males sing as a signal to other males, incompetence or inability to match the other can lead to fights or loss of territory. In species in which song is directed towards females, incompetence may prevent or delay pairing, and may result in an increased likelihood of extra-pair paternities (EPCs, Chapter 10). If being able to sing the best sort of song in the right context is so important, why don't all birds do it?

A simple answer is that producing a song is costly. As reviewed above, enhanced song content (Garamszegi & Eens 2004) and perhaps enhanced song production (DeVoogd et al. 1995) require additional commitment of neurons and synapses, which in turn require supporting tissues as well as increased supplies of oxygen and glucose. Much of the variation in song content and flexibility in its usage derives from its being learned, which in turn is a consequence of having an elaborate song system. Individuals differ in how much learning they have experienced. Some of these differences may ultimately result from heritable genetic variation (Airey et al. 2000b). Some may also result from developmental stress during the sensitive period, perhaps due to poor nutrition (Nowicki et al. 2002). In either case, these costs to males may explain why females so often assess males using song: it can give reliable clues to male quality rapidly and at a distance.

Learned song is used in many more contexts than simply attracting females, and is likely to have evolved as a consequence of other pressures as well. It facilitates individual identification – a capacity that is often used between males. It permits identification of social groups within a species – from a regional group with a common dialect to a population that uses notes in common.

3.3 Trends, directions and gaps

Several important new developments have already been referred to, such as the discoveries about neuropeptides and social behaviour in voles and estrildid finches and the insights into brain space for learned song repertoires from comparative analyses. Here we will briefly mention several others of particular importance for an understanding of social behaviour that are also receiving attention.

3.3.1 Hormones and personality types

There is increasing evidence that some of the individual differences in social behaviour in non-human animals have the hallmarks of personality types, including stability of behavioural style across contexts (Chapter 16). For example, individuals of a number of species have been found to differ consistently in ways corresponding to a bold versus shy dimension of personality (Sih *et al*. 2004). Hypotheses derived from human and other primate research about their heritability and relation to hormones (especially adrenal glucocorticoids) are now being tested in other animals. For example, bold and shy individuals have been found to differ in baseline corticosterone or cortisol, and/or in acute elevations in these hormones in response to novel or stressful situations (Koolhaas *et al*. 1999, Cockrem 2007). Such individual differences could reflect the expression of genes for the neural steroid receptors regulating peripheral hormone levels, providing a targeted approach to identifying the genetic basis of these personality types.

3.3.2 Hormones and signal honesty

One focus of current integrative research on hormones and social behaviour asks whether the hormonal mechanisms for sexually selected male behaviour

are a source of condition-dependent costs of the behaviour that help explain why such behaviour is an honest signal of the male's quality, either to other males in competitive situations or to females during mate choice. The most prevalent version of the hormone hypothesis is that the frequency and intensity of those male signals are testosterone-based, that testosterone is costly because it causes immuno-suppression, and that only males of superior genetic quality can afford to have high enough levels of testosterone to display vigorously or sing elaborately (Folstad & Karter 1992). The behaviour itself can be costly, for example, if it increases predation risk, but the immunocompetence-handicap hypothesis is that there are additional costs due to the underlying hormonal mechanism that would apply to non-behavioural male traits (such as ornamental colours) as well. Although the evidence for the hypothesis is mixed (Roberts *et al*. 2004), it has stimulated interesting integrative work on the immune systems of animals other than domestic mammals, along with an appreciation for the trade-offs that animals face between social behaviour and reproduction, on the one hand, and disease avoidance, wound healing and overall survival, on the other. Newer versions of the overall testosterone-handicap hypothesis propose other physiological costs such as increased oxidative stress (Alonso-Alvarez *et al*. 2007). Nor can the costs of the neural systems to support displays be ignored (see section 3.2.8, above).

3.3.3 Mechanisms of mating strategies and tactics

Studies of free-living vertebrates have revealed a rich array of mating strategies and tactics, some of which suggest adaptive decision making. For example, females of a number of socially monogamous birds engage in extra-pair matings as if they are seeking genes from males that will increase the fitness of their offspring (Griffith *et al*. 2002). Males have been found to allocate more sperm to a female if male competitors are present, as predicted by sperm competition theory (Birkhead & Møller 1998). Little is known about the involvement of neuroendocrine mechanisms in these kinds of decisions and allocations. Do female birds' hormone levels change following mating, and do they change differently for within-pair versus extra-pair matings in socially monogamous species? Is the brain's knowledge of the internal hormonal milieu part of the animal's assessment of its own condition that then guides its tactics? What are the mechanisms that translate the sight of another male into the number of sperm transferred to a female? There is some experimental evidence from sparrows *Melospiza melodia* and *Zonotrichia leucophrys* and dark-eyed juncos *Junco hyemalis* that activational effects of testosterone are involved in males' ranging activities, engagement in extra-pair matings, and the likelihood of being paired with more than one female, suggesting hormonal bases for species differences in mating systems as well as for variation within and between individuals in tactical decision making (Wingfield 1984, Raouf *et al.* 1997). Neuropeptides are candidate mechanisms for several reproductive strategies and tactics used by male teleost fish species (Bass & Grober 2001, Miranda *et al.* 2003).

3.3.4 Cooperative breeding and sex-role reversal

Cooperatively breeding social systems, in which young are fed by subordinate alloparents (helpers) in addition to the dominant genetic parents (Chapter 12), and sex-role reversal, in which females compete for males and males tend the young, inspire interesting questions about both ultimate and proximate causation. With respect to cooperatively breeding mammals and birds, some progress has been made in understanding species differences in whether the dominants or the subordinates have higher glucocorticoid levels (Creel 2001, Goymann & Wingfield 2004), and in viewing glucocorticoid levels as environmentally sensitive predictors of future breeding roles (Rubenstein 2007).

Studies asking whether dominants and subordinates differ in brain hormone targets and other neural mechanisms are just beginning, but are already producing some exciting discoveries. Striking differences in the sizes of several forebrain regions involved in social behaviour have been found between dominant and subordinate naked mole-rats

Heterocephalus glaber and white-browed sparrow-weavers *Plocepasser mahali* (Holmes *et al.* 2007, Voigt *et al.* 2007). The results suggest remarkable neural plasticity (dominants are former subordinates) that is independent of circulating hormone levels (which did not differ in the sparrow-weavers). This hypothesis merits experimental follow-up along with investigation of mechanisms involved in this plasticity.

The involvement of hormones in sex-role reversal has been best investigated in birds (Fivizzani *et al.* 1990, Eens & Pinxten 2000). The hypothesis that sex differences in levels of circulating sex steroids will be reversed compared to birds with conventional sex roles has been rejected. A recent study found higher expression of androgen receptor mRNA in the forebrain nucleus taeniae in female than male African black coucals *Centropus grillii*, a species in which females sing and defend territories and males provide parental care, even though males had more circulating androgens (Voigt & Goymann 2007). Nucleus taeniae is the avian homologue of one of the regions in the sheep *Ovis aries* brain where there are steroid receptor differences between males preferring males versus females as sexual partners (Roselli *et al.* 2002). Both cases raise the possibility of hormonal organisation early in life as a source of these species and individual differences.

3.3.5 Advances and needs in methods

Increased interest in the behavioural neuroendocrinology of free-living animals has contributed importantly to an integrated understanding of their lives. Even greater progress could be made if some technical limitations could be overcome. Acceptable measurement of circulating hormone levels often requires not only obtaining a blood sample, but also getting the sample within five minutes of beginning the process of catching the animal. Faecal sampling methods can sometimes be useful, especially for tracking reproductive cycles and energetic challenges, but require validation against blood measures and careful storage (Wasser *et al.* 2000, Lynch *et al.* 2003, Goymann & Jenni-Eiermann 2005). Their utility for studying social behaviour is less clear. In addition, even blood plasma assays often are not sensitive enough to measure testosterone in females or oestradiol in males. Manipulation of neurohormonal mechanisms requires treatments that can be delivered to the brain, ideally into specific sub-regions or nuclei. Because there is a pressing need to deliver these neurohormones and drugs non-invasively to human brains, we can look forward to new delivery methods that have been refined using laboratory mammal models. Non-invasive brain imaging methods for freely moving animals are not yet a reality. The closest approximations require either restraining or sedating the animal, thus precluding any social interaction (e.g. Voss *et al.* 2007), or (in the case of immunocytochemistry for the immediate early gene products that reveal where neurons were firing recently) they yield only one data point per animal, ruling out any kind of within-subject experimental design.

3.3.6 Evolution and development

On a more positive note, there is an important future for understanding the developmental mechanisms that produce evolutionary changes in social behaviour. This will require deep immersion in the neuroendocrine and other mechanisms of the brain, especially gene products, expression and regulatory interactions. It was proposed over 20 years ago that the mechanisms of song-system sexual differentiation might be the basis for evolutionary changes in singing dimorphism (Arnold *et al.* 1986). As discussed above in section 3.2.4 some progress has been made through comparative studies of song-system dimorphism. The newly available genomic resources for zebra finches will speed efforts to uncover the genetic basis of these species differences (Wada *et al.* 2006, Li *et al.* 2007). Now that some of the mechanistic bases of species differences in sociality in estrildid finches and in the mating system in microtine voles are known, a focus on development to find out at what point these gene expression differences appear and why will be important. With the sequencing of the chicken genome and the progress that has been made understanding hormonal organisation and activation of behaviour in Japanese quail, it might be possible to discover the developmental mechanisms responsible

for the frequent evolutionary changes in parental care that have occurred in the cracid family (curassows and allies) of galliform birds (Cockburn 2006). When combined with progress in understanding the selective pressures responsible for the evolution of this diversity, with advances in behavioural neurogenetics, and with better records of phylogeny as revealed by comparative genomics, we will then have a more complete picture of why and how sociality, mating systems and parental behaviour vary across species.

3.4 Conclusions and future directions

The evolution of social behaviour and its genetic basis cannot be understood by adopting a black-box approach to the brain and to neuroendocrinology, or by ignoring plasticity and learning. Integration between proximate and ultimate causation will require a more sophisticated view of hormonal and neural mechanisms that includes neurohormones, brain targets for hormones, and mechanisms for neural plasticity. Attention to mechanisms operating during early life as well as adulthood will lead to a deeper understanding of what has enabled evolutionary change and species divergence to occur, and will reveal the source of individual and sex differences as well as species differences.

Acknowledgements

The authors thank the National Science Foundation (EA-R), the National Institute of Mental Health (TJD) and the US–Hungary Joint Fund (TJD) for research support.

Suggested readings

Adkins-Regan, E. (2005) *Hormones and Animal Social Behavior*. Princeton, NJ: Princeton University Press.
Marler, P. R. & Slabbekoorn, H., eds. (2004) *Nature's Music: the Science of Birdsong*. London: Academic Press.
Pfaff, D. W., Arnold, A. P., Etgen, A. M., Fahrbach, S. E. & Rubin, R.T., eds. (2002) *Hormones, Brain and Behavior*. Amsterdam: Academic Press.

Remage-Healey, L., Maidment, N. T. & Schlinger, B. A. (2008) Forebrain steroid levels fluctuate rapidly during social interactions. *Nature Neuroscience*, **11**, 1327–1334.

Sasaki, A., Sotnikova, T. D., Gainetdinov, R. R. & Jarvis, E. D. (2006) Social context-dependent singing-regulated dopamine. *Journal of Neuroscience* **26**, 9010–9014.

References

Adkins-Regan, E. (2005) *Hormones and Animal Social Behavior*. Princeton, NJ: Princeton University Press.

Adkins-Regan, E. & Wade, J. (2001) Masculinized sexual partner preference in female zebra finches with sex-reversed gonads. *Hormones and Behavior*, **39**, 22–28.

Adkins-Regan, E., Abdelnabi, M., Mobarak, M. & Ottinger, M. A. (1990) Sex steroid levels in developing and adult male and female zebra finches (*Poephila guttata*). *General and Comparative Endocrinology*, **78**, 93–109.

Airey, D. C. & DeVoogd, T. J. (2000) Greater song complexity is associated with augmented song system anatomy in zebra finches. *Neuroreport*, **11**, 2339–2344.

Airey, D. C., Buchanan, K. L., Székely, T., Catchpole, C. K. & DeVoogd, T. J. (2000a) Song, sexual selection, and a song control nucleus (HVc) in the brains of European sedge warblers. *Journal of Neurobiology*, **44**, 1–6.

Airey, D. C., Castillo-Juarez, H., Casella, G., Pollak, E. J. & DeVoogd, T. J. (2000b) Variation in the volume of zebra finch song control nuclei is heritable: developmental and evolutionary implications. *Proceedings of the Royal Society B*, **26**, 2099–2104.

Alonso-Alvarez, C., Bertrand, S., Faivre, B., Chastel, O. & Sorci, G. (2007) Testosterone and oxidative stress: the oxidation handicap hypothesis. *Proceedings of the Royal Society B*, **274**, 819–825.

Aragona, B. J., Liu, Y., Yu, Y. J. et al. (2006) Nucleus accumbens dopamine differentially mediates the formation and maintenance of monogamous pair bonds. *Nature Neuroscience*, **9**, 133–139.

Arnold, A. P. (1975) Effects of castration and androgen replacement on song, courtship, and aggression in zebra finches (*Poephila guttata*). *Journal of Experimental Zoology*, **191**, 309–326.

Arnold, A. P. (1997) Sexual differentiation of the zebra finch song system: positive evidence, negative evidence, null hypotheses, and a paradigm shift. *Journal of Neurobiology*, **33**, 572–584.

Arnold, A. P. & Saltiel, A. (1979) Sexual difference in pattern of hormone accumulation in the brain of a songbird. *Science*, **205**, 702–705.

Arnold, A. P., Nottebohm, F. & Pfaff, D. W. (1976) Hormone concentrating cells in vocal control and other areas of the brain of the zebra finch (*Poephila guttata*). *Journal of Comparative Neurology*, **165**, 487–511.

Arnold, A. P., Bottjer, S. W., Brenowitz, E. A., Nordeen, E. J. & Nordeen, K. W. (1986) Sexual dimorphisms in the neural vocal control system in song birds: ontogeny and phylogeny. *Brain, Behavior and Evolution*, **28**, 22–31.

Ball, G. F. & Balthazart, J. (2008) Individual variation in the endocrine regulation of behaviour and physiology in birds: a cellular/molecular perspective. *Philosophical Transactions of the Royal Society B*, **363**, 1699–1710.

Balthazart, J. & Adkins-Regan, E. (2002) Sexual differentiation of brain and behavior in birds. In: *Hormones, Brain and Behavior*, ed. D. W. Pfaff, A. P. Arnold, A.M. Etgen, S. E. Fahrbach & R. T. Rubin vol. 4. Amsterdam: Academic Press, pp. 223–302.

Balthazart, J., Castagna, C. & Ball, G. F. (1997) Aromatase inhibition blocks the activation and sexual differentiation of appetitive male sexual behavior in Japanese quail. *Behavioral Neuroscience*, **111**, 381–397.

Bass, A. H. & Grober, M. S. (2001) Social and neural modulation of sexual plasticity in teleost fish. *Brain, Behavior and Evolution*, **57**, 293–300.

Bensch, S. & Hasselquist, D. (1992) Evidence for active female choice in a polygynous warbler. *Animal Behaviour*, **44**, 301–311.

Bentley, G. E., Van't Hof, T. J. & Ball, G. F. (1999) Seasonal neuroplasticity in the songbird telencephalon: a role for melatonin. *Proceedings of the National Academy of Sciences of the USA*, **96**, 4674–4679.

Bernard, D. J., Eens, M. & Ball, G. F. (1996) Age- and behavior-related variation in volumes of song control nuclei in male European starlings. *Journal of Neurobiology*, **30**, 329–339.

Birkhead, T. R. & Møller A. P., eds. (1998) *Sperm Competition and Sexual Selection*. London: Academic Press.

Bolhuis, J. J., Zijlstra, G. G. O., den Boer-Visser, A. M. & Van der Zee, E. A. (2000) Localized neuronal activation in the zebra finch brain is related to the strength of song learning. *Proceedings of the National Academy of Sciences of the USA*, **97**, 2282–2285.

Bolhuis, J. J., Hetebrij, E., den Boer-Visser, A. M., De Groot, J. H. & Zijlstra, G. G. O. (2001) Localized immediate early gene expression related to the strength of song learning in socially reared zebra finches. *European Journal of Neuroscience*, **13**, 2165–2170.

Borror, D. J. (1959) Songs of the chipping sparrow. *Ohio Journal of Science*, **59**, 347–356.

Borror, D. J. (1965) Song variation in Maine song sparrows. *Wilson Bulletin*, **77**, 5–37.

Bottjer, S. W. & Maier, E. (1991) Testosterone and the incidence of hormone target cells in song-control nuclei of adult canaries. *Journal of Neurobiology*, **22**, 512–521.

Brantley, R. K., Wingfield, J. C. & Bass, A. H. (1993) Sex steroid levels in *Porichthys notatus*, a fish with alternative reproductive tactics, and a review of the hormonal bases for male dimorphism among teleost fishes. *Hormones and Behavior*, **27**, 332–347.

Brenowitz, E. A. (1997) Comparative approaches to the avian song system. *Journal of Neurobiology*, **33**, 517–531.

Brenowitz, E. A. & Arnold, A. P. (1985) Lack of sexual dimorphism in steroid accumulation in vocal control brain regions of duetting song birds. *Brain Research*, **344**, 172–175.

Brenowitz, E. A. & Arnold, A. P. (1992) Hormone accumulation in song regions of the canary brain. *Journal of Neurobiology*, **23**, 871–880.

Brenowitz, E. A., Nalls, B., Wingfield, J. C. & Kroodsma, D. E. (1991) Seasonal changes in avian song nuclei without seasonal changes in song repertoire. *Journal of Neurobiology*, **11**, 1367–1374.

Buchanan, K. L., Spencer, K. A., Goldsmith, A. R. & Catchpole, C. K. (2003) Song as an honest signal of past developmental stress in the European starling (*Sturnus vulgaris*). *Proceedings of the Royal Society B*, **270**, 1149–1156.

Buntin, J. D. (1996) Neural and hormonal control of parental behavior in birds. In: *Parental Care: Evolution, Mechanisms, and Adaptive Significance*, ed. J. S. Rosenblatt & C. T. Snowden. Advances in the Study of Behavior, vol. 25. San Diego, CA: Academic Press, pp. 161–214.

Canady, R. A., Kroodsma, D. E. & Nottebohm, F. (1984) Population differences in complexity of a learned skill are correlated with the brain space involved. *Proceedings of the National Academy of Sciences of the USA*, **81**, 6232–6234.

Carere, C. & Balthazart, J. (2007) Sexual versus individual differentiation: the controversial role of avian maternal hormones. *Trends in Endocrinology and Metabolism*, **18**, 73–80.

Carter, C. S., DeVries, A. C. & Getz, L. L. (1995) Physiological substrates of mammalian monogamy: the prairie vole model. *Neuroscience and Biobehavioral Reviews*, **19**, 303–314.

Catchpole, C. K. (1987) Bird song, sexual selection and female choice. *Trends in Ecology and Evolution*, **2**, 94–97.

Catchpole, C. K. (2000) Sexual selection and the evolution of song and brain structure in *Acrocephalus* warblers. *Advances in the Study of Behavior*, **29**, 45–97.

Catchpole, C. K. & Slater, P. J. B. (1995) *Bird Song: Biological Themes and Variations*. Cambridge: Cambridge University Press.

Chew, S. J., Vicario, D. S. & Nottebohm, F. (1996) A large-capacity memory system that recognizes the calls and songs of individual birds. *Proceedings of the National Academy of Sciences of the USA*, **93**, 1950–1955.

Cockburn, A. (2006) Prevalence of different modes of parental care in birds. *Proceedings of the Royal Society B*, **273**, 1375–1383.

Cockrem, J. F. (2007) Stress, corticosterone responses and avian personalities. *Journal of Ornithology*, **148** (Suppl. 2), 169–178.

Creel, S. (2001) Social dominance and stress hormones. *Trends in Ecology and Evolution*, **16**, 491–497.

Crews, D. (1998) On the organization of individual differences in sexual behavior. *American Zoologist*, **38**, 118–132.

Cynx, J. & Nottebohm, F. (1992) Role of gender, season, and familiarity in discrimination of conspecific song by zebra finches (*Taeniopygia guttata*). *Proceedings of the National Academy of Sciences of the USA*, **89**, 1368–1371.

DeVoogd, T. J. & Lauay, C. (2001) Emerging psychobiology of the avian song system. In: *Developmental Psychobiology*, ed. E. Blass. New York, NY: Kluwer/Plenum, pp. 357–392.

DeVoogd, T. J., Nixdorf, B. & Nottebohm, F. (1985) Synaptogenesis and changes in synaptic morphology related to acquisition of a new behavior. *Brain Research*, **329**, 304–308.

DeVoogd, T. J., Krebs, J. R., Healy, S. D. & Purvis, A. (1993) Relations between song repertoire size and the volume of brain nuclei related to song: comparative evolutionary analyses amongst oscine birds. *Proceedings of the Royal Society B*, **254**, 75–82.

DeVoogd, T. J., Houtman, A. M. & Falls, J. B. (1995) White-throated sparrow morphs that differ in song production rate also differ in the anatomy of some song related brain areas. *Journal of Neurobiology*, **28**, 202–213.

Eales, L. A. (1985) Song learning in zebra finches: some effects of song model availability on what is learnt and when. *Animal Behaviour*, **33**, 1293–1300.

Eales, L. A. (1987) Song learning in female-raised zebra finches: another look at the sensitive phase. *Animal Behaviour*, **35**, 1356–1365.

Eens, M. & Pinxten, R. (2000) Sex-role reversal in vertebrates: behavioural and endocrinological accounts. *Behavioural Processes*, **51**, 135–147.

Eens, M., Pinxten, R. & VerHeyen, R. F. (1991) Male song as a cue for mate choice in the European starling. *Behaviour*, **116**, 210–238.

Eens, M., Pinxten, R. & Verheyen, R. F. (1993) Function of the song and song repertoire in the European starling (*Sturnus vulgaris*): an aviary experiment. *Behaviour*, **125**, 51–66.

Eriksson, D. & Wallin, L. (1986) Male bird song attracts females: a field experiment. *Behavioral Ecology and Sociobiology*, **19**, 297–299.

Fivizzani, A. J., Oring, L. W., El Halawani, M. E. & Schlinger, B. A. (1990) Hormonal basis of male parental care and female intersexual competition in sex-role reversed birds. In:. *Endocrinology of Birds: Molecular to Behavioral*, ed. M. Wada, S. Ishii & C. G. Scanes. Tokyo: Japan Scientific Societies Press; Berlin: Springer-Verlag, pp. 273–286

Folstad, I. & Karter, A. J. (1992) Parasites, bright males, and the immunocompetence handicap. *American Naturalist*, **139**, 603–622.

Forger, N. G. (2001) Development of sex differences in the nervous system. In: *Developmental Psychobiology*, ed. E. Blass. New York, NY: Kluwer/Plenum, pp. 143–198.

Frank, L. G., Glickman, S. E. & Licht, P. (1991) Fatal sibling aggression, precocial development, and androgens in neonatal spotted hyenas. *Science*, **252**, 702–704.

Fusani, L., Day, L. B., Canoine, V. *et al.* (2007) Androgen and the elaborate courtship behavior of a tropical lekking bird. *Hormones and Behavior*, **51**, 62–68.

Gahr, M. & Kosar, E. (1996) Identification, distribution, and developmental changes of a melatonin binding site in the song control system of the zebra finch. *Journal of Comparative Neurology*, **367**, 308–318.

Garamszegi, L. Z. & Eens, M. (2004) Brain space for a learned task: strong intraspecific evidence for neural correlates of singing behavior in songbirds. *Brain Research Reviews*, **44**, 187–193.

Garland, T., Bennett, A. F. & Rezende, E. L. (2005) Phylogenetic approaches in comparative physiology. *Journal of Experimental Biology*, **208**, 3015–3035.

Gentner, T. Q. & Margoliash, D. (2003) Neuronal populations and single cells representing learned auditory objects. *Nature*, **424**, 669–674.

Gentner, T. Q., Hulse, S. H., Duffy, D. & Ball, G. F. (2001) Response biases in auditory forebrain regions of female songbirds following exposure to sexually relevant variation in male song. *Journal of Neurobiology*, **46**, 48–58.

Gentner, T. Q., Hulse, S. H. & Ball, G. F. (2004) Functional differences in forebrain auditory regions during learned vocal recognition in songbirds. *Journal of Comparative Physiology A*, **190**, 1001–1010.

Goodson, J. L. (2005) The vertebrate social behavior network: evolutionary themes and variations. *Hormones and Behavior*, **48**, 11–22.

Goodson, J. L. & Bass, A. H. (2001) Social behavior functions and related anatomical characteristics of vasotocin/vasopressin systems in vertebrates. *Brain Research Reviews*, **35**, 246–265.

Goodson, J. L. & Wang, Y. (2006) Valence-sensitive neurons exhibit divergent functional profiles in gregarious and asocial species. *Proceedings of the National Academy of Sciences of the USA*, **103**, 17013–17017.

Goodson, J. L., Lindberg, L. & Johnson, P. (2004) Effects of central vasotocin and mesotocin manipulations on social behavior in male and female zebra finches. *Hormones and Behavior*, **45**, 136–143.

Goodson, J. L., Evans, A. K. & Wang, Y. (2006) Neuropeptide binding reflects convergent and divergent evolution in species-typical group sizes. *Hormones and Behavior*, **50**, 223–236.

Goymann, W. & Jenni-Eiermann, S. (2005) Introduction to the European Science Foundation technical meeting: analysis of hormones in droppings and egg yolk of birds. *Annals of the New York Academy of Sciences*, **1046**, 1–4.

Goymann, W. & Wingfield, J. C. (2004) Allostatic load, social status and stress hormones: the costs of social status matter. *Animal Behaviour*, **67**, 591–602.

Goymann, W., East, M. L. & Hofer, H. (2001) Androgens and the role of female 'hyperaggressiveness' in spotted hyenas (*Crocuta crocuta*). *Hormones and Behavior*, **39**, 83–92.

Griffith, S. C., Owens, I. P. & Thuman, K. A. (2002) Extra pair paternity in birds: a review of interspecific variation and adaptive function. *Molecular Ecology*, **11**, 2195–2212.

Gurney, M. E. (1981) Hormonal control of cell form and number in the zebra finch song system. *Journal of Neuroscience*, **1**, 658–673.

Gurney, M. E. & Konishi, M. (1980) Hormone-induced sexual differentiation of brain and behavior in zebra finches. *Science*, **208**, 1380–1383.

Hamilton, K. S., King, A. P., Sengelaub, D. R. & West, M. J. (1998) Visual and song nuclei correlate with courtship skills in brown-headed cowbirds. *Animal Behaviour*, **56**, 973–982.

Harding, C. F., Sheridan, K. & Walters, M. J. (1983) Hormonal specificity and activation of sexual behavior in male zebra finches. *Hormones and Behavior*, **17**, 111–133.

Hasselquist, D., Bensch, S. & von Schantz, T. (1996) Correlation between male song repertoire, extra-pair paternity and offspring survival in the great reed warbler. *Nature*, **381**, 229–232.

Hau, M. (2007) Regulation of male traits by testosterone: implications for the evolution of vertebrate life histories. *BioEssays*, **29**, 133–144.

Hernandez, A. M, & MacDougall-Shackleton, S. A. (2004) Effects of early song experience on song preferences and song control and auditory brain regions in female house finches (*Carpodacus mexicanus*). *Journal of Neurobiology*, **59**, 247–258.

Hill, K. M. & DeVoogd, T. J. (1991) Altered daylength affects dendritic structure in a song-related brain region in red-winged blackbirds. *Behavioral and Neural Biology*, **56**, 240–250.

Holmes, M. M., Rosen, G. J., Jordan, C. L. *et al.* (2007) Social control of brain morphology in a eusocial mammal. *Proceedings of the National Academy of Sciences of the USA*, **104**, 10548–10552.

Hultsch, H., Todt, D. (1981) Repertoire sharing an song-post distance in nightingales (*Luscinia megarhynchos* B.). *Behavioral Ecology and Sociobiology*, **8**, 183–188.

Jones, A. E., ten Cate, C. & Slater, P. J. B. (1996) Early experience and plasticity of song in adult male zebra finches (*Taeniopygia guttata*). *Journal of Comparative Psychology*, **110**, 354–369.

Kempenaers, B., Peters, A. & Foerster, K. (2008) Sources of individual variation in plasma testosterone levels. *Philosophical Transactions of the Royal Society B*, **363**, 1711–1723.

Kern, M. D. & King, J. R. (1972) Testosterone-induced singing in female white-crowned sparrows. *Condor*, **74**, 204–209.

Ketterson, E. D., Nolan, V. & Sandell, M. (2005) Testosterone in females: mediator of adaptive traits, constraint on sexual dimorphism, or both? *American Naturalist*, **166** (Suppl. 4), S85–98.

King, A. P. & West, M. J. (1983) Epigenesis of cowbird song: a joint endeavour of males and females. *Nature*, **305**, 704–706.

King, A. P., West, M. J. & White, D. J. (2003) Female cowbird song perception: evidence for plasticity of preference. *Ethology*, **109**, 865–877.

Kirn, J. R., Clower, R. P., Kroodsma, D. E. & DeVoogd, T. J. (1989) Song-related brain regions in the red-winged blackbird are affected by sex and season but not repertoire size. *Journal of Neurobiology*, **20**, 139–163.

Kirn, J. R., Alvarez-Buylla, A. & Nottebohm, F. (1991) Production and survival of projection neurons in a forebrain vocal center of adult male canaries. *Journal of Neuroscience*, **11**, 1756–1762.

Knapp, R. (2004) Endocrine mediation of vertebrate male alternative reproductive tactics: the next generation of studies. *Integrative and Comparative Biology*, **43**, 658–668.

Koolhaas, J. M., Korte, S. M., De Boer, S. F. *et al.* (1999) Coping styles in animals: current status in behavior and stress-physiology. *Neuroscience and Biobehavioral Reviews*, **23**, 925–935.

Kroodsma, D. E. (1996) Ecology of passerine song development. In: *Ecology and Evolution of Acoustic Communication in Birds*, ed. D. E. Kroodsma & E. H. Miller. Ithaca, NY: Cornell University Press, pp. 3–19.

Kroodsma, D. E. & Parker, L. D. (1977) Vocal virtuosity in the brown thrasher. *Auk*, **94**, 783–785.

Kroodsma, D. E. & Pickert, R. (1980) Environmentally dependent sensitive periods for avian vocal learning. *Nature*, **288**, 477–479.

Kruse, A. A., Stripling, R. & Clayton, D. F. (2004) Context-specific habituation of the *zenk* gene response to song in adult zebra finches. *Neurobiology of Learning and Memory*, **82**, 99–108.

Lauay, C., Gerlach, N. M., Adkins-Regan, E. & DeVoogd, T. J. (2004) Female zebra finches require early song exposure to prefer high-quality song as adults. *Animal Behaviour*, **68**, 1249–1255.

Lauay, C., Komorowski, R. W., Beaudin, A. E. & DeVoogd, T. J. (2005) Adult female and male zebra finches show distinct patterns of spine deficits in an auditory area and in the song system when reared without exposure to normal adult song. *Journal of Comparative Neurology*, **487**, 119–126.

Lefebvre L., Whittle, P., Lascaris, E. & Finkelstein, A. (1997) Feeding innovations and forebrain size in birds. *Animal Behaviour*, **53**, 549–560.

Lefebvre, L., Gaxiola, A., Dawson, S. *et al.* (1998) Feeding innovations and forebrain size in Australasian birds. *Behaviour*, **135**, 1077–1097.

Leitner, S. & Catchpole, C. K. (2004) Syllable repertoire and the size of the song control system in captive canaries (*Serinus canaria*). *Journal of Neurobiology*, **60**, 21–27.

Leitner, S., Voigt, C., Garcia-Segura, L. M., Van't Hof, T. & Gahr, M. (2001) Seasonal activation and inactivation of song motor memories in wild canaries is not reflected in neuroanatomical changes of forebrain song areas. *Hormones and Behavior*, **40**, 160–168.

Leitner, S., Nicholson, J., Leisler, B., DeVoogd, T. J. & Catchpole, C. K. (2002) Song and the song control pathway in the brain can develop independently of exposure to song in the sedge warbler. *Proceedings of the Royal Society B*, **269**, 2519–2524.

Leonard, S. L. (1939) Induction of singing in female canaries by injection of male hormone. *Proceedings of the Society for Experimental Biology and Medicine*, **41**, 229–230.

Li, X.-C., Wang, X.-J., Tannenhauser, J. *et al.* (2007) Genomic resources for songbird research and their use in characterizing gene expression during brain development. *Proceedings of the National Academy of Sciences of the USA*, **104**, 6834–6839.

Lim, M. M. & Young, L. J. (2006) Neuropeptidergic regulation of affiliative behavior and social bonding in animals. *Hormones and Behavior*, **50**, 506–517.

Lim, M. M., Wang, Z., Olazábal, D. E. *et al.* (2004) Enhanced partner preference in a promiscuous species by manipulating the expression of a single gene. *Nature*, **429**, 754–757.

Liu, W.-C. & Kroodsma, D. E. (2006) Song learning by chipping sparrows: when, where, and from whom. *Condor*, **108**, 509–517.

Lynch, J. W., Khan, M. Z., Altmann, J., Njahira, M. N. & Rubenstein, N. (2003) Concentrations of four fecal steroids in wild baboons: short-term storage conditions and consequences for data interpretation. *General and Comparative Endocrinology*, **132**, 264–271.

Maney, D. L., Goode, C. T. & Wingfield, J. C. (1997) Intraventricular infusion of arginine vasotocin induces singing in a female songbird. *Journal of Neuroendocrinology*, **9**, 487–491.

Maney, D. L., MacDougall-Shackleton, E. A., MacDougall-Shackleton, S. A., Ball, G. F. & Hahn, T. P. (2003) Immediate early gene response to hearing song correlates with receptive behavior and depends on dialect in a female songbird. *Journal of Comparative Physiology A*, **189**, 667–674.

Maney, D. L., Erwin, K. L. & Goode, C. T. (2005) Neuroendocrine correlates of behavioral polymorphism in white-throated sparrows. *Hormones and Behavior*, **48**, 196–206.

Maney, D. L., Lange, H. S., Raees, M. Q., Reid, A. E. & Sanford, S. E. (2009) Behavioral phenotypes persist after gonadal steroid manipulation in white-throated sparrows. *Hormones and Behavior*, **55**, 113–120.

Mann, P. E. & Bridges, R. S. (2001) Lactogenic hormone regulation of maternal behavior. *Progress in Brain Research*, **133**, 251–262.

Marler, P. (1956) The voice of the chaffinch and its function as a language. *Ibis*, **98**, 231–261.

Marler, P. (1997) Three models of song learning: evidence from behavior. *Journal of Neurobiology*, **33**, 501–516.

Marler, P. & Nelson, D. A. (1993) Action-based learning: a new form of developmental plasticity in bird song. *Netherlands Journal of Zoology*, **43**, 91–103.

Marler, P., Peters, S., Ball, G. F., Dufty, A. M. & Wingfield, J. C. (1988) The role of sex steroids in the acquisition and production of birdsong. *Nature*, **336**, 770–772.

Mello, C., Nottebohm, F. & Clayton, D. (1995) Repeated exposure to one song leads to a rapid and persistent decline in an immediate early gene's response to that song in zebra finch telencephalon. *Journal of Neuroscience*, **15**, 6919–6925.

Mello, C. V., Vates, G. E., Okuhata, S. & Nottebohm, F. (1998) Descending auditory pathways in the adult male zebra finch (*Taeniopygia guttata*). *Journal of Neurobiology*, **395**, 137–160.

Mennill, D. J., Ratcliffe, L. M. & Boag, P. T. (2002) Female eavesdropping on male song contests in songbirds. *Science*, **296**, 873.

Miller, D. B. (1979a) Long-term recognition of father's song by female zebra finches. *Nature*, **280**, 389–391.

Miller, D. B. (1979b) The acoustic basis of mate recognition by female zebra finches (*Taeniopygia guttata*). *Animal Behaviour*, **27**, 376–380.

Miller, J. L., King, A. P., West, M. J. (2008) Female social networks influence male vocal development in brown-headed cowbirds, *Molothrus ater*. *Animal Behaviour*, **76**, 931–941.

Miranda, J. A., Oliveira, R. F., Carneiro, L. A., Santos, R. S. & Grober, M. S. (2003) Neurochemical correlates of male polymorphism and alternative reproductive tactics in the Azorean rock-pool blenny, *Parablennius parvicornis*. *General and Comparative Endocrinology*, **132**, 183–189.

Moore, J. M., Buchan, Z. R., Székely, T. & DeVoogd, T. J. (2004) High vocal center (HVC) volumes are related to syllable repertoire sizes across a wide phylogeny of previously unstudied songbird species. *Society for Neuroscience Abstracts*, **34**, 1010.5.

Mountjoy, D. J. & Lemon, R. E. (1991) Song as an attractant for male and female European starlings, and the influence of song complexity on their response. *Behavioral Ecology and Sociobiology*, **28**, 97–100.

Nelson, D. A. (1998) External validity and experimental design: the sensitive phase for song learning. *Animal Behaviour*, **56**, 487–491.

Nelson, R. J. (2005) *An Introduction to Behavioral Endocrinology*, 3rd edn. Sunderland, MA: Sinauer Associates.

Newman, S. W. (2002) Pheromonal signals access the medial extended amygdala: one node in a proposed social behavior network. In: *Hormones, Brain and Behavior*, ed. D. W. Pfaff, A. P. Arnold, A.M. Etgen, S. E. Fahrbach & R. T. Rubin vol. 4. Amsterdam: Academic Press, pp. 17–32.

Nordeen, K. W., Nordeen, E. J. & Arnold, A. P. (1987) Estrogen accumulation in zebra finch song control nuclei: implications for sexual differentiation and adult activation of song behavior. *Journal of Neurobiology*, **18**, 569–582.

Norris, D. O. (2007) *Vertebrate Endocrinology*, 4th edn. Amsterdam: Elsevier.

Nottebohm, F. (1980) Testosterone triggers growth of brain vocal control nuclei in adult female canaries. *Brain Research*, **189**, 429–436.

Nottebohm, F. (1981) A brain for all seasons: cyclical anatomical changes in song control nuclei of the canary brain. *Science*, **214**, 1368–1370.

Nottebohm, F., Kasparian, S., Pandazis, C. (1981) Brain space for a learned task. *Brain Research*, **213**, 99–109.

Nowicki, S., Peters, S. & Podos, J. (1998) Song learning, early nutrition and sexual selection in songbirds. *American Zoologist*, **38**, 179–190.

Nowicki, S., Searcy, W. A. & Peters, S. (2002) Quality of song learning affects female response to male bird song. *Proceedings of the Royal Society B*, **269**, 1949–1954.

Ophir, A. G., Wolff, J. O. & Phelps, S. M. (2008) Variation in neural V1aR predicts sexual fidelity and space use among male prairie voles in semi-natural settings. *Proceedings of the National Academy of Sciences of the USA*, **105**, 1249–1254.

Pfaff, J. A., Zanette, L., MacDougall-Shackleton, S. A. & MacDougall-Shackleton, E. A. (2007) Song repertoire size varies with HVC volume and is indicative of male quality in song sparrows (*Melospiza melodia*). *Proceedings of the Royal Society B*, **274**, 2035–2040.

Phan, M. L., Pytte, C. L. & Vicario, D. S. (2006) Early auditory experience generates long-lasting memories that may subserve vocal learning in songbirds. *Proceedings of the National Academy of Sciences of the USA*, **103**, 1088–1093.

Phelps, S. M. & Young, L. J. (2003) Extraordinary diversity in vasopressin (V1a) receptor distributions among wild prairie voles (*Microtus ochrogaster*): patterns of variation and covariation. *Journal of Comparative Neurology*, **466**, 564–576.

Poulsen, H. (1951) Inheritance and learning in the song of the chaffinch (*Fringilla coelebs* L). *Behaviour*, **3**, 216–228.

Pröve, E. (1974) Der einfluß von kastration und testosteronsubstitutuon auf das sexualverhalten männlicher zebrafinken (*Taeniopygia guttata castanotis* Gould). *Journal of Ornithology*, **115**, 338–347.

Raouf, S. A., Parker, P. G., Ketterson, E. D., Nolan, V. & Ziegenfus, C. (1997) Testosterone affects reproductive success by influencing extra-pair fertilizations in male dark-eyed juncos (Aves: *Junco hyemalis*). *Proceedings of the Royal Society B*, **264**, 1599–1603.

Ratcliffe, L. & Otter, K. (1996) Sex differences in song recognition. In: *Ecology and Evolution of Acoustic Communication in Birds*, ed. D. E. Kroodsma & E. H. Miller. Ithaca, NY: Cornell University Press, pp. 339–355.

Rehsteiner, U., Geisser, H. & Reyer, H.-U. (1998) Singing and mating success in water pipits: one specific song element makes all the difference. *Animal Behaviour*, **55**, 1471–1481.

Reiner, A., Perkel, D. J., Bruce, L. L. *et al.* (2004) Revised nomenclature for avian telencephalon and some related brainstem nuclei. *Journal of Comparative Neurology*, **473**, 377–414.

Ribeiro, S., Cecchi, G. A., Magnasco, M. O. & Mello, C. V. (1998) Toward a song code: evidence for a syllabic representation in the canary brain. *Neuron*, **21**, 359–371.

Riebel, K. (2000) Early exposure leads to repeatable preferences for male song in female zebra finches. *Proceedings of the Royal Society B*, **267**, 2553–2558.

Riebel, K. (2003) The 'mute' sex revisited: vocal production and perception learning in female songbirds. *Advances in the Study of Behavior*, **33**, 49–86.

Riebel, K., Smallegange, I. M., Terpstra, N. J. & Bolhuis, J. J. (2002) Sexual equality in zebra finch song preference: evidence for a dissociation between song recognition and production learning. *Proceedings of the Royal Society B*, **269**, 729–733.

Roberts, M. L., Buchanan, K. L. & Evans, M. R. (2004) Testing the immunocompetence handicap hypothesis: a review of the evidence. *Animal Behaviour*, **68**, 227–239.

Roselli, C. E., Resko, J. A. & Stormshak, F. (2002) Hormonal influences on sexual partner preference in rams. *Archives of Sexual Behavior*, **31**, 43–49.

Rosenblatt, J. S. & Snowdon, C. T., eds. (1996) *Parental Care: Evolution, Mechanisms, and Adaptive Significance*, Advances in the Study of Behavior, vol. 25. San Diego, CA: Academic Press.

Rubenstein, D. R. (2007) Stress hormones and sociality: integrating social and environmental stressors. *Proceedings of the Royal Society B*, **274**, 967–975.

Schlinger, B. A. & Arnold, A. P. (1992) Circulating estrogens in a male songbird originate in the brain. *Proceedings of the National Academy of Sciences of the USA*, **89**, 7650–7653.

Schradin, C. & Anzenberger, G. (1999) Prolactin, the hormone of paternity. *News in Physiological Sciences*, **14**, 223–231.

Schwabl, H. (1993) Yolk is a source of maternal testosterone for developing birds. *Proceedings of the National Academy of Sciences of the USA*, **90**, 11446–11450.

Searcy, W. A. & Yasukawa, K. (1996) Song and female choice. In: *Ecology and Evolution of Acoustic Communication in Birds*, ed. D. E. Kroodsma & E. H. Miller. Ithaca, NY: Cornell University Press, pp. 454–473.

Sih, A., Bell, A. M., Johnson, J. C. & Ziemba, R. E. (2004) Behavioral syndromes: an integrative overview. *Quarterly Review of Biology*, **79**, 241–277.

Slater, P. J. B. & Ince, S. A. (1982) Song development in chaffinches: what is learnt and when? *Ibis*, **124**, 21–26.

Smulders, T. V., Lisi, M. D., Tricomi, E. *et al.* (2006) Failure to detect seasonal changes in the song system nuclei of the black-capped chickadee (*Poecile atricapillus*). *Journal of Neurobiology*, **66**, 991–1001.

Sockman, K. W., Gentner, T. Q. & Ball, G. F. (2002) Recent experience modulates forebrain gene-expression in response to mate-choice cues in European starlings. *Proceedings of the Royal Society B*, **269**, 2479–2485.

Spinney, L. H., Bentley, G. E. & Hau, M. (2006) Endocrine correlates of alternative phenotypes in the white-throated sparrow (*Zonotrichia albicollis*). *Hormones and Behavior*, **50**, 762–771.

Stripling, R., Volman, S. F. & Clayton, D. F. (1997) Response modulation in the zebra finch neostriatum: relationship to nuclear gene regulation. *Journal of Neuroscience*, **17**, 3883–3893.

Székely, T., Catchpole, C. K., DeVoogd, A., Marchl, Z. & DeVoogd, T. J. (1996) Evolutionary changes in a song control area of the brain (HVC) are associated with evolutionary changes in song repertoire among European warblers (Sylviidae). *Proceedings of the Royal Society B*, **263**, 607–610.

Terleph, T. A., Mello, C. V. & Vicario, D. S. (2007) Species differences in auditory processing dynamics in songbird auditory telencephalon. *Developmental Neurobiology*, **67**, 1498–1510.

Terpstra, N. J., Bolhuis, J. J. & den Boer-Visser, A. M. (2004) An analysis of the neural representation of birdsong memory. *Journal of Neuroscience*, **24**, 4971–4977.

Terpstra, N. J., Bolhuis, J. J., Riebel, K., van der Burg, J. M. M. & den Boer-Visser, A. M. (2006) Localized brain activation specific to auditory memory in a female songbird. *Journal of Comparative Neurology*, **494**, 784–791.

Theunissen, F. E. & Shaevitz, S. S. (2006) Auditory processing of vocal sounds in birds. *Current Opinon in Neurobiology*, **16**, 400–407.

Thorpe, W. H. (1957) The identification of Savi's, grasshopper and river warblers by means of song. *British Birds*, **50**, 169–171.

Thorpe, W. H. (1958) The learning of song patterns by birds, with especial reference to the song of the chaffinch *Fringilla coelebs*. *Ibis*, **100**, 535–570.

Timmermans, S., Lefebvre, L., Boire, D. & Basu, P. (2000) Relative size of the hyperstriatum ventrale is the best predictor of feeding innovation rate in birds. *Brain, Behavior and Evolution*, **56**, 196–203.

Tinbergen, N. (1963) On aims and methods of ethology. *Zeitschrift für Tierpsychologie*, **20**, 410–433.

Trainor, B. C., Bird, I. M. & Marler, C. A. (2004) Opposing hormonal mechanisms of aggression revealed through short-lived testosterone manipulations and multiple winning experiences. *Hormones and Behavior*, **45**, 115–121.

Tramontin, A. D. & Brenowitz, E. A. (1999) A field study of seasonal neuronal incorporation into the song control system of a songbird that lacks adult song learning. *Journal of Neurobiology*, **40**, 316–326.

Trumbo, S. T. (1996) Parental care in invertebrates. In: *Parental Care: Evolution, Mechanisms, and Adaptive Significance*, ed. J. S. Rosenblatt & C. T. Snowden. Advances in the Study of Behavior, vol. 25. San Diego, CA: Academic Press, pp. 3–52.

Vallet, E. & Kreutzer, M. (1995) Female canaries are sexually responsive to special song phrases. *Animal Behaviour*, **49**, 1603–1610.

Vallet, E., Beme, I. & Kreutzer, M. (1998) Two-note syllables in canary songs elicit high levels of sexual display. *Animal Behaviour*, **55**, 291–297.

Voigt, C. & Goymann, W. (2007) Sex-role reversal is reflected in the brain of African black coucals (*Centropus grillii*). *Developmental Neurobiology*, **67**, 1560–1573.

Voigt, C., Leitner, S. & Gahr, M. (2007) Socially induced brain differentiation in a cooperatively breeding songbird. *Proceedings of the Royal Society B*, **274**, 2645–2651.

Voss, H. U., Tabelow, K., Polzehl, J. *et al.* (2007) Functional MRI of the zebra finch brain during song stimulation suggests a lateralized response topography. *Proceedings of the National Academy of Sciences of the USA*, **104**, 10667–10672.

Wada, K., Howard, J. T., McConnell, P. *et al.* (2006) A molecular neuroethological approach for identifying and characterizing a cascade of behaviorally regulated genes. *Proceedings of the National Academy of Sciences of the USA*, **103**, 15212–15217.

Wade, J. (1999) Sexual dimorphisms in avian and reptilian courtship: two systems that do not play by the mammalian rules. *Brain, Behavior and Evolution*, **54**, 15–27.

Wade, J. & Arnold, A. P. (2004) Sexual differentiation of the zebra finch song system. *Annals of the New York Academy of Sciences*, **1016**, 540–559.

Wallen, K. & Baum, M. M. (2002) Masculinization and defeminization in altricial and precocial mammals: comparative aspects of steroid hormone action. In: *Hormones,*

Brain and Behavior, ed. D. W. Pfaff, A. P. Arnold, A.M. Etgen, S. E. Fahrbach & R. T. Rubin vol. 4. Amsterdam: Academic Press, pp. 385–424.

Ward, B. C., Nordeen, E. J. & Nordeen, K. W. (1998) Individual variation in neuron number predicts differences in the propensity for avian vocal imitation. *Proceedings of the National Academy of Sciences of the USA*, **95**, 1277–1282.

Wasser, S. K., Hunt, K. E., Brown, J. L. *et al.* (2000) A generalized fecal glucocorticoid assay for use in a diverse array of nondomestic mammalian and avian species. *General and Comparative Endocrinology*, **120**, 260–275.

West, M. J. & King, A. P. (1988) Female visual displays affect the development of male song in the cowbird. *Nature*, **334**, 244–246.

Whitfield-Rucker, M. G. & Cassone, V. M. (1996) Melatonin binding in the house sparrow song control system: sexual dimorphism and the effect of photoperiod. *Hormones and Behavior*, **30**, 528–537.

Wilbrecht, L. & Kirn, J. R. (2004) Neuron addition and loss in the song system: regulation and function. *Annals of the New York Academy of Sciences*, **1016**, 659–683.

Wiley, R. H., Hatchwell, B. J. & Davies, N. B. (1991) Recognition of individual males' songs by female dunnocks: a mechanism increasing the number of copulatory partners and reproductive success. *Ethology*, **88**, 145–153.

Williams, H., Kilander, K. & Sotanski, M. L. (1993) Untutored song, reproductive success and song learning. *Animal Behaviour*, **45**, 695–705.

Wingfield, J. C. (1984) Androgens and mating systems: testosterone-induced polygyny in normally monogamous birds. *Auk*, **101**, 665–671.

Wingfield, J. C., Hegner, R. E., Dufty, A. M. & Ball, G. F. (1990) The 'challenge hypothesis': theoretical implications for patterns of testosterone secretion, mating systems, and breeding strategies. *American Naturalist*, **136**, 829–846.

Wynne-Edwards, K. E. & Reburn, C. J. (2000) Behavioral endocrinology of mammalian fatherhood. *Trends in Ecology and Evolution*, **15**, 464–468.

Wynne-Edwards, K. E. & Timonin, M. E. (2007) Paternal care in rodents: weakening support for hormonal regulation of the transition to behavioral fatherhood in rodent animal models of biparental care. *Hormones and Behavior*, **52**, 114–121.

Young, L. J. & Wang, Z. X. (2004) The neurobiology of pair bonding. *Nature Neuroscience*, **7**, 1048–1054.

Young, L. J., Nilsen, R., Waymire, K. G., MacGregor, G. R. & Insel, T. R. (1999) Increased affiliative response to vasopressin in mice expressing the V1a receptor from a monogamous vole. *Nature*, **400**, 766–768.

Zera, A. J., Harshman, L. G. & Williams, T. D. (2007) Evolutionary endocrinology: the developing synthesis between endocrinology and evolutionary genetics. *Annual Review of Ecology, Evolution and Systematics*, **38**, 793–817.

In love with *Ropalidia marginata*: 34 years, and still going strong

Raghavendra Gadagkar

While interviewing potential candidates for our departmental PhD programme every year, I usually ask the candidates what they would like to work on if they had complete freedom in the matter. Some years ago an unusually determined student gave me a firm answer: he wished to work on lesser cats, asking whatever questions he might be able to and using whatever methods that might work. I tried to argue with him, reminding him that lesser cats were extremely hard to study – they were nocturnal, shy and difficult to locate, let alone observe and obtain quantitative data on. Why not work on an easier animal with which you can ask more sophisticated questions, I pleaded. No, he was adamant – lesser cats it would be, if he had any choice at all. His determination has stayed in my memory ever since. Other students have given me other kinds of answers, though I can recall none as determined as the young man in love with lesser cats. Some students gave primacy to the research field or question and were quite flexible about the study animal and methods to be employed. Others were sold on a method such as computer simulations or field biology, but were quite catholic about the exact questions or of the model organism.

No one has taught me more than students, and their various answers have given me much food for thought concerning the sociology of science. How *do* people choose what topic to study, what animal to use and what methods to employ, and how *should* they choose? As a result of much brooding spurred by the responses of students that I interview every year, I have crystallised my personal prejudice as follows: the research question should come first, and then one should choose a model organism that is best suited to the question. Methods should come last, and should be slaves at the service of the question and the animal, rather than the masters that dictate what we do.

Nevertheless, I must confess that the research question and the model animal are hard to prioritise. I think this is primarily because, though of greater importance, the question is abstract and kind of 'dead', but the study animal is alive and often rather cute. It is hard not to fall in love with your study animal. But is that a bad thing? I don't know – but I have been in love with my study animal for over 30 years, and no harm seems to have come of it so far.

I am interested in social evolution, and I study the tropical, Old World, primitively eusocial wasp, *Ropalidia marginata*. And boy, isn't it a beautiful wasp? I have been stung dozens of times but never complained. I guess that's what love does to you. I once had a letter from a fellow wasp researcher who said that he had just arrived in the Philippines, and had the great pleasure of being stung by *Ropalidia* for the first time in his life! But of course the real beauty of *R. marginata* comes from its utility as a study organism. The genus *Ropalidia* itself is unique and remarkable, comprising both primitively eusocial and highly eusocial species with unparalleled diversity in colony sizes and social biology.

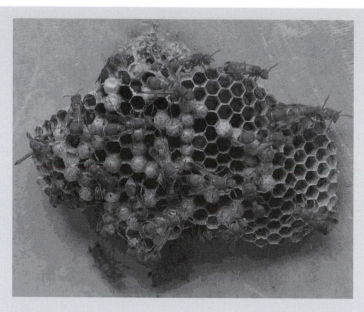

A typical nest of the primitively eusocial wasp *Ropalidia marginata*. Photo: Thresiamma Varghese.

There are two quite different ways of utilising the power of the genus *Ropalidia* to unravel the mysteries of social evolution. One is to capitalise on the diversity within the genus and undertake comparative studies of different species, a method of great power in modern evolutionary biology. The other is to concentrate on a single species and conduct detailed analyses of cooperation and conflict and assess the costs and benefits of social life. I have chosen the latter option, which is of course an important reason for my developing such an affinity for my study animal.

Indeed, *R. marginata* has turned out to be a providential choice. Its small colony size, absence of morphological caste differentiation, coexistence of single and multiple foundress associations, multiple behavioural options available to eclosing females, all make *R. marginata* ideally suited for investigating the evolutionary forces that promote social life. But what makes *R. marginata* even more special is that its tropical address makes possible a perennial indeterminate nesting cycle with mortal wasps forming potentially immortal colonies

with frequent turnover of workers and occasional turnover of queens, providing a perpetual stage for these wasps to play out their games of war and peace. If *R. marginata* has been priceless in investigating the evolutionary causes of sociality, it has been even more crucial in understanding the proximate mechanisms that make social life possible. Unlike those of other primitively eusocial wasps, queens of *R. marginata* are remarkably meek and docile individuals, raising questions about how they manage to become queens and maintain their reproductive monopoly, how they suppress worker reproduction and regulate the non-reproductive activities of their workers.

Answers to these questions are being constantly revealed, as I now have a team of students similarly smitten by the beauty of *R. marginata*. We have shown that *R. marginata* queens begin their careers as very aggressive individuals and gradually lose their aggression as they develop their ovaries and establish themselves as undisputed leaders of their colonies. This seems possible because, on the one hand, they appear to use non-volatile pheromones to suppress worker reproduction and, on the other hand, workers regulate their own non-reproductive activities in a decentralised, self-organised manner. All this raises the question of the function of aggression, which is not absent from the social life of these wasps. We may just have hit upon at least two novel functions of aggression in this remarkable species. In summary, it appears that *R. marginata* is perhaps the most advanced among the primitively eusocial wasps studied so far, providing as a bonus the insight that such characteristics of highly eusocial species as pheromonal regulation of reproduction and self-organised work regulation can arise even before increased colony size and morphological caste differentiation.

While these discoveries come in unabated, it seems most unreasonable for me to switch to the study of any other species, in spite of the lure of many fascinating species that my surroundings are endowed with. It is unlikely that I will ever find any reason to abandon my first love. I must confess that we do turn from time to time to the congeneric *Ropalidia cyathiformis* – but I keep emphasising,

much to the chagrin of my students, who devote themselves to the latter, that my only interest in *R. cyathiformis* is in using it to better understand *R. marginata*!

This claim is easy to substantiate. *R. cyathiformis* turns out to be a typical text-book example of a primitively eusocial species. Its queens are impressively aggressive, occupying the alpha position in the colony's pecking order, and appear to suppress worker reproduction through physical aggression and regulate worker foraging through centralised top-down control. The more we show the world that *R. cyathiformis* behaves like a typical primitively eusocial species even in our own hands, the more credible our unusual claims about *R. marginata* will be, thus justifying my slogan '*R. cyathiformis* in the service of *R. marginata*'.

References

Gadagkar, R. (2001) *The Social Biology of* Ropalidia marginata: *Toward Understanding the Evolution of Eusociality*. Cambridge, MA: Harvard University Press.

Evolutionary game theory

John M. McNamara and Franz J. Weissing

Overview

Evolutionary game theory may have done more to stimulate and refine research in animal behaviour than any other theoretical perspective. In this chapter, we will review some of the insights gained by applying game theory to animal behaviour. Our emphasis is on conceptual issues rather than on technical detail. We start by introducing some of the classical models, including the Hawk–Dove game and the Prisoner's Dilemma game. Then we discuss in detail the main ingredients of a game-theoretical approach: strategies, payoffs and 'solution concepts' such as evolutionary stability. It should become clear that first-generation models like the Hawk–Dove game, while of enormous conceptual importance, have severe limitations when applied to real-world scenarios. We close with a sketch of what we see as the most important gaps in our knowledge, and the most relevant current developments in evolutionary game theory.

4.1 Introduction

Social behaviour involves the interaction of several individuals. Therefore within most social contexts the best thing to do depends on what others are doing. In other words, within social contexts selection is typically frequency-dependent (Ayala & Campbell 1974, Heino et al. 1998). Game theory was originally formulated to predict behaviour when there is frequency dependence in economics, for example competition between firms (von Neumann & Morgenstern 1944, Luce & Raiffa 1957). John Maynard Smith and George Price had the fundamental insight that this theory could also be used to predict the evolutionary outcome under frequency-dependent selection within biology (Maynard Smith & Price 1973, Maynard Smith 1982). Their idea was that, rather than following the evolution of a population over time, one could use ideas from game theory to characterise the eventually stable endpoints of the evolutionary process. Their concept of an *evolutionarily stable strategy* (ESS) attempts to capture the properties of these endpoints. To understand this concept let us refer to a strategy as the *resident strategy* if almost all population members adopt this strategy. Then in intuitive terms, a given resident strategy is an ESS if no rare *mutant strategy* can invade this population under the action of natural selection. A necessary condition for this to be true is that no mutant strategy

Social Behaviour: Genes, Ecology and Evolution, ed. Tamás Székely, Allen J. Moore and Jan Komdeur. Published by Cambridge University Press. © Cambridge University Press 2010.

has greater fitness than the resident strategy. This latter condition is the familiar Nash equilibrium concept of economics (Nash 1950), with economic payoffs replaced by fitness payoffs.

The fact that an ESS corresponds to a Nash equilibrium has important conceptual implications. It implies that natural selection will shape social behaviour in such a way that it resembles the behaviour of *Homo economicus*, an agent whose decisions are guided by rational deliberations (Persky 1995). As a consequence, many insights from economic theory apply to animal behaviour, without having to assume that animals are 'rational' in any way (Hammerstein & Selten 1994). Since *Homo economicus* does not exist in our world, we may even have to face the 'rationality paradox' that economic theory describes animal behaviour better than human behaviour (Hammerstein 1996).

The 'quasi-rationality' of adaptive animal behaviour allows us to adopt many tools, ideas and insights from classical game theory. Concepts such as a payoff matrix, and examples such as the Prisoner's Dilemma game have found their way into the biological sciences. Perhaps more important is the adoption of 'strategic thinking', which led biologists to realise that important aspects of behavioural programmes may not easily be observable and that seemingly minor aspects of the interaction structure can have major implications for the evolution of behaviour. Insights like the one that in many contexts signals have to be costly in order to be reliable (the 'handicap principle': Zahavi & Zahavi 1997) had independent origins in both biology and economics (Spence 1973).

In this chapter we focus on conceptual issues rather than on technical detail (for technical reviews see van Damme 1987, Reeve & Dugatkin 1998, Gintis 2000, McGill & Brown 2007). Our goal is to introduce the simple concepts that stimulated research, and to indicate where these concepts need further refinement to reflect more of the real-world complexity of behaviour.

4.2 Setting the scene: classical models

One of the early applications of evolutionary game theory was to the evolution of levels of aggression

Table 4.1. The payoff structure of the Hawk–Dove game. Table entries give the fitness payoff to the focal player

	Opponent plays Dove	Opponent plays Hawk
Focal player plays Dove	$V/2$	0
Focal player plays Hawk	V	$(V - C)/2$

between individuals. Maynard Smith and Price (1973) considered a scenario in which two randomly selected population members contest a resource such as a mate, food item or territory. If an individual obtains the resource, the fitness of that individual is increased by an amount V. Each individual adopts one of two actions. Action 'Dove' specifies that the individual will display to opponent, but will run away if opponent attacks. Action 'Hawk' specifies that the individual will attack opponent and fight if opponent fights back. The possible outcomes are then: if both choose Dove each contestant is equally likely to obtain the resource; if one chooses Dove and the other chooses Hawk then the Hawk obtains the resource; if both choose Hawk each is equally likely to win the fight and hence the resource, but the loser has a reduction in fitness of C due to injuries sustained. The fitness consequences of the various combinations of actions are summarised in Table 4.1.

For this scenario, suppose that a strategy specifies the probability, p, that an individual plays Hawk in the contest. If the resident strategy is always to play Dove ($p = 0$) the best response for a rare mutant is to always play Hawk ($p = 1$). This is because the mutant always gets the resource in the contest since it attacks residents who then run away. In contrast, consider the situation in which the resident strategy is to always play Hawk ($p = 1$). Then if the cost of injury is greater than the value of the resource ($V < C$) the best response of a mutant is to always play Dove ($p = 0$), since this avoids the cost of injury. This illustrates the basic frequency dependence in this situation: the best thing to do depends on the actions of others. It is easy to show that when $V < C$ the strategy $p^* = V/C$ has the property that a best response to the resident strategy p^* is also to adopt strategy p^*.

In other words, p^* is a Nash-equilibrium strategy. However, this does not guarantee that p^* is an ESS. When the resident strategy is p^* any single mutant has the same fitness as a resident, and to verify that p^* is an ESS one must show that mutants are selected against when the frequency of mutants starts to increase, so that mutants can play mutants in the contest. This can be verified (Maynard Smith 1982), and it turns out that $p^* = V/C$ is the unique ESS when $V < C$, and $p^* = 1$ is the unique ESS when $V \geq C$.

Note that, although the reasoning behind an ESS suggests that a population that reaches an ESS will not evolve away from this strategy, it does not guarantee that evolution will actually lead to an ESS. This shortcoming of the original ESS concept will be discussed further below.

The Hawk–Dove game involves the competitive interaction of two population members. But the idea of an ESS can be extended to deal with n-player games – for example, to the analysis of dominance hierarchies (Chapters 7 and 14). The concept can also be used to analyse situations in which individuals 'play the field'. This term refers to situations in which the fitness of an individual depends on some overall characteristic of the resident population. For example, in analysing evolutionarily stable sex ratios, as the proportion of females in the breeding population increases the advantage to a breeding male increases for two reasons: there are more females to mate with, and fewer males to compete with. Consequently the advantage of producing sons over producing daughters depends in a non-linear way on the proportion of resident members producing sons as opposed to producing daughters (Seger & Stubblefield 2002).

The evolution of male size when there is male–male competition is another case of playing the field. Here the fitness of a male of a given size depends in a typically non-linear way on the size distribution of resident males. Because of the non-linearity the fitness of the male cannot be expressed as the sum of fitness contributions from all the pair-wise interactions with other males, so that this situation cannot be reduced to a series of independent two-player games. As we discuss further below, in many settings even the Hawk–Dove should not really be considered as a two-player game but as playing the field. Specifically, when an individual must play a series of Hawk–Dove games, fitness may not be the sum of the fitness contributions from each game.

Although all individuals in a population are maximising their fitness at an ESS, one of the important messages of game theory is that mean population fitness is not usually maximised. This is because all individuals are doing the best for themselves, and this is not necessarily the best for the population as a whole. To illustrate this point consider the Hawk–Dove game. In this game the same resources are available per pair regardless of the strategies employed by population members; one pair member gets the resource of value V, the other does not. But if fighting occurs individuals lose fitness through injury. Thus mean population fitness is maximised by avoiding fights, i.e. by all population members playing Dove. This would not evolve, however, since in such a population an individual playing Hawk would gain an advantage. The 'tragedy of the commons' also illustrates this point; if there is some common good that all individuals can share there is always selection pressure to take more than a fair share, often resulting in the overuse and demise of the common good (Hardin 1968).

As a final example of this point consider the Prisoner's Dilemma game (e.g. Axelrod & Hamilton 1981). This game is played between two opponents. Each has a choice between cooperating with their partner or defecting. The fitness payoff to an individual depends on this focal individual's choice and that of the opponent (Table 4.2). In this illustration, regardless of the choice of action by the opponent it is best to Defect (since $5 > 3$ and $1 > 0$). The opponent has an identical payoff matrix and should do likewise. Thus both players Defect at the unique ESS (and each receives a fitness payoff of 1 unit for the case illustrated). In contrast, had they both cooperated they would each have obtained a higher payoff (3 units in the case illustrated). This property of the Prisoner's Dilemma has made it a test-bed for models of the evolution of cooperation. The challenge is to understand how selfish behaviour (produced by the action of natural selection) can lead individuals to cooperate. In other words, when is it in an individual's best interests to cooperate?

Table 4.2. Illustration of the payoff structure of the Prisoner's Dilemma game. Table entries give the fitness payoff to the focal player

	Opponent cooperates	Opponent defects
Focal player cooperates	3	0
Focal player defects	5	1

Take-home messages of section 4.2

- In social contexts, selection is typically frequency-dependent.
- In the case of frequency-dependent selection, mean population fitness is usually not maximised. To predict the outcome of selection, one should not look for fitness optima but for evolutionarily stable strategies (ESS). These maximise fitness conditional on the behaviour of other population members.
- Every ESS corresponds to a Nash equilibrium and can therefore be viewed as 'quasi-rational' behaviour.

4.3 Strategies

An important insight of game theory is that of *strategic thinking*. A strategy is a rule for choosing which action to perform. For example, in the Hawk–Dove game the probabilistic rule – with probability $1 - p$ play Dove, with probability p play Hawk – is an example of a mixed strategy. Strategies are rules that are contingent on circumstances, and the choice of action can depend on an organism's state, its role, the information that it has, etc. For example, in a variant of the Hawk–Dove game two individuals contest a territory. One individual is assigned the role of territory owner, the other that of intruder. Although each player can choose to play Hawk or Dove, as in the standard game, the set of strategies is enlarged. The rule, if intruder play Dove, if owner play Hawk, is an example of a strategy that is contingent on ownership (this strategy is referred to as Bourgeois: Maynard Smith & Parker 1976). In the Repeated Prisoner's Dilemma game (e.g. Gintis 2000) two individuals play the Prisoner's Dilemma several times against each other. A strategy for this repeated game specifies the choice of action in the current round as a function of the whole history of the game up to that point. For example, the rule (known as Tit-for-Tat), choose the same action as opponent chose on the last round, is an example of a simple strategy where the action taken is contingent on the opponent's behaviour in the past.

Game-theory payoffs are assigned to the combinations of actions, but the analysis of the game is in terms of strategies and not actions. In evolutionary terms this is the right level of analysis, since genes may be viewed as 'recipes' that prescribe how an organism should act contingent on the current conditions. As we have seen before, it can be useful in social contexts to randomise one's behaviour. Strategies including an element of randomisation (for instance, play Hawk with probability 0.75 and Dove with probability 0.25) are called *mixed* strategies, whereas strategies that prescribe actions in a deterministic way (like Tit-for-Tat or Bourgeois) are called *pure* strategies.

In formulating a game, the details of the model may matter enormously for the predicted outcome; in particular, it is crucial what strategies are allowed. The Hawk–Dove game (with $V < C$) illustrates this point. In the original game a (mixed) strategy specifies the probability, p, that an individual will play Hawk. There is a unique ESS at which individuals play Hawk with probability $p^* = V/C$. In the version of the Hawk–Dove game with territorial ownership a strategy is specified by two probabilities, p_O and p_I, where p_O is the probability of playing Hawk when in the role of territory owner and p_I is the probability of playing Hawk when in the role of intruder. For the latter game the resident strategy $p_O = V/C$, $p_I = V/C$ is not evolutionarily stable (Maynard Smith & Parker 1976). Instead there are two ESSs, both of which are pure strategies. One ESS is Bourgeois, i.e. always play Hawk when owner and always play Dove when intruder ($p_O = 1$, $p_I = 0$). The other ESS is Anti-Bourgeois; i.e. always play Dove when owner and always play Hawk when intruder ($p_O = 0$, $p_I = 1$).

It is a general feature of asymmetric games that ESSs are pure strategies (Selten 1980, 1983), at least when payoffs are fixed (cf. Webb *et al.* 1999). The owner–intruder terminology suggests that there are relevant differences between the two types of players, for example with respect to fighting ability or the payoffs received. However, the above result also applies to situations where the roles are just arbitrary labels. In the absence of such labels, a mixed-strategy population is predicted, where fights occur with probability $(V/C)^2$. In the presence of an otherwise irrelevant label, a pure-strategy population will result where fights are avoided due to the strategic convention (either Bourgeois or Anti-Bourgeois). Hence a seemingly trivial change in the formulation of a game can have major implications for the evolutionary outcome.

Models of parental effort provide a second illustration of the importance of the strategic perspective (see also Chapter 11). In the parental-effort model of Houston and Davies (1985) each parent chooses its level of effort independently of the other parent. There is no variation within each sex, but males and females may differ from each other. At evolutionary stability, the effort of one parent depends on the effort expended by the other parent. Thus, if male effort increases female effort decreases, and vice versa. In this model it is implicitly assumed that parents do not respond to each other in real time. Instead, levels of effort are fixed and genetically determined, and change only occurs over evolutionary time (McNamara *et al.* 1999). This seems unrealistic; in real populations there will always be within-sex variation in effort, so that it will be advantageous to respond directly to partner's effort. Efforts will then be negotiated using response rules. Thus models should be looking at the evolution of response rules rather than of efforts. In other words, we should be taking the response rules as genetically determined rather than the efforts, and at evolutionary stability the response rule used by males will depend on the response rule used by females, and vice versa. As McNamara *et al.* (1999) show, this can mean that the effort chosen as the result of the negotiation is not the same as the best effort given the (negotiated) effort of partner.

As a third example, consider a simple game between parents in which each decides whether to care for their common young or to desert. The points we wish to make are more fully discussed by McNamara and Houston (2002). The payoff matrices for males and females are given in Table 4.3. Here the differences in payoff between males and females might arise because males are better at care than females. We consider two versions of this game. In the first version, which we refer to as the *simultaneous choice* version, each parent chooses whether to care or desert without knowing the decision of the other parent. Neither parent can change its mind once the partner's decision is revealed. In this version a male's strategy specifies the probability he will desert; similarly, a female's strategy specifies the probability she will desert. As can be seen from the payoff matrices, if the female deserts it is best for the male to care, and if the male cares it is best for the female to desert. Thus male care and female desertion are best responses to each other and are in Nash equilibrium. In fact it is easy to see that this gives the unique ESS: at evolutionary stability males always care and females always desert.

In the second version of the desertion game the male is the first to choose whether to desert. If he decides to care he stays with the young, if he decides to desert he departs. The female then decides whether to care or desert, her decision being contingent on whether the male is still present or not. In this *sequential choice* version the strategy of a male again specifies his probability of desertion. In contrast, the strategy of a female is now a contingent rule that specifies the probability of desertion if the male cares, and the probability of desertion if he deserts. Suppose that in a population the resident male strategy is for a male to always desert, and the resident female strategy is to desert if the male cares and care if he deserts. Then it can be seen from Table 4.3 that no mutant male adopting a different strategy can do better. If instead of deserting he cares, the female will desert and he will be worse off. Similarly, no mutant female adopting a different strategy can do better. Thus the population is in Nash equilibrium. Note that in this population females are never observed to desert because males never care, but the threat of partner desertion keeps the male away from caring. Thus an unobserved aspect of the female strategy is crucial to the game.

So is this resident population (males always desert and females care if the male deserts and desert if he cares) evolutionarily stable? The problem is that, since all males desert, there is no selection pressure acting on what the female would do if the male were to care. Thus the female strategy that specifies

Table 4.3. Payoffs in the parental desertion game

(a) Payoff to the male

	Female cares	Female deserts
Male cares	10	7
Male deserts	8	2

(b) Payoff to the female

	Male cares	Male deserts
Females cares	10	4
Female deserts	11	2

care under all circumstances does equally well, and can increase by drift. The resident strategy is therefore not an ESS according to the original definition of Maynard Smith and Price (1973). However, suppose that males occasionally care by mistake. Then it does matter what the female would do if the male were to care, and the female strategy of always caring is strictly worse than the strategy of caring if and only if the male deserts. Thus the population is evolutionarily stable if infrequent mistakes are assumed. As Selten (1983) emphasises, occasional mistakes can stabilise the solution of a game. Selten refers to an equilibrium that is stable under infrequent mistakes as a *limit ESS*.

In the simultaneous-choice version of the above desertion game, the payoff to the male at evolutionary stability is 7. The payoff to a male at evolutionary stability in the sequential-choice version is 8. Thus the male gains an advantage by being the first to choose. However, it is the information that each parent has when making its decision, rather than the sequence of events, that is crucial. When the female makes her decision she has reliable information on the male's action. When the male makes his decision he does not know the action of the female. It is this informational asymmetry that gives the males the advantage. Interestingly, it is just the uninformed party (the males) that profits from the information asymmetry. This is in striking contrast to (frequency-independent) optimisation problems, where extra information always provides an advantage. McNamara *et al.* (2006) explicitly consider whether it is it better to give information, to receive it or to be ignorant in a two-player game.

Similar conclusions have been drawn in 'playing the field' contexts, such as determining the evolutionarily stable sex ratio of offspring. If a mother does not make her sex-ratio decision contingent on her state or environmental conditions, she should invest equal amounts of resources into male and female offspring (*equal-allocation principle*: e.g. Seger & Stubblefield 2002). If male and female offspring are equally costly to produce, this should lead to a 50:50 sex ratio. Whenever male and female offspring are differentially affected by the mother's state or environmental conditions, the mother should make her sex-ratio decision contingent on these parameters (Trivers & Willard 1973). If she does, the population sex ratio at the ESS is no longer 50:50 (Frank & Swingland 1988), showing again that the results obtained in one type of game context cannot easily be generalised to another context, even if the differences between the models seem of minor importance. As in the desertion game considered above, information asymmetries are also of crucial importance for evolutionarily stable sex ratios. For example, Pen and Taylor (2005) show that in a queen–worker conflict over the sex ratio the workers can much better achieve their preferred sex ratio at ESS if they are not informed about the mother's decision than if they have this information. Of course, having more information can also provide an advantage. For example, Pen and Weissing (2002) show that in the conflict between the male and the female parent over the sex ratio of their offspring the informed party 'wins' the conflict.

At an ESS, individuals should make their behaviour contingent on the available information. As a consequence, it can be advantageous to manipulate the information available to an opponent. In some cases (e.g. the desertion game) a player can put an opponent at a disadvantage by giving the opponent reliable information about the player's own action (cf. Brams 1983). In other cases, it is better to hide one's intentions, or to actively deceive the opponent. It has been argued (e.g. Trivers 1985) that this intention and deception may even lead to the evolution of self-deception, since organisms can deceive their opponents more efficiently if they also deceive themselves.

In the sequential version of the desertion game, the fact that a male is not present gives the female reliable information about the male's action. This benefits the male. So can the female (who chooses second) gain an advantage by giving her partner reliable information on what she will do? In particular, suppose that the female threatens to desert if the male deserts. If this threat is credible it will give the female an advantage, since the male will be forced to care. So is the threat credible? To analyse this, consider a population in which the female strategy is to always desert regardless of the male's action, and the male strategy is always to care. These strategies are again best responses to one another. In particular, the male is forced to care by the female's threat that she will desert if he deserts. However, mistakes by the males now destabilise the equilibrium. If a male is not present (either because he makes a mistake and deserts, or because he tries to care but is killed), then it is not optimal for the female to carry out her threat. Thus a genuine threat will not evolve; i.e. the threat by the female is not credible and is not reliable information in this game.

One way to give an opponent reliable information is to handicap oneself, so limiting one's choice of options (Schelling 1960, Elster 2000). In a version of the desertion game, Barta *et al.* (2002) allow females to choose their energy reserves before they (and their mate) decide whether to care for the young or desert. Females choose reserves that are too low for them to be able to care alone. This gives the male the reliable information that the female will desert if he deserts. He is therefore forced to care.

Strategic thinking has important implications for the analysis of a game. Consider the Repeated Prisoner's Dilemma game, where the players can make their choice of action in the current round dependent on the history of the game. After one round, there are already four possible histories corresponding to the four combinations of the actions Cooperate and Defect that can be chosen by the two players in the first round. Accordingly, there are $2^4 = 16$ pure 'local' strategies prescribing the choice of action in the second round. In the third round, there are already $4^2 = 16$ possible histories and $2^{16} = 65\,536$ pure local strategies. Obviously, even in relatively simple social contexts, the strategy space can reach astronomical proportions.

Perhaps more importantly, the number of Nash equilibria can also be huge. This is formalised in the so-called Folk Theorem of game theory (e.g. van Damme 1987), which states that for almost all games *every* outcome that is feasible and 'individually rational' in the one-shot game can be realised as the Nash equilibrium outcome of the repeated version of the game, provided that the number of repetitions is sufficiently large. For the Prisoner's Dilemma game in Table 4.2, this implies that *any* payoff outcome x with $1 \leq x \leq 3$ can be realised by a Nash equilibrium. The discussion in the literature often focuses on the extreme cases, i.e. on 'uncooperative' Nash strategies like Always Defect leading to the outcome $x = 1$, and on 'cooperative' Nash strategies like Tit-for-Tat leading to the outcome $x = 3$. The Folk Theorem shows that there is much more to it. In fact, it is one of the major challenges of evolutionary game theory to single out those Nash equilibria that are most 'reasonable' from an evolutionary perspective.

Take-home messages of Section 4.3

- To understand social behaviour, one should apply *strategic thinking*, that is, focus on integrated behavioural programmes rather than on singular actions.
- In social contexts, at evolutionary stability alternative actions often have the same payoff, and the strategy of population members is to choose between the actions according to specified probabilities.
- Not all relevant aspects of a strategy may be directly observable. Strategies specify what to do under every eventuality, but in playing a game some circumstances may not be encountered because of the choice of actions by contestants. This does not mean that what a player would have done in these circumstances is irrelevant. Indeed it may be crucial to the outcome of the game, because it may be decisive in deciding whether to take actions which will lead to these circumstances.
- Seemingly irrelevant details concerning the strategic options available may matter enormously for the outcome of a social interaction. Asymmetries, even if they do not affect fighting ability or payoffs, may be crucial for solving a conflict.
- Having extra information is not always advantageous. A player can put an opponent at a disadvantage by

giving the opponent reliable information about the player's action.

- Having extra options available is not always advantageous. One way to give an opponent reliable information is to handicap oneself, so limiting one's choice of options.
- Even relatively simple social interactions will often have a huge strategy set and a huge number of Nash equilibria. The challenge is not to find one of these equilibria, but to single out those that are 'reasonable' from an evolutionary perspective.

4.4 Payoffs

Game theory is usually based on a cost–benefit analysis in which the payoff to an organism depends on its strategy and that of other population members. In classical game models payoffs are proxies for fitness. They are meant to represent how much the outcome of the game increase fitness. However, the link between outcomes and fitness is often not considered carefully or spelt out.

Fitness is a quantity assigned to strategies, not to individual actions. The fitness of a strategy is some appropriate measure of the mean number of descendants left in the future by an organism following the strategy. Technically, this can be quantified by the asymptotic growth rate of a cohort of individuals following this strategy, which corresponds to the leading eigenvalue of a so-called population projection matrix (Metz *et al.* 1992, Caswell 2001). Note, however, that the projection matrix is not usually that for the whole population. Rather it is the projection matrix for a rare mutant within the population. Fitness is then the rate of invasion of the mutant into the resident population. This fitness measure is often not intuitive and may be difficult to apply in practice (e.g. Pen & Weissing 2002). In practice, evolutionary considerations are therefore usually based on alternative measures for the evolutionary success of a strategy.

In the simplest cases, expected lifetime reproductive success (i.e. the mean lifetime number of surviving offspring produced) is a good substitute measure of fitness. However, when offspring differ in their ability to

spread the genes of their parents, this simple measure may not be adequate. For example, consider the sex-ratio problem. For this scenario a strategy for a female specifies the proportion of her offspring that are male. Just adding up the number of male and female offspring would not be an adequate fitness measure. To see this, assume that the population sex ratio in the offspring generation is male-biased. In such a situation, females are in short supply and a female offspring will on average leave more descendants (and, hence, spread its parents' genes more efficiently) than a male offspring. Adding up male and female offspring in a fitness measure would therefore be like adding up apples and oranges.

The concept of reproductive value, which was introduced by Fisher (1930), quantifies the relative evolutionary importance of individuals in different states (Grafen 2006). Reproductive values may be viewed as weighing factors that allow individuals in different states to be compared. For example, in the sex-ratio context above, the reproductive value of a male offspring is inversely proportional to the fraction s of males in the population, $v_m = 1/s$, while the reproductive value of a female offspring is inversely proportional to the fraction of females, $v_f = 1/(1-s)$. It can be shown that under many circumstances the weighted sum $W = n_m v_m + n_f v_f$ of male and female offspring, each offspring being weighted by its reproductive value, is a fitness measure that quantifies the evolutionary success of a strategy (e.g. Pen & Weissing 2002).

Reproductive values can be rigorously derived (Caswell 2001, Grafen 2006) for all kinds of situations where individuals differ in state, where 'state' may represent sex, age, body size, energy reserves, dominance status, previous actions taken in a game, and the like. For an individual, reproductive value quantifies its dependence of future descendants on current state. Under many circumstances an organism maximises its fitness by always behaving to maximise its reproductive value (McNamara 1993). The most important advantage of reproductive value is that it allows a cost–benefit analysis involving a comparison of individuals in different states. Should a mother, for example, defend her n kids if she runs a mortality risk μ but will save her kids from mortal danger with probability p? With the help of reproductive values, the answer is straightforward: nest defence will be selected if the loss in terms of reproductive value of the mother, μv_{mother}, is outweighed by the gain in terms of reproductive value of her kids, npv_{kids}.

Thus reproductive value, or some equivalent, can be used as a surrogate currency for fitness in game payoffs. We can use the Hawk–Dove game to illustrate the use of reproductive value. Suppose that males are searching for females to mate with. We assume that if a male encounters a female that is not contested by another male, he mates with her. If the female is contested by another male he must decide to play Hawk or Dove in a contest with this male. If the male wins the contest he gets to mate with the female, if he loses a Hawk versus Hawk fight he dies with probability z. In this game the payoff V for winning the contest corresponds to the value of a mating, which we can normalise to 1. Let R denote the reproductive value of the male after the contest. Then the cost of losing a fight is $C = zR$, since this is the expected loss in reproductive value as a result of losing a fight. Classical game theory would take C as given and predict an ESS probability of playing Hawk of $p^* = \min\{V/C, 1\}$. This approach may suffice for some purposes, but it is an approach that isolates each contest from its ecological and social setting, and can mislead. The problem is that R is not usually a given quantity. R corresponds to the future number of matings obtained by a male before he dies. This quantity depends on the number of uncontested females in the environment. It also depends on the fighting strategies employed by the focal male and other males in future contests, and hence depends on the solution of the game. In other words, the solution of the game depends on R, but R depends on the solution of the game! To take this complication into account, it is better not to consider each contest in isolation. Instead, one proceeds as follows (e.g. Taylor & Frank 1996, van Boven & Weissing 2004).

We consider a situation in which all population members play some given strategy in contests (the resident strategy). For such a monomorphic population, the reproductive value R can be calculated by standard means. Given this value of R, one can now check whether any alternative mutant strategy would have a higher fitness than the resident and, thus, be able to

invade. One then seeks a resident strategy that is not invadable and, hence, a Nash-equilibrium strategy and a possible ESS. For the case of the Repeated Hawk–Dove game, Houston and McNamara (1991) demonstrate that for some ecological parameters there can be two ESSs. At each, the R (and hence $C = zR$) that emerges is such that the behaviour in each contest conforms to the prediction of the classical Hawk–Dove game with $V = 1$ and this value of C. At one ESS individuals always play Hawk in contests, resulting in high mortality, low R and hence low C. This is then consistent with $p^* = 1$. At the other ESS individuals do not always fight, resulting in a higher R and hence C, and consistent with the lower value of p^* obtained.

In classical applications of game theory, the payoff parameters were usually assumed to be externally given. The above example illustrates that it is often more natural to assume that these parameters are intrinsically generated by feedbacks with the population strategy. Taking such feedbacks into account can lead to qualitatively different and sometimes surprising results (see van Boven & Weissing 2004 for an example). Many applications of game theory also neglect the ecological embedding of social interactions (Mylius & Diekmann 1995). The fitness of a resident population corresponds to the asymptotic growth rate of the population (Metz et al. 1992). In ecological equilibrium, this asymptotic growth rate has to be equal to zero, since the population would go extinct in case of a negative value and it would go to infinity in case of a positive value. In order to achieve a zero growth rate, not all payoff parameters can be fixed and externally given. In an ecologically realistic setting, at least some of the payoff parameters must be density-dependent, to allow population regulation. One might think that the way in which population regulation is achieved (e.g. by reduced survival or by reduced fecundity at high densities) is of marginal importance for the outcome of evolution. This, however, is not the case, since the mechanism of density regulation may differentially affect reproductive values and, hence, the outcome of evolutionary cost–benefit analyses. Consider, for example, a situation where density regulation acts via increased juvenile mortality at high population densities. At ecological equilibrium, the reproductive value of juveniles is relatively low, implying that adults should invest relatively much into their own survival rather than into the production and survival of offspring. The opposite would be the case if density regulation were to act via reduced survival of adults. Many examples, ranging from sex-ratio evolution (Pen & Weissing 2002) to cooperative breeding (Pen & Weissing 2000), demonstrate that neglecting the mechanism of density regulation can lead to highly misleading conclusions.

Take-home messages of section 4.4

- The payoffs assigned to strategies are proxies for fitness. In situations where individuals can differ in 'state' (e.g. sex, age, size, energy reserves, dominance status), the quantification of fitness is often difficult and not straightforward.
- In such situations, the reproductive-value concept allows a cost–benefit analysis, where individuals in different states are weighed according to their efficiency in spreading their genes to future generations.
- The solution of a game reflects the payoffs, but the payoffs often reflect the behaviour in the population and, hence, the solution of the game. Taking such feedbacks into account can strongly affect the evolutionary predictions, both quantitatively and qualitatively.
- All social interactions are embedded in an ecological context (Chapter 18). Neglecting this context and the corresponding density dependence of payoff parameters can lead to highly misleading evolutionary conclusions.

4.5 Evolutionary analysis

The evolutionary analysis of a social interaction typically starts with the specification of the set of feasible strategies. As we have seen above, the strategy set reflects assumptions on the interaction structure, the information available to the interacting agents, and the actions available in any possible situation. The strategy set also reflects all kinds of limitations and constraints at the sensory, cognitive or behavioural level. In a next step, fitness payoffs are assigned to the strategies. Since fitness is frequency-dependent in the case of social interactions, the fitness

of an organism depends not only on its own strategy p, but also on the 'population strategy' u, the distribution of strategies in the population. Hence the selective forces acting in the population are characterised by a fitness function $W(p,u)$. As we have seen above, the definition of fitness is not always obvious, and the function W will reflect life-history considerations and ecological factors such as the mechanism of density dependence. Once the fitness function has been obtained, it can be used to make predictions concerning the expected outcome of natural selection. This is, however, less straightforward than one might think.

In the case of frequency-independent selection (where fitness $W(p)$ depends only on an organism's own strategy p and not on the strategy distribution in the population), it is often useful to imagine evolution as a hill-climbing exercise on the 'fitness landscape' generated by the function W. From one generation to the next, fitness is expected to increase, until a (local) maximum is reached (Wright 1932). Such a strategy p^*, for which $W(p^*) > W(p)$ holds for all $p \neq p^*$ in the vicinity of p^*, may then be viewed as a potential outcome of evolution. The fitness-landscape metaphor can also be applied to frequency-dependent selection, but now the selective forces acting on behaviour are characterised by a bivariate function $W(p,u)$. For any given population strategy u, there is again the fitness landscape, but this landscape changes with any change of the population strategy (Fig. 4.1). Hence social evolution corresponds to a climb on a fluctuating fitness landscape, and the fluctuations themselves are the result of selection. As a consequence, the outcome of social evolution is not always obvious, and sometimes even counterintuitive.

The metaphor of a fluctuating fitness landscape explains, for example, the well-known fact that mean population fitness is usually not maximised in the case of frequency-dependent selection. Suppose that the population strategy is u_t at time t and that selection shifts the population to a new state u_{t+1}. Then the new state will typically have a higher fitness than the old state, but only with respect to the 'old' fitness landscape $W(p,u_t)$ generated by u_t. There is no a-priori reason why u_{t+1} should also have a higher fitness with respect to the new fitness landscape $W(p,u_{t+1})$. In fact, mean population fitness will often deteriorate in time, and

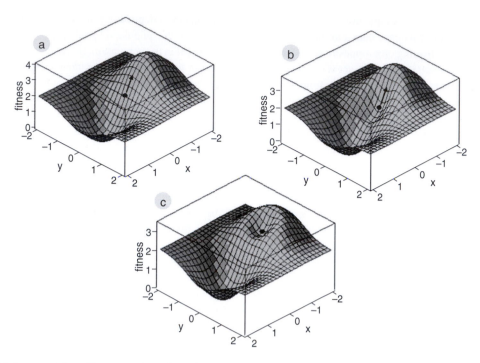

Figure 4.1 Representation of frequency-dependent selection as a climb on a fluctuating fitness landscape. The three panels depict the fitness landscape at three points in time. The corresponding population strategy u_t is indicated by a black dot. At each point of time, the population strategy changes in the direction of steepest ascent (arrow). A change in population strategy from (a) u_t to (b) u_{t+1} induces, however, a change in the fitness landscape. In the example, the fitness landscape is slightly depressed in the vicinity of the population strategy. As a consequence, the fitness of u_{t+1} in (b) is not necessarily higher than the fitness of u_t in (a). A depression of fitness near the population strategy often occurs in models where individuals with a strategy close to the established strategy in the population suffer most from intraspecific competition. In such a case, the population may even end up in a local fitness minimum (c), although the population changed in an uphill direction throughout the whole trajectory.

in some cases the population may even converge to a state where mean population fitness is minimised (as illustrated in Fig. 4.1c).

Many seemingly similar concepts have been developed in order to predict the outcome of evolution in a system where the selective forces are characterised by a frequency-dependent fitness function $W(p,u)$. Here we only mention a few, in order to indicate why a single concept does not capture all aspects. In 1973, Maynard Smith and Price introduced the concept of an evolutionarily stable strategy, which is based on the idea that the stable endpoints of evolution correspond to resident strategies that cannot be invaded by alternative 'mutant' strategies. To this end, they considered a monomorphic resident population employing strategy

p^* that is challenged by a rare mutant strategy p that occurs with a small frequency ε. Then the population strategy is given by $u_\varepsilon = (1 - \varepsilon)\, p^* + \varepsilon p$. The residents will be immune against invasion by p if their fitness $W(p^*, u_\varepsilon)$ exceeds $W(p, u_\varepsilon)$, the fitness of the mutants. Accordingly, p^* is considered an ESS if $W(p^*, (1 - \varepsilon)p^* + \varepsilon p) > W(p, (1 - \varepsilon)p^* + \varepsilon p)$ for all $p \neq p^*$ and sufficiently small mutant frequency $\varepsilon > 0$.

Taking the limit $\varepsilon \to 0$ in the above definition of an ESS, we obtain the Nash-equilibrium condition from classical game theory: $W(p^*, p^*) \geq W(p, p^*)$ for all $p \neq p^*$. In words, no strategy is better against p^* than p^* itself; p^* is a best response to itself. Alternatively, p^* corresponds to a local maximum of $W(p, p^*)$, the fitness landscape generated by p^* itself. Hence every ESS is a

Nash-equilibrium strategy. In practical applications, authors often only check the Nash condition, without demonstrating that the more stringent ESS condition of Maynard Smith and Price is also satisfied. Virtually all games considered in the literature have at least one Nash equilibrium (van Damme 1987), and specifying the Nash equilibria of a game is typically a much simpler task than specifying all ESSs. Nash-equilibrium strategies may be viewed as candidate ESSs, but one should be aware that the Nash-equilibrium condition is rather weak. In fact, many Nash equilibria are not 'reasonable' as the outcome of evolution.

As an example, consider the coordination game in Table 4.4. Two players have to choose independently between two options L and R, and they only get a positive payoff if they both choose the same option. In the human world, one might think of driving one's car on the left (L) or the right (R) side of the road. In this example, there are two Nash equilibria in pure strategies, which both happen to be an ESS: (1) always play L, or (2) always play R. However, the game also has a third Nash strategy $\tilde{p}$: play each option with probability $\frac{1}{2}$. Whenever this strategy is established in a population, it does not matter whether one chooses L or R. Whatever one's choice is, one can expect to get the payoffs 1 and 0 with probability $\frac{1}{2}$. Therefore $W(p,\tilde{p}) = \frac{1}{2}$ for all strategies p, implying $W(\tilde{p},\tilde{p}) = W(p,\tilde{p})$. Hence the Nash condition is satisfied for $\tilde{p}$ (be it in a weak sense), but it can be shown that $\tilde{p}$ is not an ESS. Intuitively, it is obvious that the corresponding population is not very stable. Whenever there is a slight majority for L in the population, it is individually advantageous to play L as well. Accordingly, one would expect a rapid evolution towards the pure strategy L. The same applies vice versa whenever there is a majority for R. This is confirmed in our human world: there are many countries where everybody drives on the left side of the road, and many other countries where everybody drives on the right side. In contrast, there are few examples where individuals decide at random on which side of the road to drive!

In contrast to the 'weak' mixed-strategy Nash equilibrium $\tilde{p}$, the two pure-strategy equilibria of the coordination game are 'strict' Nash strategies. This means that the Nash condition is satisfied in the strict sense,

Table 4.4. Payoff structure of a coordination game

	Opponent plays L	Opponent plays R
Focal player plays L	1	0
Focal player plays R	0	1

$W(p^*,p^*) > W(p,p^*)$, for all $p \neq p^*$. Strict Nash strategies have many desirable properties. In particular, every strict Nash strategy is an ESS. However, whereas all games have at least one (and often many) Nash strategies, most games do not have a strict Nash equilibrium. Moreover, most games with a rich interaction structure also do not have a single ESS *sensu* Maynard Smith and Price. For this reason, the ESS concept has been weakened in several ways, leading to concepts such as *direct ESS* or *limit ESS* (Selten 1983, van Damme 1987). Perhaps most importantly, many authors now use (often implicitly) a local definition of the Nash property and the ESS condition. For example, p^* is considered a strict Nash strategy if $W(p^*,p^*) > W(p,p^*)$ holds for all $p \neq p^*$ *in the vicinity of* p^*. Such local conditions have the advantage that they can be checked relatively easily by standard methods from differential calculus. Biologically, the local version of such stability conditions corresponds to the assumption that a resident population of p^*-strategists is only challenged by mutant strategies that differ only slightly from p^*. If all mutations have a small effect, this is indeed plausible. However, one has to be aware that this assumption is not unproblematic, since even point mutations often have a macroscopic effect on the phenotype (for further discussion see Wolf *et al.* 2008).

The example of the coordination game illustrates that the real question is often not which strategy is invasion-proof, but which of the invasion-proof strategies will actually be achieved in the course of evolution. It is rather obvious that driving on the left and on the right side of the road are alternative ESSs, but the question remains why driving on the left side is the outcome in some countries, while driving on the right side is the outcome in others. In the case of the coordination game, we already gave an intuitive answer in terms of historical contingency: whenever there is the slightest bias in one direction, it is in the self-interest of the individual to follow this bias, leading to a self-reinforcing process of evolution in the direction on the initial bias.

In systems with a simple strategic structure, arguments like this can be formalised as follows (Taylor 1996, Geritz *et al.* 1998). Take any Nash strategy p^*. The question is whether evolution will lead towards this strategy. To this end, consider a resident population with strategy $\hat{p}$ that is a small distance away from p^*. The $\hat{p}$-population will typically be not evolutionarily stable, implying that certain mutant strategies can invade. If the successful mutants are closer to p^* than $\hat{p}$, it is plausible to assume that evolution through successful invasion and replacement of the resident by the invader will eventually converge towards p^*. A strategy p^* with the property that evolution by gene substitution will converge towards p^* (because the successful invaders are closer to p^* than the former resident $\hat{p}$) will be called an *evolutionary attractor* (but there are many alternative terms for this property in the literature, including 'population stability' and 'convergence stability'). If, on the other hand, successful mutants are those that are further away from p^* than $\hat{p}$, one can assume that evolution will lead away from p^*. In such a case, p^* is called an *evolutionary repellor*.

Interestingly, the property of being evolutionarily stable against invasion attempts by mutants is, at least to a certain extent, independent of the property of being an evolutionary attractor or repellor. All four combinations are possible (Geritz *et al.* 1998). A strategy that is both an evolutionary attractor and evolutionarily stable is called a *continuously stable strategy* or CSS (Eshel 1983; see also Chapter 6). However, an ESS *sensu* Maynard Smith and Price can be an evolutionary repellor, i.e. an ESS may not be attainable by gene substitution events. Such a scenario has been dubbed 'Garden of Eden' (a desirable state that is not attainable). It is also possible that an evolutionary attractor is not evolutionarily stable. In such a case, called *evolutionary branching*, evolution will lead to a fitness minimum, which is a point of disruptive selection. Evolutionary branching plays an important role in models of sympatric speciation (Chapter 19; Dieckmann & Doebeli 1999, van Doorn *et al.* 2004). Finally, it is of course also possible that an evolutionary repellor is not evolutionarily stable. The

rich field of dynamic behaviour in the case of frequency-dependent selection has led to the emergence of a new research field called *adaptive dynamics*, which reanalyses many classical models in a more stringent and consistent way (Geritz *et al.* 1998, Diekmann 2004, McGill & Brown 2007).

The arguments given above mainly apply to contexts with a simple, one-dimensional strategy space, where a strategy p corresponds to a univariate continuous trait like a sex ratio, a switching time between activities, or a preference for a certain type of resource. In the case of social evolution, strategies are often conditional, and hence of a much more complicated structure. In such a situation, verbal or semi-quantitative arguments are usually not sufficient to predict the outcome of frequency-dependent selection. The so-called *gradient method* (also called *best response method* (McNamara *et al.* 1997, Pen *et al.* 1999) or *genetic algorithm method* (Crowley 2001, Hamblin & Hurd 2007)) is an efficient numerical technique to calculate those strategies that are plausible outcomes of evolution. Basically, this method mimics the walk uphill across the (fluctuating) fitness landscape generated by the fitness function $W(p,u)$. Starting at a population strategy u_0, this technique determines a subsequent strategy u_1 by taking a small step in the direction of steepest ascent on the fitness landscape (the fitness gradient). Repeating this procedure yields a sequence of population strategies u_t that will often converge to a Nash strategy p^*, which is both an evolutionary attractor and an invasion-proof strategy. The method can be further refined by choosing an appropriate step size and by including small errors in decision making (McNamara *et al.* 1997, van Doorn *et al.* 2003a, 2003b). Applications of the gradient method have revealed that, as in the case of univariate strategies, evolutionarily stable strategies are not necessarily dynamically attainable. It turns out that classical non-dynamical game theory has often focused on equilibria that are biologically not relevant, since they are not approached by any evolutionary trajectory (e.g. Hamblin & Hurd 2007).

The gradient method is particularly useful in the case of social interactions that, because of the underlying strategic complexity, have a multitude of Nash equilibria. Van Doorn *et al.* (2003a), for example, apply this technique to the Repeated Hawk–Dove game, which, like the Repeated Prisoner's Dilemma, has a huge number of equilibria. They start by considering the primordial situation where the interacting organisms do not make use of their memory and hence do not employ refined strategies. Under this assumption, the population will converge to $p^* = V/C$, the ESS of the one-shot Hawk–Dove game. Subsequently, van Doorn and colleagues add strategic complexity to the model in a stepwise manner, corresponding to the improvement of behavioural architecture in the course of evolution. Taking the evolutionary outcome for the previous level of complexity as their point of departure, they use the gradient method to determine the most plausible behaviour for the next level of complexity. Irrespective of the exact sequence in which strategic complexity was added, only two types of equilibria result from this type of analysis. One of these equilibria is particularly interesting, since it corresponds to the 'winner–loser' effect often observed in agonistic interactions (Chapters 7 and 14). At this equilibrium, the winners of previous fights tend to be aggressive (play Hawk) in the future, while the losers tend to be peaceful (play Dove). This is true even if winning or losing is equally likely for all individuals and hence does not reflect differences in fighting ability. Accordingly, this model provides a plausible explanation for the evolution of social dominance that does not rely on differences in payoffs, information or resource-holding potential.

Besides being a potent technique for determining potential evolutionary attractors, the gradient method has the advantage that it is a useful heuristic, since it reflects a popular way to imagine the evolutionary process. It is, however, important to realise that the metaphor of natural selection corresponding to a hill-climbing exercise on a fitness landscape has severe limitations. While virtually all methods of evolutionary game theory are based on fitness considerations, the trajectory and outcome of evolution is not solely determined by fitness differences among strategies. In sexually reproducing populations, genetic processes such as Mendelian segregation and recombination may affect the outcome of evolution in two important respects. First, genetic processes may impose constraints on the strategy combinations that are feasible in a sexual population. Consider,

for example, an ESS that can only be realised by a heterozygous genotype (a genotype Aa consisting of two different alleles A and a). Aa individuals do not transmit their genotype, but either an A-allele or an a-allele to their offspring. As a consequence, although Aa offspring are produced, so too are homozygous AA and aa offspring, even if the latter have a rather low fitness. Hence, because of Mendelian segregation, a purely heterozygous ESS population is not feasible, despite potentially strong fitness differences between genotypes. Second, genetic processes can alter the direction of evolution. Again, this is related to the fact that in a sexual population genotypes (i.e. strategies) are not directly transmitted from the parents to their offspring. Instead, the genes making up a genotype are reshuffled by recombination, and the parents only transmit half of their diploid set of genes to their offspring. Processes like meiosis and recombination have the tendency to break up coadapted sets of genes, and therefore often counteract the tendency of natural selection to increase fitness. In fact, examples can be constructed where fitness is not maximised but minimised, due to processes at the genetic level (Moran 1964).

There are various modelling approaches that attempt to integrate selection forces caused by fitness differentials and processes at the genetic level in a coherent framework. The most important ones are the approach of population genetics that directly considers allele frequency changes at the genetic level (e.g. Cressman *et al.* 1996; see also Chapters 1 and 2); the approach of quantitative genetics that is based on selection gradients and genetic variances and covariances (Taper & Case 1992); and the canonical equation of adaptive dynamics that reflects evolution by gene substitution events (Dieckmann & Law 1996). Interestingly, all these approaches, though quite different in their underlying assumptions, can be described by very similar mathematical structures (Day 2005). When applied to specific examples, it turns out that genetic detail can be of considerable importance for the outcome of evolution. For example, as a result of small differences in genetic architecture, a population can either converge to an evolutionary equilibrium or show ongoing oscillations with large amplitude (e.g. van Doorn & Weissing 2006).

Because of results like this, focusing purely on fitness considerations (as is typically done in evolutionary game theory) can be problematic (Weissing 1996). Neglecting genetic detail may indeed lead to unreliable conclusions. This, however, confronts us with three challenges. First, as we have seen, frequency-dependent selection is already an intricate process, even in the absence of complications at the genetic level. Explicitly including non-trivial genetic assumptions will often make the models intractable. Second, the same kind of fitness scenario would necessitate a different analysis for different species, since the underlying genetics can not be assumed to be the same. As a consequence, it is often difficult to distil general conclusions from models including genetic detail. Third, and most importantly, the genetics underlying social behaviour is virtually unknown (but see Chapters 1, 2, 6 and 11). Despite enormous progress in fields such as ecological genomics, we predict that this will not change fundamentally in the next few decades. Including realistic genetic assumptions into models of frequency-dependent selection is therefore not an option for years to come.

Fortunately, the situation is less bleak than it may appear at first sight. Some methods of evolutionary game theory appear rather robust and do not depend on genetic details (Leimar 2001). It can also be shown that in the limiting case of weak selection the conclusions derived from fitness considerations are quite robust (Nagylaki *et al.* 1999). Finally, it can also be argued that genetic constraints and genetic processes interfering with adaptive evolution are themselves subject to selection and, as a consequence, will disappear in a long-term perspective (Hammerstein 1996, van Doorn & Dieckmann 2006, Galis & Metz 2007).

Take-home messages of section 4.5

- In the context of frequency-dependent selection, the often-used metaphor of an adaptive landscape has to be applied with caution. The fitness landscape is not constant but fluctuates due to the influence of natural selection. As a consequence, fitness can decrease over the generations. It is even possible that a population evolves to a fitness minimum.
- There are many different concepts that all try to capture the idea of evolutionary stability. Many applications focus on Nash-equilibrium strategies. Most games have, however, a multitude of Nash equilibria, and many of these equilibria lack evolutionary stability.

- An evolutionarily stable strategy is not necessarily attainable. In fact, evolution can lead away from an ESS ('Garden of Eden'). In contrast, evolution can lead to an evolutionarily unstable strategy, a so-called branching point. Such evolutionary branching may provide an explanation for processes like sympatric speciation.

- The *gradient method* (or *genetic algorithm method*) is a useful technique to determine the attainable and evolutionarily stable Nash-equilibrium strategies of an evolutionary game.

4.6 Conclusions and future directions

Whole systems, not just components

We have noted that in the past there has been a tendency to consider simple games in isolation. An example is the parental desertion games introduced by Maynard Smith (1977). In his Model 2, each of two parents has to decide whether to desert their common young. Payoffs for desertion are given quantities, which potentially leads to a problem of consistency (Webb *et al.* 1999). The benefits of desertion for a male are meant to be in terms of re-mating opportunities. However, opportunities to re-mate necessarily depend on how many females are deserting, and hence the solution of the game. So, as with the Hawk–Dove game of Houston and McNamara (1991), payoffs determine behaviour, but behaviour feeds back to determine payoffs.

More generally, mating systems are characterised by many inherently linked games. For example, the mate-choice strategy of females should depend on both male genetic quality and male parental effort (see Chapters 10 and 18). However, if males trade off current effort against future mating opportunities, male effort should depend on female mate-choice strategies. Whether females choose to give extra-pair copulations (EPCs) should depend on how the social male reacts to loss in paternity, but this in turn should depend on his future mating opportunities and whether he can also gain

EPCs, and hence on female strategies. Of course it is always possible to consider some component such as male parental effort, holding everything else fixed. In that way it is possible to investigate whether the level of male effort makes sense given the rest of the system. However, if the objective is to predict what mating system will evolve under given circumstances, one cannot consider components in isolation. The payoffs for one component are determined by what is going on in other components, and it is necessary to specify all feedbacks and links and to solve for all aspects at the same time.

These remarks probably apply to most social systems. A holistic approach is necessary if one is to understand what systems are possible and how they depend on environmental conditions. When feedback between different components is strong we might expect that there can be more than one stable, self-maintaining system in given circumstances. However, we might also expect that only a few types of system are possible in general. If these properties hold, then models could be used to investigate how one social system flips into another system as environmental conditions change. Because reversing the change would not necessarily restore the original system, one outcome of the investigation would be to reveal which phylogenetic trees are more likely than others (see Chapter 5).

The importance of variability

From the theory of sexual selection, it is known that costly female preferences can only evolve if there is sufficient (non-adaptive) variation in male traits (Chapter 10; Andersson 1994). This is not difficult to understand. Paying the costs of being choosy can only be advantageous if these costs are balanced by benefits. Such benefits only accrue if choosy females actually 'have a choice', i.e. if there is sufficient variation among males. The same basic principle also applies to many social situations, where the variance in a behavioural trait is often also important in determining how the mean value of the trait will evolve. For example, in a version of the Repeated Prisoner's Dilemma, McNamara et al. (2004) maintain variability in a population through mutation. They show that the direction of evolution is determined by the amount of

mutation; cooperation only evolves above a critical mutation rate.

The ability to opt out of an interaction can radically change the predictions of a model. For example, in McNamara et al. (2008) individuals can break up a partnership in order to seek a more cooperative partner if their current partner is not cooperative. Whether they do so depends crucially on the variation in cooperation within the population. If future partners are all similar to the current one it is better to stick with the current partner and avoid the costs of seeking a new one, but if there is sufficient variation there are likely to be better partners and it is worth paying the cost of search. When this happens, uncooperative individuals lose their partners and must also pay the cost of seeking a new partner. Thus uncooperative individuals do badly and there will be selection for increased cooperation – so again increased variation leads to the evolution of cooperation. Note that markets of this sort tend to produce a non-random association of players even if they meet at random.

In deciding how to interact with another individual it may be possible to gain useful information on this individual by observing his or her past behaviour. However, observations waste time and energy, and so are likely to be costly. Thus if all individuals are similar it is not worth paying this cost because there is little to learn. In contrast, once there is sufficiently high variance in the trait of interest, it will be worth observing. Thus variation selects for social sensitivity. Once population members are socially sensitive this changes the selection pressure within the population: for example, individuals that are observed to be uncooperative with others may be shunned and will hence do worse.

Flexibility, personality and a complex world

Animals have to deal with a complex world. To do so they have rules of thumb which perform well on average, but are not optimal in every situation. The behavioural rule of thumb used by an individual is implemented via psychological mechanisms such as emotions and motivational states. Because of the variation that always exists in a population, different individuals are liable to have rules that are adjusted slightly differently.

Furthermore, because animals following these rules are not completely flexible, individuals will display certain predictabilities in their behaviour. In other words, different individuals will have different personalities. These non-adaptive aspects of personality pose a challenge to evolutionary game theory. They mean that the idea of subgame perfection – i.e. animals always do the best given their current situation – must be abandoned. Now, instead, previous behaviour is indicative of current behaviour, leading to the establishment of reputation and generating the need for social sensitivity, as mentioned above.

Acknowledgements

This chapter was written when JMM was Tage Erlander Guest Professor at Gothenburg University.

Suggested readings

Diekmann, O. (2004) A beginner's guide to adaptive dynamics. *Banach Center Publications*, **63**, 47–86.

Gintis, H. (2000) *Game Theory Evolving: A Problem-Centered Introduction to Modeling Strategic Interaction*. Princeton, NJ: Princeton University Press.

Houston, A. I. & McNamara, J. M. (1999) *Models of Adaptive Behaviour: An Approach Based on State*. Cambridge: Cambridge University Press.

Reeve, H. K. & Dugatkin, L. A., eds (1998) *Game Theory and Animal Behavior*. Oxford: Oxford University Press.

van Doorn, G. S., Hengeveld, G. M. & Weissing, F. J. (2003) The evolution of social dominance. *Behaviour*, **140**, 1305–1332, 1333–1358.

References

Andersson, M. (1994) *Sexual Selection*. Princeton, NJ: Princeton University Press.

Axelrod, R. & Hamilton, W. D. (1981) The evolution of cooperation. *Science*, **211**, 1390–1396.

Ayala, F. J. & Campbell, C. A. (1974) Frequency-dependent selection. *Annual Review of Ecology and Systematics*, **5**, 115–138.

Barta, Z., Houston, A. I., McNamara, J. M. & Székely, T. (2002) Sexual conflict about parental care: the role of reserves. *American Naturalist*, **159**, 687–705.

Brams, S. (1983) *Superior Beings*. New York, NY: Springer.

Caswell, H. (2001) *Matrix Population Models*, 2nd edn. Sunderland, MA: Sinauer Associates.

Cressman, R., Hofbauer, J. & Hines, W. G. S. (1996) Evolutionary stability in strategic models of single-locus frequency-dependent viability selection. *Journal of Mathematical Biology*, **34**, 707–733.

Crowley, P. H. (2001) Dangerous games and the emergence of social structure: evolving memory-based strategies for the generalized hawk–dove game. *Behavioral Ecology*, **12**, 753–760.

Day, T. (2005) Modeling the ecological context of evolutionary change: déjà vu or something new? In: *Paradigms Lost: Routes to Theory Change*, ed. K. Cuddington & B. E. Beisner. New York, NY: Academic Press, pp. 273–309.

Diekmann, O. (2004) A beginner's guide to adaptive dynamics. *Banach Center Publications*, **63**, 47–86.

Dieckmann, U. & Doebeli, M. (1999) On the origin of species by sympatric speciation. *Nature*, **400**, 354–357.

Dieckmann, U. & Law, R. (1996) The dynamical theory of coevolution: A derivation from stochastic ecological processes. *Journal of Mathematical Biology*, **34**, 579–612.

Elster, J. (2000) *Ulysses Unbound*. Cambridge: Cambridge University Press.

Eshel, I. (1983) Evolutionary and continuous stability. *Journal of Theoretical Biology*, **103**, 99–111.

Fisher, R. A. (1930) *The Genetical Theory of Natural Selection*. Oxford: Clarendon Press.

Frank, S. A. & Swingland, I. R. (1988) Sex ratio under conditional sex expression. *Journal of Theoretical Biology*, **135**, 415–418.

Galis F. & Metz J. A. J. (2007) Evolutionary novelties: the making and breaking of pleiotropic constraints. *Integrative and Comparative Biology*, **47**, 409–419.

Geritz, S. A. H., Kisdi, E., Meszena, G. & Metz, J. A. J. (1998) Evolutionarily singular strategies and the adaptive growth and branching of the evolutionary tree. *Evolutionary Ecology*, **12**, 35–57.

Gintis, H. (2000) *Game Theory Evolving: A Problem-Centered Introduction to Modeling Strategic Interaction*. Princeton, NJ: Princeton University Press.

Grafen, A. (2006) A theory of Fisher's reproductive value. *Journal of Mathematical Biology*, **53**, 15–60.

Hamblin, S. & Hurd, P. L. (2007) Genetic algorithms and non-ESS solutions to game theory models. *Animal Behaviour*, **74**, 1005–1018.

Hammerstein, P. (1996) Darwinian adaptation, population genetics and the streetcar theory of evolution. *Journal of Mathematical Biology*, **34**, 511–532.

Hammerstein, P. & Selten, R. (1994) Game theory and evolutionary biology. In: *Handbook of Game Theory with Economic Applications*, ed. R. J. Aumann & S. Hart. Amsterdam: Elsevier, Vol. 2, pp. 929–993.

Hardin, G. (1968) The tragedy of the commons. *Science*, **162**, 1243–1248.

Heino, M., Metz, J. A. J. & Kaitala V. (1998) The enigma of frequency-dependent selection. *Trends in Ecology and Evolution*, **13**, 367–370.

Houston, A. I. & Davies, N. B. (1985) Evolution of cooperation and life history in dunnocks. In: *Behavioural Ecology: the Ecological Consequences of Adaptive Behaviour*, ed. R. Sibly & R. H. Smith. Oxford: Blackwell, pp. 471–487.

Houston, A. I. & McNamara, J. M. (1991) Evolutionarily stable strategies in the repeated hawk–dove game. *Behavioral Ecology*, **2**, 219–227.

Leimar, O. (2001) Evolutionary change and Darwinian demons. *Selection*, **2**, 65–72.

Luce, R. D. & Raiffa, H. (1957) *Games and Decisions*. New York, NY: Wiley.

Maynard Smith, J. (1977) Parental investment: a prospective analysis. *Animal Behaviour*, **25**, 1–9.

Maynard Smith, J. (1982) *Evolution and the Theory of Games*. Cambridge: Cambridge University Press.

Maynard Smith, J. & Parker, G. A. (1976) The logic of asymmetric contests. *Animal Behaviour*, **24**, 159–177.

Maynard Smith, J. & Price, G. R. (1973) The logic of animal conflict. *Nature*, **246**, 15–18.

McGill, B. J. & Brown, J. S. (2007) Evolutionary game theory and adaptive dynamics of continuous traits. *Annual Review of Ecology, Evolution and Systematics*, **38**, 403–435.

McNamara, J. M. (1993) Evolutionary paths in strategy space: an improvement algorithm for life-history strategies. *Journal of Theoretical Biology*, **161**, 23–37.

McNamara, J. M. & Houston, A. I. (1996) State dependent life histories. *Nature*, **380**, 215–221.

McNamara, J. M. & Houston, A. I. (2002) Credible threats and promises. *Philosophical Transactions of the Royal Society B*, **357**, 1607–1616.

McNamara, J. M., Webb, J. N., Collins, E. J., Székely, T. & Houston A. I. (1997) A general technique for computing evolutionarily stable strategies based on errors in decision-making. *Journal of Theoretical Biology*, **189**, 211–225.

McNamara, J. M., Gasson, C. E. & Houston, A. I. (1999) Incorporating rules for responding into evolutionary games. *Nature*, **401**, 368–371.

McNamara, J. M., Barta, Z. & Houston, A. I. (2004) Variation in behaviour promotes cooperation in the prisoner's dilemma game. *Nature*, **428**, 745–748.

McNamara, J. M., Wilson, E. & Houston, A. I. (2006) Is it better to give information, receive it or be ignorant in a two-player game? *Behavioral Ecology*, **17**, 441–451.

McNamara, J. M., Barta, Z., Fromhage, L. & Houston, A. I. (2008) The coevolution of choosiness and cooperation. *Nature*, **451**, 189–192.

Metz, J. A. J., Nisbet, R. M. & Geritz, S. A. H. (1992) How should we define 'fitness' for general ecological scenarios? *Trends in Ecology and Evolution*, **7**, 198–202.

Moran, P. A. P. (1964) On the nonexistence of adaptive topographies. *Annals of Human Genetics*, **27**, 338–343.

Mylius, S. D. & Diekmann (1995) On evolutionarily stable life histories, optimization and the need to be specific about density dependence. *Oikos*, **74**, 218–224.

Nagylaki, T., Hofbauer J. & Brunovský, P. (1999) Convergence of multilocus systems under weak epistasis or weak selection. *Journal of Mathematical Biology*, **38**, 103–133.

Nash, J. (1950) Equilibrium points in *n*-person games. *Proceedings of the National Academy of Sciences of the USA*, **36**, 48–49.

Pen, I. & Taylor, P. D. (2005) Modelling information exchange in worker-queen conflict over sex allocation. *Proceedings of the Royal Society B*, **272**, 2403–2408.

Pen, I. & Weissing, F. J. (2000) Towards a unified theory of cooperative breeding: the role of ecology and life history re-examined. *Proceedings of the Royal Society B*, **267**, 2411–2418.

Pen, I. & Weissing, F. J. (2002) Optimal sex allocation: steps towards a mechanistic theory. In: *Sex Ratios: Concepts and Research Methods*, ed. I. C. W. Hardy. Cambridge: Cambridge University Press, pp. 26–45.

Pen, I., Daan, S. & Weissing, F. J. (1999) Seasonal sex ratio trend in the European kestrel: an evolutionarily stable strategy analysis. *American Naturalist*, **153**, 384–397.

Persky, J. (1995) Retrospectives: the ethology of *Homo economicus*. *Journal of Economic Perspectives*, **9**, 221–231.

Reeve, H. K. & Dugatkin, L. A., eds. (1998) *Game Theory and Animal Behavior*. Oxford: Oxford University Press.

Schelling, T. C. (1960) *The Strategy of Conflict*. Cambridge, MA: Harvard University Press.

Seger, J. & Stubblefield, J. W. (2002) Models of sex ratio evolution. In: *Sex Ratios: Concepts and Research Methods*, ed. I. C. W. Hardy. Cambridge: Cambridge University Press, pp. 1–25.

Selten, R. (1980) A note on evolutionarily stable strategies in asymmetric animal conflicts. *Journal of Theoretical Biology*, **84**, 93–101.

Selten, R. (1983) Evolutionary stability in extensive two-person games. *Mathematical Social Sciences*, **5**, 269–363.

Spence, A. M. (1973) Job market signaling. *Quarterly Journal of Economics*, **87**, 355–374.

Taper, M. L. & Case, T. J. (1992) Models of character displacement and the theoretical robustness of taxon cycles. *Evolution*, **46**, 317–333.

Taylor, P. D. (1996) Inclusive fitness arguments in genetic models of behaviour. *Journal of Mathematical Biology*, **34**, 654–674.

Taylor, P. D. & Frank S. A. (1996) How to make a kin selection model. *Journal of Theoretical Biology*, **180**, 27–37.

Trivers, R. L. (1985) *Social Evolution*. Menlo Park, CA: Benjamin/Cummings.

Trivers, R. L. & Willard, D. E. (1973) Natural selection on parental ability to vary the sex ratio of offspring. *Science*, **179**, 90–92.

van Boven, M. & Weissing, F. J. (2004) The evolutionary economics of immunity. *American Naturalist*, **163**, 277–294.

van Damme, E. (1987) *Stability and Perfection of Nash Equilibria*. Berlin: Springer-Verlag.

van Doorn, G. S. & Dieckmann, U. (2006) The long-term evolution of multilocus traits under frequency-dependent disruptive selection. *Evolution*, **60**, 2226–2238.

van Doorn, G. S. & Weissing, F. J. (2006) Sexual conflict and the evolution of female preferences for indicators of male quality. *American Naturalist*, **168**, 743–757.

van Doorn, G. S., Hengeveld, G. M. & Weissing, F. J. (2003a) The evolution of social dominance. I. Two-player models. *Behaviour*, **140**, 1305–1332.

van Doorn, G. S., Hengeveld, G. M. & Weissing, F. J. (2003b) The evolution of social dominance. II. Multi-player models. *Behaviour*, **140**, 1333–1358.

van Doorn, G. S., Dieckmann, U. & Weissing, F. J. (2004) Sympatric speciation by sexual selection: a critical re-evaluation. *American Naturalist*, **163**, 709–725.

von Neumann, J. & Morgenstern, O. (1944) *Theory of Games and Economic Behaviour*. Princeton, NJ: Princeton University Press.

Webb, J. N., Houston, A. I., McNamara, J. M. & Székely, T. (1999) Multiple patterns of parental care. *Animal Behaviour*, **58**, 983–999.

Weissing, F. J. (1996) Genetic versus phenotypic models of selection: can genetics be neglected in a long-term perspective? *Journal of Mathematical Biology*, **34**, 533–555.

Wolf, M., van Doorn, G. S., Leimar, O. & Weissing, F. J. (2008) Do animal personalities emerge? *Nature*, **451**, E9–10.

Wright, S. (1932) The roles of mutation, inbreeding, crossbreeding, and selection in evolution. *Proceedings of the Sixth International Congress of Genetics*, pp. 355–366.

Zahavi, A. & Zahavi, A. (1997) *The Handicap Principle: a Missing Piece of Darwin's Puzzle*. Oxford: Oxford University Press.

The huddler's dilemma: a cold shoulder or a warm inner glow

David Haig

My interest in huddling was aroused by the discovery that *GNAS*, the locus that encodes the G protein α stimulatory subunit (Gαs), was preferentially expressed from its maternally derived allele in brown adipose tissue of mice (Haig 2004). Since then, additional imprinted genes have been identified with effects on the recruitment and function of brown adipocytes (Haig 2008). The observation that multiple imprinted genes are expressed in brown fat – the principal site of facultative thermogenesis in young mammals – suggests that genetic conflicts over heat transfers among relatives have been a significant selective force in mammalian evolution.

Huddling together for warmth is a simple and widespread cooperative behaviour of inactive birds and mammals (Hill 1992, Forbes 2007). Huddling reduces heat loss from animals that are warmer than their environment by reducing each individual's exposed surface. Moreover, a group can raise the temperature of an enclosed space more effectively than can an individual acting alone. Savings may be substantial. For example, a 10-day-old rat pup in a group of eight consumes 37% less oxygen at 28 °C than an equivalent solitary pup (Alberts 1978).

The fuel consumed by thermogenesis is a direct personal cost to the individual generating heat, but others share in the benefit. Contributors are therefore vulnerable to exploitation by individuals who skimp on their share of the heating bill. If it pays one individual to reduce heating costs, it may pay others to do likewise, even though all would be better off by maintaining a higher body temperature (the huddler's dilemma). Heat is a public good when animals huddle, and public goods tend to be undersupplied at equilibrium, with the degree of underprovision determined by the precise balance of costs and benefits.

The temptation to defect will be particularly strong when huddlemates compete for limited resources, because individuals who contribute less to communal heating may gain a competitive advantage over individuals who contribute more. Thus, nursing pups who expend more energy than their littermates on thermogenesis may pay an additional cost of less milk obtained from their mother (poor suckers!).

Pups should reduce facultative thermogenesis in the presence of a brooding mother, and allow themselves to be passively warmed. The maternal heat source allows a pup to dedicate a greater proportion of its milk intake to growth. Why should a mother brood? The costs of keeping offspring warm are ultimately borne by the mother – whether this is via brooding or via offspring 'burning' milk – but time spent brooding means less time spent

Social Behaviour: Genes, Ecology and Evolution, ed. Tamás Székely, Allen J. Moore and Jan Komdeur. Published by Cambridge University Press. © Cambridge University Press 2010.

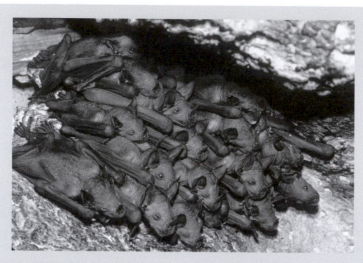

A huddling creche of greater spear-nosed bat *Phyllostomus hastatus* pups, Trinidad. Photo: Gerald S. Wilkinson.

foraging. Mothers may brood, despite this foraging cost, because offspring cannot be relied on to maintain themselves at an optimal temperature for development. Brooding by mothers avoids the huddler's dilemma, because the cost of heating is borne by a single individual who is equally related to all offspring.

Newborn altricial mammals often fail to maintain a stable body temperature in experimental settings, even though they have considerable thermogenic capacity. Thermoregulatory altriciality is often portrayed as the retention of a primitive trait, but it is probably better viewed as an adaptation whereby offspring defer the costs of staying warm to their mother while she is present in the nest (Hill 1992), and as an evolutionary response to the cruel logic of the huddler's dilemma.

The thermolability of altricial offspring is exacerbated by their lack of fur or feathers. Insulation makes adaptive sense only if individuals generate their own heat, whereas nakedness facilitates heat transfer between animals with different surface temperatures. The unfeathered incubation patch of brooding birds, and the naked skin of altricial chicks, allow parents to donate heat to offspring more effectively. Similarly, altricial mammals may have lost their fur as an adaptation

for acquiring warmth from mothers and sibs (Webb *et al*. 1990).

Many intriguing questions are raised once one starts to view thermogenesis within huddles as a problem in the evolution of cooperation. I will mention just two. Piglets huddle for warmth but compete intensely for milk (Mount 1960, Fraser & Thompson 1991). Does the huddler's dilemma explain why pigs have lost the uncoupling protein responsible for non-shivering thermogenesis (Berg *et al*. 2006)? Naked mole-rats have poor insulation and labile body temperatures, but high thermogenic capacity (Hislop & Buffenstein 1994, Daly & Buffenstein 1998). Who warms who (and when) within a mole-rat colony?

References

Alberts, J. R. (1978) Huddling by rat pups: group behavioral mechanisms of temperature regulation and energy conservation. *Journal of Comparative and Physiological Psychology*, **92**, 231–245.

Berg, F., Gustafson, U. & Andersson, L. (2006) The uncoupling protein 1 gene (*UCP1*) is disrupted in the pig lineage: a genetic explanation for poor thermoregulation in piglets. *PLoS Genetics*, **2** (8), e129.

Daly, T. J. M. & Buffenstein, R. (1998) Skin morphology and its role in thermoregulation in mole-rats,

Heterocephalus glaber and *Cryptomys hottentotus*. *Journal of Anatomy*, **193**, 495–502.

Forbes, S. (2007) Sibling symbiosis in nestling birds. *Auk*, **124**, 1–10.

Fraser, D. & Thompson, B. K. (1991) Armed sibling rivalry among suckling pigs. *Behavioral Ecology and Sociobiology*, **29**, 9–15.

Haig, D. (2004) Genomic imprinting and kinship: how good is the evidence? *Annual Review of Genetics*, **38**, 553–585.

Haig, D. (2008) Huddling: brown fat, genomic imprinting, and the warm inner glow. *Current Biology*, **18**, R172–174.

Hill, R. W. (1992) The altricial/precocial contrast in the thermal relations and energetics of small mammals.

In: *Mammalian Energetics*, ed. T. M. Tomasi & T. H. Horton Ithaca, NY: Comstock, pp. 122–159.

Hislop, M. S. & Buffenstein, R. (1994) Noradrenaline induces nonshivering thermogenesis in both the naked mole-rat (Heterocephalus glaber) and the Damara mole-rat (*Cryptomys damarensis*) despite their very different modes of thermoregulation. *Journal of Thermal Biology*, **19**, 25–32.

Mount, L. E. (1960) The influence of huddling and body size on the metabolic rate of the young pig. *Journal of Agricultural Science*, **55**, 101–105.

Webb, D. R., Fullenwider, J. L., McClure, P. A., Profeta, L. & Long, J. (1990) Geometry of maternal–offspring contact in two rodents. *Physiological Zoology*, **63**, 821–844.

5

Recent advances in comparative methods

Robert P. Freckleton and Mark Pagel

Overview

The comparative method is one of the oldest and most widely used approaches to studying evolution. The rationale is that a group of species contains more variation than can be created in an experiment or using observations on a single species, and comparisons across species can be used to test broad questions in evolutionary theory. One of the key issues in comparative analysis is the problem of phylogeny. Phylogeny can create problems through generating non-independence of data, which compromises statistical tests, but it also generates opportunity by allowing the evolution of traits to be mapped. The modern comparative method is based on modelling the evolutionary process, using models of trait evolution to generate statistical models that can fitted to trait data.

We review a range of the current models and techniques used in comparative analysis. We begin by looking at techniques for modelling continuous traits, concentrating on methods for measuring variation in the rate of evolution through time, speciational modes of evolution, constraints on traits and variable levels of phylogenetic dependence. We then look at issues of uncertainty in data and how this may be incorporated, including uncertainty resulting from phylogenetic error, measurement error and other forms of non-independence. Developments on the analysis of discrete traits are described, including the use of modern Bayesian model averaging and selection methods. Finally we describe how the links between macroevolution (speciation and extinction) and trait evolution can be uncovered.

5.1 Introduction

In evolutionary biology the most natural way to ask whether a given feature of an organism is an evolutionary adaptation is via comparison with other species. For instance, we may ask whether species with similar lifestyles possess the same adaptation, or whether all those species with a given trait have the same ecological niche. The comparative approach to studying evolution is one of the oldest and most intuitive. Indeed, comparative studies pre-date the rise of evolutionary theory with the first formal comparative study being one on mammals by Tyson in 1699 in which he used a comparison of brain structure to show that chimpanzees

Social Behaviour: Genes, Ecology and Evolution, ed. Tamás Székely, Allen J. Moore and Jan Komdeur. Published by Cambridge University Press. © Cambridge University Press 2010.

and humans were more similar to each other than to monkeys, as well as comparing the form and lifestyle of different races of humans. Since that time comparative analysis has been used both to look at the evolutionary history of groups and to ask how their adaptations meet the needs of the world in which they live.

More recently, the comparative approach has been an important tool in social and behavioural ecology. The advantage of using a comparative approach is that comparative analyses often allow much broader questions about adaptations to be asked than can be addressed using, for instance, experimental methods. Thus, a group of species contains a greater range of variation in life history, behaviour and social organisation than can be found or generated in a single species, and comparative analysis of a group can therefore offer more wide-ranging tests of evolutionary theory.

The comparative approach used today has developed in parallel with advances in genetic technology and the methodology for analysing such data to generate phylogenetic trees (e.g. Harvey 1996). The key developments in the phylogenetic literature in the past 10 years are twofold. First, a suite of methods for modelling genetic data have been developed (Page & Holmes 2000, Felsenstein 2004, Yang 2006). Second has been the adoption of Bayesian statistical methodology. Using this approach, it is possible to specify prior distributions (essentially guesses at the parameter values and variances) for the model parameters, then techniques such as Markov-chain Monte Carlo can be used to generate a distribution of parameter estimates that correspond to the Bayesian posterior, equivalent to generating a distribution of values that form some kind of 'credible' set. Bayesian methods have become commonplace in a range of areas of statistics, not just in phylogenetics. Their rise in popularity probably reflects an appreciation of their computational advantages, rather than a wide-scale conversion of statisticians and scientists to the Bayesian paradigm (e.g. Pawitan 2001).

Recent developments in comparative analysis have tracked developments in the phylogenetic literature. In essence these boil down to an increasing interest in understanding the predictions that different models make about comparative data, as well as comparative

biologists beginning to take a closer look at the techniques being used in phylogenetic analysis. For comparative biologists one of the most important consequences of the Bayesian revolution in phylogenetics is that the output of a Bayesian analysis is not a single phylogenetic tree, but is instead a distribution of trees. Different topologies are treated as alternative models, and the branch lengths (i.e. the times since evolutionary branching events occurred) of trees as individual parameters. The output of the analysis is a distribution of topologies and branch lengths. Most comparative analysis has been conducted on single phylogenies, although there are exceptions (e.g. Huelsenbeck *et al.* 2000, Lutzoni *et al.* 2001). This is an area that comparative methodology has only recently begun to embrace.

The modern comparative approach has been reviewed a number of times over the years (e.g. Harvey & Pagel 1991, Martins & Hansen 1996, Pagel 1997, 1999, Brooks & McLennan 2002, Pagel & Lutzoni 2002, Freckleton *et al.* 2003, Paradis 2006). In this chapter we do not propose to go over this ground again; rather we focus on recent developments, in the main concentrating on developments in the past 10 years and methods with which we are most familiar. We begin by looking at the methods and models available for modelling evolution in continuous trait data. We then go on to look at how new Bayesian methods can be applied to understand the evolution of discrete traits. Finally, we give an overview of recent methods for the comparative analysis of macroevolutionary patterns.

5.2 Comparative analysis of continuous data

The analysis of continuous trait data is probably the most common form of comparative analysis in the social and behavioural literature, and the method of independent contrasts (Felsenstein 1985) is the most frequently used method. The main driver of the development of this and other methods was the realisation that if species values are treated as being statistically independent then statistical analyses would likely be invalid, as species values show similarity owing to shared phylogenetic history (Harvey & Pagel 1991,

Martins & Garland 1991). Despite debates (e.g. Westoby *et al.* 1995, Harvey *et al.* 1995, Ricklefs & Starck 1996), the overwhelming majority of comparative studies use this approach.

The method of contrasts is based on a rather simple model for trait evolution, the Brownian model (Felsenstein 1973, 1985). This model makes basic assumptions about how traits evolve: traits are assumed to accrue variance continuously, with at any point in time increases or decreases in trait values being equally as likely. Furthermore, traits of different species are assumed to evolve independently. Although these assumptions are statistically convenient, such a simple model may not reflect the complex suite of processes that may be operating to shape trait evolution.

This section is organised into three parts: we begin with an outline of the state of the art in modelling traits. We then outline some alternative models and their formulation, and review evidence that such models may be warranted. Finally we look at the most

recent developments, particularly how phylogenetic uncertainty may be incorporated in studies of social behaviour.

5.2.1 Modelling continuous traits: GLS methods

The method of contrasts was initially designed to measure the correlation between a pair of continuous traits. This is analogous to fitting a regression (or correlation) in conventional non-phylogenetic analysis. In fact, it is straightforward to show that the correlation or regression slope estimated by the method of contrasts is exactly the same as would be obtained by fitting a linear regression that assumes that the residual variation is described by a particular model (Pagel 1993; Box 5.1). This is known as a generalised least squares (GLS) model (see Pagel 1997, 1999, Martins & Hansen 1997), and the method of contrasts is a computationally simple way of fitting such a model (Box 5.1; Pagel 1993, Garland *et al.* 1999).

Box 5.1 Formulation of generalised least squares (GLS) models, derivation of the variance–covariance matrix, and relationship to phylogenetically independent contrasts

The model

The basis for the approach is a simple linear model in which one trait (denoted by a vector **Y**) is modelled as a function of a set of predictors (denoted by a matrix **X**) in the following way:

$$\mathbf{Y} = \mathbf{bX} + \mathbf{E} \tag{5.1}$$

in which **b** is a list of parameter estimates, and **E** is a vector representing the error term. This is the same form as the classic linear model. In a non-phylogenetic analysis the errors are assumed to be independently normally distributed with mean of zero. In a phylogenetic analysis the errors are assumed to be correlated. This correlation is described by a variance–covariance matrix which describes the amount of similarity between species resulting from common ancestry.

Brownian variance–covariance matrix

It assumed that characters evolve according to a constant variance ('Brownian') process. Given this model of evolution, the expected variance in character state of a species is directly proportional to the time that it has evolved, whilst the covariance in character states between a pair of species is directly proportional to the amount of shared common ancestry. Consider the phylogeny below onto which the states of two characters (*X* and *Y*) have been mapped, and the variance–covariance matrix (**V**) it implies:

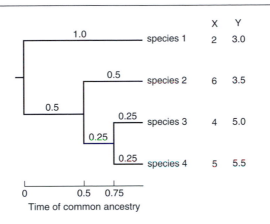

The entries of **V** are calculated as the length of time during which species coevolved until splitting. For species 1, which has evolved independently since the root of the phylogeny, the off-diagonal elements are set to zero. Species 3 and 4 shared common ancestry with species 2 for 0.5 time units, hence elements $t_{2,3}$, $t_{3,2}$, $t_{2,4}$, and $t_{2,4}$ are set to 0.5. Species 3 and 4 shared common ancestry for 0.75 time units, and elements $t_{4,3}$ and $t_{3,4}$ are set to 0.75.

Relation to independent contrasts

Given the linear model above and the assumption that traits evolve according to a Brownian model, it is straightforward to solve mathematically to generate estimates of the parameters **b**. Technically the problem with doing so is that the matrix **V** has to be inverted, which can be computationally time-consuming and mathematically numerically inaccurate. Independent contrasts were introduced by Felsenstein (1973) to enable fast and numerically accurate calculations of likelihoods in such models, and the relationship between the two is straightforward. For instance, in the case of a single trait the log-likelihood is:

$$L\left[\mu,\sigma^2,\phi\right] = -\frac{1}{2}\left(n\log\left(2\pi\sigma^2\right) + \log|\mathbf{V}| \right.$$
$$\left. + \frac{\left(\mathbf{x}-\mu\mathbf{X}\right)^T \mathbf{V}^{-1}\left(\mathbf{x}-\mu\mathbf{X}\right)}{\sigma^2} \right) \tag{5.2}$$

where μ and σ^2 are the mean and variance.

This is exactly equal to:

$$L = -\frac{1}{2}\left(n\log\left(2\pi\sigma^2\right) + \sum_{i=0}^{n}\left[\log V_i + \frac{u_i^2}{V_i\sigma^2} \right] \right) \tag{5.3}$$

where u is an unstandardised contrast and V is its variance, calculated according to the algorithm in Felsenstein (1985).

It is straightforward to extend this to the general case of a GLS model, including multiple predictors that are continuous and/or categorical in order to generate the likelihood. It is simple also to solve for the maximum likelihood using the equations for the phylogenetic contrasts.

Although the method of contrasts is a special case of GLS, there are numerous advantages to using the latter. The first is that in a GLS framework it is possible to combine continuous and categorical predictors very readily. Using contrasts this is, at best, a kludge using existing software. Second, the GLS framework is very well understood and supported statistically, so that a range of diagnostics and tools exist for analysing output from models, including analysis of variance, transformations, parameter estimates and residual diagnostics (Grafen & Hails 2004). Finally, the output from a GLS model differs in no way from a more conventional least squares regression or ANOVA, so no special reporting is required, making the results transparent and easy to interpret.

GLS methods are conventionally based on the Brownian model for trait evolution. In a regression context the assumption is that the residuals from the fitted model are distributed like a trait that has evolved according to this model. This is therefore a potential limitation of the GLS method (and of course the same is true of independent contrasts). Of course, in one respect the model fitted may be rather complex: for instance, if a trait has been modelled as a function of a set of predictors, plus this phylogenetic residual term, the overall model for trait variation may look quite complex.

A useful extension of the GLS framework is the generalised estimating equation. This is again a statistically well-developed method that was introduced for phylogenetic analysis by Paradis and Claude (2002). This method is potentially very useful, as it allows more complex assumptions about trait variance to be made, including assumptions about the distribution of the error term.

5.2.2 Alternative models

In the method of contrasts and the GLS model, the underlying model for trait evolution is the Brownian model, which assumes that variance accrues as a linear function of time, that the rate of evolution is constant, and that positive and negative changes in traits are equally likely. One approach to modelling traits is to make simple changes to these assumptions. Here we review some of the suggested modifications.

One framework was suggested by Pagel (1997, 1999), based on modelling variation in the rate of evolution through time. This approach allows the rate of evolution to vary through time via the incorporation of three parameters, κ, δ and β. The first parameter, κ, allows the rate of trait evolution to vary along individual branches. In the model, branch lengths are raised to the power κ, with $\kappa = 1$ being identical to the Brownian model. Values of $\kappa > 1$ occur when evolution speeds up on longer branches, $\kappa < 1$ occurs when evolution is faster on smaller branches, and $\kappa = 0$ indicates speciational or punctuational evolution, whereby the rate of trait evolution is independent of branch lengths (see also Garland *et al*. 1992).

The second parameter, δ, models systematic changes in the rate of evolution through time, with node heights being raised to the power δ. Thus, $\delta = 1$ corresponds to the Brownian model, $\delta < 1$ corresponds to a progressive slow-down in the rate of evolution with time, and $\delta > 1$ indicates that evolution has speeded up. This parameter is useful, for instance, in diagnosing the systematic changes in rates of evolution, as may happen for instance in adaptive radiations.

The third parameter, β, models changes in the mean value of a trait across a clade. The Brownian model assumes that across species the mean value of a trait does not change through evolutionary time, but it would seem unlikely that this assumption is generally true. In point of fact, the statistical distribution of traits will often be unaffected by the inclusion of a drift parameter (Grafen 1989). This is the case when all tips of the phylogeny are contemporaneous, and the ultimate distribution of traits will be a multivariate normal distribution defined by the phylogeny. The signature of drift can only be detected when some of the tips of the phylogeny are not contemporaneous (i.e. if some of the species are fossils or extinct).

An alternative model for trait evolution was described by Hansen (1997), who first applied the Ornstein–Uhlenbeck (OU) model to comparative data. This model includes two parameters, μ, which is an evolutionary optimum and α, which measures the strength of selection and the rate at which species move to this optimum. According to this model, random fluctuations in the environment push species' traits away from μ, but stabilising selection forces species back. The process has been likened to species' traits being on an 'elastic band', the values of the traits being pulled back as they try to move away. This model can be further refined so that in a group of species each lineage has its own optimum (Butler & King 2004; see also Hansen *et al.* 2008).

The techniques described above are essentially evolutionary models, as they can be described in terms of modifications to the rate of evolution, and fitted models can be given an evolutionary interpretation if desired and used to test evolutionary theories. Often there will be no reason to prefer one model over another, or other factors such as error in the data or the phylogeny may be suspected to play a significant role in shaping the variation in the data. For such circumstances Pagel (1997, 1999) proposed a statistic λ, which is a very useful transformation for use in a range of applications. This statistic measures how well the Brownian model fits the data, and transforms the phylogeny and variance–covariance matrix to best fit the Brownian assumptions. This is achieved by altering the proportion of shared evolution implied by the phylogeny, equivalent to lengthening (or shortening) the terminal branches of the phylogeny, and can model a continuum of trait variation between strong phylogenetic dependence and phylogenetic independence. This approach was tested by Freckleton *et al.* (2002) and shown to perform well. The advantage of using this statistic is that it can be used within a GLS framework to fit linear models to data, and to correct for the precise level of phylogenetic dependence in data when performing comparative analysis, and it is used very commonly in this way.

Tests for phylogenetic dependence are particularly important when analysing social and behavioural traits, as such variables are frequently extremely labile. For example Blomberg *et al.* (2003) examined the degree of phylogenetic dependence in a suite of traits and found that social and behavioural traits exhibited low phylogenetic dependence, lower for instance than that observed in morphological data. This is arguably to be expected, as such traits should be less constrained than morphological ones. In such circumstances the λ statistic can be used to deal with variable levels of phylogenetic dependence in statistical tests.

It seems likely that in some groups some species will evolve at faster rates than others. For instance the rate of trait change may be faster in some clades, or species with particular characteristics may accumulate trait change faster than others. Thomas *et al.* (2006) introduced a statistic θ which measures differences in evolutionary rates (see also Collar *et al.* 2005). The approach works in the following way: the rate at which traits accrue variation in the Brownian model is measured by a parameter σ^2, which is the variance in the changes in trait value per unit time. For two groups of species, the value of θ is the amount by which the rate of accumulation of traits is faster or slower for one group relative to the other. Thomas *et al.* (2006) showed how this approach could be used to measure how life-history variables determined the rate of evolution of key traits in shorebirds (Fig. 5.1).

The models described above are all formulated as extensions to the Brownian model and basically involve simple transformations of the phylogeny. In one sense these models are Brownian models on a transformed scale. The advantage of formulating models in this way is twofold. First, the Brownian represents a null model against which the data can be compared. Second, the models can be very readily fitted by maximum-likelihood methods, and parameter estimates are readily generated (see Pagel 1997, 1999, Schluter *et al.* 1997, Freckleton *et al.* 2002, Butler & King 2004, Housworth *et al.* 2004 for details of how this may be done). It should be noted, however, that maximum-likelihood estimates are frequently biased (e.g. Edwards 1972), and this may well be the case for some of the parameters described above (see Figure 2 in Freckleton *et al.* 2002 for an example). This possibility should be checked carefully by simulation before applying the methods to data (for various approaches see Freckleton *et al.* 2002, 2008, Freckleton & Harvey 2006, Thomas *et al.* 2006, Freckleton & Jetz 2009).

The disadvantage of having the Brownian model as the basis for these models is that this model is a model of continuous trait change, and the modifications to it discussed so far are essentially phenomenological. These models, for instance, do not explicitly include behavioural, ecological or social factors in their formulation. An example of how such factors may be included, and

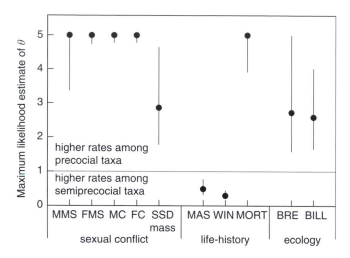

Figure 5.1 Measuring different evolutionary rates between groups of species. Thomas *et al.* (2006) examined how offspring development mode of the young (semi-precocial, i.e. fed by parents, vs. precocial, i.e. feed themselves) affected rates of evolution in a suite of traits in shorebirds. The statistic θ measures the rate in precocial species relative to semi-precocial ones. A suite of traits were tested: male and female mating system (MMS & FMS), male and female care of offspring (MC & FC), sexual size dimorphism (SSD), body mass (MAS), wing length (WIN), mortality (MORT), breeding habitat (BRE) and bill length (BILL). Shown are maximum likelihood estimates of θ, together with confidence intervals (adapted from Thomas 2004).

the possible consequences for comparative analysis, is a model by Price (1997). Price's model is one of an adaptive radiation in which traits are linked to niches. Each species is defined by a combination of a pair of traits which determine its niche. For instance, the two traits could be bill dimensions in a bird which determine which type of food (e.g. seed) that it feeds upon. According to the model, a species does not change its niche through time until a new niche arises: for instance, this could be because a new food source becomes available. When this happens the species evolves rapidly to exploit that resource, there is a divergence between the two clades exploiting the two resources, and speciation occurs. Even if simple assumptions are made about the distribution of traits (e.g. that they are distributed according to a bivariate normal distribution) the consequences of traits evolving in this way are complex. One consequence is that standard comparative methods do not perform well (Harvey & Rambaut 2000, Freckleton & Harvey 2006).

The model of Price (1997) was formulated as a model of non-Brownian trait evolution in an ecological context. However, it is entirely conceivable that such

processes could operate in social and behavioural evolution. At the heart of the model is a model of evolution where traits change at speciation, and trait change becomes more restricted as the number of species increases. Traits such as those involved in species recognition or sexual selection could easily be imagined to be subject to such a mode of trait evolution.

Indeed, it would not be surprising if the assumptions of the Brownian model were violated in the real world. Processes including variable rates of evolution, interactions between species and stabilising selection are expected to be commonplace and important. The only question is whether the data, phylogenies and statistical methods we have available to us are good enough to pick up such processes. Studies on a variety of traits from a range of species have shown clearly that the Brownian model is not sufficient on its own to describe many comparative datasets. Here we summarise some of the key results.

In the context of behavioural data, Blomberg *et al.* (2003) asked whether there was evidence that behavioural traits are more labile than non-behavioural ones. The hypothesis was that behaviour should be capable

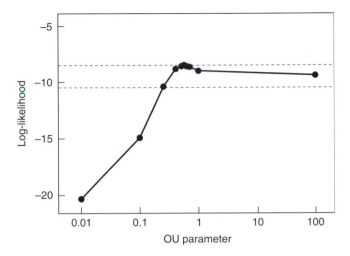

Figure 5.2 Example of fitting the Ornstein–Uhlenbeck (OU) model, adapted from Hansen (1997). The data are body size in horses; shown is the log-likelihood as a function of the OU control parameter α. The upper dashed line is the log-likelihood at the maximum likelihood estimate of α. The lower dashed line is the log-likelihood at which α differs from the maximum likelihood at the 5% level.

of evolving much faster than, for example, physiology or body parts. They found that this was indeed the case, although not explicitly considering a Brownian model, and that behavioural traits are indeed less conserved than the expectation.

Freckleton *et al.* (2002) used the λ-statistic of Pagel (1997, 1999) to ask how frequently traits used in comparative analyses of ecological data showed some degree of phylogenetic structure, and how closely this matched the Brownian model. That analysis showed that, to some degree, most traits showed phylogenetic signal. However, in most cases this signal was weaker than would be expected under the Brownian model, indicating that a modified model would better describe the data. In this vein, Hansen (1997) was the first to show such a deviation using the OU model (Fig. 5.2).

An extremely interesting comparison of evolutionary models was described by Webster & Purvis (2002). They analysed a dataset and phylogeny of extant and fossil foraminiferans. Because the dataset included both extant and fossil species, they were able to fit models using the data from extant species, then compared the predicted ancestral states with those of the fossil species in order to evaluate how good the fitted models were. The traits analysed were morphometric measures

of size and shape. The results showed that a more complex model (the Ornstein–Uhlenbeck model) predicted only a few per cent more of the variance in trait variation than the simpler Brownian model, and it seems likely that this additional explanatory power was simply the consequence of the OU model possessing an extra parameter.

As noted above, most methods work by transforming data to a Brownian scale. In order to determine whether or not the Brownian model is capable of describing data, Freckleton & Harvey (2006) developed a simple randomisation test. This test simply randomises estimated changes in trait states to generate randomised data, and asks whether randomised data and the real data have the same variance (or covariance for a pair of states). If data have evolved according to the Brownian model then this should be true, but if they have evolved according to some other process (particularly a process like the Price 1997 model), then simulated and randomised data will differ. It was found in one dataset analysed that the pattern of evolution was indeed not Brownian (despite the data showing strong phylogenetic signal), and that a process more akin to the Price model seemed likely to have generated the data. This approach is likely to yield evidence for non-Brownian trait evolution when analysing small groups of closely related species. In the context of behavioural and social data such tests could be used to look at whether key traits are tied to the diversification process.

5.2.3 Uncertainty

The models described above make a number of general assumptions about data and phylogenies. First, it is assumed that the phylogeny is known without error. Second, there is an assumption that the data are measured without error. And finally, there is an assumption that the main driver of trait variation is phylogenetically related trait variation, i.e. that rates of evolution are primarily a function of phylogenetic distance. In reality the data may violate one or more of these assumptions, and here we review how modifications to all three have been made.

It is only relatively recently that phylogenetic uncertainty has been accounted for formally in comparative analyses (Lutzoni *et al.* 2001, Pagel & Lutzoni 2002, Thomas & Székely 2005, Pagel *et al.* 2004, Pagel & Meade 2006). As noted above, the output of using Bayesian phylogenetic techniques is a distribution of phylogenetic trees. One simple way of dealing with phylogenetic uncertainty is to use this set of trees as the basis for the comparative analysis, rather than conduct the analysis on just a single tree. This approach has been taken, for example, by Huelsenbeck *et al.* (2000). The one downside of using this approach is that, although it takes phylogenetic uncertainty into account, it does not account for uncertainty in the parameters of the comparative model. Thus one set of parameters is estimated per phylogeny, although in a fully Bayesian analysis the parameters would also be random variables (Pagel *et al.* 2004, Pagel & Meade 2006; see Link & Barker 2006 for a discussion of this in an ecological setting). The latter approach has also been implemented by Organ *et al.* (2007) in a regression setting. Software implementing the Bayesian approach to the GLS model that these authors used is available from www.evolution.rdg.ac.uk.

Most comparative analyses use a single value for each species. This ignores the fact that species can be intraspecifically extremely variable, or that species'

values are estimates which may be subject to error. This is important in two respects: first, error in a trait erodes the signal from the phylogeny; second, in linear models errors in the predictors can lead to problems with regression analyses. Several approaches to this have been taken. For example, Martins and Hansen (1996) suggest how the GLS method may be modified to include observation error in the data, and recently Garamszegi and Møller (2007) have applied this to comparative data. The λ statistic of Pagel should be a reasonable method when the errors are identically distributed across species. Felsenstein (2004) suggested the use of migration matrices to include intraspecific phylogenies within a multi-species comparative framework. More recently Ives *et al.* (2007) have developed several methods for including intraspecific variation within comparative analysis. Importantly, they point out that statistics based on data containing error in the predictors may well be biased, if error in the predictors is ignored owing to the statistical phenomenon of attenuation (see Freckleton in press for a discussion of this in the context of social and behavioural data).

In most comparative analyses it is recognised that non-independence of data may arise as a consequence of phylogenetic relatedness of species, and this is normally corrected for using methods like the ones described above. However, other sources of non-independence may exist, and they may go unrecognised. One potentially important source of non-independence results from spatial dependence: observations taken from two locations close together may be expected to be more similar because of environmental effects and physical constraints, and a huge literature exists on spatial analysis (see Haining 1990 for an overview). This is important because advances in geographical information systems (GIS) technology, as well as the collation of large geo-referenced datasets on species' distributions and traits (e.g. Davies *et al.* 2007, Orme *et al.* 2006, Jetz *et al.* 2007). In such datasets there may be a large element of trait variation that is generated not by phylogenetic effects but by spatial processes, and this can potentially be a large source of noise in data.

Recently Freckleton & Jetz (2009) have combined models for spatial and phylogenetic variation in comparative data. According to this method, trait variation is described by two variance–covariance matrices. The first is given by phylogenetic relatedness (as in Box 5.1). The second is a variance–covariance matrix based on geographic distances. The analysis works by measuring the contribution of one matrix relative to the other. It was found that for some traits, particularly relating to environmental tolerances and distributions, spatial effects were stronger than phylogenetic ones, showing that a combined approach to modelling such data is required. In the context of analysing social and behavioural data, the important contribution that an approach of this sort can make is to test the degree to which behavioural and social traits are shaped by the environment (space) versus historical factors (phylogeny).

5.3 Modelling the evolution of discrete traits

The evolution of continuous traits has proved reasonably straightforward to model, as the Brownian model is relatively easy to parameterise and modify. Depending on the form of analysis used, it is simple either to estimate ancestral states via weighted averaging, or to specify the expected distribution of traits at the tips. The evolution of discrete traits is somewhat more tricky to model, mainly because the evolutionary changes in the trait state have to be modelled. Maximum likelihood can be used (e.g. Pagel 1994), but this is time-consuming and for complex traits success cannot be guaranteed. Another approach is to employ parsimony (or some other heuristic method), then to use randomisation to put confidence intervals on rates of state change for hypothesis testing and comparative analysis (Reynolds *et al.* 2002). However, this is less satisfactory as it relies on a single reconstruction of the evolution of the trait to estimate rates of transition between states. Moreover, both approaches rely on a single phylogeny, whereas in reality the phylogeny will also be estimated with some error.

Comparative analysis of discrete traits is, for these reasons, ideally suited to analysis with Bayesian methods. To summarise, the problem is threefold: (1) the

parameters determining the rates of change between states have to be estimated, along with standard errors; (2) there is a range of possible models for the transitions between states (unless the trait is a binary trait); (3) there are potentially many trees across which to search.

To address this problem Pagel and Meade (2006) developed a method based on reversible jump Markov-chain Monte Carlo (RJMCMC). RJMCMC is a technique ideally suited for analysing data when there are a number of candidate models. To illustrate how the method works, consider the example of modelling the evolution of a pair of binary traits. Individually the two traits may be in either of two states (0 or 1), so that there are four possible co-states {0,1}, {1,1}, {1,0} and {0,0}. Figure 5.3a shows a general model for the transitions between the possible states. This model is defined by eight parameters measuring the rate of transition between states. These are denoted q_{ij}, the rate of transition from state i to state j.

The model shown in Figure 5.3a is a general case that covers a range of possible models. For instance, it could be assumed that all rate parameters are identical to each other, so that changes between states are all equally likely. In this case there would be just a single parameter to estimate. Or it could be assumed that the rates of change between states are different, but that forward and reverse changes are equally likely. In this case there would be four parameters to estimate, with $q_{ij} = q_{ji}$. For a general model of this sort there are a large number of possible simpler models (4140 in total) that describe a wide range of evolutionary possibilities (Pagel & Meade 2006). These include various forms of independent transitions between traits, as well as models in which transitions depend on the state of the traits. For example, in Figure 5.3a, if $q_{12} \neq q_{34}$ then that implies that the rate of transition of character 2 from 0 to 1 depends on whether character 1 is in state 0 or in state 1.

The method of Pagel & Meade (2006) is to move between different models in the model space by proposing new parameters and models, and asking whether these are an improvement over the current model. A new model is accepted if it improves the fit to data, or, if not, the new model is accepted with a

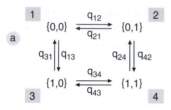

	from			
	1	2	3	4
1	-	4.9	3.7	-
2	4.2	-	-	2.3
3	0.0	-	-	0.1
4	-	4.6	3.5	-

to

Figure 5.3 Analysis of discrete traits using a Bayesian modelling approach (adapted from Pagel & Meade 2006). (a) A model for two discrete traits, each of which can exist in one of two states (1 or 0). The rate parameters (q) measure the transitions between states. (b) The model represented as a transition matrix. The numbers shown are estimates of rates for transitions between mating systems and oestrus in primates: 1, lack of oestrous advertisement and single-male mating system; 2, lack of oestrous advertisement and multi-male mating system; 3, oestrous advertisement and single-male mating system; 4, oestrous advertisement and multi-male mating system.

probability proportional to the ratio of its likelihood to that of the existing model. The proposal of new models is determined by algorithms that allow models of differing complexity to be included in the sampling (jumped between). By moving among models, the RJMCMC algorithm samples models in proportion to their posterior probabilities. To determine which models describe best the data, it is a simple matter to query this posterior sample.

As an example of social and behavioural evolution, Pagel & Meade (2006) analysed the evolution of two traits (oestrus displays and mating systems) in primates, and Figure 5.3b shows the estimated rate matrix. This analysis shows that changes from the ancestral state (lack of oestrous advertising and single-male mating system) to the derived co-state (oestrous advertising and multi-male mating system) occurred mainly through the intermediate state

of multi-male mating system without oestros advertising. The interpretation is that the mating system changed first, followed by changes in female display strategy.

The approach of Pagel and Meade (2006) has the advantage that it allows phylogenetic, model and parameter uncertainty to be simultaneously included, whilst extracting the signal for the data. A range of other applications could be envisaged, including more complex models and to test between specific classes of evolutionary models.

5.4 Macroevolution

In the majority of cases comparative analysis is used to ask what factors have shaped trait evolution for a given phylogeny of species. The phylogeny is regarded as fixed and trait variation is analysed upon it. Even if a distribution of phylogenetic trees is assumed, the assumption is that the data are conditional upon the tree. It is however entirely possible that the phylogeny is not fixed and independent of the traits, but that trait variation plays a role in shaping the phylogeny (see Chapter 19). The potential for such effects is well known: for example, key innovations have been hypothesised to account for the diversification of a range of groups (Mitter *et al.* 1988, Farrell *et al.* 1991, Marzaluff & Dial 1991, Barraclough *et al.* 1995, Parker & Partridge 1998, Owens *et al.* 1999, de Queiroz 2002, Ree 2005). However, to some extent theories for the diversification of groups as a consequence of key innovations can be based on ad hoc arguments and correlations (so-called story-telling, *sensu* Gould & Lewontin 1979). Recent years have seen the development of a variety of methods for measuring how closely species traits are related to tree structure. To simplify matters, we group these into two classes of test, the first analysing asymmetry and imbalance in the structure of trees, the second looking at rates of diversification. We concentrate here on how these can be used within a comparative framework. We realise of course that there are further methods for analysing and measuring diversification that we are not able to cover here; Ricklefs (2007) provides a useful review of some of these methods. The methods we discuss have largely been developed in the macroevolutionary literature during the last 10 years. We describe them here to highlight the existence of these approaches. In analysing social and behavioural data the methods we describe can be used to ask how groups of species evolve as a consequence of differences in their traits, so students of social behaviour could use these to ask how social and behavioural traits affect large-scale evolutionary processes.

5.4.1 Null model

The simplest models for the evolution of phylogenetic trees are the constant-birth model (also called the Yule model) in which lineages are added to an existing phylogeny at a constant rate b per lineage, or the birth–death model in which species also become extinct at a rate d per lineage. These are very simple models, and the techniques exist with which to analyse phylogenies and to fit these models to data.

Figure 5.4 shows examples of trees evolved according to the constant-birth model (Fig. 5.4a), and according to the birth–death model before (Fig. 5.4b) and after (Fig. 5.4c) pruning out the extinct lineages. According to the pure birth model the number of lineages increases exponentially with time, so that the majority of the nodes are concentrated near to the tips. In comparison, there are more deep nodes in the tree evolved according to the birth–death process. Notably, in the case of the birth–death model extinction of lineages eradicates much of the evolutionary history of the clade, such that there is little resemblance between the actual tree (Fig. 5.4b) and the observed tree of extant species (Fig. 5.4c). One consequence is that one should be cautious about inferring historical patterns and processes in phylogenies in which extinction rates are high (see Ricklefs 2007).

In terms of comparative data, the key element of these models is that any extant lineage is equally as likely as any other to give rise to a new lineage, or to become extinct. This results in phylogenies evolving according to this model having statistically predictable properties. These include predictable distributions of branch lengths, node ages and shapes of tree. Given this, it is possible to determine whether real

phylogenies show systematic deviation from these predictions. What is clear is that whenever tree shape and topology are examined, real phylogenies do not look like the Yule trees generated by constant-birth models.

5.4.2 Diversification rates

In a comparative analysis the obvious way to ask whether traits shape trees is to attempt to measure diversification rate and to link this to species traits. In one of the first papers to do this directly, Harmon *et al.* (2003) constructed lineages through time (LTT) plots and correlated the rate of accumulation of lineages in these with the rate of accumulation of trait variation. They compared these measures with the rate at which trait variation accrued randomly on the same phylogeny using data simulated according to a Brownian model. Their test then permits the degree of correspondence between the rate of accumulation of trait variation and the rate of accumulation of lineages to be estimated relative to a null model.

A more sophisticated approach was developed by Paradis (2005; see also Paradis 2008), who developed a model for phylogenetic tree growth based on the pure birth process in which the speciation parameter b is a direct function of a trait. Based on this simple model, Paradis developed a maximum-likelihood approach for estimating the speciation rate and its correlation with traits. This method is set within a regression modelling framework, thus permitting complex analyses of diversification. For instance, Paradis (2005) shows how the method can be used to relate diversification rate to body size in primates, and how this relationship varies between clades.

One of the problems with the method of Paradis (2005) is an apparent sensitivity to extinction rate, with the power of the approach suffering with increasing extinction rate. Freckleton *et al.* (2008) offer an alternative method which is a simple approach based on GLS. The latter method measures the speciation (or diversification) rate of a lineage as the number of nodes between the root and the tip. This measure is calculated for each lineage of the phylogeny, and these values are correlated with the values of a continuous

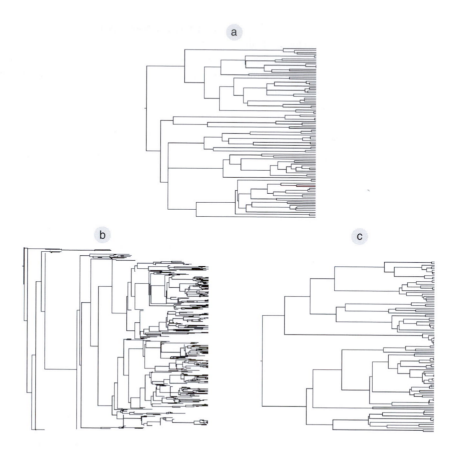

Figure 5.4 Examples of phylogenies simulated under different models of diversification. (a) A phylogeny simulated under a constant-birth model (i.e. with no extinction). (b) A phylogeny simulated under a birth–death process in which the death rate is 0.8 times the birth rate. (c) The same phylogeny as shown in (b), but with extinct species pruned out. In all three cases there are 100 extant tips.

trait (or even multiple traits). This method is simple and is readily implemented with existing statistical packages.

5.4.3 Evidence

What is the evidence that speciation and phylogenetic tree structure are linked to each other? Several studies cited above have shown strong correlates between diversification rates and species' traits. For example, in replicated radiations of *Anolis* lizards Harmon *et al.*

(2003) found that there is a close association between the rate at which trait variation accumulated and the rate at which lineages accumulate. At higher taxonomic levels Phillimore *et al.* (2006, 2007) found that family and subspecies richness in birds could be explained by ecological traits. At the species level, both Paradis (2005) and Freckleton *et al.* (2008) showed that the rate of diversification is linked to comparative traits including behavioural and social traits; for instance, Freckleton *et al.* (2008) found that group size was a significant predictor of diversification rate in primates (Fig. 5.5).

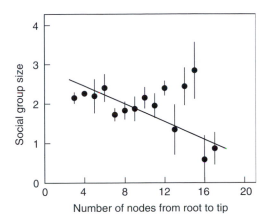

Figure 5.5 Speciation rate and group size in primates (adapted from Freckleton *et al.* 2008). Social group size is plotted against the number of nodes linking the root to the tip. The number of nodes from root to tip is an estimate of speciation rate. The regression shown (corrected for phylogeny) is statistically significant.

5.5 Conclusions and future directions

We have reviewed some of the most promising recent techniques for analysing comparative data in social and behavioural ecology. These can be used to examine the evolution of traits, how traits relate to the evolution of phylogenies, or simply to correct statistical tests for non-independence. Comparative methods are tracking changes in the techniques used to analyse phylogenetic data, and the next few years are likely to see an increase in the number of studies that simultaneously fit models for the phylogeny and for the evolution of traits. This will open up many avenues for studying social evolution and behaviour, as the techniques should permit the development and testing of more sophisticated evolutionary models. Equally, it should prove easier to link social and behavioural traits to macroecological and ecological data and hence to develop evolutionary theories that link ecology, evolution and behaviour more closely. There are of course limits to what can be achieved using a purely comparative approach, but these are exciting times in evolutionary biology – and we are only starting to consider what is possible using the data and methods that are becoming available.

Acknowledgements

RPF is funded by a Royal Society University Research Fellowship and by NERC (NE/C004167/1). MP acknowledges funding from NERC and the Leverhulme Trust.

Suggested readings

Freckleton, R. P. (2009) The seven deadly sins of comparative analysis. *Journal of Evolutionary Biology*, **22**, 1367–1375.

Freckleton, R. P., Harvey, P. H. & Pagel, M. (2002) Phylogenetic dependence and ecological data: a test and review of evidence. *American Naturalist*, **160**, 716–726.

Garland, T., Midford, P. E. & Ives, A. R. (1999) An introduction to phylogenetically-based statistical methods with a new method for confidence intervals on ancestral values. *American Zoologist*, **39**, 374–388.

Pagel, M. (1999) Inferring the historical patterns of biological evolution. *Nature*, **401**, 877–884.

Paradis, E. (2006) *Analysis of Phylogenetics and Evolution with R*. New York, NY: Springer.

References

Barraclough, T. G., Harvey, P. H. & Nee, S. (1995) Sexual selection and taxonomic diversity in passerine birds. *Proceedings of the Royal Society B*, **259**, 211–215.

Blomberg, S. P., Garland, T. & Ives, A. R. (2003) Testing for phylogenetic signal in comparative data: behavioral traits are more labile. *Evolution*, **57**, 717–745.

Brooks, D. R. & McLennan, D. A. (2002) *The Nature of Diversity: an Evolutionary Voyage of Discovery*. Chicago, IL: University of Chicago Press.

Butler, M. A. & King, A. A. (2004) Phylogenetic comparative analysis: a modeling approach for adaptive evolution. *American Naturalist*, **164**, 683–695.

Collar, D. C., Near, T. J. & Wainwright, P. C. (2005) Comparative analysis of morphological diversity: does disparity accumulate at the same rate in two lineages of centrarchid fishes? *Evolution*, **59**, 1783–1794.

Davies, R. G., Orme, C. D. L., Olson, V. *et al.* (2007) Topography, energy and the global distribution of bird species richness. *Proceedings of the Royal Society B*, **274**, 1189–1197.

de Queiroz, A. (2002) Contingent predictability in evolution: key traits and diversification. *Systematic Biology*, **51**, 917–929.

Edwards, A. W. F. (1972) *Likelihood*. Cambridge: Cambridge University Press.

Farrell, B., Dussord, D. E. & Mitter, C. (1991) Escalation of plant defence: do latex and resin canals spur plant diversification? *American Naturalist*, **138**, 881–900.

Felsenstein, J. (1973) Maximum-likelihood estimation of evolutionary trees from continuous characters. *American Journal of Human Genetics*, **25**, 471–492.

Felsenstein, J. (1985) Phylogenies and the comparative method. *American Naturalist*, **126**, 1–25.

Felsenstein, J. (2004) *Inferring Phylogenies*. New York, NY: Sinauer.

Freckleton, R. P. (in press) Dealing with colinearity in behavioral and ecological data: model averaging and the problems of measurement error. *Behavioral Ecology and Sociobiology*, in press.

Freckleton, R. P. & Harvey, P. H. (2006) Detecting non-Brownian trait evolution in adaptive radiations. *PLoS Biology*, **4** (11), e373.

Freckleton, R. P. & Jetz, W. (2009) Space versus phylogeny: disentangling phylogenetic and spatial signals in comparative data. *Proceedings of the Royal Society B*, **276**, 21–30.

Freckleton, R. P., Harvey, P. H. & Pagel, M. (2002) Phylogenetic dependence and ecological data: a test and review of evidence. *American Naturalist*, **160**, 716–726.

Freckleton, R. P., Harvey, P. H. & Pagel, M. (2003) Comparative methods for adaptive radiations. In: *Macroecology: Concepts and Consequences*, ed. T. M. Blackburn & K. J. Gaston. Oxford: Blackwell, pp. 391–407.

Freckleton, R. P., Phillimore, A. B. & Pagel, M. (2008) Relating traits to diversification: a simple test. *American Naturalist*, **172**, 102–115.

Garamszegi, L. Z. & Møller, A. P. (2007) Prevalence of avian influenza and host ecology. *Proceedings of the Royal Society B*, **274**, 2003–2012.

Garland, T. J., Harvey, P. H. & Ives, A. R. (1992) Procedures for the analysis of comparative data using phylogenetically independent contrasts. *Systematic Biology*, **41**, 18–32.

Garland, T., Midford, P. E. & Ives, A. R. (1999) An introduction to phylogenetically-based statistical methods with a new method for confidence intervals on ancestral values. *American Zoologist*, **39**, 374–388.

Gould, S. J. & Lewontin, R. (1979) The spandrels of San Marco and the Panglossian paradigm: a critique of the adaptationist programme. *Proceedings of the Royal Society B*, **205**, 581–598.

Grafen, A. (1989) The phylogenetic regression. *Philosophical Transactions of the Royal Society B*, **326**, 119–157.

Grafen, A. & Hails, R. S. (2004) *Modern Statistics for the Life Sciences*. Oxford: Oxford University Press.

Grenfell, B. T., Pybus, O. G., Gog, J. R. *et al.* (2004) Unifying the epidemiological and evolutionary dynamics of pathogens. *Science*, **303**, 327–332.

Haining, R. (1990) *Spatial Data Analysis in the Social and Environmental Sciences*. Cambridge: Cambridge University Press.

Hansen, T. F. (1997) Stabilizing selection and the comparative analysis of adaptation. *Evolution*, **51**, 1341–1351.

Hansen, T. F. & Martins, E. P. (1996) Translating between microevolutionary process and macroevolutionary patterns: the correlation structure of interspecific data. *Evolution*, **50**, 1404–1417.

Hansen, T. F, Pienaar, J. & Orzack, S. H. (2008) A comparative method for studying adaptation to a randomly evolving environment. *Evolution*, **62**, 1965–1977.

Harmon, L. J., Schulte, J. A., Losos, J. B. & Larson, A. (2003) Tempo and mode of evolutionary radiation in iguanian lizards. *Science*, **301**, 961–964.

Harvey, P. H. (1996) Phylogenies for ecologists. *Journal of Animal Ecology*, **65**, 255–263.

Harvey, P. H. & Pagel, M. D. (1991) *The Comparative Method in Evolutionary Biology*. Oxford: Oxford University Press.

Harvey, P. H. & Rambaut, A. (2000) Comparative analyses for adaptive radiations. *Philosophical Transactions of the Royal Society B*, **355**, 1599–1606.

Harvey, P. H., Read, A. F. & Nee, S. (1995) Why ecologists need to be phylogenetically challenged. *Journal of Ecology*, **83**, 535–536.

Housworth, E. A., Martins, E. & Lynch, M. (2004) The phylogenetic mixed model. *American Naturalist*, **163**, 84–96.

Huelsenbeck, J. P., Rannala, B. & Masly, J.P. (2000) Accommodating phylogenetic uncertainty in evolutionary studies. *Science*, **288**, 2349–2350.

Ives, A. R., Midford, P. E. & Garland, T. (2007) Within-species variation and measurment error in phylogenetic comparative methods. *Systematic Biology*, **56**, 252–270.

Jetz, W., Wilcove, D. S. & Dobson, A. P. (2007) Projected impacts of climate and land-use change on the global diversity of birds. *PLoS Biology*, **5** (6), e157.

Kimura, M. (1991a) Recent development of the neutral theory viewed from the Wrightian tradition of theoretical population genetics. *Proceedings of the National Academy of Sciences of the USA*, **88**, 5969–5973.

Link, W. A. & Barker, R. J. (2006) Model weights and the foundations of multimodel inference. *Ecology*, **87**, 2626–2635.

Lutzoni, F., Pagel, M. & Reeb, V. (2001) Major fungal lineages are derived from lichen symbiotic ancestors. *Nature*, **411**, 937–940.

Martins, E. P. & Garland, T. (1991) Phylogenetic analyses of the correlated evolution of continuous characters: a simulation study. *Evolution*, **45**, 534–557.

Martins, E. P. & Hansen, T. F. (1996) The statistical analysis of interspecific data: a review and evaluation. In: *Phylogenies and the Comparative Method in Animal Behaviour*, ed. E. P. Martins. Oxford: Oxford University Press, pp. 22–75.

Martins, E. P. & Hansen, T. F. (1997) Phylogenies and the comparative method: a general approach to incorporating phylogenetic information into the analysis of interspecific data. *American Naturalist*, **149**, 646–667.

Marzaluff, J. M. & Dial, K. P. (1991) Life history correlates of taxonomic diversity. *Ecology*, **72**, 428–439.

Mitter, C., Farrell, B. & Wiegmann, B. (1988) The phylogenetic study of adaptive zones: has phytophagy promoted insect diversification? *American Naturalist*, **132**, 107–128.

Organ, C., Shedlock, A., Meade, A., Pagel, M. & Edwards, E. (2007) Origin of avian genome size and structure in non-avian dinosaurs. *Nature*, **446**, 180–184

Orme, C. D. L., Davies, R. G., Olson, V. A. et al. (2006) Global patterns of geographic range size in birds. *PLoS Biology*, **4** (7), e208.

Owens, I. P. F., Bennett, P. M. & Harvey, P. H. (1999) Species richness among birds: body size, life history, sexual selection or ecology? *Proceedings of the Royal Society B*, **266**, 933–939.

Page, R. D. M. & Holmes, E. C. (2000) *Molecular Evolution: a Phylogenetic Approach*. Oxford: Blackwell.

Pagel, M. (1993) Seeking the evolutionary regression coefficient: an analysis of what comparative methods measure. *Journal of Theoretical Biology*, **164**, 191–205.

Pagel, M. (1994) Detecting correlated evolution on phylogenies: a general method for the comparative analysis of discrete characters. *Proceedings of the Royal Society B*, **255**, 37–45.

Pagel, M. (1997) Inferring evolutionary processes from phylogenies. *Zoologica Scripta*, **26**, 331–348.

Pagel, M. (1999) Inferring the historical patterns of biological evolution. *Nature*, **401**, 877–884.

Pagel, M. & Lutzoni, F. (2002) Accounting for phylogenetic uncertainty in comparative studies of evolution and adaptation. In: *Biological Evolution and Statistical Physics*, ed. M. Laessig and A. Valleriani. Berlin: Springer Verlag, pp. 151–164.

Pagel, M. & Meade, A. (2006) Bayesian analysis of correlated evolution of discrete characters by reversible-jump Markov chain Monte Carlo. *American Naturalist*, **167**, 808–825.

Pagel, M., Meade, A. & Barker, D. (2004) Bayesian estimation of ancestral character states on phylogenies. *Systematic Biology*, **53**, 673–684.

Paradis, E. (2005) Statistical analysis of diversification with species traits. *Evolution*, **59**, 1–12.

Paradis, E. (2006) *Analysis of Phylogenetics and Evolution with R*. New York, NY: Springer.

Paradis, E. (2008) Asymmetries in phylogenetic diversification and character change can be untangled. *Evolution*, **62**, 241–247.

Paradis, E. & Claude, J. (2002) Analysis of comparative data using generalized estimating equations. *Journal of Theoretical Biology*, **218**, 175–185.

Parker, G. & Partridge, L. (1998) Sexual conflict and speciation. *Proceedings of the Royal Society B*, **353**, 261–274.

Pawitan, Y. (2001) *In All Likelihood: Statistical Modelling and Inference Using Likelihood*. Oxford: Oxford University Press.

Phillimore, A. B., Freckleton, R. P., Orme, C. D. L. & Owens, I. P. F. (2006) Ecology predicts large-scale patterns of phylogenetic diversification in birds. *American Naturalist*, **168**, 220–229.

Phillimore, A. B., Orme, C. D. L., Davies, R. G. et al. (2007) Biogeographical basis of recent phenotypic divergence among birds: a global study of subspecies richness. *Evolution*, **61**, 942–957.

Price, T. (1997) Correlated evolution and independent contrasts. *Philosophical Transactions of the Royal Society B*, **352**, 519–529.

Ree, R. H. (2005) Detecting the historial signature of key innovations using stochastic models of character evolution and cladogenesis. *Evolution*, **59**, 257–265.

Reynolds, J. D., Goodwin, N. B. & Freckleton, R. P. (2002) Evolutionary transitions in parental care and live bearing in vertebrates. *Philosophical Transactions of the Royal Society B*, **357**, 269–281.

Ricklefs, R. E. (2007) History and diversity: explorations at the intersection of ecology and evolution. *American Naturalist*, **170**, S56–70.

Ricklefs, R. E. & Starck, J. M. (1996) Application of phylogenetically independent contrasts: a mixed progress report. *Oikos*, **77**, 167–172.

Schluter, D., Price, T., Mooers, A. Ø. & Ludwig, D. (1997) Likelihood of ancestor states in adaptive radiation. *Evolution*, **39**, 396–404.

Thomas, G. H. (2004) Sexual conflict, ecology and breeding systems of shorebirds: phylogenetic analyses. Unpublished PhD Thesis, University of Bath, UK.

Thomas, G. H. & Székely, T. (2005) Evolutionary pathways in shorebird breeding systems: Sexual conflict, parental care, and chick development. *Evolution*, **59**, 2222–2230.

Thomas, G. H., Freckleton, R. P. & Székely, T. (2006) Comparative analyses of the influence of developmental mode on phenotypic diversification rates in shorebirds. *Proceedings of the Royal Society B*, **273**, 1619–1624.

Tyson, E. (1699) *Orang-outang, sive, Homo sylvestris: or, the anatomy of a pygmie compared with that of a monkey and ape and a man*. London: printed for Thomas Bennet.

Webster, A. J. & Purvis, A. (2002) Testing the accuracy of methods for reconstructing ancestral states of continuous characters. *Procedings of the Royal Society B*, **269**, 143–149.

Westoby, M., Leishman, M. R. & Lord, J.M. (1995) On misinterpreting the 'phylogenetic correction'. *Journal of Ecology*, **83**, 531–534.

Yang, Z. (2006) *Computational Molecular Evolution*. Oxford: Oxford University Press.

Multi-component signals in ant communication

Bert Hölldobler

What the fruit fly is for classical genetics and the squid axon for neurobiology, the insect society is for experimental sociobiology. Many of the sociobiological concepts and hypotheses proposed more than 40 years ago were confirmed, modified, revised or advanced by empirical studies with social insects during the past quarter-century.

The remarkable ecological success of social insects, and in particular of ants, is largely based on two key features of insect societies: cooperation and communication. In fact, a central element of any social behaviour is communication (see Chapter 8). The study of communication behaviour is at the core of any attempt to analyse social organisations. Without communication, social interactions and cooperation of any kind are impossible, be they interactions between genes in a genome, between organelles inside a cell, interactions of cells and organs in organisms, or cooperation among individuals in societies.

From early on in my scientific career I was interested in decoding communication mechanisms in social insects, particularly in ants, and I was fascinated by the comparative exploration of the evolutionary origin, function, diversity and complexity of social systems. I was, and continue to be, intrigued by the universal observation that wherever social life in groups evolved on this planet, we encounter (with only a few exceptions) a striking correlation:

the more tightly organised within-group cooperation and cohesion, the stronger the between-group discrimination and hostility. Ants, again, are excellent model systems for studying the transition from primitive eusocial systems, characterised by considerable within-group reproductive competition and conflict, and poorly developed reciprocal communication and cooperation, and little or no between-group competition, on one side, to the ultimate superorganisms (such as the gigantic colonies of the *Atta* leafcutter ants) with little or no within-group conflict, pronounced caste systems, elaborate division of labour, complex reciprocal communication, and intense between-group competition, on the other side (Hölldobler & Wilson 2008).

These are some of the key research topics that I attempt to investigate, both from the behavioural mechanistic and adaptation perspectives, with the ultimate goal of understanding the evolutionary pathways and selection forces that transform primitive insect societies to 'superorganisms'. In the following paragraphs I present a few 'snapshots' of this diverse research programme, with the emphasis not on details, but on concepts.

Ants are masters in chemical communication. In the early stages of the study of chemical communication in animals, scientists assumed that in insects behavioural responses are released by single chemical substances, whereas in vertebrates, and in particular in mammals, chemical signals are complex blends of substances, mediating inter-individual recognitions and interactions. However, most insect pheromones (semiochemicals) have proven to consist of several compounds, whereby different components of complex pheromones may have different effects on the receiver, or specific blends of compounds may identify group members, rank, or individuals. Thus, with respect to the sophistication of their chemical communication systems, vertebrates and insects do not differ greatly. The properties of complex chemical signals may be clarified by drawing an analogy from the field of artificial intelligence, which is concerned (among other things) with programming computers to distinguish among different types of objects. As such discriminations are comparable to those made by insects, this analogy seems not inappropriate. In the technique known as object-oriented programming, objects are characterised by both class variables and instance variables.

Instance variables are specific to each object, while a class variable is common to all members of the same class. In addition, classes may themselves be instances of a higher class, that is, a higher class is characterised by all the class and instance variables contained in its component classes. However, just as each instance differs from the others in the same class, the class variables of each component class differ from those of other members. When we employ this principle to multi-component chemical signals we begin to understand the anonymity and specificity of animal signals. We define anonymous properties of a signal as those which identify the signaller as a member of a class or organisational level, but do not distinguish it from other instances in the same class or level. Anonymous cues or signals are uniform or invariant among all instances of a class. The specific properties are those which vary, identifying the signaller as a particular instance of its class, or as belonging to one class among others which together comprise a higher class. Clearly these terms are relative, and their application depends on the level under examination.

The application of these principles has led to a completely new understanding of the complexity of multi-component communication in social insects. As a brief example, consider an ant following a chemical recruitment trail. At the species level, it orients with respect to the species-specific trail substance, and (usually) does not respond to trails of other species. At the colony level, this response may be anonymous – that is, a trail laid by any conspecific will be followed – or it may be colony-specific. At the individual level, no distinction may be made among the anonymous trails of different nestmates, or each individual may specifically recognise its own trail. Many other such analyses have revealed similar patterns that exhibit anonymity and specificity in chemical communication in ants and other social insects. These studies demonstrate that chemical communication in ants is at least as complex as any other mode of animal communication. The recognition of this organising principle in chemical communication also led to new insights, and new approaches in the study of the evolution of chemical communication.

It is also well known that communication can work through several sensory channels, that is, a signal can be composed of distinct physical components, transmitted simultaneously or in tightly paced sequence. Such multimodal perception of composite signals has been investigated particularly well in human and non-human primates, and in birds, and in fact was recognised by Charles Darwin in his book *The Expression of the Emotions in Man and Animals* (1872), where he noted that the intensity of communication by language is much enhanced by 'the expressive movements of face and body'. I think we have, for a long time, underestimated the complexity of communication signals in ants, having focused our analysis on one (or the other) sensory channel through which signals are perceived and processed. However, in a series of studies that began in the 1970s and continue to date, we discovered that multimodal communication is paramount in ants. The drumming, knocking, stridulation, antennation, tapping and waggling, shaking and jerking movements are not just insignificant by-products, but rather serve as communication specifiers and modulators that affect the response threshold to chemical signals, or, in some cases, can even have behaviour-releasing function independent of chemical signals.

Another example of multi-component chemical communication is the recognition cue contained in the cuticular hydrocarbon blends in social insects. They are wonderful examples illustrating how complex communication cues can arise through the evolutionary process of 'ritualisation'. The primary function of cuticular hydrocarbons is to provide resistance to desiccation and cuticle injuries, but they also have the potential for containing information through recognisable quantitative and qualitative differences of the blends of compounds. For example, changes in cuticular hydrocarbons correlate with colony differences, suggesting they may be used as cues for nestmate recognition. Even more strikingly, particular hydrocarbon profiles in numerous ant species reliably correlate with changes in reproductive ability. As an individual becomes reproductively active, it can be identified by changes in the cuticular hydrocarbon blends. If an individual 'turns on' its fertility at the wrong time and thereby risks reducing colony efficiency, this individual will be policed by nestmates. There is almost no escape from being policed, because the hydrocarbon cues appear to be 'honest signals'. Their production is intimately linked with the development of the ovaries and oocytes.

Such multi-component chemical recognition cues are often combined with behavioural motor displays, such as dominance and submission behaviour, ritualised duelling consisting of antennal bouts, body postures and locomotor patterns. These signals and behaviours regulate reproductive division of labour within 'primitive' eusocial colonies. In such societies queens and workers have almost the same size and reproductive potential. In some cases we found up to 60–80% of the workers being mated. Mated workers can replace the queen. Such egg-laying, mated workers are called gamergates. Obviously, in such societies worker individuals should resist worker specialisation, and they should continuously monitor the fertility status of the reproductive individuals. If fertility of such individuals wanes, young mated workers may dislodge the ageing reproductive queen, and take over her role as dominant reproductive. Such hierarchical organisations are characterised by frequent bouts of dominance interactions, poor division of labour and poor reciprocal communication. Within-colony friction and competition is pronounced, and because these colonies invariably are relatively small, there are no significant territorial interactions between conspecific neighbouring colonies.

Cooperation and reciprocal communication typically is much more elaborate in species with large colony size, which usually also exhibit a pronounced caste dimorphism between queen and workers. When ecological and genetic factors advance a society to near the upper extreme of the superorganism continuum, subsequent selection may result in complete loss of costly physiological structures involved in within-group competition. In other words, when advanced eusocial species have reached the 'point of no return', i.e. a point at which the capacity for selfishness has become insignificant because the underlying organs (e.g. ovaries and spermatheca) important for within-group competition degenerate or become completely lost, they are unlikely to be restored in a single mutational step. Thus, at this advanced eusocial status, within-colony competition is weak or non-existent, but between-colony competition is often intense, because these large colonies compete for limited resources. In such advanced eusocial organisations the colony effectively becomes a main target of selection, i.e. it is a coherent 'extended phenotype' of the genes within colony members. Each colony

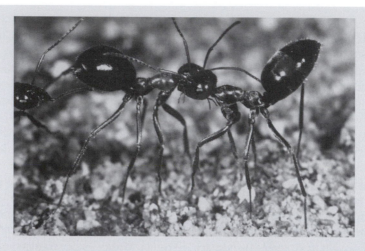

Two honey ants (*Myrmecocystus mimicus*) engaged in a ritualised tournament display. Photo: Bert Hölldobler.

consists of many genotypes coding for many pheno-types that together produce the colony phenotype. Selection therefore optimises caste demography, patterns of division of labour and communication systems at the colony level. For example, colonies that employ the most effective recruitment system to retrieve food, or that exhibit the most powerful colony defence against enemies and predators, will be able to raise the largest number of reproductive females and males every year and thus will have the greatest fitness within the population of colonies. Ultimately, of course, the evolutionary process entails selection on the genotypes of the found-ing females of the colony and their mates, acting through colony traits determined by the genotypes of the worker offspring.

Striking examples of colony phenotypes are the nest architectures and the territorial strategies. The design of territories is based on the distribu-tion of limited resources for which neighbouring conspecific colonies compete. Game-theory mod-els (see Chapter 4) predict that where fights endan-ger reproductive success or survival, individuals should monitor the quality of the resource and the resource-holding potential (RHP) of their oppon-ent. If they might lose the ensuing conflict, they should withdraw without escalating the contest.

As behavioural ecologists have frequently noted, if RHPs of opponents are similar, the contestants engage in an elaborate ritualised communication behaviour, the signals of which do not provide reli-able information, and the contests therefore can go on for extended periods. In animal species that live in social groups, groups of individuals com-pete as a unit for limited resources. This is true of many social mammals, where groups communi-cate resource-holding potential.

Ant territories are defended cooperatively by the usually sterile worker castes, and because of the division of labour between reproductive indi-viduals and workers, fatalities caused by territor-ial contest have a different qualitative significance for social insects as compared to solitary animals or groups of individuals in which each member has full reproductive potential. The death of a ster-ile worker represents an energy and labour debit, rather than the destruction of a reproductive agent. In fact, worker death might more than offset its costs by bringing or maintaining resources and colony security.

Nevertheless, ritualised combat is also known to exist in a few ant species. Its ecological significance has been analysed in greater depth in the honey ant *Myrmecocystus mimicus*. These ants conduct tournaments in which tens to hundreds of ants can be involved, but almost no physical fights occur. Instead, individual ants engage each other in highly stereotyped aggressive displays (see photo). During these tournaments spatiotemporal territories are defended, and simultaneously opposing colonies seem to assess each others' strength. Depending on the outcome of this mutual assessment, the opponents either continue to fight a ritualised combat in which the tournament site may be shifted towards the nest of the weaker colony, thus interfering with the foraging activity of that colony, or, if one colony is considerably stronger the contest will quickly escalate into the raiding, and possibly the enslavement, of the weaker colony. We postulated that numerous threat displays between individual workers at the tournament site are integrated into a massive group display between opposing colonies. In parallel to the procedure followed by solitary animals, the groups' 'strategic decision' whether to retreat, to recruit reinforcements in order to continue to fight by display, or to launch an escalated attack, depends on information about the strength of the opposing colony, and this information is obtained during the ritualised combats at the tournament site. The behaviour patterns involved suggest that it is based on complex multimodal communication.

Ritualised combats involve communication both within and between colonies. By means of chemical trails and motor displays, nestmates are summoned to the tournament site, and during encounters and confrontations with other ants, they use colony-specific chemical cues for recognition of nestmates and opponents. The emergent property of the *Myrmecocystus* superorganism, comprising division of labour and communication, is the extended phenotype of the ant colony's collective membership. The territorial strategy is part of the behavioural phenotype of this superorganism. The tournamenting ants are for the *Myrmecocystus* superorganism what the antlers are for a deer.

References

Darwin, C. (1872/1965) *The Expression of the Emotions in Man and Animals*. Chicago, IL: University of Chicago Press.

Hölldobler, B. & Wilson, E. O. (2008) *The Superorganism*. New York, NY: Norton.

6

Social evolution theory: a review of methods and approaches

Tom Wenseleers, Andy Gardner and Kevin R. Foster

Overview

Over the past decades much progress has been made in understanding the evolutionary factors that can promote social behaviour. Nevertheless, the bewildering range of methods that have been employed leave many confused. Here we review some of the major approaches that can be used to model social evolution, including the neighbour-modulated fitness, inclusive fitness and multilevel selection methods. Through examples we show how these different methodologies can yield complementary insight into the evolutionary causes of social behaviour, and how, for a wide range of problems, one method can be translated into the other without affecting the final conclusion. We also review some recent developments, such as the evolution of cooperation in spatial settings and networks, and multilocus extensions of the theory, and discuss some remaining challenges in social evolution theory.

6.1 The puzzle of altruism

Individuals sometimes give up resources to benefit their neighbours, to the extent that this helping lowers the individual's reproductive fitness. Such altruistic traits (Table 6.1) pose a difficulty for Darwin's theory of natural selection, which emphasises the spread of individually advantageous traits (Darwin 1859). Yet altruism abounds in the natural world, and is observed in settings as diverse as bacteria (Chapter 13), multicellular organisms with specialised non-reproductive tissues (Michod 1999, Strassmann & Queller 2007), social insects with a sterile worker caste (Bourke & Franks 1995, Ratnieks *et al.* 2006, Ratnieks & Wenseleers 2008),

and, of course, human society (Chapter 15; Gintis *et al.* 2005). Thus, altruism poses a major problem for evolutionary theory.

Formal attempts to solve the puzzle of altruism have a long history, going back at least to Darwin (reviewed in Dugatkin & Reeve 1994, Gardner & Foster 2008). The major breakthrough in cracking the problem, however, only came in the 1960s with the formulation of Hamilton's (1963, 1964) theory of inclusive fitness (later dubbed kin selection: Maynard Smith 1964). This showed that altruism is selectively favoured if $b.r > c$, where c is the personal fitness cost to the actor, b is the personal fitness benefit to the recipient, and r is the genetic relatedness between actor and recipient, an

Social Behaviour: Genes, Ecology and Evolution, ed. Tamás Székely, Allen J. Moore and Jan Komdeur. Published by Cambridge University Press. © Cambridge University Press 2010.

Table 6.1. A classification of social behaviours, based on Hamilton (1964, 1970) and West *et al.* (2007a, 2007b). Fitness impact means the impact on direct fitness, which is the fitness that comes from personal reproduction

	Fitness impact on recipient	
	+	−
Fitness impact +	Mutual benefit	Selfishness
on actor −	Altruism	Spite
	Cooperation	Competition

inequality that later become known as Hamilton's rule. The intuitive explanation is that when altruists help relatives reproduce this results in the indirect propagation of copies of the altruists' own genes, thereby enabling a gene for altruism to spread (Hamilton 1963, Dawkins 1976). Independently from Hamilton, however, others have taken a different approach and tried to solve the puzzle of altruism in terms of opposing selection within and between groups (Price 1972, Wilson 1975; for two early attempts see Wright 1945, Williams & Williams 1957). These multilevel selection approaches later turned out to be just a different way of looking at the same problem, and in all cases resulted in the same conclusion as kin-selection models (Hamilton 1975, Wade 1980, Crow & Aoki 1982, Queller 1992a, Dugatkin & Reeve 1994, Wenseleers *et al.* 2003, Lehmann *et al.* 2007a). Unfortunately, this fact still does not seem to be universally acknowledged, as it is still all too common to see kin and group selection incorrectly being pitted against each other, and being presented as two different mechanisms that can promote cooperation (e.g. Gintis 2000a, Gintis *et al.* 2003, Fehr & Fischbacher 2003, Wilson & Hölldobler 2005, Nowak 2006, Traulsen & Nowak 2006, Taylor & Nowak 2007).

Even within the kin-selection tradition, some confusion remains, partly because Hamilton derived his theory from two different perspectives, based either on the concepts of neighbour-modulated fitness, which was just classical Darwinian fitness but taking explicit account of the social neighbourhood, and inclusive fitness, which extends the notion of Darwinian fitness to non-descendent offspring (Hamilton 1964, Taylor *et al.* 2007a, Gardner & Foster 2008). These two perspectives,

although generally giving the same result, differ in their interpretation of the benefit of altruism and of relatedness, which leads to the confusing situation that when people mention Hamilton's rule they do not always mean exactly the same thing (Frank 1997a). A large body of literature also exists on the appropriate definition of the cost, benefit and relatedness terms that make Hamilton's rule work in a population genetic sense (Michod & Hamilton 1980, Queller 1984, 1992b, Frank 1997b).

The aim of this chapter is to show the formal relationship among the neighbour-modulated fitness, inclusive fitness and multilevel selection methods, and to show how, for a wide range of problems, one method can be translated into the other, without affecting the final conclusion. In addition, we will review some of the recent developments and remaining challenges in social evolution theory.

6.2 Social evolution theory: methods and approaches

6.2.1 The Price equation

Ultimately, given that evolution at its simplest level is a change in allele frequencies over time, all evolutionary theory has its basis in population genetics. Thus the traditional way of analysing social evolutionary models is to determine conditions, in terms of model parameters, for which genes encoding social traits can spread in the population (Cavalli-Sforza & Feldman 1978, Charnov 1978, Uyenoyama & Feldman 1980, Feldman & Cavalli-Sforza 1981, Gayley 1993). Although this population genetic approach remains the gold standard, it has several disadvantages. First, it is tedious, involving processes such as the construction of mating tables, writing down recurrence equations and determining the conditions for gene spread – usually via matrix algebra (Bulmer 1994, Kokko 2007, Otto & Day 2007). Second, such models generally require very specific assumptions, e.g. regarding the underlying genetic architecture of the trait, and hence they lack generality. Therefore there has been a need for the development of shortcut methods, which are both easier to apply and more general, but which are still solidly founded in population genetic theory. As we will show, a population genetic theorem known as the Price equation (Price 1970, 1972, 1995) provides the basis for several such shortcut methods. It also provides the foundation for a universally applicable theory of selection (Frank 1995a, Price 1995).

To start, consider a population containing n entities indexed by j. These entities will usually be taken to be individuals, but as we will see they can also be genes within diploid genomes, cells, social groups or even species. Let w_j be the absolute fitness of the jth entity, i.e. how many successful offspring entities it leaves in the next generation (this may also be a function of the probability of itself surviving to the next time period), and v_j the fitness relative to the population average $(w_j, \bar{w})$. In its simplest form, Price's theorem (Price 1970, 1972) states that the average change in the value of some trait z $(\Delta\bar{z})$ from one generation to the next is given by

$$\Delta\bar{z} = \text{cov}\left(\frac{w_j}{\bar{w}}, z_j\right) + E\left(\frac{w_j}{\bar{w}}\Delta z_j\right) = \text{cov}(v_j, z_j) + E(v_j \Delta z_j)$$

(6.1)

Here, the terms cov and E denote covariance (a measure of the statistical non-independence of two quantities; here, v_j and z_j) and expectation (arithmetic average), both taken over all the entities in the population. The term Δz_j is simply the change in the entity's trait value z_j across a generation, i.e. between parent (z_j) and offspring (z_j'), where $\Delta z_j = z'_j - z_j$. In the standard case, the first term in equation 6.1 corresponds to the effects of selection (Price 1970, Frank 1995a, 1997b, 1998, Okasha 2006). To better understand this, we can, without loss of generality, decompose the covariance term into two separate components: a least-squares linear regression coefficient and a statistical variance $(\text{cov}(v_j, z_j) = \beta_{vz} \cdot V_z)$. Note that this transformation does not require that the relationship between the trait and relative fitness actually be linear. Instead, Price's great insight here was that a linear regression can be used to determine the net direction of change upon a trait across generations. Now, one can clearly see the effects of selection. The regression terms describe whether the trait of interest z will

increase or decrease the relative fitness v of the focal entity, and the trait-variance term gives us the rate at which selection can act. This is intuitive: the more variability in the focal trait, the more fodder for the process of selection. The second term in equation 6.1, $E(v_j \Delta z_j)$, captures systematic biases in the transmission of the trait, for example due to biased mutation (see below).

Price's selection equation is very general (Price 1995, Frank 1995a), and applications are not limited to population genetics. Price's equation has been successfully applied to problems in epidemiology (Day & Gandon 2007) and ecology (Loreau & Hector 2001, Fox 2006), and even beyond the biological sciences. In economics, for example, w_j might be the growth rates of businesses and z_j some predictor of the firm's growth. In this case, the covariance term would describe selection among competing firms, and processes such as innovation could generate a positive covariance term and lead to positive selection (Andersen 2004). Many other applications exist, and links to standard population and quantitative genetic theory are given by Queller (1992b), Frank (1995a, 1997b, 1998), Wolf et al. (1999), Rice (2004), Okasha (2006) and Gardner et al. (2007). Page and Nowak (2002) also show how other equations for modelling evolutionary change – including the quasispecies equation, the replicator equation and the replicator–mutator equation – are all special cases of the Price equation.

For our purposes, however, we are interested in the genetic evolution of social behaviour (cultural evolution will be considered in section 6.3.5). In this instance the entities under consideration are normally individuals, w is biological fitness, i.e. the number of successful offspring or gametes produced, and z is usually defined as individual allele frequency g at the locus that controls the social behaviour, or more formally breeding value. The concept of breeding value comes from quantitative genetics and is defined as the linear combination of the alleles across loci that best predicts an individual's phenotype (Falconer 1981, Crow & Aoki 1982, Frank 1998). It is useful because not all effects of alleles will be inherited when there are interactions between focal alleles and the environment or alleles at other loci that may not be co-inherited (Chapters 1 and 2).

If we ignore mutation and genetic drift, and if we assume that in the case of diploid organisms meiosis is fair, the second term in equation 6.1, $E(v_j \Delta z_j)$, will be zero. Hence, the Price equation states that a gene coding for a social trait would spread when

$$\Delta \bar{g} = \beta_{vg} \cdot V_g > 0 \qquad (6.2)$$

where the covariance is again written as the product of a regression (β) and a variance (V). Before Price, this equation was independently derived by Robertson (1966, 1968), who termed it the 'secondary theorem of natural selection'. Given that genetic variance (V_g) is always non-negative, equation 6.2 simply states that any response to selection will always be in the same direction as the regression of relative fitness on breeding value (β_{vg}) and, because mean fitness will generally be a positive quantity ($\bar{w} > 0$), the condition for selection to favour an increase in average breeding value of the trait of interest can be written as $\beta_{wg} > 0$. That is, genetic variance only affects the rate of selection, not its direction, so one can focus simply on the effects of a trait on fitness to predict whether the trait will be favoured by natural selection.

6.2.2 Three equivalent methods for modelling social evolution

The condition that β_{wg} should be greater than zero provides a formal basis for explaining standard Darwinian adaptations, in which traits are selected for when they increase the fitness of their bearer. But how can it account for the evolution of altruistic behaviour that decreases individual fitness? As we will see, there are three main solutions to this problem: the neighbour-modulated fitness and inclusive fitness approaches that form the basis of kin selection theory, and also a levels-of-selection approach (Fig. 6.1). In many cases, these methods can be used interchangeably; they simply provide alternative ways for describing net gene frequency change.

The neighbour-modulated fitness approach

A first solution to the puzzle of altruism is based on the concept of neighbour-modulated fitness, first introduced by Hamilton (1964, 1970, 1975; see also

Queller 1992b, Taylor 1996, Taylor & Frank 1996, Frank 1998, Rousset 2004, Taylor *et al.* 2007a). This captures the way in which a focal individual's personal fitness is a function of its own genotype (direct fitness effect) and also the genotypes of its social partners (indirect fitness effect), as illustrated in Figure 6.1a. That is, all fitness accounting is done through the effects on this focal individual, such that the fitness of an average recipient of the behaviour (w) is expressed as a function of that individual's genotype or breeding value (g, Falconer 1981) and the genotype of its social neighbours (g'). The neighbour-modulated fitness approach has often been referred to as an analysis of 'direct fitness', because of the way that fitness accounting is done through the effects on the personal reproduction of an average bearer of the altruistic genes. This makes it clear that a gene for altruism can only spread if the direct fitness of an average bearer increases.

First, assume that individuals interact in pairs, and that both individuals are identical in every respect other than their genotypes for the trait in question (Queller 1992b, Grafen 2006; extensions for interactions between individuals of different classes will be treated in section 6.3.1). In this case, an individual's neighbour-modulated fitness can be written as

$$w = \bar{w} + \beta_{wg \cdot g'} \cdot (g - \bar{g}) + \beta_{wg' \cdot g} \cdot (g' - \bar{g}) \qquad (6.3)$$

where $\bar{w}$ and $\bar{g}$ are the average fitness and the average allele frequency of the individuals in the population, and the terms $(g - \bar{g})$ and $(g' - \bar{g})$ describe how the two individuals' genotypes depart from the population mean. The $\beta_{wg \cdot g'}$ and $\beta_{wg' \cdot g}$ terms separate out how these two genotypes affect the focal individual's fitness. Specifically, they are the least-squares partial regressions of the individual's fitness on its own and its partner's breeding values (Queller 1992b), where $\beta_{wg \cdot g'}$ means the effect of g on w, when g' is held constant.

Substituting equation 6.3 into equation 6.1, for $z = g$, and neglecting changes in 'transmission', one obtains

$$\Delta \bar{g} = [\beta_{wg \cdot g'} \operatorname{cov}(g, g) + \beta_{wg' \cdot g} \operatorname{cov}(g', g)] / \bar{w} \qquad (6.4)$$

Hence the condition for an increase in the average breeding value of the trait of interest ($\Delta g > 0$) is:

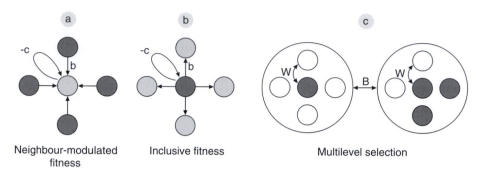

Figure 6.1 Three alternative but equivalent methods for solving the puzzle of altruism, via three different concepts. (a) *Neighbour-modulated fitness*: an average bearer of the altruistic genotype (lighter circle) will receive benefits (b, straight arrows) from other carriers of the altruistic genotype who express the trait in the individual's social neighbourhood (darker circles); if the individual itself expresses the altruistic genotype it will experience a direct fitness cost (–c, curved arrow). (b) *Inclusive fitness*: an individual that expresses the altruistic genotype (darker circle) will experience a direct fitness cost (–c, curved arrow) but cause fitness benefits to its social neighbours (b, straight arrows), some of whom may be more likely than chance to be carriers of the altruistic genotype. (c) *Levels of selection*: cooperators (open circles) experience a within-group disadvantage against cheats (filled circles), leading to a negative within-group selection component W, but groups with more cooperators end up being more productive, leading to a positive between-group selection component B.

$$\beta_{wg.g'} + \beta_{wg'.g} \cdot \beta_{g'g} > 0 \qquad\qquad (6.5)$$

This inequality is Hamilton's rule, $-c + b.r > 0$, in its neighbour-modulated fitness form where $r = \beta_{g'g}$ = cov$(g',g)/$cov(g,g) is the coefficient of relatedness, which is defined as the least-squares regression of social-partner breeding value on one's own breeding value (Michod & Hamilton 1980, Grafen 1985), $\beta_{wg.g'}$ $= -c$ is the cost of carrying the genes for the social behaviour, and $\beta_{wg'.g} = b$ is the benefit one receives when one's social partners carry the genes for social behaviour.

From a neighbour-modulated fitness perspective, then, altruism can be favoured when $r > 0$, or, more specifically, when the direct fitness cost c to the actor is outweighed by the benefit $b.r$ of associating with neighbours who also carry genes for the social trait. The intuitive explanation is that with positive relatedness, altruistic individuals will tend to associate with other altruistic individuals that help them back. Meanwhile, non-altruistic individuals will associate with other non-altruists, and they will do badly. Relatedness (r) measures the extent to which other individuals are more likely than chance to carry the same genes, and, as we have said, it is formally defined as a regression

coefficient $(\beta g'g)$. Nevertheless, regression relatedness is usually well approximated by genealogical relatedness under the assumption of weak selection, in which case it can be directly calculated from pedigrees (Michod & Hamilton 1980, Grafen 1985). An exception where relatedness does not strictly correspond to genealogical relatedness, even for weak selection, is when it is caused by a phenotype-matching mechanism whereby cooperators directly recognise each other and preferentially interact (green-beard mechanisms: Hamilton 1964, Dawkins 1976, Traulsen & Schuster 2003, Axelrod *et al.* 2004, Lehmann & Keller 2006a, Gardner & West 2010), or if the cooperator gene has a pleiotropic effect on habitat preference, so that individuals with cooperative genotypes would tend to assort together (Hamilton 1975). Nevertheless, both these mechanisms may be quite rare in nature (Lehmann & Keller 2006a).

The neighbour-modulated-fitness approach to kin selection closely mirrors recent methodological developments in the theory of indirect genetic effects (IGEs, Chapter 2): both examine the consequences of genes carried by the focal individual and by the individual's social partners. However, kin-selection theory is typically concerned with between-individual genetic interactions at the fitness level only, and the pheno-typic traits of key interest are usually assumed to be controlled by a single individual, whereas researchers working on IGEs are mostly motivated by phenotypic traits other than fitness, which are determined by genes carried by multiple individuals (Bijma & Wade 2008).

Although Hamilton (1964) originally used individual genotypes as predictors of fitness, one could also express neighbour-modulated fitness as a function of an individual's and its social partner's phenotypes y and y' (Frank 1998). This leads to the following phenotypic version of Hamilton's rule:

$$\beta_{wy.y'} + \beta_{wy'.y}.(\beta_{y'g}/\beta_{yg}) > 0 \qquad (6.6)$$

in which costs and benefits are now defined as $\beta_{wy.y'}$ and $\beta_{wy'.y}$ and $r = \beta_{y'g} / \beta_{yg}$ is interpreted as a measure of assortative interaction (Orlove & Wood 1978) that measures the extent to which individuals carrying the altruistic genotype tend to interact with social partners with a cooperative phenotype (Eshel & Cavalli-Sforza 1982, Nee 1989, Frank 1997a, Pepper 2000, Gardner & West 2004, Fletcher & Zwick 2006).

One problem, however, with using phenotypic fitness predictors is that this would change the way that social behaviours are classified (Table 6.1), and result in the erroneous classification of reciprocal altruism (Trivers 1971) as true altruism (Foster *et al.* 2006a, West *et al.* 2007b), which is defined as coming at a cost to the actor's lifetime fitness (Hamilton 1964). Consider, for example, a strategy whereby individuals only cooperate with others if they cooperated with them during a previous encounter (this is known as Tit-for-Tat in the literature: Axelrod & Hamilton 1981). Here, there is a positive assortment between cooperators on a per-interaction basis, even if the interacting individuals are not genetic relatives (Nee 1989, Fletcher & Zwick 2006). Assuming a large number of rounds of interaction, $\beta_{y'g}/\beta_{yg}$ in this case turns out to be equal to p, the likelihood that two players meet again, leading to the condition that Tit-for-Tat is an evolutionary equilibrium when $p.b > c$ (Axelrod & Hamilton 1981). Similarly, if individuals have information about the likely behaviour of social interactants, e.g. based on reputation (indirect reciprocity: Nowak & Sigmund 1998), then $\beta_{y'g}/\beta_{yg}$ measures the probability

q of knowing someone else's reputation (Suzuki & Toquenaga 2005). Positive values of $\beta_{y'g}/\beta_{yg}$ can even arise in interspecific interactions (Frank 1994a, Foster & Wenseleers 2006), due to conditional (Tit-for-Tat-like) behaviour (Nee 1989, Fletcher & Zwick 2006) or due to cooperative pairs gaining fitness benefits and staying together across multiple generations (Frank 1994a, Foster & Wenseleers 2006).

Although some would find it pleasing that the relatedness coefficient $\beta_{y'g}/\beta_{yg}$ in expression 6.6 brings out positive assortment as a key mechanism that can promote cooperation (Frank 1994a, Hamilton 1995, Skyrms 1996, Griffin & West 2002, Fletcher & Doebeli 2006), it has the disadvantage that it would misclassify behaviours that have delayed direct benefits as being truly altruistic. To avoid such confusion, we will use the genotypic version of Hamilton's rule (inequality 6.5) throughout the remainder of this chapter. That said, if phenotypes are not conditional on the social partner's behaviour and if phenotypes linearly map onto genotype (additive genetics: Chapter 1), then one does not need to make a distinction between expressions 6.5 and 6.6, as they will then be fully equivalent (McElreath & Boyd 2007).

The regression-analysis form of Hamilton's rule outlined above has the benefit of allowing huge generality. The downside is that it can be awkward to analyse particular models in this way. Nevertheless, under the assumption that genetic variation is vanishingly small (i.e. if we are considering the spread of a rare mutant) and that mutants differ only slightly from the wild type (weak selection), one can switch from statistical, least-squares-regression analysis to methodology involving simpler expected-fitness functions that can be analysed using powerful calculus approaches (Box 6.1). This is because if there is vanishingly little genetic variation and variation in fitness, then the population occupies only a small segment of the function that relates genotype and phenotype, and hence the least-squares regressions of fitness on breeding value can be approximated by the tangent to the expected-fitness curve at the population-average breeding value, i.e. $\beta_{wg} \rightarrow dw/dg \mid_{g = \bar{g}}$, as var$(g)$ and var$(w) \rightarrow 0$. Making this transition from least-squares partial regressions to partial derivatives, expression 6.5 can be rewritten in differential-calculus form as

$$\frac{\partial w}{\partial g} + \frac{\partial w}{\partial g'}\frac{dg'}{dg} > 0 \qquad (6.7)$$

where $\partial w/\partial g = -c$ is the cost of carrying genes for the social behaviour, $\partial w/\partial g' = b$ is the benefit of one's social partners carrying genes for the social behaviour, and $dg'/dg = r$ is the coefficient of genetic relatedness. This method forms the basis of a powerful maximisation approach to finding the evolutionarily stable strategy (ESS: Chapter 4) in social evolutionary models, which has truly revolutionised the field (Taylor & Frank 1996, Taylor 1996, Frank 1997a, 1998, Taylor *et al.* 2007a; Box 6.1). As with the regression approach, extensions for class-structured populations are also readily made (Taylor & Frank 1996, Taylor *et al.* 2007a, Frank 1998; see section 6.3.1).

The inclusive fitness approach

The neighbour-modulated fitness approach focuses attention on a particular 'recipient' individual, and is concerned with how that individual's personal fitness is determined by the genes that it carries (direct fitness effects) and by the genes carried by its social partners (indirect fitness effects) (Fig. 6.1a). An alternative formulation, inclusive fitness, introduced by Hamilton (1964), instead focuses on how a random actor affects the fitness of others (Fig. 6.1b). Relatedness in this case measures the value of the recipient in transmitting copies of the actor's own genes, leading to an elegant gene-centered view of evolutionary change (Hamilton 1963, Dawkins 1976).

Formulating the selection of social traits in this way was a great breakthrough as it analyses gene frequency change entirely from the perspective of the actors that actually express the behaviour. In this way, it better captures the apparent agenda underlying organismal behaviour (Hamilton 1995, Grafen 2006, Gardner *et al.* 2007, Gardner & Foster 2008, Gardner & Grafen 2009). Organisms are expected to behave as if they value the reproductive success of their neighbours –

devalued according to their genetic relatedness – as well as their own reproductive success. In short, they behave as if they are trying to maximise their inclusive fitness (Grafen 2006).

In our example, the inclusive fitness approach differs only from the neighbour-modulated fitness approach in the fact that the benefit term in Hamilton's rule is now calculated as the benefit *to* social partners ($\beta_{w'g\cdot g'}$), rather than as the benefit of receiving help *from* social partners ($\beta_{wg'\cdot g}$) (Fig. 6.1a,b). Thus, the net inclusive fitness effect of an actor carrying a certain gene is calculated as

$$\beta_{wg\cdot g'} + \beta_{w'g\cdot g}\cdot\beta_{g'g} > 0 \qquad (6.8)$$

Because we assume no class structure, so that individuals are identical in all respects other than their genes for the social trait of interest (strategic equivalence: Grafen 2006), the impact of the focal individual's variant gene on the fitness of her social partner ($\beta_{w'g\cdot g'}$) is equal to the impact on the focal individual's fitness that would occur if the social partner carried the variant gene ($\beta_{wg'\cdot g}$), and hence the conditions described by expressions 6.5 and 6.8 are equivalent. As in the neighbour-modulated fitness framework, the inclusive fitness effect is composed of two parts, a direct and indirect fitness effect, which are due to the effect of the actor's genotype on its own fitness and on the fitness of others, respectively (West *et al.* 2007a, 2007b). Whilst the direct fitness component retains the same meaning in both neighbour-modulated fitness and inclusive fitness approaches, the indirect fitness term describes the effect of social-partner genes on own fitness in the neighbour-modulated fitness view and the effect of own genes on social-partner fitness (weighted by relatedness) in the inclusive fitness view.

As before, when selection is weak and the population is nearly monomorphic, the partial regression coefficients in inequality 6.8 can be approximated using partial derivatives (see Box 6.1 for an example). In addition, as with the neighbour-modulated fitness approach to social evolution, the inclusive fitness approach can also be readily applied to class-structured populations (Taylor 1990, 1996; see section 6.3.1).

The levels-of-selection approach

Price's (1970) theorem, which underpins the most general derivation of Hamilton's rule (Hamilton 1970), has also been applied to levels of selection in evolution (Price 1972, Hamilton 1975). Instead of separating individual fitness into direct and indirect components, this approach phrases social evolution in terms of selection within and between groups (Fig. 6.1c). Some researchers greatly prefer thinking in terms of this partition over the direct/indirect partition (Wilson 1975, 1983, Wade 1980, Sober & Wilson 1998), and in recent years there has been much renewed interest in this theory (Keller 1999, Henrich 2004, Okasha 2006). Some of the earliest theoretical treatments of the evolution of altruism were also explicitly phrased in terms of opposing selection between and within groups (Wright 1945, Williams & Williams 1957), and Darwin used both kinship and group-level arguments to explain social insect workers (Gardner & Foster 2008). The combination of kin and group arguments used by Darwin reflects the fact that choosing a multilevel methodology over kin-selection thinking is just a question of how to phrase the problem. Sadly, however, there is a continuing tendency to mistakenly assume that switching between the methods also means that different biological processes are at play (e.g. Wilson 1975, Colwell 1981, Sober & Wilson 1998, Gintis 2000a, Gintis *et al.* 2003, Fehr & Fischbacher 2003, Wilson & Hölldobler 2005, Nowak 2006, Traulsen & Nowak 2006, Taylor & Nowak 2007; see also Edward O. Wilson's profile). We feel this is misguided, given that the Price-equation derivations we use here show the compatability that allows results from one framework to be rephrased in terms of the other (see also Box 6.1).

Analysing social evolution in terms of opposing levels of selection is straightforward. Recall that the Price equation can be applied to describe selection among any type of entity. What we do first, then, is to take the standard form of the Price equation (equation 6.1) and use it to capture the effects of a change in the mean gene frequency on the mean fitness of individuals within a given group, rather than the effects of a change in individual genotype on absolute individual fitness as we did above. This requires a slight change in notation only, and we will now use subscripts i and ij to refer to the ith group and the jth individual within group i respectively. Now we can write the evolutionary change in the average gene frequency g as a function of the mean fitness and mean gene frequency in the ith group as

$$\bar{w}\Delta\bar{g} = \mathrm{cov}(w_i, g_i) + E_i(w_i \Delta g_i) \qquad (6.9)$$

Equation 6.9 describes selection on the groups in our population. But what about selection on individuals within each group? This is the clever part. Price (1972) noticed that one can expand the expectation term $E_i(w_i \Delta g_i)$ to capture the full effects of within-group selection because

$$E_i(w_i \Delta g_i) = E_i(\mathrm{cov}_i(w_{ij}, g_{ij}) + E_{j.i}(w_{ij} \Delta g_{ij})) \qquad (6.10)$$

where the right-hand side is a second version of the standard Price equation, but this time one level lower in the selective hierarchy, i.e. it describes within-group selection. Substituting this equation into equation 6.9 yields:

$$\bar{w}\Delta\bar{g} = \mathrm{cov}(w_i, g_i) + E_i(\mathrm{cov}_i(w_{ij}, g_{ij}) \\ + E_{j.i}(w_{ij} \Delta g_{ij})) \qquad (6.11)$$

where the expectations and covariances are taken over their subscripts, with i standing for groups, ij standing for individual j of group i, and $j.i$ for individuals j for a specified group i. That is, the first covariance term captures the effects of the gene on group success, the second covariance term captures the effect of the gene on the relative success of individuals within a group, and the final term accounts for any deviations due to processes other than selection. This idea of expanding the Price equation to include multiple levels of selection can be continued until all relevant levels are included (e.g. the intragenomic level in the case of meiotic drive). Doing so, and disregarding mutation, the last term $(E_{ji}(w_{ij} \Delta g_{ij}))$ can be set to zero. Noting that mean fitness w is always greater than zero, it is then clear that a gene for a social trait is selected for when

$$\text{cov}(w_i, g_i) + E_i(\text{cov}_i(w_{ij}, g_{ij})) = \beta_{w_i g_i}.V_{g_i} + \beta_{w_{ij} g_{ij.i}}.V_{g_{ij.i}} > 0$$

$$(6.12)$$

where, as we did above, the covariances have been broken up into their constituent regression and variance terms. In this inequality, the two sets of terms reflect between-group and within-group (among-individual) selection respectively. Each level of selection entails a selective response equal to an intensity of selection (how the mean gene frequency at a certain level affects the relative fitness of that level) weighed by the genetic variance present at that level. The between- and within-group genetic variances can be calculated using the techniques of classic population genetics, namely Wright's hierarchical F-statistics (Yang 1998). Importantly, however, they can also be expressed as a function of genetic relatedness, which links everything back to kin selection (Hamilton 1975, Breden 1990). To see this, one can multiply top and bottom of equation 6.12 by the total genetic variance in the population, V_t, yielding

$$V_t \cdot \left(\beta_{w_i g_i} \cdot \frac{V_{g_i}}{V_t} + \beta_{w_{ij} g_{ij.i}} \right) \cdot \frac{V_{g_{ij.i}}}{V_t} > 0 \qquad (6.13)$$

where V_{g_i}/V_t is known as Wright's intraclass correlation coefficient R (Falconer 1981, Crow & Aoki 1982; Box 6.1). Since $V_t = V_{g_i} + V_{g_{ij.i}}$ and is always positive, the inequality simplifies to

$$\beta_{w_i g_i}.R + \beta_{w_{ij} g_{ij.i}}.(1 - R) > 0 \qquad (6.14)$$

where, for a group size of n, Wright's intraclass correlation coefficient R equals $(1/n) + ((n-1)/n).r$, with r being the pair-wise genetic relatedness between group members (Hamilton 1975). As in the neighbour-modulated fitness and inclusive fitness approaches, when selection is weak and the population is nearly monomorphic, the partial regression coefficients in inequality 6.14 can be approximated using partial derivatives (see Box 6.1).

In group-selection models, positive between-group genetic variance often arises from limited migration (Crow & Aoki 1982, Traulsen & Nowak 2006). For example, under Wright's island-population model, it has been shown that the ratio of the within- to

between-group genetic variance $(1 - R)/R$ equals two times the number of migrant diploid organisms per generation (Wright 1951, Hamilton 1975, Crow & Aoki 1982). This leads to the condition that if within-group and between-group selection terms are of equal magnitude ($\beta_{w_i g_i} = \beta_{w_{ij} g_{ij.i}}$), between-group selection can override within-group selection only when less than one migrant is exchanged every two generations (Crow & Aoki 1982, Leigh 1983). Taking a kin-selection approach, this would be interpreted as limited migration increasing relatedness and causing greater cooperation.

Expression 6.14 is very useful for conceptualising the potential tension between the within-group interests of individuals and the needs of the group as a whole (Hamilton 1975), and provides a formal foundation upon which to rest group-selection analyses. In particular, the among- and within-group genetic variances R and $1 - R$ determine the extent to which the group and the individual within the group can be considered units of selection (Wenseleers *et al.* 2003), and the signs of the β coefficients tell us whether a trait either benefits or harms the group ($\beta_{w_i g_i} > 0$ or < 0), and increases or decreases the fitness of individuals relative to other individuals within the same group ($\beta_{w_{ij} g_{ij.i}} > 0$ or < 0). This allows for a classification of social behaviours similar to that in the inclusive fitness scheme (Table 6.1). The classification, however, is not completely identical, since even with zero relatedness, investment in an individually costly trait ($\beta_{w_{ij} g_{ij.i}} < 0$) could result in a net increase in absolute individual fitness when it results in a sufficiently large feedback benefit to the whole group (specifically, this occurs when $\beta_{w_i g_i} > \beta_{w_{ij} g_{ij.i}} / (n - 1)$). Such traits are referred to as weakly altruistic, to differentiate them from true strong altruism, which entails direct fitness costs to individuals expressing the trait (Wilson 1990, Foster *et al.* 2006b).

Expression 6.14 clarifies that the kin selection and group selection approaches to social evolution are entirely interchangeable, and are not competing hypotheses about how social evolution occurs, as was often been claimed. Instead, group selection – as formalised by the multilevel Price equation – and the direct or inclusive fitness methods are simply alternative fitness accounting schemes that lead to the same net selective result (Hamilton 1975, Wade 1980, Crow & Aoki 1982, Queller 1992a, Dugatkin & Reeve 1994, Wenseleers *et al.* 2003, Lehmann *et al.* 2007a). To see this, take the example of altruism between a pair of interacting individuals, where the fitness of the two individuals is given by $w_{i1} = \bar{w} - c.(g_{i1} - \bar{g}) + b.(g_{i2} - \bar{g})$ and $w_{i2} = \bar{w} - c.(g_{i2} - \bar{g}) + b.(g_{i1} - \bar{g})$. The mean fitness of the pair $w_i = \bar{w} + (b - c).(g_i - \bar{g})$, and since $g_i = (g_{i1} + g_{i2})/2$, individual fitness can be written as $w_{ij} = \bar{w} - c.(g_i - \bar{g}) + b.(2g_i - g_{ij} - \bar{g})$. Nothing that $\beta_{w_i g_i} = \partial w_i / \partial g_i = b - c$, $\beta_{w_{ij} g_{ij},i} = \partial w_{ij} / \partial g_{ij} = -(b + c)$ and $R = (1 + r)/2$, and substituting these terms into inequality 6.14, shows that increased altruism is selected for when $(b - c)(1 + r)/2 - (b + c)(1 - r)/2 > 0$, which indeed just simplifies to Hamilton's rule, $b.r > c$ (Hamilton 1975, Wade 1980, Queller 1992a).

One drawback of the multilevel framework is that in principle, it applies only to strictly hierarchically nested populations, and usually requires that all individuals are equivalent and equally likely to express the trait under study. Hence it cannot easily deal with situations where the individuals affected by the altruistic behaviour belong to different sex or age classes. This is in contrast to kin selection theory, where the impact of class structure has been given a very general treatment. (Taylor 1990, Taylor & Frank 1996, Taylor *et al.* 2007a; see section 6.3.1). A general theory of class structure for multilevel selection models is currently lacking. However, multilevel selection analysis of class structured models has been made possible by using the number of grand offspring as a proxy for fitness (Wilson & Colwell 1981, Frank 1986), by including the genetic variance present in different classes of individuals affected by a social trait in the between-group genetic variance (Wenseleers *et al.* 2003) or even by using inclusive fitness theory to partition selection in components that owe to fitness differences between groups and between individuals within groups (Ratnieks & Reeve 1992).

In addition, some have argued that the multilevel Price equation does not always properly capture people's intuitive notion of group selection. For example, it has been suggested that it is problematic that one could have between-group selection even in contexts not involving social traits (reviewed by Okasha 2006). For example, if good eyesight enhances individual fitness in a straightforward way, then some groups will be fitter than others simply because they contain, by chance, better-sighted individuals (Hamilton 1975). However, it is equally intuitive to identify group selection as the part of natural selection that owes to fitness differences between groups, whether or not social behaviour is involved. Furthermore, it is Price's between-group selection that is identified as the driver of group-level adaptation in superorganism theory (Wilson & Sober 1989, Gardner & Grafen 2009), and this provides further justification for terming this part of natural selection "group selection".

An alternative approach aimed at remedying some of these perceived problems is 'contextual analysis' (Heisler & Damuth 1987). This mirrors the neighbour-modulated fitness approach discussed above, and describes individual fitness as a function of its own genes or behaviour (g_{ij}) and the mean gene frequency or behaviour (g_i) or other characteristics of its group. Next, the selection for the social trait is decomposed as

$$\beta_{w_{ij} g_{ij} . g_i} . \beta_{g_{ij} g_{ij}} + \beta_{w_{ij} g_i . g_{ij}} . \beta_{g_i g_{ij}} = \beta_{w_{ij} g_{ij} . g_i} + \beta_{w_{ij} g_i . g_{ij}} . R > 0$$

$$(6.15)$$

where $\beta_{w_{ij} g_i g_{ij}}$ is the impact of the group character on individual fitness, and is taken to be a measure of group selection, and R is Wright's intraclass correlation coefficient $R = (1/n) + ((n - 1)/n).r$, where r is the pair-wise genetic relatedness between group members (Hamilton 1975). Although contextual analysis avoids the diagnosis of group selection in the hypothetical example of good eyesight, it has its own difficulties (Heisler & Damuth 1987, Goodnight *et al.* 1992). For example, if we consider again the selection for individual eyesight, but now assume soft selection (Goodnight *et al.* 1992, Okasha 2006) is in operation so that every group is constrained to have the same total productivity, then an individual with particularly strong group mates would tend to have lower fitness than it would in another group. Contextual analysis would diagnose group selection in this scenario, because individual fitness depends on the group environment. However, the general consensus is that group selection should require fitness differences between groups, so there appears to be a mismatch between the formalism and the fundamental process that it was intended to capture (West *et al.* 2008). We emphasise that this is not necessarily a failing of the levels-of-selection or contextual-analysis approaches, but rather a failure to find a match between the theory and semantics of group selection.

On a final note, it should be mentioned that species-level selection is distinct from the multilevel theory outlined above, as it is not concerned with gene frequency change, but with rates of speciation or species extinction. For example, the evolution of asexuality in multicellular organisms appears to be associated with low species persistence times, i.e. multicellular asexuals are particularly prone to extinction and this makes them relatively rare in nature. Such processes do not directly affect the evolution of the trait itself – as is the case for within- or between-group selection – but rather the frequency of the trait in the natural world. Despite this, species-level selection is still often referred to as a multilevel selection problem (Heisler & Damuth 1987), and it can also be analysed using the Price equation (equation 6.1) by taking w_j as the rate with which a species j speciates or tends to go extinct as a function of some characteristic g_j (say geographic range) (Arnold & Fristrup 1982, Okasha 2006). In this case, the covariance would measure species-level selection, and the expectation the fidelity of transmission of the trait to daughter species (Arnold & Fristrup 1982, Okasha 2006). Interestingly, it has recently been shown that species-level selection can potentially reduce the mean level of selfishness observed among species. As with asexuals, there is some evidence that more selfish species are more prone to extinction than more cooperative species (Parvinen 2005, Rankin & López-Sepulcre 2005, Rankin 2007, Rankin *et al.* 2007). The prediction then is that while natural selection may frequently favour the evolution of selfish strategies within a species, species-level selection may counter this. If correct, this will mean that cooperative species are more common in nature than would be predicted by within-species processes alone.

Box 6.1 The different ways of analysing social evolution

To illustrate the different methods, we here analyse Frank's (1994b, 1995b) 'tragedy of the commons' model, which has been successfully applied to a variety of biological problems (Frank 1994b, Foster 2004, Wenseleers *et al.* 2003, 2004a, 2004b). The tragedy of the commons states that each individual would gain by claiming a greater share of the local resources, but that the group would perish if all local resources were exhausted (Hardin 1968). Frank's model captures this tension between group and individual interests by writing individual fitness as

$$w_{ij} = (1 - g_i).(g_{ij} / g_i) \tag{6.B1}$$

where g_{ij} and g_i are the individual and group mean breeding values for a behaviour that causes individuals to selfishly grab local resources (normalised to go from 0 to 1). In this simple model, $1 - g_i$ is the group's productivity, which declines as the average level of selfishness g_i increases (we assume linearly, but this can easily be relaxed: Foster 2004) and g_{ij} / g_i is the relative success of an individual within its group. Similarly, we can write the fitness of another member in the group as

$$w' = (1 - g_i).(g'/ g_i) \tag{6.B2}$$

where g' is the average level of selfishness of these other individuals. Note that with a group size of n, $g_i = (1/n)g_{ij} + ((n-1)/n)g')$, which we can substitute into equations 6.B1 and 6.B2.

From a neighbour-modulated fitness perspective, a rare mutant that is slightly more selfish than the wild type is favoured when

$$\partial w_{ij} / \partial g_{ij} + \partial w_{ij} / \partial g'.r > 0 \tag{6.B3}$$

because an individual carrying the mutation would experience a direct cost $\partial w_{ij} / \partial g_{ij}$ but with probability r would be paired with group mates that also carry the mutation, hence resulting in a return benefit of $\partial w_{ij} / \partial g'$.

Similarly, from an inclusive fitness perspective, a rare, slightly more selfish mutant is favoured when

$$\partial w_{ij} / \partial g_{ij} + (n-1).\partial w'/\partial g_{ij}.r > 0 \tag{6.B4}$$

because an individual actor that expresses the mutant behaviour would experience a direct cost $\partial w_{ij} / \partial g_{ij}$ but impose a cost of $\partial w' / \partial g$ to each of its $n - 1$ group mates, which with probability r would carry copies of its own mutant gene. It is easily checked that since $\partial w' / \partial g = (\partial w / \partial g')(g' / g_{ij})/(n - 1)$, and since mutations have small effect so that $g' \cong g_{ij}$, $(n - 1).\partial w'/\partial g_{ij} = \partial w_{ij} / \partial g'$, and inequalities 6.B3 and 6.B4 are therefore equivalent.

Finally, from a levels-of-selection perspective, selection would be partitioned into components that are due to the differential fitness of groups with different mean levels of selfishness and the differential success of more versus less selfish individuals within groups. Specifically, if we call G group productivity and I individual fitness relative to other group members, we have $G = w_i = (1-g_i)$, $I = w_{ij}/w_i = g_{ij}/g_i$ and individual fitness $w_{ij} = G.I$. From equation 6.12 it is clear that a more selfish mutant will be selected for when positive within-group selection balances with negative among-group selection:

$$\partial w_{ij} / \partial g_{ij}.(1 - R) > -\partial w_i / \partial g_i.R \tag{6.B5}$$

where R and $1 - R$ are proportional to the between- and within-group genetic variances and $R = (1/n) + ((n - 1)/n).r$ is known as Wright's intraclass correlation coefficient. Note that the among- and within-group selection components are also sometimes calculated in an equivalent way as $\partial w_{ij} / \partial G.dG / dg_{ij} = I.\partial G / \partial g_i.dg_i / dg_{ij} = I.\partial G / \partial g_i.R$ and $\partial w_{ij} / \partial I.dI / dg_{ij} = G.(\partial I / \partial g_{ij}.dg_{ij} / dg_{ij} + \partial I / \partial g_i.dg_i / dg_{ij}) = G.(\partial I / \partial g_{ij} + \partial I / \partial g_i.R)$ (cf. Ratnieks & Reeve 1992), which has the advantage that these only require the calculation of derivatives, and do not involve variances.

Differently still, using contextual analysis (inequality 6.15), we can see that a more selfish mutant can invade when

$$\beta_{w_{ij}g_{ij}.g_i} + \beta_{w_{ij}g_i.g_{ij}}.R > 0 \tag{6.B6}$$

Reassuringly, the evaluation of the partial derivatives in equations 6.B3 to 6.B6 for the case where $g_{ij} \approx g' \approx g_i \approx g$ shows that, no matter how we partition social evolution, the net selective effect is the same, and that an equilibrium is reached when $g^* = 1 - R$, i.e. the equilibrium level of selfishness decreases as relatedness, or more specifically, the intraclass correlation coefficient, increases. At this equilibrium, no mutant that behaves slightly differently can invade in the population (Maynard Smith 1982). In addition, it can be checked that the equilibrium is evolutionarily stable, i.e. a fitness maximum, since the derivatives of the above fitness gradients D (equations 6.B3–6.B6) with respect to g_{ij} are negative. Finally, an additional stability criterion, convergence stability, specifies whether the equilibrium is an attractor or not, and is therefore attainable, and requires that the fitness gradient is positive when evaluated for g slightly below g^* and

> **Box 6.1** Continued
>
> negative when g is slightly higher than g^*. Formally, this occurs when $\partial D/\partial g^*\big|_{g_{ij}=g'=g_i=}$ $_{g^*} < 0$ (Eshel & Motro 1981, Taylor 1996). A strategy that is simultaneously evolutionarily and convergence stable is termed a continuously stable strategy (CSS: Eshel 1983, Christiansen 1991), and it can be checked that the equilibrium in our example is indeed a CSS. Strategies that are convergence stable but not evolutionarily stable, however, are also possible, and can lead to disruptive selection and evolutionary branching (Metz *et al.* 1992, Geritz *et al.* 1998). Evolutionary branching points are interesting, as they provide us with the conditions under which continuous or mixed-strategy ESSs would be expected to evolve towards discrete-strategy ESSs (see section 6.3.1 and Doebeli *et al.* 2004 for an example).

6.2.3 Which method is best?

As we have demonstrated, for a wide variety of problems it is possible to analyse social evolution in an equivalent way based on the concepts of neighbour-modulated fitness, inclusive fitness or multilevel selection (Fig. 6.1, Box 6.1). These methods are simply different fitness accounting schemes, which in all cases lead to the same net gene frequency change. Neighbour-modulated fitness is perhaps closest to how natural selection actually works, and analyses social evolution in terms of correlated interaction, whereby individuals carrying a gene for a social trait would tend to interact more ($r > 0$) or less ($r < 0$) likely than chance with other individuals expressing the social trait. In recent years, neighbour-modulated fitness has emerged as one of the most popular methods for modelling kin selection (e.g. Frank 1998, Gandon 1999, Day 2001, Leturque & Rousset 2003, Wild & Taylor 2005, Pen 2006). Inclusive fitness instead adds up the effects of the actor's social behaviour on all recipients, using relatedness as the value of each recipient in helping to propagate copies of the actor's own genes. Inclusive fitness, in tracking the various fitness effects of a single individual's behaviour, mirrors the way that most evolutionary biologists think, particularly within the discipline of animal behaviour, and, likely for that reason, remains the preferred mode of analysis for most biologists. Finally, a levels-of-selection perspective takes explicit account of the hierarchical nature of biological systems, and analyses social evolution in terms of opposing selection within and among groups. This tells us to what extent evolution will favour maximal group success, or maximal individual success, relative to other group members (Sober & Wilson 1998). The contextual-analysis approach makes a similar partition of individual and group effects that can be useful for understanding the causal mechanisms of social evolution.

Which of these methods is preferable is partly a matter of taste, as each of them offers certain advantages, and may be more intuitive for any particular problem (Queller 1992a, Dugatkin & Reeve 1994, Foster 2006). In addition, all of these frameworks have led to unique, original insights (West *et al.* 2007b, 2008, Wilson & Wilson 2007, Wilson 2008). On the other hand, at a technical level, it is fair to say that the kin-selection approach (neighbour-modulated and inclusive fitness methods) has been developed to a much greater extent than the group-selection approaches (levels of selection and contextual analysis), and is the only method that can easily take into account class structure (Frank 1998, Rousset 2004, West *et al.* 2008; also section 6.3.1 and Chapter 12, but see Frank 1986, Ratnieks & Reeve 1992, Wenseleers *et al.* 2003). Furthermore there is some controversy over whether or not the levels-of-selection and contextual analysis approaches succeed in capturing the process of group selection for which they were originally devised (Okasha 2006, Wilson & Wilson 2007, West *et al.* 2008). Finally, Gardner & Grafen (2009) have argued that only inclusive fitness theory provides a clear adaptationist interpretation of the action of natural selection, with the dynamics of gene frequency change formally corresponding to the design objective of inclusive-fitness maximization (Grafen 2006). In contrast, there is no formal justification for regarding groups as fitness-maximizing agents, unless within-group selection can be considered negligible (Gardner & Grafen 2009). As a corollary, however, one could say that levels of selection theory also provides a maximand of selection, but one which within that framework would be a weighted average of group and relative, individual success. This suggestion, however, still remains to be formalized.

Whatever one's opinion of the different methodologies, it is clear that all have led to important and interesting insights. The prominence of genetic relatedness in kin-selection models has led to numerous tests that confirm its importance. These include considerable evidence from the social insects that patterns of kin structure within colonies are central to the balance between cooperation and conflict (Wenseleers & Ratnieks 2006b, Ratnieks et al. 2006, Ratnieks & Wenseleers 2008; Box 6.2, Fig. 6.2), data from social vertebrates that relatedness is linked to helping behaviour (Griffin & West 2003) and a growing body of evidence that genetic relatedness is important in microbial groups (Chapter 13). Meanwhile, consideration of the potential for group selection has led to a series of experiments that show the differential productivity of groups, and even communities, can strongly affect evolutionary trajectories (Chapter 2; Wade 1976, 1977, Wilson 1997, Wade & Goodnight 1998, Swenson et al. 2000, Bijma & Wade 2008). Group selection logic has also had practical applications (Bijma & Wade 2008): selecting chickens (*Gallus gallus domesticus*) for productivity at the level of groups in cages increases yield more than selecting for individual egg-laying ability (Muir 1996, 2005, Craig & Muir 1996).

6.3 Complexities in modelling social evolution

In the sections above we introduced the general approaches by which social evolution can be modelled, and illustrated these using a few very simple examples. In practice, however, several complications may arise. While it is not our intention to show how all of these can be dealt with, we will provide some key pointers to the relevant literature.

6.3.1 Multiple classes of individuals

The most common complication is that a social trait affects not just the individual's own age or sex class, but also that of one or more other classes of individuals, which usually do not themselves express the trait. The problem, then, is to correctly calculate the average fitness consequences of carrying the gene for such a trait across all classes (in a neighbour-modulated fitness scheme), or, from an actor's point of view, to correctly value a member of each class of recipients in mediating gene frequency change (in an inclusive fitness scheme). For example, it is clear that a sexually mature individual should be valued differently than an aged individual that is about to die.

One can account for the differences in value among classes in a neighbour-modulated fitness model using something appropriately called the class reproductive value c_k (Taylor 1990, Taylor & Frank 1996, Taylor et al. 2007a), which is the product of the number of individuals u_k in a given class k and each of its members' reproductive value v_k, which measures the ability of an individual of class k to contribute to the future gene pool (Fisher 1930). Another way to think about c_k is to recall that in a neighbour-modulated fitness model, one must determine the average effect of a gene coding for a social trait in a random carrier, such that picking a random carrier would mean picking an individual of a certain class with relative probability c_k (Taylor 1990, Taylor & Frank 1996, Taylor et al. 2007a). More technically, if we write the transmission probabilities between the different classes of individuals in a stable population (i.e. in the absence of selection) as a matrix A, then $c = v.u$, and u and v are the dominant right and dominant left eigenvectors of A (Taylor & Frank 1996). For an age-structured population, A is known as the Leslie matrix (Bulmer 1994).

To give an example, Wenseleers et al. (2003) discussed the case of stingless bees of the genus *Melipona* where female larvae can control their own caste development and gain a fitness advantage by increasing their probability of developing into queens rather

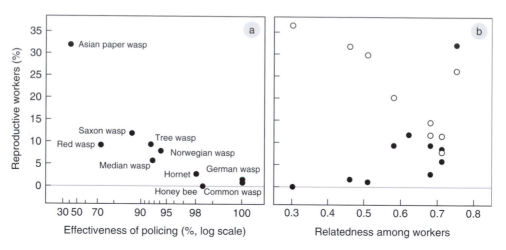

Figure 6.2 Testing social evolution theory: the effect of policing efficiency and relatedness on male production by workers in the eusocial Hymenoptera (see Box 6.2). (a) A comparative analysis of nine wasp species and the honey bee *Apis mellifera* shows that significantly fewer workers attempt to reproduce when the eggs they lay are more effectively killed or 'policed' by nestmates. (b) The effect of worker relatedness on worker male production. Here one must distinguish between colonies with a queen and those without a queen. In colonies with a queen, worker policing occurs, and this is what drives the frequency of laying workers. Moreover, and for reasons we have not discussed (see Ratnieks & Wenseleers 2008 for a review), the strength of policing correlates negatively with relatedness. This means that, somewhat paradoxically, more workers reproduce in species with a queen (filled circles) when workers are more related to each other. In queenless colonies (open circles), however, the relationship is reversed and, as predicted by Hamilton's rule, workers are more altruistic and fewer lay eggs in the species where they are more related to each other. Data from Wenseleers and Ratnieks (2006b).

than workers. Colony productivity, however, would go down as more larvae chose to develop into queens, due to the resultant shortage of workers, and this would reduce both male production and the production of new daughter swarms. Similar to Frank's tragedy of the commons model (Box 6.1), this situation was captured by assuming that male production is given by $W_m = 1 - g_i$ and that the relative success of a female larva (the relative probability that she heads the swarm, multiplied by the likelihood of it being produced) is given by $W_f = (g_{ij}/g_i)(1 - g_i)$, where g_{ij} and g_i are the individual and colony average probabilities with which larvae turn into queens, and with $g_i = (1/n)g_{ij} + ((n-1)/n)g_{ij}')$, where n are the number of competing female larvae and g_{ij}' is the average genetic value of the social partners of the focal individual ij. Following a neighbour-modulated fitness logic, a mutant that makes larvae develop into queens with a slightly higher probability is favoured when $c_f(\partial W_f/\partial g_{ij} + \partial W_f/\partial g'.r_f) + c_m.\partial W_m/\partial g_i.$

$r_m > 0$, where c_f and c_m are the class reproductive values of queens and males, and r_f and r_m are the regression relatedness values of larvae to sisters and males reared in the colony. From this, it is readily shown that when n is large, the ESS is for larvae to develop into queens with a probability of $(1- r_f)/(1 + (c_m/c_f).r_m)$. For the case where colonies are headed by a single once-mated queen and where all males are produced by the queen, this results in an ESS in which 20% of the females should develop into queens, since due to haplodiploidy $c_m/c_f = 1/2$, $r_f = 3/4$ and $r_m = 1/2$ (Hamilton 1972, Bourke & Franks 1995), a result that in fact is quite close to empirically observed ratios (Wenseleers & Ratnieks 2004).

This same result can be recovered from an inclusive fitness analysis, illustrating the equivalence of approaches. The inclusive fitness effect of an increase in queen development probability of a focal female larva is given by $\partial W_f/\partial g_{ij} v_f + (n - 1).\partial W_f/\partial g_{ij} v_f r_f + m.\partial W_m/\partial g_{ij} v_m.r_m,$ where $W'_f = (1 - g_i)(g'_{ij}/g_i)$ is the fitness of another female larva in the colony, $W'_m = (1 - g_i)$ is the fitness of a male in the colony, m are the number of males produced over a colony's lifetime, v_f and v_m are the individual reproductive value of female larvae and males, and r_f and r_m are the regression relatedness to them, respectively. Simplifying by dividing everything by v_f yields $\partial W_f/\partial g_{ij} + (n-1).\partial W'_f/\partial g_{ij}.R_f + m.\partial W'_m/\partial g_{ij}.R_m$, where $R_f = r_f$ and $R_m = r_m.(v_m/v_f)$ are the life-for-life relatedness to females and males, which are defined as the product of regression

relatedness and relative reproductive value (Hamilton 1972, Taylor & Frank 1996, Taylor et al. 2007a). Observing that $(v_m/v_f) = (c_m/c_f).(u_f/u_m) = (c_m/c_f).(n/m)$ and setting the inclusive fitness effect to zero and solving for $g_{ij} = g'_{ij} = g_i = g = g^*$ obtains the ESS $g^* = (1 - r_f)/(1 + (c_m/c_f).r_m)$.

Other examples of class-structured kin selection models involving interactions between different age classes are discussed by Charlesworth and Charnov (1981), Taylor and Frank (1996) and Taylor et al. (2007a).

Box 6.2 A model and an empirical test: worker male production in the social insects

In order to illustrate the predictive power of social evolution theory, we here describe a model and associated data for a classic problem in sociobiology: the evolution of worker sterility. Specifically, we are focusing on the evolution of male production by workers. The eusocial Hymenoptera (bees, wasps and ants) are haplodiploid: males are haploid and females are diploid. This means that unmated workers in many species are able to lay unfertilised, haploid eggs that would develop into males if reared. Nevertheless, despite this ability workers in many species appear to refrain from laying eggs. Why is this so?

Wenseleers et al. (2004a, 2004b) analysed this problem using an inclusive fitness model. Specifically, they asked what are the factors that determine the frequency of workers that attempt to lay eggs in insect societies. We review the model here because its specific predictions have subsequently been shown to hold in real systems. Let n be the number of workers in the colony, p the probability that a worker-laid male egg is removed by another individual (the queen and workers remove or 'police' worker-laid eggs in many species: Wenseleers & Ratnieks 2006a), and q the fecundity of the queen relative to a single reproductive worker in terms of laying male eggs. Assume that a focal worker j in colony i activates her ovaries to lay eggs with probability g_{ij} and that each of its $n - 1$ nestmates activates her ovaries with probability g'_{ij}, so that the colony contains ng_i egg-laying workers where g_i is the average probability with which workers activate their ovaries, $g_i = (1/n)g_{ij} + ((n - 1)/n)g'_{ij}$. We can now write the total number of males produced by this focal worker and by each nestmate worker as $W_{mw} = G(g_i).g_{ij}(1 - p)/(ng_i(1 - p) + q)$ and $W'_{mw} = G(g_i).g'_{ij}(1 - p)/(ng_i(1 - p) + q)$, where $G(g_i)$ is the colony productivity (total number of males reared) as a function of how many laying workers there are in the colony (egg-laying workers generally perform less work and so decrease total colony productivity) and the terms following G represent the proportion of all males that are workers' sons. That is, the total number of sons of the focal and other workers that survive policing, divided by all surviving males, which includes both workers' sons $((ng_i(1 - p))$ and queen's sons, laid in proportion to the relative rate q at which these are produced. For simplicity, we will assume that worker reproduction linearly reduces colony productivity, i.e. $G = 1 - g_i$, because fewer workers will work when more reproduce.

By a similar argument, the total number of males produced by the queen is $W_{mq} = G(g_i).q/(ng_i(1 - p) + q)$.

Box 6.2 Continued

Finally, the total amount of female reproduction by the colony (winged queens, or swarms for swarm-founding species such as honey bees *Apis mellifera*) is also a decreasing function of g_i. For simplicity, we assume that worker reproduction reduces queen and male production equally. Hence, the total number of queens or swarms produced is $W_f = G(g_i) = 1 - g_i$.

The inclusive fitness effect of increasing the probability of becoming a laying worker for a focal individual is given by $\partial W_{mw}/\partial g_{ij}.v_m.r_{son} + (n-1).(\partial W'_{mw}/\partial g_{ij}).v_m.r_{nephew} + (\partial W_{mq}/\partial g_{ij}).v_m.r_{brother} + (\partial W_f/\partial g_{ij}).v_f r_{sister}$.

Finally, in haplodiploids, one must make adjustments for the fact that males only carry half the genes of females, i.e. males will often have a lower reproductive value than females (reviewed in Bourke & Franks 1995). This gives so-called 'life-for-life relatedness coefficients' of $R_{son} = r_{son}.v_m = 1.v_m$, $R_{nephew} = r_{sister}.v_m$ and $R_{brother} = r_{brother}.v_m = (1/2).v_m$, where v_m is the relative reproductive value of males to females, which is $1/2(2-\psi)$ where ψ is the population-wide proportion of males that are workers' sons (Pamilo 1991). In our case, it can be seen that $\psi = ng(1-p)/(ngS+q)$, where g is the average proportion of laying workers in an average colony in the population. Setting the inclusive fitness effect to zero and solving for $g_{ij} = g'_{ij} = g_i = g = g^*$ obtains the ESS:

$$g^* = \frac{-B + \sqrt{B^2 - 4AC}}{2A}$$

with $A = 2n^2(1-p)^2(1+r_{sister})$ (6.B7)

$B = 2(1-p)(q(1+n-r_{sister}+4nr_{sister}) + (n-1)n(1-r_{sister})(1-p))$

$C = q(q(1+4r_{sister}) - n(1-p))$

The solution makes a number of predictions (Wenseleers *et al.* 2004a, 2004b) but here we will focus on two main insights. Firstly, species with the strongest policing, in which the queen or other workers efficiently remove worker eggs, should have the lowest proportion of laying workers. Intuitively, this is because the benefit to a worker of laying $(\partial W_{mw}/\partial g_{ij})$ declines when fewer of her eggs are reared. Second, in the absence of egg removal by policing, the proportion of laying workers should decrease with increased relatedness among workers, because high sister–sister relatedness decreases the relatedness gain of replacing nephews with sons (Bourke 1988). Empirical data from wasps and bees have been shown to support both of these predictions (Wenseleers & Ratnieks 2006b; Fig. 6.2).

6.3.2 Non-additive fitness interactions and frequency-dependent selection

In many situations the fitness consequences of the cooperative behaviour of actors and recipients do not simply add up (Queller 1984, 1985, 1992b). For example, consider a scenario where individuals interact in pairs in which each social partner chooses whether to cooperate or defect, and with cooperation carrying a personal cost C to the actor, giving a benefit B to the recipient, and additionally giving an extra benefit D if the other individual also cooperates, in addition to a baseline fitness of 1. The quantity D has been described as the 'synergy' effect, and might be positive (benefit) or negative (cost) (Queller 1984, 1985).

If the cooperation phenotype is controlled in a probabilistic way, and a focal individual's genes encode a strategy value g such that the individual cooperates with probability g and defects with probability $1 - g$, then we can express fitness as

$$w = 1 - C.g + B.g' + D.g.g' \qquad (6.16)$$

where g' is the social partner's breeding value for the cooperation trait. If we make the assumption that g is a quantitative character with vanishing variation around the population average of $\bar{g}$, then we can employ the usual derivation approach to determine the costs and benefits of cooperation in Hamilton's rule (Box 6.1; Taylor & Frank 1996, Frank 1998), yielding the result that an increase in the level of cooperation will be selected for when

$$\frac{\partial w}{\partial g} + \frac{\partial w}{\partial g'}.r = (-C + D.\bar{g}) + (B + D.\bar{g}).r > 0 \qquad (6.17)$$

This identifies an equilibrium point at $g^* = (C - Br)/(D(1 + r))$ which, when it takes an intermediate value (between 0 and 1) is unstable for $D > 0$ and stable for $D < 0$ (Grafen 1979, Queller 1984, Wenseleers 2006). Note that while the cooperation and defection phenotypes have selective value that is frequency-dependent, the minor genetic variants that alter the probabilistic expression of these phenotypes are governed by selection that is frequency-independent.

Alternatively, the cooperation phenotype of an individual might be fully determined by its genotype, with some individuals carrying a cooperation allele ($g = 1$) and others carrying a defection allele ($g = 0$; for simplicity, we assume haploidy). In this case, the assumptions underlying the differentiation approach fail, and so we use the more general version of Hamilton's rule instead (inequality 6.5), $\beta_{wg.g'} + \beta_{wg'.g}\beta_{g'g} > 0$, where the costs and benefits of cooperation are defined as the partial regression coefficients $\beta_{wg.g'}$ and $\beta_{wg'.g}$ (Gardner et al. 2007). These coefficients are defined so that fitness is predicted as a linear function of one's own and one's social partner's breeding value:

$$\hat{w} = \bar{w} + \beta_{wg.g'}(g - \bar{g}) + \beta_{wg'.g}(g' - \bar{g}) \qquad (6.18)$$

and where mean fitness $w = f_{10}\, w_{10} + f_{11}\, w_{11} + f_{01}\, w_{01} + f_{00}\, w_{00}$, f_{XY} is the frequency of XY pairs in the population, and w_{XY} is the fitness of an individual playing strategy X against an individual playing strategy Y. The

proportion of fitness variance that is not explained by the linear model is given by the average squared residual $S = \sum_{X,Y} f_{XY}(w_{XY} - \hat{w}|_{g=X,g'=Y})^2$. We obtain the partial regression coefficients by the usual method of least squares, i.e. the values of $\beta_{wg.g'}$ and $\beta_{wg'g}$ that minimise S and for which $\partial S/\partial \beta_{wg.g'} = \partial S/\partial \beta_{wg'g} = 0$, and Gardner et al. (2007) show that these are equal to

$$\beta_{wg.g'} = -c = -C + \frac{r + (1-r)\bar{g}}{1+r} D \qquad (6.19)$$

$$\beta_{wg'.g} = b = B + \frac{r + (1-r)\bar{g}}{1+r} D \qquad (6.20)$$

Hence in this case cooperation spreads when $-c + b.r = -C + B.r + D.(r + (1-r)\bar{g}) > 0$, a condition that can be verified using a standard population-genetic approach (Grafen 1979, Queller 1984). The three parts in this equation split up additive and non-additive effects on fitness. Increasing one's level of cooperation incurs a cost $-C$ but also results in a benefit $B.r$ as a result of the cooperation received from neighbours. In addition, increasing one's level of cooperation will incur an extra non-additive benefit D insofar as one's partner is also a cooperator, which will be the case in a proportion $(r + (1-r)\bar{g})$ of all interactions. This third effect is due to the combined action of own and social-partner genes, the former being of relative importance 1 (the association between own genes and own phenotype) and the latter being of relative importance r (the association between own genes and partner's phenotype), and so a proportion $1/(1+r)$ of the effect is attributed to own genes and a proportion $r/(1+r)$ is attributed to partner's genes. Hence the direct fitness effect is $-c = -C + (1/(1+r)).(r + (1-r)\bar{g}).D$, and the indirect fitness effect is $b.r = B.r + (r/(1+r)).(r + (1-r)\bar{g}).D$. Thus, in contrast to what has sometimes been claimed (Queller 1984, Bulmer 1994, Wenseleers 2006), Hamilton's rule $-c + b.r > 0$ does hold for situations where strategies are discrete and selection is strong (major as opposed to minor genetic variants), provided that the fitness effects b and c are calculated according to their proper least-square-regression definitions (Gardner et al. 2007).

In contrast to typical models of kin selection, which assume that selection is weak and hence frequency-independent (Hamilton 1995, Rousset 2004, 2006,

Ross-Gillespie *et al.* 2007), allowing for discrete strategies and strong selection generates frequency-dependent kin selection. In the above example, selection acting upon the cooperation gene ($g = 1$) depends on the frequency of this gene in the population ($\bar{g}$). If the synergy term D is positive, then selection is positively frequency-dependent: either cooperation or defection or both cooperation and defection are evolutionarily stable, depending on parameter values, and there is no stable polymorphism between the two alleles. However, if the synergy term D is negative, then selection is negatively frequency-dependent, and depending on parameter values the population will evolve either towards complete cooperation, complete defection, or a stable polymorphism between the two whereby cooperation is maintained at intermediate frequency $g^* = (C - (B + D)r)/(D(1 - r))$ (Grafen 1979, Queller 1984, Wenseleers 2006).

In principle, the same approach as outlined above could be used to deal with frequency dependence in an inclusive fitness or a levels-of-selection framework (Breden 1990). Nevertheless, it is fair to say that more work remains to be done on frequency dependence in social evolution models (see Grafen 2006, 2007a and commentaries on Lehmann & Keller 2006a). This is perhaps surprising, given that in economics, game theory (Chapter 4) is almost entirely concerned with frequency-dependent interaction, even though, in contrast to kin-selection models, interactions are usually assumed to occur among non-relatives (Gintis 2000b).

6.3.3 Multilocus models and non-additive gene action

Both kin selection (equations 6.4 and 6.6) and multi-level selection (equation 6.11) have often been formulated so that the fitness predictors g refer to the frequency of an allele in individuals at a single locus (Hamilton 1964, Wade 1980). This has led many to conclude that these methods are unrealistic, for clearly a social trait would unlikely be controlled by just a single locus. This criticism, however, is not well founded. First, if one considers the evolution of continuous or probabilistically expressed traits (Box 6.1), where one looks at the repeated invasion of mutants of small effect,

then although each invasion event would consider the spread of a single allele at a single locus, the wild type in each case could be controlled by any number of loci. In addition, in recent years, there has been a tendency to define g, as in quantitative genetics, as the breeding value (additive genetic value) for a given trait, which is a linear combination of the frequency of any number of alleles at any number of loci that best predicts an individual's phenotype (Falconer 1981, Crow & Aoki 1982, Frank 1998). Either way, it is not assumed that social traits are under the control of a single locus.

A fully general and more explicit multilocus social evolution theory was recently also developed by Billiard and Lenormand (2005), Roze and Rousset (2005, 2008) and Gardner *et al.* (2007), based on the multilocus methodology of Barton and Turelli (1991) and Kirkpatrick *et al.* (2002). This theory, which was formulated from a neighbour-modulated fitness perspective, takes explicit account of the fact that the natural selection operating upon one genetic locus can potentially spill over onto associated loci and indirectly drive changes in gene frequencies. Within the multilocus framework, such genetic hitchhiking is measured by the association between genes within individuals (i.e. linkage disequilibrium), and relatedness arises in a similar way as the association between genes in different individuals (Gardner *et al.* 2007). These methods are important, as they allow the coevolution between different traits in the same or in different sets of individuals (e.g. parents and offspring) to be examined, taking explicit account of the fact that some of the genes involved in the traits may be linked, and taking account of any type of non-additive gene interaction (dominance or epistasis). When selection is weak and the genes for the different traits are unlinked, however, coevolutionary problems may also be analysed more simply using the maximisation methods discussed in Box 6.1 (see Frank 1995b).

6.3.4 Complex demographics and spatially explicit models

A frequent complication is that social interactions do not occur within family groups that reform in each generation, but instead occur locally among individuals that tend to stay near their natal patch. Hamilton (1964, 1972) suggested that such population viscosity could favour cooperation because limited dispersal would result in interacting individuals tending to be relatives. However, Wilson et al. (1992) later showed, using an explicitly spatial cellular automaton model, that in a simple-case scenario this argument does not hold. The reason is that limited dispersal also results in local competition, the consequence of which is that patches of altruists would be unable to export their higher productivity to the rest of the population. In the model of Wilson et al. (1992) these two factors exactly cancelled, so that population viscosity had negligible influence on the evolution of cooperation. The same year, Taylor was also able to confirm analytically, using a kin-selection approach, that the effect of increased competition between relatives exactly cancels out with the effect of increased relatedness if the spatial scale of competition is the same as the spatial scale of dispersal (Taylor 1992, reviewed by Queller 1992c, West et al. 2002). Since then, a number of theoretical models have examined the extent to which more complex and possibly biologically realistic assumptions can reduce the problem of local competition, and lead to limited dispersal favouring altruism (Kelly 1992, 1994, van Baalen & Rand 1998, Mitteldorf & Wilson 2000, Taylor & Irwin 2000, Gardner & West 2006, Lehmann et al. 2006, 2008a). For example, Gardner and West (2006) and Lehmann et al. (2006) show that the effect of local competition can be partly overcome if individuals disperse in groups or buds, while van Baalen and Rand (1998) also show how the invasion condition for a small cluster of altruists in a cellular automata-type model reduces to a form of Hamilton's rule. Recent analyses using evolutionary graph theory, whereby individuals interact in social networks (Chapter 9; Ohtsuki et al. 2006, Ohtsuki & Nowak 2006), have been shown to similarly fall under the remit of inclusive fitness theory (Grafen 2007b, Lehmann et al. 2007b, Taylor et al. 2007b).

Typical for most models involving complex demographies is that relatedness is not just a fixed genetic parameter, but instead depends on population demographic processes such as migration and birth/death dynamics (Taylor 1992, van Baalen & Rand 1998, Gardner & West 2006, Lehmann et al. 2006). Taylor et al. (2007c) present a recursive method for calculating relatedness as a function of population demographic parameters, and Rousset (2004) also presents general methods for analysing inclusive fitness models under complex population demographies.

6.3.5 Social and individual learning

In some situations, particularly in humans (Chapter 15), it is likely that social traits are not purely genetically determined but are also affected by norms and beliefs that are culturally transmitted through imitation and social learning (Cavalli-Sforza & Feldman 1981, Boyd & Richerson 1985). Dawkins, by analogy with genes, refers to such cultural beliefs as memes (Dawkins 1976), and they may be either discrete in nature (e.g. whether or not one advocates a particular religion) or continuously varying traits (e.g. hunting skill: Boyd & Richerson 1985, Henrich 2004). Using the above methods, the spread of cultural beliefs can be modelled in much the same way as the spread of genes within populations, although there are some important qualifications. First, biological fitness (w) is usually redefined as cultural fitness, which is the extent to which an individual can affect the proportional representation of a cultural trait in the next generation or time step (Henrich 2004). Second, mutation sometimes requires to be taken into account, since cultural traits are liable to mutate and change at a much faster rate than genes. This can be done by retaining the transmission bias term of the Price equation (equation 6.1; for an example see Frank 1998, p. 55).

Models of cultural evolution have been constructed within both the group-selection and inclusive-fitness traditions. From a group-selection perspective, it has been noted that in cultural evolution among-group differences tend to be much larger than in genetic models, since individuals that migrate to other groups are frequently forced to adopt the customs and norms of the group they join (conformist transmission: Boyd & Richerson 1985, Henrich 2004). This can favour cooperative behaviour via cultural group selection (Boyd et al. 2003, reviewed in Henrich 2004), although it is an open question as to whether cultural transmission will in general promote or hinder cooperation relative to genetic transmission (Lehmann et al. 2008b, 2008c).

From an inclusive fitness perspective, Allison (1992) noted that the concept of genetic relatedness can be readily extended to cultural relatedness, which is defined as the likelihood that two interacting individuals are more likely than chance to share the same cultural belief. Allison (1992) showed that if cultural beliefs are copied from a limited set of individuals in the group (e.g. a tribal chief), as would be the case in conformist transmission, cultural relatedness can be very high, and that this could promote cooperation (see also Lehmann *et al.* 2007c). Using recurrence equations, equilibrium levels of cultural relatedness under various vertical, oblique and horizontal transmission schemes were also provided. Clearly, the inclusive-fitness optimisation method may well be a promising approach for gaining a better understanding of cultural evolution, particularly if cultural change occurs relatively slowly (i.e. if cultural variants have small effects and mutate slowly). The notion of reproductive value would also be readily applicable, given that human groups generally contain different classes of individuals (e.g. leaders and followers, teachers and students) that have a different influence in causing future cultural change. When cultural variants have large effects, however, it may be easier to resort to a traditional population-genetic approach (Cavalli-Sforza & Feldman, 1981, Boyd & Richerson 1985, Feldman *et al.* 1985).

While models of the social learning of culture bring added realism to social evolution in humans and derived vertebrates, they tend, like genetic models, to assume that individuals inherit simple and relatively fixed strategies by cultural means. Many economists, however, instead emphasise the impressive ability of humans to modify their social behaviours by trial-and-error learning or reasoning (Rubinstein 1998). Such individual learning can again be modelled using evolutionary logic. Nevertheless, the full impact of incorporating individual learning into genetic and cultural models remains to be determined (Lehmann *et al.* 2008c).

6.4 Conclusions and future directions

Close to 50 years after Hamilton's seminal papers (1963, 1964), the evolution of cooperation and altruism remains one of the most active areas of study in

evolutionary biology. Indeed, it is considered to be one of the most important unsolved questions in science (Pennisi 2005). This is not to say we have not made great progress already. The available methods now allow complex demographies to be analysed (Taylor 1992, Rousset 2004, Lehmann *et al.* 2006, Gardner & West 2006), spatial, age and sex structure to be explicitly incorporated (Taylor & Frank 1996, van Baalen & Rand 1998, Lehmann & Keller 2006a, Lehmann *et al.* 2007b, Grafen 2007b, Taylor *et al.* 2007a, 2007b), the effects of synergy and frequency dependence to be assessed (Queller 1984, Wenseleers 2006, Lehmann & Keller 2006b, Gardner *et al.* 2007), multilocus and non-additive genetics to be incorporated (Billiard & Lenormand 2005, Roze & Rousset 2005, 2008, Gardner *et al.* 2007), the conditions to be determined under which disruptive selection and evolutionary branching will occur (Taylor 1996, Doebeli *et al.* 2004), and cultural evolution to be analysed in much the same way as genetic evolution (Allison 1992, Frank 1997b, Henrich 2004, Lehmann *et al.* 2007c). In addition, results can often be obtained in equivalent ways within the frameworks of neighbour-modulated fitness, inclusive fitness or levels of selection.

Nevertheless, important challenges remain. For example, many of the derivations require weak selection (e.g. in the calculation of reproductive value, relatedness and between- and within-group genetic variances), inclusive fitness theory requires strategic equivalence (i.e. all actors being equivalent: Grafen 2006), and better methods to deal with frequency dependence in inclusive fitness models remain to be developed (Wenseleers 2006, Grafen 2006, 2007a). Levels-of-selection approaches still suffer from semantic difficulties that would be desirable to fix (Okasha 2006, Wilson & Wilson 2007), and as yet they struggle somewhat to properly incorporate class structure (West *et al.* 2008). Lastly, much work remains to be done on cultural evolution (Cavalli-Sforza & Feldman 1981, Boyd & Richerson 1985, Lehmann *et al.* 2007c). It is clear that social evolution theory will remain a fruitful topic for years to come.

Acknowledgements

We thank the FWO-Flanders (TW), the Royal Society (AG) and the National Institute of General Medical

Sciences Center of Excellence (KRF) for financial support.

Suggested readings

Frank, S. A. (1998) *The Foundations of Social Evolution*. Princeton, NJ: Princeton University Press.

Kokko, H. (2007) *Modelling for Field Biologists and other Interesting People*. Cambridge: Cambridge University Press.

McElreath, R. & Boyd, R. (2007) *Mathematical Models of Social Evolution: a Guide for the Perplexed*. Chicago, IL: University of Chicago Press.

Okasha, S. (2006) *Evolution and the Levels of Selection*. Oxford: Oxford University Press.

Rousset, F. (2004) *Genetic Structure and Selection in Subdivided Populations*. Princeton, NJ: Princeton University Press.

References

Allison, P. D. (1992) Cultural relatedness under oblique and horizontal transmission rules. *Ethology and Sociobiology*, **13**, 153–169.

Andersen, E. S. (2004) Population thinking, Price's equation and the analysis of economic evolution. *Evolutionary and Institutional Economics Review*, **1**, 127–148.

Arnold, A. J. & Fristrup, K. (1982) The theory of evolution by natural selection: a hierarchical expansion. *Paleobiology*, **8**, 113–129.

Axelrod, R. & Hamilton, W. D. (1981) The evolution of cooperation. *Science*, **211**, 1390–1396.

Axelrod, R., Hammond, R. A. & Grafen, A. (2004) Altruism via kin-selection strategies that rely on arbitrary tags with which they coevolve. *Evolution*, **58**, 1833–1838.

Barton, N. H. & Turelli, M. (1991) Natural and sexual selection on many loci. *Genetics*, **127**, 229–255.

Bijma, P. & Wade, M. J. (2008) The joint effects of kin, multi-level selection and indirect genetic effects on response to genetic selection. *Journal of Evolutionary Biology*, **21**, 1175–1188.

Billiard, S. & Lenormand, T. (2005) Evolution of migration under kin selection and local adaptation. *Evolution*, **59**, 13–23.

Bourke, A. F. G. (1988) Worker reproduction in the higher eusocial Hymenoptera. *Quarterly Review of Biology*, **63**, 291–311.

Bourke, A. F. G. & Franks, N. R. (1995) *Social Evolution in Ants*. Princeton, NJ: Princeton University Press.

Boyd, R. & Richerson, P. J. (1985) *Culture and the Evolutionary Process*. Chicago, IL: University of Chicago Press.

Boyd, R., Gintis, H., Bowles, S. & Richerson, P. J. (2003) The evolution of altruistic punishment. *Proceedings of the National Academy of Sciences of the USA*, **100**, 3531–3535.

Breden, F. (1990) Partitioning of covariance as a method for studying kin selection. *Trends in Ecology and Evolution*, **5**, 224–228.

Bulmer, M. (1994) *Theoretical Evolutionary Ecology*. Sunderland, MA: Sinauer Associates.

Cavalli-Sforza, L. L. & Feldman, M. W. (1978) Darwinian selection and altruism. *Theoretical Population Biology*, **14**, 268–280.

Cavalli-Sforza, L. L. & Feldman, M. W. (1981) *Cultural Transmission and Evolution*. Princeton, NJ: Princeton University Press.

Charlesworth, B. & Charnov, E. L. (1981) Kin selection in age-structured populations. *Journal of Theoretical Biology*, **88**, 103–119.

Charnov, E. L. (1978) Evolution of eusocial behavior: offspring choice or parental parasitism? *Journal of Theoretical Biology*, **75**, 451–465.

Christiansen, F. B. (1991) On conditions for evolutionary stability for a continuously varying character. *American Naturalist*, **138**, 37–50.

Colwell, R. K. (1981) Group selection is implicated in the evolution of female biased sex ratios. *Nature*, **290**, 401–404.

Craig, J. V. & Muir, W. M. (1996) Group selection for adaptation to multiple-hen cages: behavioral responses. *Poultry Science*, **75**, 1145–1155.

Crow, J. F. & Aoki, K. (1982) Group selection for a polygenic behavioral trait: a differential proliferation model. *Proceedings of the National Academy of Sciences of the USA*, **79**, 2628–2631.

Darwin, C. (1859) *On the Origin of Species by Means of Natural Selection*. London: John Murray.

Dawkins, R. (1976) *The Selfish Gene*. Oxford: Oxford University Press.

Day, T. (2001) Population structure inhibits evolutionary diversification under competition for resources. *Genetica*, **112/113**, 71–86.

Day, T. & Gandon, S. (2007) Applying population-genetic models in theoretical evolutionary epidemiology. *Ecology Letters*, **10**, 876–888.

Doebeli, M., Hauert, C. & Killingback, T. (2004) The evolutionary origin of cooperators and defectors. *Science*, **306**, 859–862.

Dugatkin, L. A. & Reeve, H. K. (1994) Behavioral ecology and levels of selection – Dissolving the group selection controversy. *Advances in the Study of Behavior*, **23**, 101–133.

Eshel, I. (1983) Evolutionary and continuous stability. *Journal of Theoretical Biology*, **103**, 99–111.

Eshel, I. & Cavalli-Sforza, L. L. (1982) Assortment of encounters and evolution of cooperativeness. *Proceedings of the National Academy of Sciences of the USA*, **79**, 1331–1335.

Eshel, I. & Motro, U. (1981) Kin selection and strong evolutionary stability of mutual help. *Theoretical Population Biology*, **19**, 420–433.

Falconer, D. S. (1981) *Introduction to Quantitative Genetics*, 2nd edn. London: Longman.

Fehr, E. & Fischbacher, U. (2003) The nature of human altruism. *Nature*, **425**, 785–791.

Feldman, M. W. & Cavalli-Sforza, L. L. (1981) Further remarks on Darwinian selection and altruism. *Theoretical Population Biology*, **19**, 251–260.

Feldman, M. W., Cavalli-Sforza, L. L. & Peck, J. R. (1985) Gene–culture coevolution: models for the evolution of altruism with cultural transmission. *Proceedings of the National Academy of Sciences of the USA*, **82**, 5814–5818.

Fisher, R. A. (1930) *The Genetical Theory of Natural Selection*. Oxford: Clarendon Press.

Fletcher, J. A. & Doebeli, M. (2006) How altruism evolves: assortment and synergy. *Journal of Evolutionary Biology*, **19**, 1389–1393.

Fletcher, J. A. & Zwick, M. (2006) Unifying the theories of inclusive fitness and reciprocal altruism. *American Naturalist*, **168**, 252–262.

Foster, K. R. (2004) Diminishing returns in social evolution: the not-so-tragic commons. *Journal of Evolutionary Biology*, **17**, 1058–1072.

Foster, K. R. (2006) Balancing synthesis with pluralism in sociobiology. *Journal of Evolutionary Biology*, **19**, 1394–1396.

Foster, K. R. & Wenseleers, T. (2006) A general model for the evolution of mutualisms. *Journal of Evolutionary Biology*, **19**, 1283–1293.

Foster, K. R., Wenseleers, T., Ratnieks, F. L. W. & Queller, D. C. (2006a) There is nothing wrong with inclusive fitness. *Trends in Ecology and Evolution*, **21**, 599–560.

Foster, K. R., Wenseleers, T. & Ratnieks, F. L. W. (2006b) Kin selection is the key to altruism. *Trends in Ecology and Evolution*, **21**, 57–60.

Fox, J. W. (2006) Using the Price Equation to partition the effects of biodiversity loss on ecosystem function *Ecology*, **87**, 2687–2696.

Frank, S. A. (1986) Hierarchical selection theory and sex-ratios. 1. General solutions for structured populations. *Theoretical Population Biology*, **29**, 312–342.

Frank, S. A. (1994a) Genetics of mutualism: the evolution of altruism between species. *Journal of Theoretical Biology*, **170**, 393–400.

Frank, S. A. (1994b) Kin selection and virulence in the evolution of protocells and parasites. *Proceedings of the Royal Society B*, **258**, 153–161.

Frank, S. A. (1995a) George Price's contributions to evolutionary genetics. *Journal of Theoretical Biology*, **175**, 373–388.

Frank, S. A. (1995b) Mutual policing and repression of competition in the evolution of cooperative groups. *Nature*, **377**, 520–522.

Frank, S. A. (1997a) Multivariate analysis of correlated selection and kin selection, with an ESS maximization method. *Journal of Theoretical Biology*, **189**, 307–316.

Frank, S. A. (1997b) The Price equation, Fisher's fundamental theorem, kin selection, and causal analysis. *Evolution*, **51**, 1712–1729.

Frank, S. A. (1998) *The Foundations of Social Evolution*. Princeton, NJ: Princeton University Press.

Gandon, S. (1999) Kin competition, the cost of inbreeding and the evolution of dispersal. *Journal of Theoretical Biology*, **200**, 345–364.

Gardner, A. & Foster, K. R. (2008) The evolution and ecology of cooperation: history and concepts. In: *Ecology of Social Evolution*, ed. J. Korb & J. Heinze. Berlin, Heidelberg: Springer, pp. 1–36.

Gardner, A. & Grafen, A. (2009) Capturing the superorganism: a formal theory of group adaptation. *Journal of Evolutionary Biology* **22**, 659–671.

Gardner, A. & West, S. A. (2004) Cooperation and punishment, especially in humans. *American Naturalist*, **164**, 753–764.

Gardner, A. & West, S. A. (2006) Demography, altruism, and the benefits of budding. *Journal of Evolutionary Biology*, **19**, 1707–1716.

Gardner, A. & West, S. A. (2010) Greenbeards. *Evolution*, **64**, 25–38.

Gardner, A., West, S. A. & Barton, N. H. (2007) The relation between multilocus population genetics and social evolution theory. *American Naturalist*, **169**, 207–226.

Gayley, T. (1993) Genetics of kin selection: the role of behavioral inclusive fitness. *American Naturalist*, **141**, 928–953.

Geritz, S. A. H., Kisdi, E., Meszéna, G. & Metz, J. A. J. (1998) Evolutionarily singular strategies and the adaptive growth and branching of the evolutionary tree. *Evolutionary Ecology*, **12**, 35–57.

Gintis, H. (2000a) Strong reciprocity and human sociality. *Journal of Theoretical Biology*, **206**, 169–179.

Gintis, H. (2000b) *Game Theory Evolving: A Problem-Centered Introduction to Modelling Strategic Interaction*. Princeton, New Jersey: Princeton University Press.

Gintis, H., Bowles, S., Boyd, R. & Fehr, E. (2003) Explaining altruistic behavior in humans. *Evolution and Human Behavior*, **24**, 153–172.

Gintis, H., Bowles, S., Boyd, R. T. & Fehr, E. (2005) *Moral Sentiments and Material Interests: the Foundations of Cooperation in Economic Life*. Cambridge, MA: MIT Press.

Goodnight, C. J., Schwartz, J. M. & Stevens, L. (1992) Contextual analysis of models of group selection, soft selection, hard selection, and the evolution of altruism. *American Naturalist*, **140**, 743–761.

Grafen, A. (1979) The hawk–dove game played between relatives. *Animal Behaviour*, **27**, 905–907.

Grafen, A. (1985) A geometric view of relatedness. *Oxford Surveys in Evolutionary Biology*, **2**, 28–89.

Grafen, A. (2006) Optimization of inclusive fitness. *Journal of Theoretical Biology*, **238**, 541–563.

Grafen, A. (2007a) The formal Darwinism project: a mid-term report. *Journal of Evolutionary Biology*, **20**, 1243–1254.

Grafen, A. (2007b) An inclusive fitness analysis of altruism on a cyclical network. *Journal of Evolutionary Biology*, **20**, 2278–2283.

Griffin, A. S. & West, S. A. (2002) Kin selection: fact and fiction. *Trends in Ecology and Evolution*, **17**, 15–21.

Griffin, A. S. & West, S. A. (2003) Kin discrimination and the benefit of helping in cooperatively breeding vertebrates. *Science*, **302**, 634–636.

Hamilton, W. D. (1963) The evolution of altruistic behaviour. *American Naturalist*, **97**, 354–356.

Hamilton, W. D. (1964) The genetical evolution of social behaviour, I & II. *Journal of Theoretical Biology*, **7**, 1–52.

Hamilton, W. D. (1970) Selfish and spiteful behaviour in an evolutionary model. *Nature*, **228**, 1218–1220.

Hamilton, W. D. (1972) Altruism and related phenomena, mainly in social insects. *Annual Review of Ecology and Systematics*, **3**, 193–232.

Hamilton, W. D. (1975) Innate social aptitudes in man: an approach from evolutionary genetics. In: *Biosocial Anthropology*, ed. R. Fox. New York, NY: Wiley, pp. 133–155.

Hamilton, W. D. (1995) *Narrow Roads of Gene Land. Volume 1. Evolution of Social Behaviour*. New York, NY: W.H. Freeman.

Hardin, G. (1968) The tragedy of the commons. *Science*, **162**, 1243–1244.

Heisler, I. L. & Damuth, J. (1987) A method for analyzing selection in hierarchically structured populations. *American Naturalist*, **130**, 582–602.

Henrich, J. (2004) Cultural group selection, coevolutionary processes and large-scale cooperation. *Journal of Economic Behavior and Organization*, **53**, 3–35.

Keller, L. (1999) *Levels of Selection in Evolution*. Princeton, NJ: Princeton University Press.

Kelly, J. K. (1992) Restricted migration and the evolution of altruism. *Evolution*, **46**, 1492–1495.

Kelly, J. K. (1994) The effect of scale dependent processes on kin selection: mating and density regulation. *Theoretical Population Biology*, **46**, 32–57.

Kirkpatrick, M., Johnson, T. & Barton, N. H. (2002) General models of multilocus evolution. *Genetics*, **161**, 1727–1750.

Kokko, H. (2007) *Modelling for Field Biologists (and Other Interesting People)*. Cambridge: Cambridge University Press.

Lehmann, L. & Keller, L. (2006a) The evolution of cooperation and altruism: a general framework and a classification of models. *Journal of Evolutionary Biology*, **19**, 1365–1376.

Lehmann, L. & Keller, L. (2006b) Synergy, partner choice and frequency dependence: their integration into inclusive fitness theory and their interpretation in terms of direct and indirect fitness effects. *Journal of Evolutionary Biology*, **19**, 1426–1436.

Lehmann, L., Perrin, N. & Rousset, F. (2006) Population demography and the evolution of helping behaviors. *Evolution*, **60**, 1137–1151.

Lehmann, L., Keller, L., West, S. & Roze, D. (2007a) Group selection and kin selection: two concepts but one process. *Proceedings of the National Academy of Sciences of the USA*, **104**, 6736–6739.

Lehmann, L., Keller, L. & Sumpter, D. J. T. (2007b) The evolution of helping and harming on graphs: the return of the inclusive fitness effect. *Journal of Evolutionary Biology*, **20**, 2284–2295.

Lehmann, L., Rousset, F., Roze, D. & Keller, L. (2007c) Strong reciprocity or strong ferocity? A population genetic view of the evolution of altruistic punishment. *American Naturalist*, **170**, 21–36.

Lehmann, L., Ravigne, V. & Keller, L. (2008a) Population viscosity can promote the evolution of altruistic sterile helpers and eusociality. *Proceedings of the Royal Society B*, **275**, 1887–1895.

Lehmann, L., Feldman, M. W. & Foster, K. R. (2008b) Cultural transmission can inhibit the evolution of altruistic helping. *American Naturalist*, **172**, 12–24.

Lehmann, L., Foster, K. R., Borenstein, E. & Feldman, M. W. (2008c) Social and individual learning of helping in humans. *Trends in Ecology and Evolution*, **23**, 664–671.

Leigh, E. G. (1983) When does the good of the group override the advantage of the individual? *Proceedings of the National Academy of Sciences of the USA*, **80**, 2985–2989.

Leturque, H. & Rousset, F. (2003) Joint evolution of sex ratio and dispersal: Conditions for higher dispersal rates from good habitats. *Evolutionary Ecology*, **17**, 67–84.

Loreau, M. & Hector, A. (2001) Partitioning selection and complementarity in biodiversity experiments. *Nature*, **412**, 72–76.

Maynard Smith, J. (1964) Group selection and kin selection. *Nature*, **201**, 1145–1147.

Maynard Smith, J. (1982) *Evolution and the Theory of Games*. Cambridge: Cambridge University Press.

McElreath, R. & Boyd, R. (2007) *Mathematical Models of Social Evolution: a Guide for the Perplexed*. Chicago, IL: University of Chicago Press.

Metz, J. A. J., Nisbet, R. & Geritz, S. A. H. (1992) How should we define 'fitness' for general ecological scenarios? *Trends in Ecology and Evolution*, **7**, 198–202.

Michod, R. E. (1999) *Darwinian Dynamics: Evolutionary Transitions in Fitness and Individuality*. Princeton, NJ: Princeton University Press.

Michod, R. E. & Hamilton, W. D. (1980) Coefficients of relatedness in sociobiology. *Nature*, **288**, 694–697.

Mitteldorf, J. & Wilson, D. S. (2000) Population viscosity and the evolution of altruism. *Journal of Theoretical Biology*, **204**, 481–496.

Muir, W. M. (1996) Group selection for adaptation to multiple-hen cages: selection program and direct responses. *Poultry Science*, **75**, 447–458.

Muir, W. M. (2005) Incorporation of competitive effects in forest tree or animal breeding programs. *Genetics*, **170**, 1247–1259.

Nee, S. (1989) Does Hamilton's rule describe the evolution of reciprocal altruism? *Journal of Theoretical Biology*, **141**, 81–91.

Nowak, M. A. (2006) Five rules for the evolution of cooperation. *Science*, **314**, 1560–1563.

Nowak, M. A. & Sigmund, K. (1998) Evolution of indirect reciprocity by image scoring. *Nature*, **393**, 573–577.

Ohtsuki, H. & Nowak, M. A. (2006) Evolutionary games on cycles. *Proceedings of the Royal Society B*, **273**, 2249–2256.

Ohtsuki, H., Hauert, C., Lieberman, E. & Nowak, M. A. (2006) A simple rule for the evolution of cooperation on graphs and social networks. *Nature*, **441**, 502–505.

Okasha, S. (2006) *Evolution and the Levels of Selection*. Oxford: Oxford University Press.

Orlove, M. J. & Wood, C. L. (1978) Coefficients of relationship and coefficients of relatedness in kin selection: covariance form for the Rho formula. *Journal of Theoretical Biology*, **73**, 679–686.

Otto, S. P. & Day, T. (2007) *A Biologist's Guide to Mathematical Modeling in Ecology and Evolution*. Princeton, NJ: Princeton University Press.

Page, K. M. & Nowak, M. A. (2002) Unifying evolutionary dynamics. *Journal of Theoretical Biology*, **219**, 93–98.

Pamilo, P. (1991) Evolution of colony characteristics in social insects 1. Sex allocation. *American Naturalist*, **137**, 83–107.

Parvinen, K. (2005) Evolutionary suicide. *Acta Biotheoretica*, **53**, 241–264.

Pen, I. (2006) When boys want to be girls: effects of mating system and dispersal on parent-offspring sex ratio conflict. *Evolutionary Ecology Research*, **8**, 103–113.

Pennisi, E. (2005) How did cooperative behavior evolve? *Science*, **309**, 93.

Pepper, J. W. (2000) Relatedness in trait group models of social evolution. *Journal of Theoretical Biology*, **206**, 355–368.

Price, G. R. (1970) Selection and covariance. *Nature*, **227**, 520–521.

Price, G. R. (1972) Extension of covariance selection mathematics. *Annals of Human Genetics*, **35**, 455–458.

Price, G. R. (1995) The nature of selection. *Journal of Theoretical Biology*, **175**, 389–396 [written circa 1971].

Queller, D. C. (1984) Kin selection and frequency-dependence: a game theoretic approach. *Biological Journal of the Linnean Society*, **23**, 133–143.

Queller, D. C. (1985) Kinship, reciprocity and synergism in the evolution of social behaviour. *Nature*, **318**, 366–367.

Queller, D. C. (1992a) Quantitative genetics, inclusive fitness, and group selection. *American Naturalist*, **139**, 540–558.

Queller, D. C. (1992b) A general model for kin selection. *Evolution*, **46**, 376–380.

Queller, D. C. (1992c) Does population viscosity promote kin selection? *Trends in Ecology and Evolution*, **7**, 322–324.

Rankin, D. J. (2007) Resolving the tragedy of the commons: the feedback between intraspecific conflict and population density. *Journal of Evolutionary Biology*, **20**, 173–180.

Rankin, D. J. & López-Sepulcre, A. (2005) Can adaptation lead to extinction? *Oikos*, **111**, 616–619.

Rankin, D. J., López-Sepulcre, A., Foster, K. R. & Kokko, H. (2007) Species-level selection reduces selfishness through competitive exclusion. *Journal of Evolutionary Biology*, **20**, 1459–1468.

Ratnieks, F. L. W. & Reeve, H. K. (1992) Conflict in single-queen hymenopteran societies: the structure of conflict and processes that reduce conflict in advanced eusocial species. *Journal of Theoretical Biology*, **158**, 33–65.

Ratnieks, F. L. W. & Wenseleers, T. (2008) Altruism in insect societies and beyond: voluntary or enforced? *Trends in Ecology and Evolution*, **23**, 45–52.

Ratnieks, F. L. W., Foster, K. R. & Wenseleers, T. (2006) Conflict resolution in insect societies. *Annual Review of Entomology*, **51**, 581–608.

Rice, S. H. (2004) *Evolutionary Theory: Mathematical and Conceptual Foundations*. Sunderland, MA: Sinauer Associates.

Robertson, A. (1966) A mathematical model of the culling process in dairy cattle. *Animal Production*, **8**, 95–108.

Robertson, A. (1968) The spectrum of genetic variation. In: *Population Biology and Evolution*, ed. R. C. Lewontin. Syracuse, NY: Syracuse University Press, pp. 5–16.

Ross-Gillespie, A., Gardner, A., West, S. A. & Griffin, A. S. (2007) Frequency dependence and cooperation: theory and a test with bacteria. *American Naturalist*, **170**, 331–342.

Rousset, F. (2004) *Genetic Structure and Selection in Subdivided Populations*. Princeton, NJ: Princeton University Press.

Rousset, F. (2006) Separation of time scales, fixation probabilities and convergence to evolutionarily stable states under isolation by distance. *Theoretical Population Biology*, **69**, 165–179.

Roze, D. & Rousset, F. (2005) Inbreeding depression and the evolution of dispersal rates: a multilocus model. *American Naturalist*, **166**, 708–721.

Roze, D. & Rousset, F. (2008) Multilocus models in the infinite island model of population structure. *Theoretical Population Biology*, **73**, 529–542.

Rubinstein, A. (1998) *Modeling Bounded Rationality*. Cambridge, MA: MIT Press.

Skyrms, B. (1996) *Evolution of the Social Contract*. Cambridge: Cambridge University Press.

Sober, E. & Wilson, D. S. (1998) *Unto Others: the Evolution of Altruism*. Cambridge, MA.: Harvard University Press.

Strassmann, J. E. & Queller, D. C. (2007) Altruism among amoebas. *Natural History*, **116**, 24–29.

Suzuki, Y. & Toquenaga, Y. (2005) Effects of information and group structure on evolution of altruism: analysis of two-score model by covariance and contextual analyses. *Journal of Theoretical Biology*, **232**, 191–201.

Swenson, W., Wilson, D. S. & Elias, R. (2000) Artificial ecosystem selection. *Proceedings of the National Academy of Sciences of the USA*, **97**, 9110–9114.

Taylor, C. & Nowak, M. A. (2007) Transforming the dilemma. *Evolution*, **61**, 2281–2292.

Taylor, P. D. (1990) Allele-frequency change in a class-structured population. *American Naturalist*, **135**, 95–106.

Taylor, P. D. (1992) Altruism in viscous populations: an inclusive fitness model. *Evolutionary Ecology*, **6**, 352–356.

Taylor, P. D. (1996) Inclusive fitness arguments in genetic models of behaviour. *Journal of Mathematical Biology*, **34**, 654–674.

Taylor, P. D. & Frank, S. A. (1996) How to make a kin selection model. *Journal of Theoretical Biology*, **180**, 27–37.

Taylor, P. D. & Irwin, A. J. (2000) Overlapping generations can promote altruistic behavior. *Evolution*, **54**, 1135–1141.

Taylor, P. D., Wild, G. & Gardner, A. (2007a) Direct fitness or inclusive fitness: how shall we model kin selection? *Journal of Evolutionary Biology*, **20**, 301–309.

Taylor, P. D., Day, T. & Wild, G. (2007b) Evolution of cooperation in a finite homogeneous graph. *Nature*, **447**, 469–472.

Taylor, P. D., Day, T. & Wild, G. (2007c) From inclusive fitness to fixation probability in homogeneous structured populations. *Journal of Theoretical Biology*, **249**, 101–110.

Traulsen, A. & Nowak, M. A. (2006) Evolution of cooperation by multilevel selection. *Proceedings of the National Academy of Sciences of the USA*, **103**, 10952–10955.

Traulsen, A. & Schuster, H. G. (2003) Minimal model for tag-based cooperation. *Physical Review E*, **68**, 046129.

Trivers, R. L. (1971) The evolution of reciprocal altruism. *Quarterly Review of Biology*, **46**, 35–57.

Uyenoyama, M. & Feldman, M. W. (1980) Theories of kin and group selection: a population genetics perspective. *Theoretical Population Biology*, **17**, 380–414.

Van Baalen, M. & Rand, D. A. (1998) The unit of selection in viscous populations and the evolution of altruism. *Journal of Theoretical Biology*, **193**, 631–648.

Wade, M. J. (1976) Group selection among laboratory populations of *Tribolium*. *Proceedings of the National Academy of Sciences of the USA*, **73**, 4604–4607.

Wade, M. J. (1977) An experimental study of group selection. *Evolution*, **31**, 134–153.

Wade, M. J. (1980) Kin selection: its components. *Science*, **210**, 665–667.

Wade, M. J. & Goodnight, C. J. (1998) Perspective. The theories of Fisher and Wright in the context of metapopulations: when nature does many small experiments. *Evolution*, **52**, 1537–1553.

Wenseleers, T. (2006) Modelling social evolution: the relative merits and limitations of a Hamilton's rule-based approach. *Journal of Evolutionary Biology*, **19**, 1419–1422.

Wenseleers, T. & Ratnieks, F. L. W. (2004) Tragedy of the commons in *Melipona* bees. *Proceedings of the Royal Society B*, **271**, S310–312.

Wenseleers, T. & Ratnieks, F. L. W. (2006a) Comparative analysis of worker reproduction and policing in eusocial Hymenoptera supports relatedness theory. *American Naturalist*, **168**, E163–E179.

Wenseleers, T. & Ratnieks, F. L. W. (2006b) Enforced altruism in insect societies. *Nature*, **444**, 50.

Wenseleers, T., Ratnieks, F. L. W. & Billen, J. (2003) Caste fate conflict in swarm-founding social Hymenoptera: an inclusive fitness analysis. *Journal of Evolutionary Biology*, **16**, 647–658.

Wenseleers, T., Hart, A. G. & Ratnieks, F. L. W. (2004a) When resistance is useless: Policing and the evolution of reproductive acquiescence in insect societies. *American Naturalist*, **164**, E154–E167.

Wenseleers, T., Helanterä, H., Hart, A. G. & Ratnieks, F. L. W. (2004b) Worker reproduction and policing in insect societies: an ESS analysis. *Journal of Evolutionary Biology*, **17**, 1035–1047.

West, S. A., Pen, I. & Griffin, A. S. (2002) Cooperation and competition between relatives. *Science*, **296**, 72–75.

West, S. A., Griffin, A. S. & Gardner, A. (2007a) Evolutionary explanations for cooperation. *Current Biology*, **17**, R661–672.

West, S. A., Griffin, A. S. & Gardner, A. (2007b) Social semantics: altruism, cooperation, mutualism, strong reciprocity and group selection. *Journal of Evolutionary Biology*, **20**, 415–432.

West, S. A., Griffin, A. S. & Gardner, A. (2008) Social semantics: how useful has group selection been? *Journal of Evolutionary Biology*, **21**, 374–385.

Wild, G. & Taylor, P. D. (2005) A kin-selection approach to the resolution of sex-ratio conflict between mates. *Journal of Theoretical Biology*, **236**, 126–136.

Williams, G. C. & Williams, D. C. (1957) Natural selection of individually harmful social adaptations among sibs with special reference to social insects. *Evolution*, **11**, 32–39.

Wilson, D. S. (1975) A theory of group selection. *Proceedings of the National Academy of Sciences of the USA*, **72**, 143–146.

Wilson, D. S. (1983) The group selection controversy: history and current status. *Annual Review of Ecology and Systematics*, **14**, 159–187.

Wilson, D. S. (1990) Weak altruism, strong group selection. *Oikos*, **59**, 135–140.

Wilson, D. S. (1997) Biological communities as functionally organized units. *Ecology*, **78**, 2018–2024.

Wilson, D. S. (2008) Social semantics: toward a genuine pluralism in the study of social behaviour. *Journal of Evolutionary Biology*, **21**, 368–373.

Wilson, D. S. & Colwell, R. K. (1981) Evolution of sex-ratio in structured demes. *Evolution*, **35**, 882–897.

Wilson, D. S. & Sober, E. (1989) Reviving the Superorganism. *Journal of Theoretical Biology*, **136**, 337–356.

Wilson, D. S. & Wilson, E. O. (2007) Rethinking the theoretical foundation of sociobiology. *Quarterly Review of Biology*, **82**, 327–348.

Wilson, D. S., Pollock, G. B. & Dugatkin, L. A. (1992) Can altruism evolve in purely viscous populations? *Evolutionary Ecology*, **6**, 331–341.

Wilson, E. O. & Hölldobler, B. (2005) Eusociality: origin and consequences. *Proceedings of the National Academy of Sciences of the USA*, **102**, 13367–13371.

Wolf, J. B., Brodie, E. D. & Moore, A. J. (1999) Interacting phenotypes and the evolutionary process. II. Selection resulting from social interactions. *American Naturalist*, **153**, 254–266.

Wright, S. (1945) Tempo and mode in evolution: a critical review. *Ecology*, **26**, 415–419.

Wright, S. (1951) The genetical structure of populations. *Annals of Eugenics*, **15**, 323–354.

Yang, R. C. (1998) Estimating hierarchical F-statistics. *Evolution*, **52**, 950–956.

What's wrong with this picture?

Sarah B. Hrdy

Research on wild primates was still a relatively new endeavour in the USA when I entered graduate school in 1970. Courses on primate behaviour were primarily taught in anthropology departments. I was drawn to the field because Japanese researchers had reported that adult male monkeys sometimes killed infants in a species of South Asian monkey known as the Hanuman langur *Semnopithecus entellus*, and I wanted to find out why. The summer after my first year in graduate school I went to Mount Abu, in Rajasthan, with this question in mind. At the time I had no special interest in female behaviour, which frankly struck me as boring.

According to the only available article on the subject, entitled 'The female primate', 'Her primary focus, a role which occupies more than 70 percent of her life, is motherhood … A female raises one infant after another for her entire adult life … Dominance interaction is usually minimal' (Jay 1963). This narrow view of female natures was the result of a combination of factors, including Victorian social biases left over from Darwin's day, the fact that earlier observations had focused on captive animals, often consisting of mothers caged individually with their young, and evolutionary theory itself. As then formulated, Darwin's remarkably original and quite powerful theory of sexual selection left out many sources of variation affecting the differential reproductive success of females.

Darwin's theory that members of one sex (almost always males) were competing among themselves for access to the other (i.e. females) did a good job of explaining why langur males who usurped control of breeding females sought to eliminate unweaned infants sired by their competitors. The incoming male was essentially cancelling the last choice those mothers had made and, in doing so, reducing the time before he himself might have a chance to sire offspring. Except for specifying their role in choosing the 'best' male, however, sexual selection theory did not then ascribe active roles to females. They were viewed as essentially passive pawns in a brutal system. Yet the more I learned, the more interested I became in the females. Partly this was because, as a female myself, I could not help but empathise (Hrdy 1986). Here was a mother, and every 27 months on average some male, weighing almost twice as much as she did, equipped with canine weapons she did not have, would arrive in her troop intent on killing her baby. The more I watched them, the more fascinated I became by the flexible and often quite innovative strategies females employed to cope with the challenges posed by males.

The accompanying portrait of an 'all-male band,' 13 monkeys on a rocky crag, reminds me

Social Behaviour: Genes, Ecology and Evolution, ed. Tamás Székely, Allen J. Moore and Jan Komdeur. Published by Cambridge University Press. © Cambridge University Press 2010.

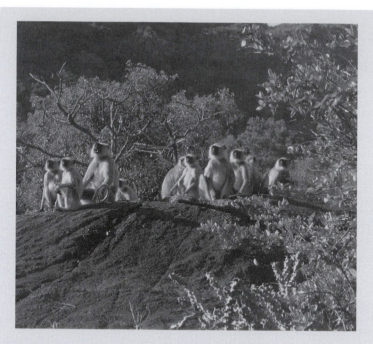

Portrait of a Hanuman langur 'all-male' band. Photo: S. B. Hrdy/AnthroPhoto.

of my own dawning awareness of how opportunistic females can be. Hanuman langurs live in breeding troops composed of overlapping generations of females accompanied by one or more adult males who enter the troop from outside. The home ranges of these troops are traversed by all-male bands, containing anywhere from two to 60 or more males of all ages (Hrdy 1977). In the picture, the male I nicknamed 'Split-ear', longtime resident in the 'Toad Rock troop', grinds his teeth as he sits with eight juvenile and subadult males from his former troop, who like him have been driven out by a new male. For months, Split-ear and these possible-sons continued to skulk about their former home range. But take a closer look. The langur on the far right is a multiparous female. In her arms she holds her 13-month-old daughter. To her left, back to the camera, sits another female holding her infant. What were these females doing in what I assumed was an 'all-male band'?

Beginning with my first field season, I had occasionally seen females outside of their troops. But lacking any theoretical framework for interpreting their behaviour, I failed to attach any significance to them. As it happened, the very first wild langur I ever got a close look at was a lone female who had temporarily left the troop I had been searching for, and had probably (though I did not realise this at the time) gone off to solicit males in one of the roving all-male bands. Such polyandrous tendencies, it turns out, are typical of female primates, including langurs.

The highest incidence of extra-troop sexual solicitations was recorded for a troop in which an unusually successful alpha male had managed to remain in residence for many years. Since some females in his troop were likely daughters, there was a genetic rationale (inbreeding avoidance) for their extra-troop solicitations. However, on other occasions I saw females that I knew to be pregnant solicit unfamiliar males. Furthermore, I learned that instead of being strictly cyclical, as non-human primates were assumed to be, langurs were capable of what I called 'situation-dependent' sexual receptivity. Unlike savanna baboons and some other monkeys, langurs do not advertise mid-cycle ovulation with conspicuous pink 'sexual swellings'. The only visible sign is their behaviour, presenting their rumps while frenetically shaking their heads. Only the resident male living with females month in and month out seemed to be much good at discriminating actual ovulation from non-fertile solicitations. Since langur males do not attack the offspring of females with whom they have previously mated, I hypothesised that females might be taking out an insurance policy in case one of these males usurped her troop one day, manipulating the information available to him about possible paternity.

The females 'out of place' in this photograph were pursuing yet another strategy. Shortly after this photograph was taken, one of the females left her partially weaned daughter in the band with the tolerant ousted males and returned to her former troop alone. This tactic for keeping her daughter safe might have worked, except that the daughter found her way back and rejoined her mother, and was attacked by the new male. The infant's wounds from the first attack were only superficial, but I feared she was doomed. Then, even though still years away from sexual maturity, the 13-month-old began to solicit the usurping male. Although rump-presentation was a usual posture for a subordinate to assume before a dominant animal, combining it with frenetic head-shaking was not. It was as if this infant, at the margin of the age when an unweaned infant would be killed, strove to remind the new male 'I am a potential mate, not worth your killing'. Thereafter, his attacks ceased.

Decades later, my research still focuses on variation between females, and increasingly also between infants, and on how Darwinian selection acts on them (e.g. Hrdy 1999). I date my interest in maternal reproductive strategies to the days when I was puzzled by seeing females where they 'did not belong'.

References

Hrdy, S. B. (1977) *The Langurs of Abu: Female and Male Strategies of Reproduction*. Cambridge, MA: Harvard University Press.

Hrdy, S. B. (1986, reprinted 2006) Empathy, polyandry and the myth of the coy female. In: *Conceptual Issues in Evolutionary Biology*, ed. E. Sober. Cambridge, MA: MIT Press, pp. 131–159.

Hrdy, S. B. (1999) *Mother Nature: A History of Mothers, Infants and Natural Selection*. New York, NY: Pantheon.

Jay, P. (1963) The female primate. In: *The Potential of Woman*, ed. S. Farber and R. Wilson. New York, NY: McGraw Hill, pp. 3–47.

Themes

7

Aggression: towards an integration of gene, brain and behaviour

Robert Huber and Edward A. Kravitz

Overview

Aggression ranks among the most misunderstood concepts in the behavioural sciences. Commonly viewed as an aberrant form of behaviour, situations of conflict are pictured in the context of unfavourable or stressful circumstances, brought about by amoral urges, in critical need of our cognitive control, and with negative consequences for all involved. Such a view fundamentally misunderstands the biological significance of all behaviours that occur in the context of attack, defence or threat. Deeply routed in the demands of the natural world, the ability to assert oneself represents a critical solution to any individual's need for self-preservation, defence of its interests or resource competition. Examples of aggression are found throughout the entire animal kingdom, regardless of its bearer's specific neural or cognitive faculties, phylogenetic origins or sociobiological circumstances. It has become abundantly clear that aggressive traits have been shaped by evolution like any other behavioural phenotypes, and a range of underlying mechanisms in the causation of aggression are now being unravelled.

This chapter aims to present a comprehensive overview of the issues that are encountered when trying to understand the *how*s and *why*s as individuals oppose each other. The chapter focuses special attention on delineating distinct behavioural phenomena such as aggressive tendencies, dominance or violence. Game-theoretical considerations offer a powerful theoretical framework to assess the evolutionary consequences of different behavioural strategies. A discussion of proximate mechanisms attempts to link these behavioural heterogeneities to the functioning of underlying neural and endocrine control systems. Three case studies review powerful interdisciplinary approaches, which uniquely bridge multiple levels of organisation. First, the application of recombinant DNA technologies and behavioural genetics to the aggressive behaviour of fruit flies *Drosophila* spp. has produced novel insights into the behaviour's essential brain circuitry. This approach may allow us to image the functional roles of embedded neurons in living animals as these respond to behaviourally meaningful cues. Second, recent evidence, linking violence or lack of impulse control to amine metabolism in primates, illustrates the social and endocrine conditions in which aggression and fierce behaviours may be appropriate and selected

Social Behaviour: Genes, Ecology and Evolution, ed. Tamás Székely, Allen J. Moore and Jan Komdeur. Published by Cambridge University Press. © Cambridge University Press 2010.

for. Third, efforts to select for enhanced levels of aggression in distinct genetic strains in dogs and mice generally produce, within a few generations, animals with levels of aggressive behaviour that greatly exceed those of controls. This chapter thus aims to integrate a diverse range of approaches into a better understanding of aggression, its functional roles, and its neural and hormonal causes.

7.1 Introduction

Aside from sex, few animal acts match aggression's ability to attract and hold our attention. Actions during conflict feature some of the most spectacular and dramatic behaviours of a species' repertoire. Imagine two northern elephant seal *Mirounga angustirostris* bulls locked in mortal combat on a deserted, rocky, windswept beach, copious amounts of blood flowing into the churned-up sea, with a harem of on-looking females desperate to escape the mayhem developing around them. Although cases of such unbridled social hostility are relatively rare, the basic tendency towards aggression appears almost ubiquitous. Aside from aggression's general prevalence, fundamental rules governing combat seem to be just as natural and widespread. In most species, aggression relies mostly on highly visual and elaborately ritualised displays, which effectively channel aggression, govern the conflict's resolution, and structure how individuals interact (Lorenz 1963, Archer 1988, Nelson 2005).

As we witness animals engaged in situations of conflict, we cannot help but be drawn in by the behaviour's inherent relevance to our own biological roots. Demanding attention from generations of behavioural scientists across a wide range of disciplines, interests include proximate, neural or endocrine causes of aggression, alongside the role social roots play in its expression. We explore the eye-catching behaviours that make up social encounters, analyse the effectiveness of different strategies, advance powerful predictors that eventually help settle them, and assess the social consequences that emerge in their wake.

7.2 Evolutionary perspectives

Conflicts are energetically costly and inherently carry a wide range of risks. Natural selection offers a powerful conceptual tool, as it is expected to refine behavioural decisions and strategies so that they maximise beneficial outcomes for each individual involved (see Chapter 6). The meeting of two clawed crustaceans, for example the American lobster *Homarus americanus* or its crayfish cousins, matched in size and willing to do battle, epitomises a typical scenario for highly structured fighting (Huber & Kravitz 1995). Opponents engage in a sequence of hostilities where intensity increases in discrete steps as long as the fight lasts. Serving to illustrate constituent concepts of aggression and how these may relate to one another, the encounter begins as one individual approaches another intent on attack (Fig. 7.1). The threatened crustacean, depending on its own aggressive state, may respond in kind. Combatants advance towards each other with vigorous whips of the antennae that signal readiness to step up the encounter to the next intensity. In an escalating sequence of behaviours, opponents first touch with wide-open claws, grab and hold in attempts to displace each other with pushes, pulls and lifts, and finally resort to unrestrained use of their weapons. During such escalating encounters, combatants are able to assess each other's relative abilities and strengths in a stepwise fashion. Despite the presence of potentially lethal weapons in many taxa, their use is largely restricted to fights among closely matched opponents, where a series of earlier stages had failed to yield a clear winner (Hofmann & Schildberger 2001).

7.2.1 Aggressive state

Not all individuals are equally likely to engage an opponent, and intensities vary greatly from a restrained, delicate threat display to fierce, unbridled charges. Such individual differences in attack tendencies are ascribed to an animal's aggressiveness or aggressive state. As in other forms of arousal and

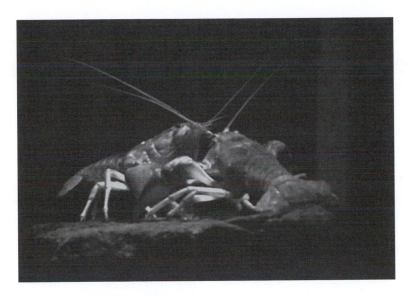

Figure 7.1 Fighting crayfish *Astacus astacus*. Photo: Robert Huber.

motivation, this term is used purely as an intervening variable (i.e. a hypothetical, helpful construct), which justifies its use only in those instances in which it effectively simplifies our understanding of the observed behavioural phenotypes. It makes no claims, however, to accurately represent the true number and nature of internal factors that feed into it. We must acknowledge that if we had a truly comprehensive understanding of how an aggressive behaviour was produced, we would have no need for this term at all. Contingent on social conditioning and past events, and influenced by a variety of neural, endocrine and genetic factors, aggressive state represents a top-down effort to operationally characterise behavioural variation until we can offer a better understanding of its actual causation. Despite these limitations, concepts of motivation help us to understand which brain systems mediate the psychological processes that guide real behaviour (Berridge 2004).

7.2.2 Fight strategies

In most scenarios, ritualised displays take the place of unchecked, aggressive interactions, as all-out fighting between members of a species is rarely in anyone's long-term interest. Game theory provides a powerful and formal understanding of why animals only tend to fight with great ferocity when a resource of exceptional value is at stake (see Chapter 4; Dugatkin & Reeve 2000). The Hawk–Dove game explores conditions that optimise the beneficial consequences during resource-centred conflicts (Maynard Smith 1982). The behavioural strategy of a Hawk is to readily use its weapons during the fight until either it sustains an injury or its opponent retreats. A Dove, in contrast, contests the interaction with displays only. If faced with a Hawk, a Dove will retreat immediately as the opponent threatens to use its weapons. A formal payoff matrix shows the different players' consequences for all possible combinations of strategies (see Chapter 4), where each individual would prefer to win, prefer to tie rather than lose, and prefer to lose rather than receive injury. In encounters between Hawks, the winner gains control over the value of the resource while the losing Hawk sustains an injury. Expectations from this model demonstrate that in situations where the cost of injury exceeds the benefit of winning, populations are expected to adjust to balanced proportions of the two strategies – the great majority of individuals will fight in highly restrained fashion, while a small number of Hawks persists. In rare cases where the value of an exceptional resource exceeds the cost of injury, a Hawk strategy will be widespread as it always carries an advantage over Doves, replacing the latter completely. Fighting, for instance, is particularly intense in elephant seals, because in this case a victorious male monopolises a section of the shore, along with sole reproductive access to a group of females who reside on that part of the beach. In the great majority of instances, however, resources are rarely worth the risk of being injured, and competing individuals will do best by resolving conflicts with ritualised displays only (see Chapter 4; Maynard Smith 1974).

Additional strategies for signalling and assessment in fighting exist within War of Attrition scenarios (Maynard Smith 1982). As fighting slowly progresses through levels of increasing intensity, both individuals gain detailed, cheat-proof information about their opponent, while they grind down the opponent's defences by inflicting continued small damages. There is no fixed cost associated with losing or contesting but, as the encounter wears on, each player accumulates incremental costs. When an individual decides to back down, it effectively relinquishes access to the contested resource, rather than continue to sustain further insults. The emergence of structured fighting behaviour thus clearly represents a favourable option for all parties, and has given rise to the evolution of encounters that are conducted with a stepwise comparison of signals.

Skill in assessing the relative strength of an opponent is key for navigating the demands, risks and opportunities of social living. Selection will favour those with an ability to effectively anticipate their chances well in advance, and to choose the most beneficial strategies. When an animal is bested by an opponent, it is always far better to adopt submissive behaviour and accept subordinate status, rather than risk something far worse. Decisions to retreat come suddenly and often without warning, as a combatant begins to regard its chances of winning as increasingly slim. Game theory also confirms that opponents should only signal strength while hiding any intentions to eventually withdraw

(Maynard Smith 1974, Számadó 2008). A wide range of attributes decides between victory and defeat. In invertebrates, where individuals generally pursue a solitary existence, physical superiority is often the primary determinant of an interaction's eventual outcome. With prominent asymmetries in the size of body or weapons, or in sex or reproductive status, most fights are resolved quickly. In vertebrates, aggressive success depends to a great extent on the ability to form successful alliances, to harness cognitive skills, or to inherit status from high-ranking kin. In addition to size and strength, success is contingent on the development of social competence (Suomi 1997).

Natural selection enhances overall effectiveness in aggression, rather than absolute amounts of it. High-ranking individuals will most likely display a favourable combination of strength along with ability to titre their levels of aggression, to pick fights that are winnable, and to compete only in those that are worth it. Hyper-aggression (see Chapter 14) describes behaviours that appear to greatly exceed the most effective norm – individuals who readily launch the initial attack even in situations where they ought not to, who are overly eager to escalate or retaliate, who show a willingness to follow an excessively physical trajectory even when an opponent has already withdrawn, or who fail to back down in situations where there is little prospect of winning. Such behaviours rarely make for an effective strategy, as they coincide with greater risk of injury or death, or, in the best-case scenario, gaining a low rank.

7.2.3 Dominance

When winning one or more prior encounters produces a lasting polarity in the outcome of future bouts between a given pair of individuals, a dominance relationship has been established (see Chapter 14). In its most common form, the past loser will be less likely to initiate further bouts against the winner, or will retreat quickly if confronted (Chase *et al.* 1994). Most instances of dominance rely on individual recognition or familiarity, which establishes learned, pair-wise relationships. Alternatively, the recognition of an opponent's aggressive state, or of signals that indicate past success, may serve similar roles. Memories of past social encounters also impact future behaviour regardless of the opponent. These are collectively grouped into winner/loser effects, and recent winners often become likely to win again even when faced with a novel opponent, while general chances for success further decline in former losers (see Chapter 14; Dugatkin 1997). Such effects rarely impact actual fighting abilities, but rather seem to alter an animal's aggressive state or self-assessment of future outcomes. In general, the relative magnitude of loser effects often exceeds those of winner effects and is frequently longer-lasting (Chase *et al.* 1994). Moreover, loser effects by themselves are often sufficient for maintaining stable hierarchical relationships and social structure (Hock & Huber 2006). Empirical evidence for the existence of winner and loser effects derives from a wide range of taxa, yet the mechanisms that underlie them are still poorly understood (Hsu & Wolf 2000). Current evidence suggests that proximate causes for winner and loser effects reside in behavioural–neuroendocrine feedback loops for aggression (see below and Chapter 17).

As individuals repeatedly meet and interact with others, higher-order social organisation emerges through a series of sequential dyadic interactions among the group members. Individuals of many species, including humans, tend to arrange themselves in linear social hierarchies (Wilson 1975, Hemelrijk 1999). Although relatively fixed individual characteristics such as size, strength or agility often determine their owner's rank, these characteristics are more often overshadowed by contextual factors and chance events (Chase *et al.* 2002). Experiments in which identical groups are repeatedly reconstituted result in similar overall hierarchical structures, although individuals show surprising variation in the final ranks they occupy (Chase *et al.* 2002). Moreover, the ranks that individuals establish is highly dependent on the order in which they join the group. Prior residence effects confers significant advantages to those members who establish themselves early (Huntingford & Garcia de Leaniz 1997). With future

success contingent on past interaction histories through social conditioning, the emergence of social rank is critically governed by a host of dynamic, self-structuring properties. The importance of self-assembly in structuring a web of dominance relationships within the group is supported by a host of empirical evidence (Theraulaz *et al.* 1995, Bonabeau *et al.* 1997, Goessmann *et al.* 2000, Beacham 2003). Theoretical models explore the outcome of situations in which initially similar entities perform a series of self-reinforcing dominance interactions (Dugatkin & Dugatkin 2007). Ranks differentiate as individuals lose to an opponent early and are consequently slated for lower ranks than those who won during the critical, initial stages. The stability and precise structure of hierarchies thus represent an automatic consequence of the progressive polarisation in dominance status (Hock & Huber 2006). As some individuals become multiple losers, their aggressiveness further declines along with any opportunities to engineer future rank reversals. Ranks may be evenly spaced, or biased towards a few very dominant or subordinate individuals. The self-reinforcing effects of winning and losing may also extend to bystanders, where unrelated third individuals automatically either submit to a winner or dominate a loser (Grosenick & Fernald 2007).

7.2.4 Human aggression

Human ingenuity for inflicting intentional harm is without equal, although warring tendencies may already be rooted in a deep, pre-human past (see Chapter 15; Wrangham & Peterson 1996). Instances of violence have been documented for a range of non-human apes and may arguably have been wired into our genes when aggressive ancestors shoved the nice guys aside, seized the females, and reproduced. Humans, however, with their searing capacity for cruelty, killing, torture and rape, are clearly in a category of their own when basic, violent tendencies combine with a burning intellect that excels at harnessing novel techniques and implements. Aside from an unprecedented potential for carnage and destruction, we are at the same time also capable of the most remarkable instances of compassion, understanding and peaceful negotiation. The direction depends on each individual's ethical codes and moral norms, driven by societal expectations, good parenting or social contexts (Pinker 2007). A clear vision has emerged where 'natural' tendencies for aggression appear to be ubiquitous, but so too are a plethora of sophisticated mechanisms that keep conflicts in check, channel aggression, negotiate fighting signals, resolve conflicts, and ultimately govern social group structure.

7.3 Definitions, misconceptions and solutions

It is quite remarkable that, despite this wealth of empirical and theoretical attention, a comprehensive synthesis of aggression and of its biological roots has stubbornly remained elusive. A central explanation for this paradox resides in the lack of a unified, operational definition of aggression across disciplines, and of a general agreement on what the term actually includes. For instance, psychologists define aggression as 'all behaviour that is intended to cause bodily harm' (Krahé 2001). Moyer's (1968) widely adopted classification of aggression recognises multiple subtypes, including competition between males, a mother's efforts to protect her offspring, and fighting as a learned response to cope with a particular situation. Biologists regard a definition that focuses solely on injury as inadequate, because it excludes a wide range of threat behaviours directed at rivals – birds that challenge their adversaries with song, an impala's exaggerated strutting as a signal of strength, or a resident's territorial claims through scent markings. Moreover, there is little agreement on whether a predator's hunting behaviour is included – a lion chasing and killing a gazelle undoubtedly inflicts injury, but it is debatable whether this represents aggression any more than a cow cropping the top off a clump of grass. Efforts to define animal aggression with a broader focus on all behaviours of attack, defence and threat have proven considerably more practical (Immelmann & Beer 1992).

Disagreements on terminology combine with common misconceptions that treat aggression as a single, unitary concept. The latter, either explicitly or tacitly, views different study approaches simply as separate perspectives on the same underlying phenomenon. Many concepts seem so intimately related that we are tempted to view them with much overlap or even synonymously, including the occurrence of fighting, effectiveness in a contest, or an ability to socially dominate others (Francis 1988). A more compelling view acknowledges aggression's multidimensional nature and uses the term simply as an overarching term for an entangled complex of multiple, distinct components, causes and functions. Behaviour during aggressive encounters always involves the relative strengths of contrasting impulses for attack with a tendency to flee – rarely is either present entirely alone. To acknowledge a difficulty of separating these components, the term *agonistic behaviour* has been introduced. The term specifically addresses the balance of forces for both attacking and fleeing, and it accommodates all instances of attack, threat or defence (i.e. offensive agonistic behaviour) alongside escape and submission (i.e. defensive agonistic behaviour). The most comprehensive and practical definition of aggression has arguably emerged from an evolutionary viewpoint (Alcock 2005). In this context, aggression includes all behaviour directed at increasing an attacker's reproductive prospects at the expense of the attacked or threatened rival. Interspecific contests also focus to a greater extent on competitive interactions, rather than on predator–prey scenarios.

Attempts to search for proximate mechanisms underlying aggression critically require us to characterise aggression's natural building blocks, to recognise the various factors that control them, and to effectively label their behavioural expression in the form of consistent and reliable behavioural phenotypes. A quantitative characterisation of agonistic behaviour usually commences with a compiled list of behaviours and analyses that report observed frequencies, rates and durations. Unfortunately, measures of behaviour that focus on *'what'* an animal does are intrinsically sensitive to the variability inherent in behavioural systems. A focus on '*how*' individuals conduct their fighting examines the higher-order structure present within behavioural frameworks and offers a substantially better alternative than descriptions of any particular instance. It thereby centres on behaviour as a series of structured rules which remain largely constant across a wide range of scenarios. Estimates for the rate at which opponents escalate the encounter are surprisingly stable even across fights that vary widely in the particular behaviour patterns used, the duration of the encounters, or the intensity with which combatants conduct themselves (Huber *et al.* 2002). Reliance on the encounter's structural characteristics assesses behaviour in the form of particular fighting strategies rather than accounting for activity on a minute-to-minute basis. Structural features are used to provide estimates for an individual's intrinsic aggressive tendencies, to identify their particular attack strategies, and to determine the rules that govern decisions for escalation and retreat (Chen *et al.* 2002).

A willingness to submit to an opponent may also depend on the perceived value of the resource at stake (Dugatkin & Dugatkin 2007). With significant prior investments in it, a mother will be likely to defend her young even when faced with a superior foe, a resident may not be willing to give up a shelter containing its food stores without a fight, or a male with reproductive access to a harem of mates may not relinquish it easily. As such instances make for striking observations, these different situations are frequently regarded as distinct, fundamental subtypes of aggression. Although this view may be tempting, shared fundamental scenarios in which knowledge about the salient value of a resource constrains the available options may not, in fact, warrant this. Moreover, instances of unusually heightened aggressive state show considerable, but poorly defined, overlap with similar higher-order concepts, including impulsivity, risk-taking, lack of behavioural control, violence, or detrimental consequences of stress (Dugatkin & Dugatkin 2007).

7.4 Case studies

7.4.1 The fruit fly fight club

Model behavioural systems have been widely used for the study of aggression. These allow detailed examination of the behaviour, addressing essentially all the features highlighted above, but now being performed in artificial settings designed to simulate real-world situations. They offer additional great advantages, however, in being able to control the rearing, handling and social experience of animals from conception, and in the ability to subsequently ask what is happening in the nervous system underlying the behaviour. An ideal organism for exploring the roots of aggression would allow precise examination of the genetic, environmental and hormonal factors contributing to the aggressiveness of individual animals. The animals should be willing to compete over desired resources in an experimental arena with sufficient ethological constraints built in to allow any results obtained to be related to real-world situations. Ultimately one might want to map the brain circuitry essential to the behaviour, and possibly image the involved neurons while they function in living animals responding to behaviourally meaningful cues. Finding a single experimental model that will satisfy all these criteria is a tall order for most of the models that have been used thus far in the study of aggression. One recently developed model using fruit flies, however, comes close to meeting these demands.

Historical background

It was not well known until recently that common strains of male and female fruit flies show agonistic behaviour in same-sex pairings. This despite the fact that aggression between male fruit flies had been described in the larger Hawaiian species (Spieth 1968, 1974, Boake *et al.* 1998) as well as in a much earlier paper on sexual selection (Sturtevant 1915). In addressing situations in which two males are courting the same female, Sturtevant wrote: 'In such cases they [males] may sometimes be seen to spread their wings, run at each other, and apparently butt heads. One of them soon gives up and runs away. If the other then runs at him again within the next few minutes he usually makes off without showing fight.' A study of the effects of light on mating of ebony and light strains of *Drosophila melanogaster* (Jacobs 1960) reported that male flies showed what he termed 'territorial behaviour'. Jacobs also described components of the behaviour, demonstrated that bouts between flies varied widely in duration, and showed that the behaviour itself was not seen in male flies during the first day after emerging. When marked male and female flies were placed together in a competitive situation, interactions between flies were mainly aggressive or sexual (Dow & von Schilcher 1975). The authors also described the behavioural components of wing threat, charging and boxing. In addition, great variability was seen in the numbers of times individual males were found on the food surface, attacked or were attacked, won or lost fights or copulated. These results suggested that dominant males won most of their fights and had the greatest success in mating behaviour. The most complete studies of fighting and territorial behaviour in common *Drosophila* species (*D. melanogaster*, *D. simulans*), prior to the studies from the Kravitz laboratory (Chen *et al.* 2002, Nilsen *et al.* 2004) came in 1987 (Hoffmann 1987). Following up on earlier studies (Dow & von Schilcher 1975), and using a similar experimental protocol, the components that made up fighting behaviour were defined, the proportions of time flies showed the different patterns were measured, and factors that influenced the outcome of fights were identified (Hoffmann 1987). These studies were in a complex social situation, however, in which six virgin male flies were placed in a chamber with three mated females and the ensuing social interactions were continuously videotaped for eight hours. Despite the complexity, these investigations provided a firm basis for the existence of territorial aggression in *D. melanogaster*. Even less well known was that female *D. melanogaster* also showed same-sex aggression (Ueda & Kidokoro 2002). This was confirmed when the Kravitz laboratory carried out a

quantitative analysis and a comparison of male and female aggression, highlighting the similarities and the differences in same-sex fighting behaviour in *D. melanogaster* (Nilsen *et al.* 2004).

A quantitative analysis of aggression

An examination of the genetic roots of aggression begins with an examination of the behaviour. Without understanding the 'normal' patterns of aggression in any species, including flies, it is extremely difficult to identify the consequences of any genetic perturbations that are carried out. To analyse the behaviour, a simplified arena was designed that allowed examination of agonistic encounters between pairs of animals. The arena offered resources (food, potential mates in some cases, and light to attract the flies to a central area in the arena), but also allowed room for the flies to escape from each other. Since all fly fights are different, despite the extensive inbreeding of fly lines, large sample sizes were needed to generate stable 'snapshots' of average male and female fly fights (Chen *et al.* 2002, Nilsen *et al.* 2004). For this purpose, standard methods of behavioural analyses were used, involving the generation of ethograms and the examination of how likely it was that any given behaviour changed into any other behaviour.

The results allowed a comparison of male and female patterns of aggression and showed that some behavioural patterns were shown by both males and females (approach, fencing), some were male-specific (lunge, boxing, extended wing threat), and some were female-specific (shove and head-butt). The most common patterns in the latter two categories (lunge, shove and head-butt) were subsequently used in genetic studies to characterise aggression as male-like or female-like. The flies used in the studies characterising the above behaviours were isolated in individual test tubes as pupae and therefore emerged as adults in isolation. They remained singly in tubes for 3–5 days, after which they were size-matched and paired for fights. Thus, the first time adult male or female flies encountered another fly in competition for resources was when they were paired for fights.

All of the patterns of aggression of which flies are capable are seen in these first pairings, and in all cases the behaviours and the responses of opponents are appropriate to the situation. This and other evidence not described here suggest that the establishment of the highly complex patterns of behaviour seen during aggression is largely governed by the genetic profile of the flies.

Learning and memory during fly fights

Genetics is not the whole story, however, as experience moulds the patterns of behaviour shown by winners and losers of fights during and after the time that hierarchical relationships have been established between male flies (Yurkovic *et al.* 2006). The final winner in male fights is the first fly to perform a lunge as the opponent retreats. It is as if an operant learning situation is established where one fly learns that a strategy has worked (the opponent runs away) and then uses that strategy more and more during subsequent encounters. At the end of a 30-minute fight a winner is lunging approximately 30% of the time. Losers by contrast never lunge after a decision has been made in a fight. Retreat behaviour shows a converse pattern, with losers retreating more and more as the fight progresses, while winners never retreat after a decision is reached. After a 30-minute separation period, when loser flies are paired with familiar and unfamiliar winners or with naive flies that have not fought before, the losers fight differently against familiar and non-familiar opponents. They rarely lunge against familiar opponents, but will lunge against unfamiliar opponents. Despite this difference, losers will lose all subsequent fights against all opponents except against other losers, where they can win in a small percentage of cases if they lunge against an opponent. Thus, while genes play a major role in establishing the behavioural patterns shown by flies during fights, the usage of these patterns can be modified by experience. Recent unpublished work from our laboratory suggests that the training protocol (one long fight against a single opponent versus several shorter fights against different opponents) will influence how long flies remember that they have lost a fight. Multiple short trials are far more effective at preserving the strength of loser effects that had developed from the first fight than one long trial.

Single genes specify both how flies court and how they fight

A major reason for selecting an animal like *Drosophila* for the study of aggression, however, relates to the wealth of genetic tools that are available for use. Traditional mutants are readily available for most of the genes in the fruit fly nervous system. However, one of the most powerful tools available is the Gal4/UAS system (Brand & Perrimon 1993). This method and its variations essentially allow one to manipulate any gene desired (add foreign gene, knock out gene, change levels of gene), any place desired in the fly including within subtypes of neurons in the nervous system, and any time desired in development (up to and including inducing changes in behaving adult flies). Moreover, the genes involved in the early stages of sex determination in flies have already been identified (Billeter *et al.* 2006). These include genes that code for several splicing factors (*sex lethal* and *transformer*) and ultimately for two families of transcription factors (members of the *doublesex* and *fruitless* families) that are differentially spliced in male and female flies. The transcripts derived from the most distal promoter of the complex *fruitless* gene are spliced into sex-specific variants. In males, transcription and translation results in the formation of three or more protein forms (collectively called Fru^M), while in females the splice variants of *fruitless* are not translated into proteins. Fru^M variants are expressed in approximately 20 clusters of neurons in male fly nervous systems, which together account for approximately 2% of the total neurons in the *Drosophila* nervous system. When Fru^M is expressed in female brains, female flies are generated that court other females and that fight using male patterns of aggression (they lunge and box, but do not show the normal female shove and head-butt patterns) – the complete description of the behavioural patterns seen in male and female fights is found in Nilsen *et al.* (2004). On the other hand, generation of the female splice variants of *fruitless* in male flies leads to males that show female patterns of aggression (Vrontou *et al.* 2006). The extended wing threat behaviour, usually a male-limited behaviour, is still only displayed by males after these manipulations. Genes involved in establishing wing threat, therefore, must be under the control of a gene (or genes) other than *fruitless*. The Gal4 system can be used to alter the sex of all or of subgroups of neurons in the nervous systems of flies (sex is cell autonomous in fruit flies) through expression of *transformer* in male flies, where it usually is not expressed, or by elimination of *transformer* expression in females (Chan & Kravitz 2007). When this is done, the same aggression phenotype is observed as when *fruitless* is altered, but, in addition, it is possible to separate clusters of Fru^M-expressing neurons into some that are essential to heterosexual courtship behaviour and some that are essential to whether flies fight like males or females. Finally, by eliminating the amine neurotransmitter (or neurohormone) octopamine (the invertebrate equivalent of norepinephrine), or by changing the sex of only the three neurons in the male-fly nervous system that normally express Fru^M and octopamine, it is possible to influence the behavioural choice between courtship and aggression (Certel *et al.* 2007).

Summary of genetic studies with
D. melanogaster

Thus, in *D. melanogaster*, splice variants of the *fruitless* gene play essential roles in determining both how flies court and how flies fight. Therefore, in flies at least, a close relationship exists between these two usually mutually exclusive behaviours. Other genes undoubtedly will be discovered that are important to these behaviours (Dierick & Greenspan 2006, Edwards *et al.* 2006), including *doublesex*, the second transcription factor that is alternatively spliced in male and female flies. With one key gene already identified, however, a

world of new experimental approaches to the study of behaviour has been opened up through the use of this experimental model system.

7.4.2 Impulsive violence and serotonin neurochemistry in primates

Primates, including humans, are generally gregarious. Embedded in complex social hierarchies, individuals prosper with an ability to forge alliances, nurture affiliations, and enlist reliable support from fellow group members (Silverberg & Gray 1992). In many primates, high-ranking individuals are able to seize a disproportionate share of the spoils, and affirm their position with increased aggression; they initiate fights, display with attack gestures and vocalisations, and often harass subordinates. The latter tend to respond with submissive acts and calls, while they cower or flee from dominants. This is particularly true for aggressive species, such as rhesus macaques *Macaca mulatta*, where heightened impulsiveness and risk-taking may contribute to their ability to spread across inhospitable habitats and marginal conditions (Maestripieri 2007). Groups form rigid hierarchies, dominance is enforced with ferocious aggression, and opponents rarely reconcile following a fight. After the initial burst of overt aggressive activity, individuals quickly settle into their respective ranks as social structure forms and stabilises. Unambiguous hierarchies may thereby play an essential part in reducing the chronic tensions inherent to group living and, with it, a variety of stress-related pathologies (Thierry *et al.* 2004).

Most individuals of structured social groups readily cope with the need for negotiated conflict resolution (Aureli & De Waal 2000). However, a small number of juvenile males frequently attracts attention with excessive impulsive behaviour, extreme risk-taking, a distinct unwillingness to submit to stronger group members, or with displays of inappropriate aggression (Mehlman *et al.* 1994, Higley *et al.* 1996). An extensive literature across a variety of experimental scenarios supports the notion that dysfunction in serotonin neuromodulation is associated with the occurrence of abnormally high levels of overt physical aggression, suicide attempts, a lack of impulse control, social ostracism, early migration, and a wide range of other psychiatric diagnoses and early mortality (Maes & Coccaro 1998). These behavioural pathologies of hyper-aggression strongly cluster with a range of altered measures of serotonin system function, including low titres of serotonin metabolites, reduced enzymatic activity in amine turnover, lowered serotonin receptor sensitivity, and decreased activity of serotonergic reuptake systems (see Chapter 17; Ferrari *et al.* 2005).

Despite the general association between serotonin dysfunction and inability to control violent behaviour, explanations that simply focus on absolute levels alone have failed to produce a consistent picture. Although this suggests that caution may be necessary in discussing putative links between amine neuromodulators and behaviour in general, it more likely reflects the essential constraints and properties of a dynamic modulatory system. Embedded in highly fluid networks, compensatory mechanisms constantly adjust the effectiveness of amine neuromodulators with respect to inherent set-points. Determinants of the resulting behavioural phenotype presumably reside in synaptic changes, in the magnitude, duration and temporal pattern of release, rates of inactivation, and neuromodulator ratios. The power of arousal mechanisms is thus not in determining, or producing, a behaviour. Rather, neural substrates are altered to make the emergence of a particular act more likely; neurochemical axes modulate the animal's behaviour towards adaptive responses (Libersat 2004).

Several genetic risk factors for abnormal aggression provide surprisingly strong predictability in humans and non-human primates, including a set of autosomal dominant polymorphisms in genes for the serotonin transporter and monoamine oxidase A (Retz *et al.* 2004, Wendland *et al.* 2006). As is true of behavioural and personality traits, measures of serotonin function and metabolism are strongly heritable in many primates. The serotonin transporter protein actively recycles the signalling molecule into internal sites, thereby clearing neurotransmitter from its targets. In this way it regulates synaptic serotonin concentrations and modulates the

duration of serotonergic activity (Brown & Hariri, 2006). The serotonin transporter gene in humans and rhesus macaques contains length polymorphisms in the upstream promoter region. Carriers of the short allele exhibit reduced transcriptional activity for the serotonin transporter gene, two fold lower measures of serotonin uptake, and blunted central serotonin function (Bennett *et al.* 2002). Aggression scores are also significantly higher, and an overrepresentation of the short variant is found among violent individuals (Zalsman *et al.* 2001). Hyper-aggression shows comorbidity with a range of abnormal personality traits and neurological disorders (Haberstick *et al.* 2006, Zalsman *et al.* 2006).

Consistent differences between individuals with such length polymorphisms are already observed in early infant temperament, and become more exaggerated when the individual is exposed to bad parenting and general deprivation (Newman *et al.* 2005). Illustrating the interacting influence of genotype and early rearing experiences of the developing hyper-aggressive phenotype, serotonin systems play an integral, although not yet fully understood, role.

7.4.3 Breeding lines for aggressive phenotypes

A particular trait can be transformed over time, if (1) the trait is at least partially heritable, (2) individuals exhibit variation in it, and (3) there is enhanced reproductive success associated with some variants. Charles Darwin's knowledge of the effects of selective breeding was crucial to his articulation of natural selection as a structuring process (Darwin 1859). The view that selection is as applicable to behaviour as to any morphological trait would form the basis of a bitter nature-versus-nurture argument that pitted ethologists, who endorsed the idea, against behaviourists, who denied its role (see Chapter 1; Bolhuis & Giraldeau 2004). Aside from this controversy, the presence of distinct genetic strains with enhanced levels of aggression has long been noted within a wide range of species of insects, birds, dogs, fish and mice (see Chapter 2; Sandnabba 1996). Efforts to further enhance such behaviours through selective breeding have generally managed to produce, within a few generations, animals with levels of aggressive behaviour that greatly exceed those of controls (Nelson 2005). Our ability to create pedigrees with distinct, aggressive phenotypes represents an important tool for the analysis of genotypic variation. In addition to such selected lines, attempts to map or identify genes for aggressive behaviour have relied on outbred, inbred and recombinant inbred lines.

Arguably, no breeding programme has been maintained longer than that from which our current breeds of dogs emerged as a domesticated subspecies of the wolf *Canis lupus* (Wayne & Ostrander 2007). At least since the late Pleistocene, some 17 000 years ago, humans have continued to select dogs for qualities that make them useful as well as pleasant companions (Serpell 1995). Aimed at individuals with an overrepresentation of juvenile characteristics, such as big eyes or a playful nature, our selective control has enhanced a wide range of paedomorphic traits. Even breeds where largely adult morphologies are needed to cope with demanding work tasks, such as St Bernards or salukis, exhibit a youthful temperament that has toned down or stylised aggressive behaviour. Aggressive behaviours like barking, herding or compulsive fighting have been retained in some breeds that are commonly used for guard duties, such as rottweilers, German shepherds, German shorthair pointers and Chesapeake Bay retrievers. These are generally dominant and protective breeds, and high levels of aggression often limit their popularity within a family context. Aggressive traits are even more prominent in breeds selected for attacking prey and fighting, such as pit bull terriers (Scott 1972). The need for proper socialisation in order to prevent the emergence of problematic behaviours and human-directed aggression has contributed to the recommendation that many of these breeds should only be kept by experienced owners. In contrast, selection for demands that combine general hunting tasks with a close integration into human social companionship has given rise to breeds with calm dispositions, such as beagles, Brittanys and Labrador retrievers. In addition to such broader trends, the correlation between dog aggression directed at other dogs and attacks on humans is relatively low, suggesting that these traits utilise, at least in part, different genetic backgrounds (Liinamo *et al.* 2007).

In mice *Mus musculus*, long-term selective breeding efforts have produced genetic lines with both altered amounts and characteristics of aggressive behaviour. A highly aggressive line of Swiss albino mice has been obtained by selecting males who scored high in an isolation-induced, inter-male aggression paradigm at 60 days of age (Turku Aggressive). Mating partners were the sisters of high-scoring males. A complementary line (Turku Non-Aggressive) has propagated only individuals with the lowest scores in the same test (Lagerspetz & Lagerspetz 1971). Although selected only for high and low aggression towards other males, behaviour varied more broadly between the lines, including measures in alternative paradigms of male aggression, territorial signalling and sexual activity, brain morphology and neurochemistry, as well as nursing competence, enhanced maze learning, and some measures of aggression in mothers.

Other breeding lines, descended from a feral population, were selected bidirectionally with attack latency as the criterion (Sluyter *et al.* 1996). Agonistic encounters between male mice occur naturally during the patrol of territorial borders, and the tests aimed to create such a context for behavioural assessment. Test males were allowed to occupy and acquired a sense of ownership of the test cage. They were then confronted with a standard, novel, male opponent who elicited offensive agonistic behaviours by his mere presence but did not initiate any attacks himself. Attack latency represents a robust behavioural measure which reliably separates individuals who attack rapidly from those who hesitate to confront the intruder. In this paradigm aggressive mice exhibit an active response towards a challenging situation, whereas non-aggressive ones cope more passively. Assigning an aggressive phenotype is to some degree contingent on the precise behavioural measure used. Even in the same paradigm, somewhat different subsets of aggressive individuals emerge if the primary measure focuses instead on the number of attacks, or on accumulated attack time. In all of these selection efforts, significant differences between the breeding lines were obtained beginning with the second generation, and they have persisted ever since. As with other complex traits, aggression is most likely influenced by multiple genes (Plomin *et al.* 1994), although single gene effects have been noted (see below).

Increased aggression has, for instance, been linked to altered levels of expression of genes coding for amine receptors (e.g. 5-HT1B) or monoamine oxidase A (Brunner 1993). In the latter case, a rodent model demonstrates that monoamine oxidase A deficits lead to severe developmental abnormalities with an unusual aggression phenotype (Upton *et al.* 1999). In humans, possibly, one manifestation of this might be the impulsive aggression shown by males carrying a mutant form of the gene. The temptation to refer to these as mean or aggression genes should be avoided, however, because aggression is definitely not the only behavioural parameter that is altered. The ability to manipulate levels of aggression, combined with evidence from twin and adoption studies (Bartels *et al.* 2003), illustrates that links between individual differences in aggressive behaviour and genetic inheritance are contributing factors in the aetiology of aggression.

7.5 Conclusions and future directions

Attempts to define, characterise and explain aggression have generally met with considerable difficulty. This chapter has examined our current understanding of the behavioural phenomena within the context of all forms of attack, defence or threats. We have reviewed the significance of aggression in light of explanatory concepts that range from proximate to ultimate viewpoints. In summary, aggression is rarely an aberrant form of behaviour with negative consequences for all involved but, in its common expression, allows individuals to assert themselves in competition for resources. Examples of aggression span the entire animal kingdom, and its traits have been shaped by evolution like that of any other behavioural phenotype.

Aggression is clearly not a single, monolithic, behavioural category. Any attempt at explanation will critically depend on a thorough characterisation of its elemental building blocks, and it requires us to recognise the factors that control them. A better understanding of aggression will demand that we overcome the inherent difficulties in capturing the essence of an inherently multifaceted behaviour, and begin to unravel underlying elements of motivation that are not readily observed or elicited. Moreover, additional research is needed both to understand and to discover new treatments for all pathologic expressions of aggression and violence. Targeted gene deletions, RNA interference, or the generation of inducible and brain-region-specific mutants are just some of the exciting new experimental approaches for studying the role of genes, environment and their interaction in the causation of aggression. Regardless of the precise experimental protocol employed, however, success will ultimately depend on our ability to assess, precisely delineate and account for all of aggression's underlying behavioural and neural components.

Acknowledgements

We thank members of the Huber and Kravitz laboratories for their commentary and helpful discussions. We thank the members of the Kravitz laboratory for conducting most of the experiments described in the fruit fly section of the article. This work was supported by grants from the National Institute of General Medical Sciences (GM074675 and GM067645) and the National Science Foundation (IDS-075165) to EAK, and from the National Institute on Drug Abuse (NIH/NIDA 1 R21 DA016435–01A1) to RH.

Suggested readings

Chase, I. D., Tovey, C., Spangler, D. & Manfredonia, M. (2002) Individual differences versus social dynamics in the formation of animal dominance hierarchies. *Proceedings of the National Academy of Sciences of the USA*, **99**, 5744–5749.

Goessmann, C., Hemelrijk, C. & Huber, R. (2000) The formation and maintenance of crayfish hierarchies: behavioral and self-structuring properties. *Behavioral Ecology and Sociobiology*, **48**, 418–428.

Kravitz, E. A. (2000) Serotonin and aggression: insights gained from a lobster model system and speculations on the role of amine neurons in a complex behavior like aggression. *Journal of Comparative Physiology A*, **186**, 221–238.

Nelson, R. J. (2005) *Biology of Aggression*. Oxford: Oxford University Press.

Nilsen, S. P., Chan, Y.-B., Huber, R. & Kravitz, E. A. (2004) Gender-selective patterns of aggressive behavior in *Drosophila melanogaster*. *Proceedings of the National Academy of Sciences of the USA*, **101**, 12342–12347.

Silverberg, J. & Gray, J. P. (1992) *Aggression and Peacefulness in Humans and Other Primates*. Oxford: Oxford University Press.

Vrontou, E., Nilsen, S., Demir. E., Kravitz, E. A. & Dickson, B. J. (2006) *fruitless* regulates aggression and dominance in *Drosophila*. *Nature Neuroscience*, **9**: 1469–1471.

References

Alcock, J. (2005) *Animal Behavior: an Evolutionary Approach*, 8th edn. Sunderland, MA: Sinauer Associates.

Archer, J. (1988) *The Behavioural Biology of Aggression*. Cambridge: Cambridge University Press.

Aureli, F. & De Waal, F. B. M. (2000) *Natural Conflict Resolution*. Berkeley, CA: University of California Press.

Bartels, M., Van den Berg, M., Sluyter, F., Boomsma, D. I. & de Geus, E. J. (2003) Heritability of cortisol levels: review and simultaneous analysis of twin studies. *Psychoneuroendocrinology*, **28**, 121–37.

Beacham, J. (2003) Models of dominance hierarchy formation: effects of prior experience and intrinsic traits. *Behaviour*, **140**, 1275–1303.

Bennett, A. J., Lesch, K. P., Heils, A. *et al.* (2002) Early experience and serotonin transporter gene variation interact to influence primate CNS function. *Molecular Psychiatry*, **7**, 118–122.

Berridge, K. C. (2004) Motivation concepts in behavioral neuroscience. *Physiology and Behavior*, **81**, 179–209.

Billeter, J.-C., Rideout, E. J., Dornan, A. J. & Goodwin, S. F. (2006) Control of male sexual behavior in *Drosophila* by the sex determination pathway. *Current Biology*, **16**, R766–776.

Boake, C. R. B., Price, D. K. & Andreadis, D. K. (1998) Inheritance of behavioral differences between two infertile, sympatric species *Drosophila sylvestris* and *D. heteroneura*. *Heredity*, **80**, 642–650.

Bolhuis, J. J. & Giraldeau, L.-A. (2004) *The Behavior of Animals: Mechanisms, Function and Evolution*. Oxford: Blackwell.

Bonabeau, E., Theraulaz, G., Deneubourg, J. L., Aron, S. & Camazine, S. (1997) Self-organization in social insects. *Trends in Ecology and Evolution*, **12**, 188–193.

Brand, A. H. & Perrimon, N. (1993) Targeted gene expression as a means of altering cell fates and generating dominant phenotypes. *Development*, **118**, 401–415.

Brown, S. M. & Hariri, A. R. (2006) Neuroimaging studies of serotonin gene polymorphisms: exploring the interplay of genes, brain, and behavior. *Cognitive, Affective and Behavioral Neuroscience*, **6**, 44–52.

Brunner, H., Nelen, M., Breakefield, X., Ropers, H. & van Oost, B. (1993) Abnormal behavior associated with a point mutation in the structural gene for monoamine oxidase A. *Science*, **262**, 578–580.

Certel, S. J., Savella, M. G., Schlegel, D. C. F. & Kravitz, E. A. (2007) Modulation of *Drosophila* male behavioral choice. *Proceedings of the National Academy of Sciences of the USA*, **104**, 4706–4711.

Chan, Y. B. & Kravitz, E. A. (2007) Specific subgroups of Fru^M neurons control sexually dimorphic patterns of aggression in *Drosophila melanogaster*. *Proceedings of the National Academy of Sciences of the USA*, **104**, 19577–19582.

Chase, I., Bartolomeo, C. & Dugatkin, L. (1994) Aggressive interactions and inter-contest interval: how long do winners keep winning? *Animal Behaviour*, **48**, 393–400.

Chase, I., Tovey, C., Spangler-Martin, D. & Manfredonia, M. (2002) Individual differences versus social dynamics in the formation of animal dominance hierarchies. *Proceedings of the National Academy of Sciences of the USA*, **99**, 5744–5749.

Chen, S., Lee, A. Y., Bowens, N., Huber, R. & Kravitz, E. A. (2002) Fighting fruit flies: a model system for the study of aggression. *Proceedings of the National Academy of Sciences of the USA*, **99**, 5664–5668.

Darwin, C. (1859) *On the Origin of Species by Means of Natural Selection*. London: John Murray.

Dierick, H. A. & Greenspan, R. J. (2006) Molecular analysis of flies selected for aggressive behavior. *Nature Genetics*, **38**, 1023–1032.

Dow, M. A. & von Schilcher, F. (1975) Aggression and mating success in *Drosophila melanogaster*. *Nature*, **254**, 511–512.

Dugatkin LA (1997) Winner and loser effects and the structure of dominance hierarchies. *Behavioral Ecology*, **8**, 583–587.

Dugatkin, L. A. & Dugatkin, A. D. (2007) Extrinsic effects, estimating opponents' RHP, and the structure of dominance hierarchies. *Biology Letters*, **3**, 614–616.

Dugatkin, L. A. & Reeve, H. K. (2000) *Game Theory and Animal Behavior*. Oxford: Oxford University Press.

Edwards, A. C., Rollmann, S. M., Morgan, T. J. & MacKay, T. F. C. (2006) Quantitative genomics of aggressive behavior in *Drosophila melanogaster*. *PLoS Genetics*, **2** (9), e154.

Ferrari, P. F., Palanza, P., Parmigiani, S., de Almeida, R. M. M. & Miczek, K. A. (2005) Serotonin and aggressive behavior in rodents and nonhuman primates: Predispositions and plasticity. *European Journal of Pharmacology*, **526**, 259–273.

Francis, R. C. (1988) On the relationship between aggression and social dominance. *Ethology*, **78**, 223–237.

Goessmann, C., Hemelrijk, C. & Huber, R. (2000) The formation and maintenance of crayfish hierarchies: behavioral and self-structuring properties. *Behavioral Ecology and Sociobiology*, **48**, 418–428.

Grosenick, L., Clement, T. & Fernald, R. D. (2007) Fish can infer social rank by observation alone. *Nature*, **445**, 429–432.

Haberstick, B. C., Smolen, A. & Hewitt, J. K. (2006) Family-based association test of the 5HTTLPR and aggressive behavior in a general population sample of children. *Biological Psychiatry*, **59**, 836–843.

Hemelrijk, C. K. (1999) An individual-oriented model of the emergence of despotic and egalitarian societies. *Proceedings of the Royal Society B*, **266**, 361–369.

Higley, J. D., Mehlman, P. T., Higley, S. B. *et al.* (1996) Excessive mortality in young free-ranging male nonhuman primates with low cerebrospinal fluid 5-hydroxyindoleacetic acid concentrations. *Archives of General Psychiatry*, **53**, 537–543.

Hock, K. & Huber, R. (2006) Modeling the acquisition of social rank in crayfish: winner and loser effects and self-structuring properties. *Behaviour*, **143**, 325–346.

Hoffmann, A. A. (1987) A laboratory study of male territoriality in the sibling species *Drosophila melanogaster* and *D. simulans*. *Animal Behaviour*, **35**, 807–818.

Hofmann, H. & Schildberger, K. (2001) Assessment of strength and willingness to fight during aggressive encounters in crickets. *Animal Behaviour*. **62**, 337–348.

Hsu, Y. & Wolf, L. L. (2000) The winner and loser effect: what fighting behaviours are influenced? *Animal Behaviour*, **61**, 777–786.

Huber, R. & Kravitz, E. A. (1995) A quantitative study of agonistic behavior and dominance in juvenile American lobsters (*Homarus americanus*). *Brain, Behavior and Evolution*, **46**, 72–83.

Huber, R., Daws, A., Tuttle, S. B. & Panksepp, J. B. (2002) Quantitative behavioral techniques for the study of crustacean aggression. In: *The Crustacean Nervous System*, ed. K. Wiese. Berlin: Springer, pp. 186–201.

Huntingford, F,. & Garcia de Leaniz, C. (1997) Social dominance, prior residence and the acquisition of profitable feeding sites in juvenile Atlantic salmon. *Journal of Fish Biology*, **51**, 1009–1014.

Immelmann, K. & Beer, C. (1992) *A Dictionary of Ethology*. Cambridge, MA: Harvard University Press.

Jacobs, M. E. (1960) Influence of light on mating of *Drosophila melanogaster*. *Ecology*, **41**, 182–188.

Krahé, B. (2001) *The Social Psychology of Aggression*. Hove: Psychology Press.

Lagerspetz, K. M. J. & Lagerspetz, K. Y. H. (1971) Changes in aggressiveness of mice resulting from selective breeding, learning and social isolation. *Scandinavian Journal of Psychology*, **12**, 241–248.

Libersat, F. (2004) Monoamines and the orchestration of behavior. *Bioscience*, **54**, 17–25

Liinamo, A.-E., van den Berg, L., Leegwater, P. A. J. *et al.* (2007) Genetic variation in aggression-related traits in golden retriever dogs. *Applied Animal Behaviour Science*, **104**, 95–106

Lorenz, K. (1963) *On Aggression*. San Diego, CA: Harcourt Brace.

Maes, M. & Coccaro, E. F. (1998) *Neurobiology and Clinical Views on Aggression and Impulsivity*. New York, NY: Wiley.

Maestripieri, D. (2007) *Macachiavellian Intelligence: How Rhesus Macaques and Humans Have Conquered the World*. Chicago, IL: University of Chicago Press.

Maynard Smith, J. (1974) Theory of games and the evolution of animal conflicts. *Journal of Theoretical Biology*, **47**, 209–221

Maynard Smith, J. (1982) *Evolution and the Theory of Games*. Cambridge: Cambridge University Press.

Mehlman, P. T., Higley, J. D., Faucher, I. *et al.* (1994) Low CSF 5-HIAA concentrations and severe aggression and impaired impulse control in nonhuman primates. *American Journal of Psychiatry*, **151**, 1485–1491.

Moyer, K. E. (1968) Kinds of aggression and their physiological basis. *Communications in Behavioral Biology*, **2**, 65–87.

Nelson, R. J. (2005) *Biology of Aggression*. Oxford: Oxford University Press, p. 528.

Newman, T. K., Syagailo, Y. V., Barr, C. S. *et al.* (2005) Monoamine oxidase A gene promoter variation and rearing experience influences aggressive behavior in rhesus monkeys. *Biological Psychiatry*, **57**, 167–172

Nilsen, S. P., Chan, Y.-B., Huber, R. & Kravitz, E. A. (2004) Gender-selective patterns of aggressive behavior in *Drosophila melanogaster*. *Proceedings of the National Academy of Sciences of the USA*, **101**, 12342–12347.

Pinker, S. (2007) A history of violence. *The New Republic*, March 19, 2007.

Plomin, R., Owen, M. J. & McGuffin, P. (1994) The genetic basis of complex human behaviors. *Science*, **264**, 1733–1739

Retz, W., Retz-Junginger, P., Supprian, T., Thome, J. & Rösler, M. (2004) Association of serotonin transporter promoter gene polymorphism with violence: relation with personality disorders, impulsivity, and childhood ADHD psychopathology. *Behavioral Sciences and the Law*, **22**, 415–425.

Sandnabba, N. K. (1996) Selective breeding for isolation-induced intermale aggression in mice: associated responses and environmental influences. *Behavior Genetics*, **26**, 477–488.

Scott, J. P. (1972) *Animal Behavior*. Chicgao, IL: University of Chicago Press.

Serpell, J. (1995) *The Domestic Dog: its Evolution, Behaviour, and Interactions with People*. Cambridge: Cambridge University Press.

Silverberg, J. & Gray, J. P. (1992) *Aggression and Peacefulness in Humans and Other Primates*. Oxford: Oxford University Press.

Sluyter, F., van Oortmerssen, G. A., de Ruiter, A. J. H. & Koolhaas, J. M. (1996) Aggression in wild house mice: current state of affairs. *Behavior Genetics*, **26**, 489–496.

Spieth, H. T. (1968) The evolutionary implications of sexual behavior in *Drosophila*. *Evolutionary Biology*, **2**, 157–191.

Spieth, H. T. (1974) Courtship in *Drosophila*. *Annual Review of Entomology*, **19**, 385–405

Sturtevant, A. H. (1915) Experiments on sex recognition and the problem of sexual selection in *Drosophila*. *Journal of Animal Behavior*, **5**, 351–366.

Suomi, S. (1997) Early determinants of behaviour: evidence from primate studies. *British Medical Bulletin*, **53**, 170–184

Számadó, S. (2008) How threat displays work: species-specific fighting techniques, weaponry and proximity risk. *Animal Behaviour*, **76**, 1455–1463.

Theraulaz, G., Bonabeau, E. & Deneubourg, J. (1995) Self-organization of hierarchies in animal societies: the case of the primitively eusocial wasp *Polistes dominulus*. *Journal of Theoretical Biology*, **174**, 313–323

Thierry, B., Singh. M, & Kaumanns, W. (2004) *Macaque Societies: a Model for the Study of Social Organization*. Cambridge: Cambridge University Press.

Ueda, A. & Kidokoro, Y. (2002) Aggressive behaviours of female *Drosophila melanogaster* are influenced by their social experience and food resources. *Physiological Entomology*, **27**, 21–28.

Upton, A. L., Salichon, N., Lebrand, C. *et al.* (1999) Excess of serotonin (5HT) alters the segregation of ipsilateral and contralateral retinal projections in monoamine oxidase A knock-out mice: possible role of 5HT uptake in retinal ganglion cells during development. *Journal of Neuroscience*, **19**, 7007–7024.

Vrontou, E., Nilsen, S., Demir, E., Kravitz, E. A. & Dickson, B. J. (2006) *fruitless* regulates aggression and dominance in *Drosophila*. *Nature Neuroscience*, **9**, 1469–1471.

Wayne, R. K. & Ostrander, E. A. (2007) Lessons learned from the dog genome. *Trends in Genetics*, **23**, 557–567

Wendland, J. R., Lesch, K. P., Newman, T. K. *et al.* (2006) Differential functional variability of serotonin transporter and monoamine oxidase A genes in macaque species displaying contrasting levels of aggression-related behavior. *Behavior Genetics*, **36**, 163–172.

Wilson, E. O. (1975) *Sociobiology: the New Synthesis*. Cambridge, MA: Harvard University Press.

Wrangham, R. & Peterson, D. (1996) *Demonic Males*. Boston, MA: Houghton Mifflin.

Yurkovic, A., Wang, O., Basu, A. C. & Kravitz, E. A. (2006) Learning and memory associated with aggression in *Drosophila melanogaster*. *Proceedings of the National Academy of Sciences of the USA*, **103**: 17519–17524.

Zalsman, G., Frisch, A., Bromberg, M. *et al.* (2001) Family-based association study of serotonin transporter promoter in suicidal adolescents: no association with suicidality but possible role in violence traits. *American Journal of Medical Genetics*, **105**, 239–245.

Zalsman, G., Huang, Y. Y., Oquendo, M. A. et al. (2006) Association of a triallelic serotonin transporter gene promoter region (5-HTTLPR) polymorphism with stressful life events and severity of depression. *American Journal of Psychiatry*, **163**, 1588–1593.

From behavioural observations, to genes, to evolution

Laurent Keller

My interest in social behaviour probably stems from me belonging to a species where social interactions rule our lives. As a teenager I was very interested in psychiatry, and I also recall spending hours observing the human-like attitudes of chimpanzees and gorillas in the zoo. Accordingly, while studying biology at university, I seriously considered the option of studying chimpanzees. But at the time of graduating I had come to realise that this was not an easy task. Either one would conduct studies in the field with the only hope to collect sparse observational data, or one could study chimpanzees in enclosures, but the very contrived and artificial environment makes it difficult to understand how behaviour might have been modulated by natural selection. I therefore started to think about other social organisms that could be easily observed and, importantly, where it was possible to experimentally manipulate key components of social organisation. This paved the way for my interest in myrmecology.

My first work in the field of myrmecology (the ant world) was primarily concerned with understanding the evolution of multiple-queen colonies, which at that time was seen as a major problem for kin selection theory. During my PhD and postdoc I conducted many experiments, which, together with the work of some colleagues, allowed us to solve the apparent paradox of reduced relatedness stemming from colonies containing several reproductive queens. After completing my PhD, I decided to work on the fire ant *Solenopsis invicta*, because this species exhibits two types of social organisation, a monogyne form in which colonies have a single queen and a polygyne form where colonies contain a large number of queens. As in many other ants, this difference in queen number is associated with differences in a host of reproductive and social traits, including queen phenotype and breeding strategy, mode of colony reproduction, and pattern of sex allocation (Ross & Keller 1995). My plan was to conduct cross-garden experiments to show that social environment could influence the phenotype of queens and their breeding opportunities.

I conducted such an experiment together with my colleague Ken Ross, and we found that social environment indeed affected the phenotype of queens (Keller & Ross 1993a). However, a population-genetic study revealed that, while the two social forms had similar allele frequencies at most loci studied, they differed in allele frequencies at the enzyme-encoding gene *Pgm-3* (*Phosphoglucomutase-3*) (Ross 1992). Even more surprising, there was a strong departure from Hardy–Weinberg distribution at the locus, with one class of homozygotes (*Pgm-3^{AA}*) being completely absent among reproductive queens in polygyne, but not monogyne, colonies.

Social Behaviour: Genes, Ecology and Evolution, ed. Tamás Székely, Allen J. Moore and Jan Komdeur. Published by Cambridge University Press. © Cambridge University Press 2010.

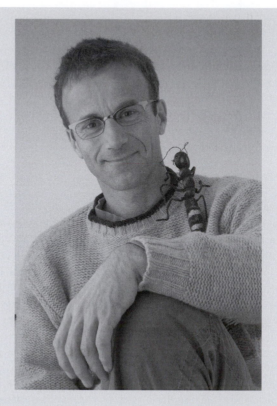

Laurent Keller. Photo: University of Lausanne.

This prompted us to design experiments to test hypotheses (e.g. that *Pgm-3* is associated with a dispersal polymorphism) that might explain why *Pgm-3^{AA}* queens never become reproductively active in polygyne colonies. Our experiments disproved all but one of the hypotheses. We found that the genotype at the locus *Pgm-3* was strongly associated with morphological and physiological differences between queens, as well as with their probability of being accepted by workers in established polygyne colonies. *Pgm-3^{AA}* queens were selectively killed by workers when they initiated reproduction in polygyne colonies (Keller & Ross 1993b). Intriguingly, *Pgm-3^{AA}* queens are heavier and more fecund than queens with alternative genotypes, raising the question of why workers selectively destroy them.

The answer was to come some years later with the finding that selection acts on another locus. In the monogyne form, all queens were found to be homozygous for allele *B* at the locus *Gp-9* (*general protein-9*), while almost all reproductive queens were *Gp-9^{Bb}* heterozygotes in the polygyne form. The genomic region marked by *Gp-9^{b}* was found to be deleterious, with most *Gp-9^{bb}* females dying prematurely as adults (Ross 1997). Moreover, there is almost no recombination between *Gp-9* and *Pgm-3*, and all the known phenotypic and behavioural effects associated with *Gp-9* and *Pgm-3* can be accounted for by the genomic region marked by *Gp-9* (Keller & Ross 1999). By conducting experiments we also found why polygyne colonies only host *Gp-9^{Bb}* queens. The genomic region marked by *Gp-9^{b}* behaves as a green-beard gene that induces workers carrying one allele in that genomic region to selectively kill queens that do not bear it (Keller & Ross 1998).

Interestingly, the genomic region marked by Gp-9 also determines the existence of the monogyne and polygyne social forms (Ross & Keller 1998). Monogyne colonies are always headed by Gp-9^{BB} queens mated with a Gp-9^{B} male, and the Gp-9^{BB} workers in such colonies never accept additional queens (regardless of their Gp-9 genotype). However, when the proportion of Gp-9^{Bb} workers is greater than about 10% (which is always true in polygyne colonies), workers readily accept several queens, but only those carrying at least one copy of the genomic region marked by Gp-9^{b} (Ross & Keller 2002). Hence, social organisation in fire ants depends on whether or not colonies contain a given proportion of Gp-9^{Bb} workers.

This work on fire ants led me to realise that if one is to understand ultimate questions about why an animal behaves in a particular way, one has to also address the proximate mechanisms at work. For example, we would never have been able to understand why workers eliminate the larger and more fecund Pgm-3^{AA} queens in polygyne colonies if we had not provided experimental evidence that this behaviour was the outcome of a selfish gene. Similarly, all the conflict theory in social Hymenoptera is based on their having a haplodiploid system of sex determination, yet an increasing number of studies show that the modes of reproduction in social insects can follow different rules, with even some species where both males and females reproduce by clonal reproduction (e.g. Helms Cahan & Keller 2003, Fournier *et al.* 2005, Pearcy *et al.* 2004, Ohkawara *et al.* 2006).

With the advent of new technologies, it starts to be possible to conduct genetic studies in non-model organisms. For example, we recently developed a microarray for the fire ant (Wang *et al.* 2007) to investigate how the social behaviour of fire ant workers is determined by the interaction of their own Gp-9 genotype and the Gp-9 genotypic composition of other workers in the colony (Wang *et al.* 2008). The use of genetic tools in non-model organisms will, I believe, drastically change the way we study social behaviour in the near future. Instead of collecting data that, in aggregation, allow us to become more confident in the predictions we can derive from evolutionary theory, we should soon be able to identify how natural selection has acted on the genes affecting behaviour.

References

Fournier, D., Estoup, A., Orivel, J. *et al.* (2005) Clonal reproduction by males and females in the little fire ant. *Nature*, **435**, 1230–1234.

Helms Cahan, S. & Keller, L. (2003) Complex hybrid origin of genetic caste determination in harvester ants. *Nature*, **424**, 306–309.

Keller, L. & Ross, K. G. (1993a) Phenotypic plasticity and 'cultural transmission' of alternative social organizations in the fire ant *Solenopsis invicta*. *Behavioral Ecology and Sociobiology*, **33**, 121–129.

Keller, L. & Ross, K. G. (1993b) Phenotypic basis of reproductive success in a social insect: genetic and social determinants. *Science*, **260**, 1107–1110.

Keller, L. & Ross, K. G. (1998) Selfish genes: a green beard in the red fire ant. *Nature*, **394**, 573–575.

Keller, L. & Ross, K. G. (1999) Major gene effects on phenotype and fitness: the relative roles of Pgm-3 and Gp-9 in introduced populations of the fire ant *Solenopsis invicta*. *Journal of Evolutionary Biology*, **12**, 672–680.

Ohkawara, K., Nakayama, M., Sato, A., Trindl, A. & Heinze, J. (2006) Clonal reproduction and genetic caste differences in a queen-polymorphic ant, *Vollenhovia emeryi*. *Biology Letters*, **2**, 359–363.

Pearcy, M., Aron, S., Doums, C., Keller, L. (2004) Conditional use of sex and parthenogenesis for worker and queen production in ants. *Science*, **306**, 1780–1783.

Ross, K. G. (1992) Strong selection on a gene that influences reproductive competition in a social insect. *Nature*, **355**, 347–349.

Ross, K. G. (1997) Multilocus evolution in fire ants: effects of selection, gene flow, and recombination. *Genetics*, **145**, 961–974.

Ross, K. G. & Keller, L. (1995) Ecology and evolution of social organization: insights from fire ants and other highly eusocial insects. *Annual Review of Ecology and Systematics*, **26**, 631–656.

Ross, K. G. & Keller, L. (1998) Genetic control of social organization in an ant. *Proceedings of the National Academy of Sciences of the USA*, **95**, 14232–14237.

Ross, K. G. & Keller, L. (2002) Experimental conversion of colony social organization by manipulation of worker genotype composition in fire ants (*Solenopsis invicta*). *Behavioral Ecology and Sociobiology*, **51**, 287–295.

Wang, J., Jemielity, S., Uva, P. *et al.* (2007) An annotated cDNA library and microarray for large-scale gene-expression studies in the ant *Solenopsis invicta*. *Genome Biology*, **8**, R9.

Wang, J., Ross, K. G. & Keller, L. (2008) Genome-wide expression patterns and the genetic architecture of a fundamental social trait. *PLoS Genetics*, **4** (7), e1000127.

8

Social influences on communication signals: from honesty to exploitation

Mark E. Hauber and Marlene Zuk

Overview

Communication is at the core of understanding sociality as an interface between behaviours and phenotypes, and their evolutionary trajectories. Central to communication research is gaining an understanding of the information content of signals and the ecological, social and physiological factors that influence their format. It is clear that individuals which benefit from social exchange can critically influence what information is transmitted, how it is transmitted and whether it is scrambled to prevent eavesdropping. Less clear is how the physical channels through which signals are emitted and received might influence the extent to which they are prone to errors, dishonesty and manipulation. Here we show how sensory systems, perceptual physiology, cognitive decision rules and evolutionary trajectories produce the broad range of signalling modalities and contents that we see in nature. Our overview

suggests that experimental evidence on the meaning, honesty and selective benefits of communication for signallers and receivers across invertebrates and vertebrates can provide a taxonomically broad but conceptually similar set of examples. This is not surprising, since studies across diverse lineages have demonstrated that the mechanism and function of communication systems both critically shape social behaviour and are being shaped by sociality. In particular, functional investigations of the sensory systems of vocal communication in songbirds, visual signals in trap-building predators, and chemical signalling in arthropods, have established clear examples of the limits to perception and discrimination of signal design. Together, such multilevel approaches pose new or understudied questions regarding our understanding of the evolution of honest and deceptive signals.

8.1 Introduction

Communication, by definition, involves two or more participants in the exchange of information (Hauser 1997). To narrow such a broad definition

requires specifying whether the exchange is intentional and whether it is beneficial to one or more participants, and identifying the physical and sensory mode of transmission that is utilised (Bradbury & Vehrencamp 1998). For example, the definition of

Social Behaviour: Genes, Ecology and Evolution, ed. Tamás Székely, Allen J. Moore and Jan Komdeur. Published by Cambridge University Press. © Cambridge University Press 2010.

reliable or deceitful communication would contain detailed predictions about the role and evolutionary function of signal production and reception (Searcy & Nowicki 2005). In this chapter we take a general approach, and consider communication systems to involve all types of information exchange between individuals in the course of animals' interactions.

Social interactions can vary dramatically in both space and time. For example, pheromones and sounds will carry their respective messages over long distances relative to the scale of body size of the emitter, especially in gaseous or aquatic media under environmental, physical and biological conditions that favour long-distance signal transmission (e.g. downstream in a river or during silent nights: Symonds & Elgar 2008). In contrast, communication signals emitted in the same modalities but in still or loud environments will fail to reach the receiver at distances beyond just a handful of body lengths of the emitter (Symonds & Elgar 2004). How do individuals then cope with such physical and social uncertainty in communication systems (Wiley 2006), and solve the reliability of message reception?

Recent observations suggest, and experiments confirm, that anthropogenic noise can provide a significant context to interfere with the sound transmission of urban songbirds, including great tits *Parus major*, blackbirds *Turdus merula* and song sparrows *Melospiza melodia* (Slabbekoorn & Peet 2003, Wood & Yezerinac 2006, Slabbekoorn & Ripmeester 2008). The loud and variable low-frequency vibrations of machinery (Katti & Warren 2004) can mask critical low-frequency components of acoustic intraspecific communication signals, including avian mate attraction songs and calls. To escape this constraint, singers respond by consistently increasing the amplitude and/or the fundamental frequency of their calls compared to individuals calling in more quiet habitats (Patricelli & Blickley 2006).

However, shifting song frequencies to escape background sounds, as well as increasing the amplitude of vocalisations produced in noisy environments, are not at all novel responses for vocally communicating taxa. Natural sources of loud sounds, including streams and rivers, present frequent environmental constraints on auditory perception, and several species of birds, including chaffinches *Fringilla coelebs* (Brumm & Slater 2006), have evolved to accommodate these acoustic constraints by altering the frequency and amplitude of their vocal outputs. Furthermore, the auditory physiology of many vocal-learner songbirds has adapted to escape the constraints imposed by loud external noise sources by delaying the sensitive period of song imprinting (Patricelli & Blickley 2006), and most avian species can also regenerate damaged hair-cells critical for sound perception of the voices of others and of self during vocal learning and display (Woolley *et al.* 2001).

How do animals then respond to such perturbations and fluctuations in the reliability of environmental transmission channels? For example, ultraviolet spectra of sunlight can amplify visual display cues in white web silk of *Nephila clavipes* spiders in forest clearings better than the yellow silk used for the web of conspecifics weaving their orbs under the more limited light spectra under the tropical forest canopy (Craig *et al.* 1996). In turn, more UV reflectance can attract visually oriented prey items to increase the spiders' foraging success (Hauber 1998).

One frequently considered aspect of potentially derailed communication is the exploitation of signal transmission channels by predators and parasites. An overview of signalling modality and exploitation risk later in this chapter shows that some modalities of sensory exchange are indeed more prone to eavesdropping and appropriation by unintended recipients than others: for example, in arthropods, mating calls and visual signals are often perceived or turned into lures by predators and parasitoids, whereas similar eavesdropping and hijacking of conspecific communication channels are less frequently seen in pheromonal signals. Recent research on Australian wasp-mimetic tongue orchids *Cryptostylis* spp. clearly illustrates the strength and cost of visual trickery: the colour and shape resemblance of female wasps is so close to the real thing that males ejaculate to deposit sperm on the deceptive flowers (Gaskett *et al.* 2008).

Thus, sensory exploitation *sensu stricto* can be the basis of coevolutionary arms races between the increasingly private (i.e. heterospecifically

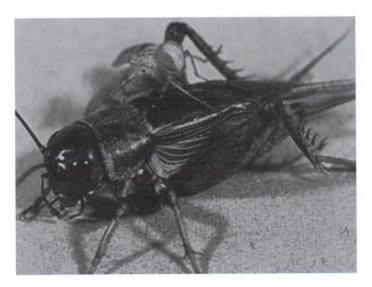

Figure 8.1 The Pacific field cricket *Teleogryllus oceanicus* is native to Australasia and has been introduced to Hawaii, where it is subject to an acoustically orienting parasitoid fly. The parasitised populations show many changes in behaviour and morphology, apparently in response to selection by the fly. Photo: R. Hoy.

hard-to-perceive) communication channels between conspecifics and the greater elaboration of the sensory physiology of the exploiters (Arnqvist 2006). For example, the auditory system of parasitoid *Ormia* flies has evolved not to perceive conspecific communication signals but to eavesdrop on the typical frequencies and to decipher the direction of the mating calls of their cricket hosts, despite the acoustic challenge imposed on directional hearing by small size (Mason *et al.* 2001). In turn, host crickets *Teleogryllus* parasitised by these flies have evolved to change their daily calling cycle, to call less or not at all overall, and to become more phonotactic, through more frequent approach behaviour to cricket call playbacks, in sympatry with acoustically oriented parasitoids (Fig. 8.1; Cade 1981, Zuk *et al.* 1993, 2006).

Additional complexity in the design and content of communication systems is imposed by social contexts of negotiating the relative fitness trade-offs of sending, receiving or eavesdropping on signals that carry information about the sender, including its internal and external environment (Searcy & Nowicki 2005). Such social conflicts can be illustrated through the classic example of the signalling

systems of nestling birds seeking parental provisioning and the attending parents deciding how much to provision (Kilner & Johnstone 1997, Wright & Leonard 2002), and this will be described in the next section.

8.2 Begging: a framework for the study of communication

8.2.1 The begging game

Imagine an adult American robin *Turdus migratorius* taking care of its newly hatched young huddled up in a cup nest halfway up a tree sapling. The young appear to be helpless, with eyes still shut and the naked skin barely covered by natal down. Yet, at the moment when the adult lands on its nest, suddenly causing it to shake and casting a shadow, these young birds immediately raise their necks, extend their legs, open their beaks, loudly call, and jostle for positions to await food to be deposited in their gapes (McRae *et al.* 1993). Once one or two of the chicks are fed, the parent departs, and the chicks settle down, both in posture and in calls (Smith & Montgomery 1991).

From the perspectives of the mechanism and adaptive function of such a communication system, the scenario of begging by nestling robins requires several explanations. In particular, how are the dynamics of such a complex set of displays and decisions altered when the chicks are not the genetic progeny of the adults, and are not necessarily related to each other (Briskie *et al.* 1994, Hauber & Ramsey 2003)?

The complexities of parent–offspring communication cues have provided a rich and successful, and still puzzling, source for scientific research (Dearborn & Lichtenstein 2002). Much theoretical work has focused on variation in signal strength emitted by avian chicks regarding (1) how it reflects short- and long-term need of the young and (2) whether there exists some cooperation between nestlings to minimise inclusive fitness costs paid by underfed related nestmates and exhausted genetic parents (Kilner & Johnstone 1997). Empirical work in turn has shown that short- and long-term physiological needs are both encoded in the begging displays of nestling birds: the hungrier and faster-growing the chick, especially in sexually dimorphic species, the more extensive the display (Hauber & Ramsey 2003). Furthermore, loud and intensive begging displays by chicks appear to be not only costly with respect to reduced growth of the chicks (Kilner 2001), but also regarding the attraction of acoustically oriented predators to noisy broods (Haskell 1994, Dearborn 2000).

Finally, chicks from broods with lower overall relatedness owing to extra-pair copulations by their mothers (Chapter 10) are observed to be more competitive and to beg more intensely compared to broods from more monogamous pairs with greater potential inclusive fitness benefits (Briskie *et al.* 1994). Unsurprisingly, interspecific patterns of chick vocalisations also correlate with the extent of maternal programming of the developing embryos. For instance, in species with higher rates of extra-pair parentage, and thus lower intra-brood relatedness, females invest more testosterone in egg yolk, which modulates begging behaviour (Schwabl *et al.* 2007). In contrast, brood parasites do not modulate the testosterone in the yolk of their eggs, contrary to predictions of maternal-investment theory (Fig. 8.2; Hauber & Pilz 2003, Pilz *et al.* 2005). Future work requires detailed physiological analyses of the mechanisms by which brood-parasitic young successfully compete with unrelated nestmates for parental provisioning.

8.2.2 Socioecological contexts of begging

In parallel with these theoretical and empirical advances, the search continues for the recognition cues that reliably allow early parental identification of extra-pair or parasitic young in the nest, arising either from extra-pair parentage or from intra- and interspecific parasitism – although a surprising number of experimental studies reported negative results (Sherman *et al.* 1997). Furthermore, because negative results can reflect either experimental design flaw and/or biological reality, which limits the conclusions (and, importantly, makes the work difficult to publish: Hauber & Pilz 2003), critical alternative tests are lacking (Goth & Hauber 2004, Campbell *et al.* 2009).

For instance, three specific scenarios of the socioecological contexts of begging-call displays have yet to be fully understood. First, in many seabirds and tropical bird species, brood sizes of one are not uncommon (Fig. 8.3). In the absence of potential competitors for parental provisioning, it remains unclear whether signalling rules for single chicks, and the benefits and costs of begging displays, should be altered. Under predictions of honesty of chick physiological needs, brood size should have limited influence on the relationship between begging-call volume and chick hunger (Lotem 1998). This is especially relevant for many seabirds, which nest in remote locations in large colonies where the predatory costs of begging vocalisations are probably minimal, compared to broods of vulnerable mainland-nesting passerines. In contrast, under scenarios of kin selection and inclusive fitness restraint on begging displays, single-chick broods should be less loud but more honest on a per capita basis than broods of several variably related chicks (Briskie *et al.* 1999, Hauber 2003). Empirical tests and experimental evaluations of these alternatives should form fruitful areas of future research in the tropics and in non-passerine avian begging signals.

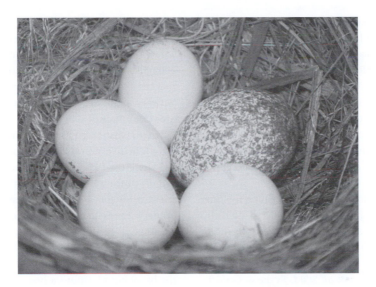

Figure 8.2 Brood-parasitic chicks of the brown-headed cowbird *Molothrus ater* typically beg more intensively than host chicks. Yet maternally deposited androgen levels are not consistently higher in eggs of obligate brood parasites than their hosts. Here a maculated cowbird egg is found in the nest of an eastern phoebe *Sayornis phoebe*. Photo: M. Hauber.

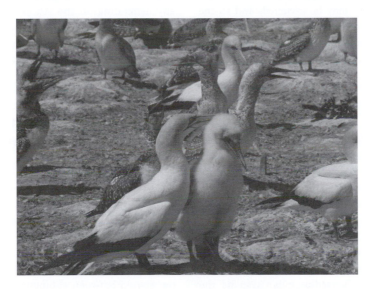

Figure 8.3 Chicks of the Australasian gannet *Morus serrator* typically grow up alone, yet display for food conspicuously to parents. How do selection pressures on signal structure and information content vary between avian broods with single or multiple chicks? Photo: C. Daniel.

Second, a handful of studies on signal variability and its relation to growth differences between female and male chicks have already provided empirical examples that require new theory to be developed for sex-specific benefits of parent–offspring signalling (Hauber & Ramsey 2003). For example, when faced with the superior size and competitive abilities of the obligate brood parasitic brown-headed cowbird's

Molothrus ater chicks, female song sparrow nestlings seem unable to beg to secure sufficient parental provisioning, which causes sex-biased mortality and a male bias in the fledgling sex ratio of host chicks from parasitised broods (Zanette *et al.* 2005). In turn, begging behaviours also vary between the size-dimorphic cowbird chicks (Hauber & Ramsey 2003), so that smaller female chicks suffer and grow more slowly when hatching synchronously with host eggs compared to larger and faster-growing male chicks (Tonra *et al.* 2008).

With more and more research describing the finer scales of embryonic programming (e.g. sex determination, yolk steroid and carotenoid concentrations, incubation patterns) by female birds to influence the developing embryo's ultimate phenotype (Komdeur *et al.* 1997, Forstmeier *et al.* 2004, Pryke & Griffiths 2009), the empirical constraints of whether chicks themselves are able and need to assess relatedness to nestmates and other competitive contexts of the brood's social milieu may be lessened, and so the theoretical conflict regarding the difference between selfish and nepotistic offspring signalling behaviours may be an epiphenomenon of maternal effects (Smiseth *et al.* 2007).

Third, most altricial birds' chicks continue begging after they leave the spatial and perhaps acoustic constraints of the nest. Little theoretical and empirical work has compared signal design and honesty between the nestling and fledgling stages of begging, despite the divergent social (brood division, dispersal or loss of brood mates), ecological (predation), physical (acoustic and spatial), and physiological (growth, mobility, transition to independent foraging) factors influencing the cost/benefit factors of begging displays (Hauber & Ramsey 2003).

Although the overwhelming majority of begging-display research has focused on avian systems, the generality of both theory and signal ecology awaits testing in taxonomically diverse non-avian taxa. For example, altricial young that require parental and helper provisioning in communally breeding mammals have already served as evolutionarily independent but ecologically parallel tests of begging-display theory. More studies should also be forthcoming

on the information content of begging displays of tadpoles in parental frog species, including the Taiwanese tree frog *Chirixalus eiffingeri* (Kam & Yang 2002). Similarly, there is much work to be done on the complexity of prenatal communication signals between embryos and adults in crocodiles and lizards (Main & Bull 1996).

There is also ongoing research on parent–offspring signals in invertebrates. Vibrational signals transmitted along the branches of the host plant by juvenile broods of the phloem-feeding treehopper *Umbonia crassicornis* guarded by their mothers covary with predation pressure by wasps (Cocroft 1999). This has led to phylogenetic studies of signal design in treehoppers, as such signals have design constraints arising from the need for efficient transmission along the branches of different host plant species (Cocroft *et al.* 2006). Need-based, truthful signalling has been studied also in the burying beetle *Nicrophorus vespilloides*. Larval begging signals differ in intensity depending on the sex of the attending parent (Smiseth & Moore 2007). Such studies are likely only the first handful of many future examples of novel experimental work on parent–offspring communication in invertebrate systems.

8.3 Cognitive capacity and social signalling: from sensory systems to perceptual decoding

Successful communication requires that signals carry meaning that can be both perceived and subsequently decoded by the receiver. Many communication modalities are prone to both evolutionary privacy and hijacking. Communication channels (i.e. physiological modalities of signal carriers) that are not shared between competitors, for instance, may undergo rapid specialisation to create private modalities of communication that cannot be perceived and thus decoded by competitors (Goth & Hauber 2004).

Among rodents, for example, ultrasonic communication efficiently eliminates detection by avian predators, because raptorial bird ears do not perceive high-frequency sounds (Wilson & Hare 2004).

Rodents are not, however, completely free of predation pressure from birds: during daytime, urine marks deposited by voles reflect ultraviolet light, which in turn is perceived and recognised by avian predators, including the rough-legged buzzard *Buteo lagopus*, in search of mammalian prey (Koivula & Viitala 1999). In contrast, at night the physiologically sophisticated auditory and nervous system of barn owls *Tyto alba* serves to pinpoint the presence of rodents using noisy footsteps generated by movement through the leaf litter (Knudsen & Konishi 1979). Thus, even though ultrasounds are not audible to birds and could therefore form a private communication channel (Stowers *et al.* 2002), the unavoidable ecological contexts of ultraviolet spectra of sunlight and noisy movement through dry leaves provide an inescapable opportunity for detection by predators and constraint for escape by prey.

Predator–prey communication can also provide examples of increasingly complex social behaviours, owing to evolutionary interactions between distantly related taxa. A dramatic example is the antipredatory behaviour of California ground squirrels *Spermophilus beecheyi* in response to rattlesnakes *Crotalus oreganus* that detect infrared spectra (Rundus *et al.* 2007). Given the poor vision of these snakes, their prey appear to have evolved an ability to indicate the detection of the predators using thermal signals. Specifically, there is increased heat emitted from the elevated tail of the ground squirrel that is easily perceived by the rattlesnakes. Squirrels do not increase the heat in their tails in response to harmless gopher snakes *Pituophis melanoleucus*. Further experimental work is still required to decode the meaning of this signal: do squirrels signal to the predators in a selfish manner (to reduce predation attempts on themselves) or are these signals of predator detection nepotistic, for instance, to attract the predator's attention away from more vulnerable family members (Sherman 1985)? With the design of a robotic squirrel with a wire that can be heated running through its artificial tail (Rundus *et al.* 2007), researchers are preparing to conduct critical tests of these alternatives.

In contrast to studies based on decoding the communication context and signal content of unique behavioural displays, a recent line of research on complex insect societies illustrates the concept that researcher innovation and willingness to explore seemingly difficult-to-decipher signals can result in the discovery of a general pattern in social communication signals. For example, facial markings of females across different species in the group-living paper wasp genus *Polistes* can signal species identity (Tibbetts & Dale 2007), condition and fighting ability (Tibbetts & Dale 2004) or individual identity (Tibbetts *et al.* 2008), depending on the extent of social complexity characterised at the species and the colony level (Tibbetts 2004). In turn, species with larger colonies, and with longer-lasting memories for familiar social companions (Sheehan & Tibbetts 2008), have similar brain sizes but more complex neural structures within the antennal lobe and mushroom body subcompartments of the brain (Gronenberg *et al.* 2008). Though such comparative data are by definition correlational, they can pinpoint the substrate for fruitful future physiological and neuroimaging research in non-model organisms for studies on complex social cognition (Hauber & Sherman 2001).

8.4 Ontogeny and communication: how experience shapes meaning and response

Perhaps the greatest puzzle of communication-system theory is how to reconcile the apparent evolutionary stability of signal design and information content with the observed ontogenetic unpredictability and plasticity of signal production, perception and decoding. A classic example of this evolutionary conundrum is sexual imprinting (Irwin & Price 1999). All sexually reproducing organisms must successfully identify and mate with conspecifics if they are to avoid the costs of hybridisation (Fisher 1958). Yet, in both invertebrates and vertebrates, including spiders and birds, early social experience with conspecifics of a particular phenotype is critical for subsequent mate choice to discriminate between preferred or suitable sexual partners (ten Cate *et al.* 1993, Hauber & Sherman 2001). In female wolf spiders (Araneae: Lycosidae), for example, mating preferences are exhibited through

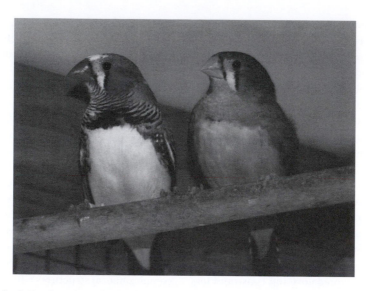

Figure 8.4 The zebra finch *Taeniopygia guttata* has become a model species for the vocal, visual and neurobiological analyses of the development and mechanism of conspecific recognition systems and the development of the production of
species-specific communication signals. Photo: A. & D. Campbell.

both the propensity of females to mate with males
with differently coloured foreleg hairs and the cannibalism of males with the less-preferred coloration
(Hebets 2003). Manipulation of the social experience
of subadult female wolf spiders by exposing them to
one of two types of males, painted within the natural
range of black or brown male colours, revealed that the
females preferentially mated with conspecific males
of the familiar phenotype. Interestingly, in contrast
to the sexual imprinting on suitable male phenotypes
illustrated above (ten Cate *et al.* 2006), there is no parallel evidence for filial imprinting (Lorenz 1937) or a
password-like recognition system (Hauber *et al.* 2001),
as the experience-dependent social preference of conspecific male phenotypes does not extend to developmental flexibility of interspecific recognition in the
wolf spider *Schizocosa uetzi* (Hebets 2005, 2007).

Such long-term memory for specific colour patterns of social partners across moults is not unusual
among arthropods, but the study on wolf spiders
was the first that paralleled a large body of similar
work on sexual imprinting in birds (Irwin & Price
1999). For instance, extensive experimental work
has shown that zebra finches *Taeniopygia guttata*

preferentially mate with individuals which share the
phenotype of familiar individuals from the period
of early social development, including plumage and
song traits (Clayton 1988, Campbell & Hauber 2009).
Recent experiments, however, demonstrate that this
preference for the familiar phenotype can also serve
as a starting point of preference for sexually exaggerated traits (ten Cate *et al.* 2006): young female
zebra finches exposed to males with bills varying in
brightness prefer males whose phenotype lies at the
brighter extreme of what was experienced and familiar during development (Fig. 8.4).

In the face of the often limiting (or debilitating)
costs of hybridisation and mating with otherwise
genetically mismatched individuals, why should the
learning of the phenotypic traits of social companions during ontogeny shape communication signals
that are relevant for species recognition? The answer
may come from an unexpected source: signal redundancy (Hauber *et al.* 2000). The idea that multiple signals should encode the same information is not novel.
Yet the heritability of recognition templates necessary
for the successful identification of conspecifics may
impose energetic or genetic costs that are simply too

high for taxa with ecological unpredictability in the outcome of gene–environment interactions (Lotem 1993). Accordingly, from an evolutionary perspective, selection will favour a decision rule that assures reliability through the redundancy of incorporating multiple communication signals that, together, encode a more reliable set of phenotypic templates of suitable social partners (Hauber *et al.* 2000). The learning of a suite of phenotypic traits, rather than single passwords (Hauber *et al.* 2001), may be more error-proof, and thus can become the norm of conspecific recognition systems and mate-choice signalling, across taxonomically and ecologically widespread taxa. Indeed, in female spiders both seismic and visual displays (i.e. multiple sensory modalities or multimodal signals) are required for successful courtship (Elias *et al.* 2005), while in zebra finches the interaction of colour and song are necessary precursors of eventual mating decisions by females (Campbell & Hauber 2008).

8.5 Manipulation or communication: why are some channels more susceptible for eavesdropping?

Almost any signal is, by definition, conspicuous – and when the signaller is a potential prey item or a host for parasitism, an opportunity is provided for the signal to be exploited by an unintended receiver. Signals used to attract mates or signal status, including colourful plumage and vigilance, or those performing a social function, including alarm calls and aggregation pheromones, are particularly subject to such eavesdropping. Anecdotes about the risks of display from the perspective of the eavesdropper have been in the literature since at least the seventeenth century; Erasmus Darwin, the grandfather of Charles Darwin, described frogs attacking glowing coal that they apparently mistook for fireflies (Zuk & Kolluru 1998). In contrast, eavesdropping on male territorial contest calls in black-capped chickadees *Poecile atricapillus* leads to potentially adaptive allocation of extra-pair parentage by females, given that they are more likely to seek extra-pair fertilisations after their own mate is successfully challenged by the invisible

calls of an experimentally simulated intruder male (Mennill *et al.* 2002). Such signal exploitation is distinct from mates, conspecifics, predators or parasites simply being extremely sensitive to inadvertent indications of a host or prey animal's location or identity, as when a mosquito detects a host by the presence of carbon dioxide or other compounds in its sweat.

Exploitation can be either general or specific. General cases might involve a variety of vertebrate predators being attracted to the call of a frog, or the flash of orange in the scales of a male guppy *Poecilia reticulata*. In such situations, selection on the signal itself is not likely to be intense, and the predators do not exclusively rely on the signaller for food. In contrast, tachinid flies from the tribe Ormiini obligately parasitise singing insects by locating the song of calling males; female flies deposit larvae on and around the male, and they burrow into the host's body cavity to complete their development (Zuk *et al.* 1993).

Signals in all modalities – including visual, acoustic and olfactory – are subject to exploitation. Although visual signals such as colourful feathers or skin are often assumed to be particularly susceptible to detection by predators (Alcock 1984), relatively few examples of exploitation of visual signals have been documented. In an experimental test of the conspicuous-coloration hypothesis, great tit fledglings' leg bands were not more likely to be recovered at the roosts of visually oriented birds of prey when the young birds' plumage had been painted red over the species-typical yellow, but instead the birds ended up being fatter, perhaps owing to more parental provisioning (Gotmark & Olsson 1997). It is possible that predation on visual signals is simply more difficult to demonstrate because they are produced continuously, in a variety of contexts, and because they are under selection by other forces, such as thermoregulation, territorial display, and even crypsis against some backgrounds (Zuk & Kolluru 1998).

Notable exceptions where exploitation does occur include the male guppy orange coloration that attracts predatory fish (Endler & Houde 1995) and the conspicuous flashing of fireflies (Lloyd 1997). Among the latter, the best known is probably the *Photinus–Photuris* complex, in which predatory female *Photuris* mimic the flash response patterns of the other genus, luring in male *Photinus* that are then eaten as prey. Recent work on *Photinus* showed that the fitness cost of the energetic investment in flashes is minimal compared with the fitness cost via the risk of predation by the mimics (Woods *et al.* 2007). This finding is particularly intriguing, given the role that in theory an inherent high cost of signalling is assumed to play in the evolution of communication through reliable and honest indicator signals (de Crespigny & Hosken 2007).

Acoustic mating signals, unlike visual ones, can be produced only at discrete times. They are also easy to localise, travel quickly over long distances, and can be detected at night as well as during the day (Sakaluk 1990). These characteristics make their transmission easy, but they also make mating songs produced by animals such as frogs or orthopteran insects prone to detection by a variety of invertebrate and vertebrate natural enemies. Acoustic signal exploitation has been examined from a mechanistic standpoint, as in the studies of the phonotactic fly parasitoid ear morphology (Robert & Gopfert 2002), or of the avoidance of bat predation by noctuid moths and other insects (Windmill *et al.* 2006). From an evolutionary perspective, Ryan and colleagues have examined the tungara frog *Physaleaemus pustulosus* and its acoustically orienting bat predator (Ryan 1985). As in the guppy studies, work on the tungara frog has revealed the compromise between sexual and natural selection that can result from mating-signal exploitation.

In contrast to visual and acoustic displays, olfactory signals, such as pheromones, seem to be less often exploited by predators and parasites. A few types of egg parasitoids are attracted to noctuid moths at oviposition, and aggregating bark beetles also produce pheromones that attract predators (Noldus *et al.* 1991). Other parasitoid wasps exploit host aggregation and sex pheromones, plant compounds induced by egg deposition or host feeding, or short-range contact cues derived from the adult host or the host plant (Fatouros *et al.* 2008). Egg parasitoids also have evolved the ability to use so-called 'chemical espionage' in combination with hitchhiking on the adult host when it disperses, to compensate for the parasitoid's

limited flight capability and to gain access to freshly laid host eggs (Fatouros *et al.* 2008). In some of these cases, exploitation may be inadvertent, as with the mosquito detecting host odour described above, so that the parasitoids evolved sensitivity to cues that accompany host life-history stages.

In a specialised case of exploitation of odours, the slave-making ant parasite *Polyergus rufescens* integrates into its host colony by modifying its cuticular hydrocarbon profile to match that of the rearing species and thus avoids detection (D'Ettorre *et al.* 2002). The parasite is capable of self-referencing its olfactory environment (Hauber & Sherman 2001), and adapting its own chemical signature to its several potential host species (D'Ettorre *et al.* 2002).

Nevertheless, few experimental examples of odour detection by predators or parasitoids exist, particularly with respect to the exploitation of sex pheromones, compared with exploitation of, for example, acoustic signals (Zuk & Kolluru 1998). Why might this be the case?

One answer may lie in a distinction that Maynard Smith (1991) drew between signals that are 'notices' and those that are 'advertisements'. If signaller and receiver interests are not the same, costly advertisements are more likely to evolve, like the ads by companies (signallers) exhorting consumers (receivers) to buy a product that may or may not be the best for the consumers' needs. Most sexual signals fall into this category, because male and female interests rarely coincide (Arnqvist & Rowe 2005). Other signals (Maynard Smith uses railway timetables as an example), however, are not expected to be costly because both parties benefit when information is accurately transferred. Numerous researchers have suggested that sex pheromones, at least those produced by Lepidoptera, are energetically not costly (Greenfield 2002, Cardé and Baker 2004), and indeed they are emitted at very low concentrations and hence low intensity. This quantitative lack of conspicuousness would then be less detectable by natural enemies. In a related argument, it has been suggested that predators might find it more difficult to exploit odours because of the precise chemical composition and strong canalisation of most pheromones. This seems unlikely, given the ability of natural enemies to detect specialised acoustic or visual signals, but it cannot be ruled out. In reality, little is known about the energetic or other physiological costs of producing odour communication signals.

Indeed, a recent review of chemical communication in mate choice suggests that chemical signals are not unlike other forms of communication in their function and evolution (Johansson & Jones 2007). Pheromones can be used for more than simply species identification, and show both sufficient intraspecific variability and high enough heritability to function in much the same way as visual and acoustic signals (Johansson & Jones 2007). The diversity of pheromones and the generation of new signals via new blends of previously used chemicals can also lend itself to diversification of the populations using each pheromone variant, and potentially to reproductive isolation (Symonds & Elgar 2008).

Finally, signals produced in multiple modalities may make their bearers particularly vulnerable to eavesdropping. In *Schizocosa ocreata* wolf spiders, females respond more to males that display using both visual and seismic signals (Roberts *et al.* 2007). A predatory jumping spider also responded with greater alacrity to wolf spider signals that combined the two forms (Roberts *et al.* 2007). Such vulnerability may provide much of the counter selection against increased exaggeration of multimodal communication signals.

8.6 Conclusions and future directions

Any exploration of the complexity of communication systems associated with social behaviours, as indicated consistently by our examples, should not be limited to intraspecific interactions in general and parent–offspring interactions in particular. Instead, the functional diversity and sociality of vocal, visual and mechanical alarm call signals makes testable predictions about signal design, intensity and sensory modality within both inter- and intraspecifically antagonistic (i.e. predatory, parasitic or competitive) contexts.

We may ask, for example from the point of view of the American robin's young, how do the chicks know that the sudden movement of the nest is related to parental food delivery and not predation? Does the parent emit a specific begging solicitation call to signal its arrival, and call with a different sound when a predator is lurking nearby (Otter *et al.* 2007)? How would the nestling birds tell the difference between these two call types (Platzen & Magrath 2005)? Are the chicks themselves displaying to the parent, and do parents respond to chicks in proportion to physiological needs (Kilner & Johnstone 1997)? Most surprisingly, recent data from the nutritional ecology of begging house sparrows *Passer domesticus* suggest that being fed by parents when the chicks beg less near satiation is wasted parental effort, because full chicks more often refuse to take food (Grodzinski & Lotem 2007) and what they ingest is in turn digested with poorer efficiency (Grodzinski *et al.* 2009). On the other hand, from the point of view of the parent, how does it decide which chick to feed and which one to ignore among all the ones that are begging? Can adult robins perceive and, thus, efficiently rely on the relative and absolute levels of the intensity of the begging display, including loudness, the rate of the calling, the height of the neck raised, and the angle and the colour of the open gape, to assess the proximate and long-term physiological needs of each of their chicks?

Indeed, the appeal of the study of communication systems is that it is both theory-driven and empirically rich, because communication theory makes parallel predictions about signal design, efficiency, perception and content, across shared functional, ecological and social contexts against diverse ecological, genetic and phylogenetic backgrounds. Accordingly, by contrasting the physiological and evolutionary benefits of sensory system diversity and information content, these studies also contribute towards novel insights and make critical predictions for future research into coevolutionary networks between the genetic and ontogenetic controls of signalling behaviour, and the extent to which perception in particular, and cognition in general, can be shaped by social and ecological constraints and opportunities (Hauber & Kilner 2007).

Acknowledgements

We thank many students and colleagues for critical collaborations and valuable discussions, and the University of Auckland Hood Fellowship Fund, the Human Frontier Science Program, the National Geographic Society and NSF for funding.

Suggested readings

Bradbury, J. W. & Vehrencamp, S. L. (1998) *Principles of Animal Communication*. Sunderland, MA: Sinauer Associates.

Hauser, M. D. (1997) *The Evolution of Communication*. Cambridge, MA: MIT Press.

Maynard Smith, J. & Harper, D. (2003) *Animal Signals*. New York, NY: Oxford University Press.

Searcy, W. A. & Nowicki, S. (2005) *The Evolution of Animal Communication: Reliability and Deception in Signaling Systems*. Princeton, NJ: Princeton University Press.

References

Alcock. J. (1984) *Animal Behavior: an Evolutionary Perspective*. Sunderland, MA: Sinauer Associates.

Arnqvist. G. (2006) Sensory exploitation and sexual conflict. *Philosophical Transactions of the Royal Society B*, **361**, 375–386.

Arnqvist, G. & Rowe, L. (2005) *Sexual Conflict*. Princeton, NJ: Princeton University Press.

Bradbury, J. W. & Vehrencamp, S. L. (1998) *Principles of Animal Communication*. Sunderland, MA: Sinauer Associates.

Briskie, J. V., Naugler, C. T. & Leech, S. M. (1994) Begging intensity of nestling birds varies with sibling relatedness. *Proceedings of the Royal Society B*, **258**, 73–78.

Briskie, J. V., Martin, P. R. & Martin, T. E. (1999) Nest predation and the evolution of nestling begging calls. *Proceedings of the Royal Society B*, **266**, 2153–2159.

Brumm, H. & Slater, P. (2006) Ambient noise, motor fatigue, and serial redundancy in chaffinch song. *Behavioral Ecology and Sociobiology*, **60**, 475–481.

Cade, W. (1981) Alternative male strategies: genetic differences in crickets. *Science*, **212**, 563–564.

Campbell, D. L. M. & Hauber, M. E. (2008) Dissecting and validating the salience of recognition cues used by female zebra finches to discriminate con- and heterospecific

males. In: *Proceedings of the 6th Measuring Behavior Conference*, Maastricht, the Netherlands, 2008, p. 332.

Campbell, D. L. M. & Hauber, M. E. (2009) Disassociation of visual and acoustic conspecific cues decreases discrimination by female zebra finches (*Taeniopygia guttata*). *Journal of Comparative Psychology*, **123**, 310–315.

Campbell, D. L. M., Weiner, S. A., Starks, P. T. B. & Hauber, M. E. (2009) Context and control: behavioural ecology experiments in the laboratory. *Annales Zoologici Fennici*, **46**, 112–123.

Cardé, R. T. & Baker, T. C. (2004) *Chemical Ecology of Insects*. New York, NY: Chapman and Hall.

Clayton, N. S. (1988) Song discrimination learning in zebra finches. *Animal Behaviour*, **36**, 1016–1024.

Cocroft, R. B. (1999) Offspring–parent communication in a subsocial treehopper (Hemiptera: Membracidae: *Umbonia crassicornis*). *Behaviour*, **136**, 1–21.

Cocroft, R. B., Shugart, H. J., Konrad, K. T. & Tibbs, K. (2006) Variation in plant substrates and its consequences for insect vibrational communication. *Ethology*, **112**, 779–789.

Craig, C. L., Weber, R. S. & Bernard, G. D. (1996) Evolution of predator-prey systems: spider foraging plasticity in response to the visual ecology of prey. *American Naturalist*, **147**, 205–229.

Dearborn, D. C. (2000) Brown-headed cowbird nestling vocalizations and the risk of nest predation. *Auk*, **116**, 448–457.

Dearborn, D. C. & Lichtenstein, G. (2002) Begging behaviour and host exploitation in parasitic cowbirds. In: *The Evolution of Begging: Competition, Cooperation and Communication*, ed. J. Wright & M. L. Leonard. Dordrecht: Kluwer, pp. 361–387.

de Crespigny, F. E. C. & Hosken, D. J. (2007) Sexual selection: signals to die for. *Current Biology*, **17**, R853–R855.

D'Ettorre, P., Tofilski, A., Heinze, J. & Ratnieks, F. L. W. (2002) Non-transferable signals on ant queen eggs. *Naturwissenschaften*, **93**, 136–140.

Elias, D. O., Hebets, E. A., Mason, A. C. & Hoy, R. R. (2005) Seismic signals are crucial for male mating success in a visual specialist jumping spider (Araneae: Salticidae). *Animal Behaviour*, **69**, 931–938.

Endler, J. A. & Houde, A. E. (1995) Geographic variation in female preferences for male traits in *Poecilia reticulata*. *Evolution*, **49**, 456–468.

Fatouros, N. E., Dicke, M., Mumm, R., Meiners, T. & Hilker, M. (2008) Foraging behavior of egg parasitoids exploiting chemical information. *Behavioral Ecology*, **19**, 677–689.

Fisher, R. A. (1958) *The Genetical Theory of Natural Selection*, 2nd edn. New York, NY: Dover.

Forstmeier, W., Coltman, D. W. & Birkhead, T. R. (2004) Maternal effects influence the sexual behaviour of sons and daughters in the zebra finch. *Evolution*, **58**, 2574–2583.

Gaskett A. C., Winnick, C. G. & Herberstein, M. E. (2008) Orchid sexual deceit provokes ejaculation. *American Naturalist*, **171**, E206–212.

Goth, A. & Hauber, M. E. (2004) Ecological approaches to species recognition in birds through studies of model and non-model species. *Annales Zoologici Fennici*, **41**, 823–842.

Gotmark, F. & Olsson, J. (1997) Artificial colour mutation: do red-painted great tits experience increased or decreased predation? *Animal Behaviour*, **53**, 83–91.

Greenfield, M. D. (2002) *Signalers and Receivers: Mechanisms and Evolution of Arthropod Communication*. Oxford: Oxford University Press.

Grodzinski, U. & Lotem, A. (2007) The adaptive value of parental responsiveness to nestling begging. *Proceedings of the Royal Society B*, **274**, 2449–2456.

Grodzinski, U., Hauber, M. E. & Lotem, A. (2009) The role of feeding regularity and nestling digestive efficiency in parent–offspring communication: an experimental test. *Functional Ecology*, **23**, 569–577

Gronenberg, W., Ash, L. A. & Tibbetts, E. A. (2008) Correlation between facial pattern recognition and brain composition in paper wasps. *Brain, Behavior and Evolution*, **71**, 1–14.

Haskell, D. (1994) Experimental evidence that nestling begging behaviour incurs a cost due to nest predation. *Proceedings of the Royal Society B*, **257**, 161–164.

Hauber, M. E. (1998) Web decorations and alternative foraging tactics of the spider *Argiope appensa*. *Ethology, Ecology and Evolution*, **10**, 47–54.

Hauber, M. E. (2003) Lower begging responsiveness of host vs. cowbird nestlings is related to species identity but not to early social experience in parasitized broods. *Journal of Comparative Psychology*, **117**, 24–30.

Hauber, M. E. & Kilner, R. M. (2007) Who mimics whom? Communication, co-evolution, and chick mimicry in parasitic finches. *Behavioral Ecology and Sociobiology*, **61**, 497–503.

Hauber, M. E. & Pilz, K. M. (2003) Yolk testosterone levels are not consistently higher in the eggs of obligate brood parasites than their hosts. *American Midland Naturalist*, **149**, 354–362.

Hauber, M. E. & Ramsey, C. K. (2003) Honesty in host-parasite communication signals: the case for begging by fledgling brown-headed cowbirds (*Molothrus ater*). *Journal of Avian Biology*, **34**, 339–344.

Hauber, M. E. & Sherman, P. W. (2001) Self-referent phenotype matching: theoretical possibilities and empirical tests. *Trends in Neurosciences*, **10**, 609–616.

Hauber, M. E., Sherman, P. W. & Paprika, D. (2000) Self-referent phenotype matching in a brood parasite: the armpit effect in brown-headed cowbirds (*Molothrus ater*). *Animal Cognition*, **3**, 113–117.

Hauber, M. E., Russo, S. A. & Sherman, P. W. (2001) A password for species recognition in a brood parasitic bird. *Proceedings of the Royal Society B*, **268**, 1041–1048.

Hauser, M. D. (1997) *The Evolution of Communication*. Cambridge, MA: MIT Press.

Hebets, E. A. (2003) Subadult experience influences adult mate choice in an arthropod: exposed female wolf spiders prefer males of a familiar phenotype. *Proceedings of the National Academy of Sciences of the USA*, **100**, 13390–13395.

Hebets, E. A. (2005) Attention-altering interactions among signals in multimodal wolf spider courtship displays. *Behavioral Ecology*, **16**, 75–82.

Hebets, E. A. (2007) Subadult experience does not influence species recognition in the wolf spider *Schizocosa uetzi* Stratton 1997. *Journal of Arachnology*, **35**, 1–10.

Irwin, D. E. & Price, T. (1999) Sexual imprinting, learning and speciation. *Heredity*, **82**, 347–354.

Johansson, B. J. & Jones, T. M. (2007) The role of chemical communication in mate choice. *Biological Reviews of the Cambridge Philosophical Society*, **82**, 265–289.

Kam, Y.-C. & Yang, H.-W. (2002) Female–offspring communication in a Taiwanese tree frog, *Chirixalus eiffingeri* (Anura: Rhacophoridae). *Animal Behaviour*, **64**, 881–886.

Katti, M. & Warren, P. S. (2004) Tits, noise and urban bioacoustics. *Trends in Ecology and Evolution*, **19**, 109–110.

Kilner, R. M. (1997) Mouth colour is a reliable signal of need in begging canary nestlings. *Proceedings of the Royal Society B*, **264**, 963–968.

Kilner, R. M. (2001) A growth cost of begging in captive canary chicks. *Proceedings of the National Academy of Sciences of the USA*, **98**, 11394–11398.

Kilner, R. M. & Johnstone, R. A. (1997) Begging the question: are offspring solicitation behaviours signals of need? *Trends in Ecology and Evolution*, **12**, 11–15.

Koivula, M. & Viitala, J. (1999) Rough-legged buzzards use vole scent marks to assess hunting areas. *Journal of Avian Biology*, **30**, 329–332.

Komdeur, J., Daan, S., Tinbergen, J. & Mateman, C. (1997) Extreme adaptive modification in sex ratio of the Seychelles warbler's eggs. *Nature*, **385**, 522–525.

Knudsen, E. l. & Konishi, M. (1979) Mechanisms of sound localization in the barn owl (*Tyto alba*). *Journal of Comparative Physiology*, **133**, 13–21.

Lloyd, J. E. (1997) Firefly mating ecology, selection and evolution. In: *The Evolution of Mating Systems in Insects and Arachnids*, ed. J. C. Choe & B. J. Crespi. Cambridge: Cambridge University Press, pp. 184–192.

Lorenz, K. (1937) The companion in the bird's world. *Auk*, **54**, 245–273.

Lotem, A. (1993) Learning to recognize nestlings is maladaptive for cuckoo *Cuculus canorus* host. *Nature*, **362**, 743–745.

Lotem, A. (1998) Differences in begging behaviour among barn swallow (*Hirundo rustica*) nestlings. *Animal Behaviour*, **55**, 809–818.

Main, A. R. & Bull, C. M. (1996) Mother–offspring recognition in two Australian lizards, *Tiliqua rugosa* and *Egernia stokesii*. *Animal Behaviour*, **52**, 193–200.

Mason, and A.C., Oshinsky, M. L. & Hoy, R. R. (2001) Hyperacute directional hearing in a microscale auditory system. *Nature*, **410**, 686–690.

Maynard Smith, J. (1991) Honest signalling: the Philip Sidney game. *Animal Behaviour*, **42**, 1034–1035.

McRae, S. B., Weatherhead, P. J. & Montgomerie, R. (1993) American robin nestlings compete by jockeying for position. *Behavioral Ecology and Sociobiology*, **33**, 101–106.

Mennill, D. J., Ratcliffe, L. M. & Boag, P. T. (2002) Female eavesdropping on male song contests in songbirds. *Science*, **296**, 873.

Noldus, L. P. J. J., van Lenteren, J. C. & Lewis, W. J. (1991) How *Trichogramma* parasitoids use moth sex pheromones as kairomones: orientation behavior in a wind tunnel. *Physiological Entomology*, **16**, 313–327.

Otter, K. A., Atherton, S. E. & van Oort, H. (2007) Female food solicitation calling, hunger levels and habitat differences in the black-capped chickadee. *Animal Behaviour*, **74**, 847–853.

Patricelli, G. L. & Blickley, J. L. (2006) Avian communication in urban noise: causes and consequences of vocal adjustment. *Auk*, **123**, 639–649.

Pilz, K. M., Smith, H. G. & Andersson, M. (2005) Brood parasitic European starlings do not lay high-quality eggs. *Behavioral Ecology*, **16**, 507–513.

Platzen, D. & Magrath, R. D. (2005) Adaptive differences in response to two types of parental alarm call in altri-cial nestlings. *Proceedings of the Royal Society B*, **272**, 1101–1106.

Pryke, S. R. & Griffith, S. C. (2009) Genetic incompatibility drives sex allocation and maternal investment in a polymorphic finch. *Science*, **323**, 1605–1607.

Robert, D. & Gopfert, M. C. (2002) Antennal acoustic sensitivity in flies. *Physiological Entomology*, **48**, 189–196.

Roberts, J. A., Taylor, P. W. & Uetz, G. W. (2007) Consequences of complex signaling: predator detection of multimodal cues. *Behavioral Ecology*, **18**, 236–240.

Rundus, A. S., Owings, D. H., Joshi, S. S., Chinn, E., Giannini, N. (2007) Ground squirrels use an infrared signal to deter rattlesnake predation. *Proceedings of the National Academy of Sciences of the USA*, **104**, 14372–14376.

Ryan, M. J. (1985) *The Túngara Frog: a Study in Sexual Selection and Communication*. Chicago, IL: University of Chicago Press.

Sakaluk, S. K. (1990) Sexual selection and predation: balancing reproductive and survival needs. In: *Insect Defenses: Adaptive Mechanisms and Strategies of Prey and Predators*, ed. D.L. Evans and J.O. Schmidt. Albany, NY: SUNY Press, pp. 63–90.

Schwabl, H., Palacios, M. G. & Martin, T. E. (2007) Selection for rapid embryo development correlates with embryo exposure to maternal androgens among passerine birds. *American Naturalist*, **170**, 196–206.

Searcy, W. A. & Nowicki, S. (2005) *The Evolution of Animal Communication: Reliability and Deception in Signaling Systems*. Princeton, NJ: Princeton University Press.

Sheehan, M. J. & Tibbetts, E. A. (2008) Robust long-term social memories in a paper wasp. *Current Biology*, **18**, R851–852.

Sherman, P. W. (1985) Alarm calls of Belding's ground squirrels to aerial predators: nepotism or self-preservation? *Behavioral Ecology and Sociobiology*, **17**, 313–323.

Sherman, P. W., Reeve, H. K. & Pfennig, D. W. (1997) Recognition systems. In: *Behavioural Ecology: an Evolutionary Approach*, 4th edn, ed. J. R. Krebs & N. B. Davies. Oxford: Blackwell, pp. 69–96.

Slabbekoorn, H. & Peet, M. (2003) Birds sing at a higher pitch in urban noise. *Nature*, **424**, 267.

Slabbekoorn, H. & Ripmeester, E. A. P. (2008) Birdsong and anthropogenic noise: implications and applications for conservation. *Molecular Ecology*, **17**, 72–83.

Smiseth, P. T. & Moore, A. J. (2007) Signalling of hunger by senior and junior larvae in asynchronous broods of a burying beetle. *Animal Behaviour*, **74**, 699–705.

Smiseth, P. T., Lennox, L. & Moore, A. J. (2007) Interaction between parental care and sibling competition: parents

enhance offspring growth and exacerbate sibling competition. *Evolution*, **61**, 2331–2339.

Smith, H. G. & Montgomerie, R. (1991) Nestling American
robins compete with siblings by begging. *Behavioral
Ecology and Sociobiology*, **29**, 307–312.

Stowers, L., Holy, T., Meister, M., Dulac, C. & Koetnges. G.
(2002) Loss of sex discrimination and male-male aggression in mice deficient in TRP2. *Science*, **295**, 1493–1500.

Symonds, M. R. E. & Elgar, M. A. (2004) The mode of pheromone evolution: evidence from bark beetles. *Proceedings
of the Royal Society B*, **271**, 839–846.

Symonds, M. R. E. & Elgar, M. A. (2008) The evolution of
pheromone diversity. *Trends in Ecology and Evolution*, **23**,
220–228.

ten Cate, C., Vos, D. R. & Mann, N. (1993) Sexual imprinting
and song learning: two of one kind? *Netherlands Journal of
Zoology*, **43**, 34–45.

ten Cate, C., Verzijden, M. N. & Etman, E. (2006) Sexual
imprinting can induce sexual preferences for exaggerated
parental traits. *Current Biology*, **16**, 1128–1132.

Tibbetts, E. A. (2004) Complex social behavior can select for
variable visual features: a case study in *Polistes* wasps.
Proceedings of the Royal Society B, **271**, 1955–1960.

Tibbetts, E. A. & Dale, J. (2004) A socially enforced signal of
quality in paper wasp. *Nature*, **432**, 218–222.

Tibbetts, E. A. & Dale, J. (2007) Individual recognition: it is
good to be different. *Trends in Ecology and Evolution*, **22**,
529–537.

Tibbetts, E. A., Sheehan, M. J. & Dale, J. (2008) A testable definition of individual recognition. *Trends in Ecology and
Evolution*, **23**, 356.

Tonra, C. M., Hauber, M. E., Heath, S. K. & Johnson, M. D. (2008)
Ecological correlates and sex differences in early development of a generalist brood parasite. *Auk*, **125**, 205–213.

Wiley, R. H. (2006) Signal detection and animal communication. *Advances in the Study of Behavior*, **36**, 217–247.

Wilson, D. R. & Hare, J. F. (2004) Ground squirrel uses ultrasonic alarms. *Nature*, **430**, 523.

Windmill, J. F. C., Jackson, J. C., Tuck, E. J. & Robert, D. (2006)
Keeping up with bats: dynamic auditory tuning in a moth.
Current Biology, **16**, 2418–2423.

Wood, W. E. & Yezerinac, S. M. (2006) Song sparrow
(*Melospiza melodia*) song varies with urban noise. *Auk*,
123, 650–659.

Woods, W. A., Hendrickson, H., Mason, J. & Lewis, S. M.
(2007) Energy and predation costs of firefly courtship signals. *American Naturalist*, **170**, 702–708.

Woolley, S. M. N., Wissman, A. M. & Rubel, E. W. (2001) Hair
cell regeneration and recovery of auditory thresholds following aminoglycoside ototoxicity in Bengalese finches.
Hearing Research, **153**, 181–195.

Wright, J. & Leonard, M. L., eds. (2002) *The Evolution of
Begging: Competition, Cooperation and Communication*.
Dordrecht: Kluwer.

Zanette, L., MacDougall-Shackleton, E., Clinchy, M. &
Smith, J. N. M. (2005) Brown-headed cowbirds skew host
offspring sex ratios. *Ecology*, **86**, 815–820.

Zuk, M. & Kolluru, G. R. (1998) Exploitation of sexual signals
by predators and parasitoids. *Quarterly Review of Biology*,
73, 415–438.

Zuk, M., Simmons, L. W. & Cupp, L. (1993) Calling characteristics of parasitized and unparasitized populations of
the field cricket *Teleogryllus oceanicus*. *Behavioral Ecology
and Sociobiology*, **33**, 339–343.

Zuk, M., Rotenberry, J. T. & Tinghitella, R. M. (2006) Silent
night: adaptive disappearance of a sexual signal in a
parasitized population of field crickets. *Biology Letters*, **2**,
521–524.

Reputation can make the world go round – or why we are sometimes social

Manfred Milinski

Reciprocity is the secret of our success, even though two unrelated individuals sometimes find it difficult to cooperate. They may mutually reciprocate help, if they know they will meet again. However, there is always the temptation not to return the help to the donor. Using a strategy such as Tit-for-Tat (see Chapter 4) can minimise the risk of being the sucker in the end, but there is no guarantee. To achieve cooperation seems hopeless when groups of three or more unrelated individuals need to cooperate in order to maintain a common resource: the resource is usually overused and collapses, as do fish populations as a consequence of over-fishing, and the global climate as a consequence of unrestricted use of fossil energy. The latter is regarded as the greatest challenge to humankind. The *tragedy of the commons*, as Hardin (1968) called this kind of social dilemma (see Chapter 6), appears inevitable – free access to a public resource brings ruin to all.

The so-called Public Goods game has been invented as a paradigm to study tragedy of the commons situations experimentally. For example, a group of four volunteers is asked to supply one euro each to a public pool, which is then doubled and redistributed among the four players irrespective of whether they have contributed. If all contribute, each has a net gain of one euro. However, a single defector has a net gain of 1.50 euro whereas each of the three contributors gains only 50 cents. Why should you cooperate? From your own euro invested you receive only 50 cents back (1 euro × 2 / 4 = 50 cents). So the rational strategy in a Public Goods game is not to contribute anything, and instead to rely on the stupidity of your co-players. Public Goods games usually start unexpectedly cooperatively, but cooperation collapses within a few rounds, thus fulfilling Hardin's destructive vision. Are there conditions under which each individual profits from investing in the public good? Directly punishing defectors after each round disciplines free-riders, but the cost of punishing and being punished destroys almost all gains from enhanced cooperation (Rockenbach & Milinski 2006).

For me it had been a great challenge to find a way to solve the dilemma in a more gentle way than by allowing people to punish their potential cooperators. I thought that the interaction between the Public Goods game and another game in which you need a good reputation to receive something could at least reduce the decline of cooperation in the Public Goods game: you might not dare to demolish your reputation by never giving in the Public Goods game. A game in which reputation matters is Indirect Reciprocity: 'give and you shall receive', as the Bible tells us. You give to those who have helped others, i.e. you help those who have a reputation of being good guys. This worked in computer simulations of evolution (Nowak & Sigmund 1998), and

Social Behaviour: Genes, Ecology and Evolution, ed. Tamás Székely, Allen J. Moore and Jan Komdeur. Published by Cambridge University Press. © Cambridge University Press 2010.

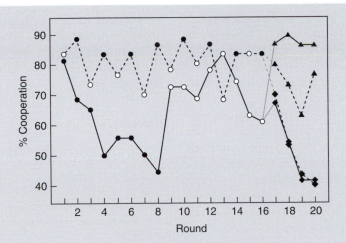

Percentage of cooperation ('yes') per group of six subjects in each round of the Public Goods game (filled symbols) and in each round of the Indirect Reciprocity game (open symbols). In one treatment (dashed line), the groups alternated between rounds of Indirect Reciprocity and rounds of Public Goods until round 16. In the other treatment (solid line), groups started with eight consecutive rounds of the Public Goods game and continued with eight rounds of the Indirect Reciprocity game. In rounds 17–20, groups of both treatments played the Public Goods game, which was either announced, 'from now on only this type of game until the end' (diamonds), or not announced (triangles). Adapted from Milinski *et al.* (2002).

in experiments with human subjects (Wedekind & Milinski 2000): players indeed helped those who had a reputation of being generous to others. Being a good guy pays off.

In our experiments, people are anonymous, but are recognisable as players by their pseudonyms, e.g. Despina, Japetus, Ananke, etc. Would Ananke dare to free-ride in a Public Goods round when she knows that someone, e.g. Japetus, is asked later to give her money which is doubled by the experimenter? We did this experiment in two treatments with students from the University of Hamburg in Germany. We had 10 groups with six students each who at first played eight consecutive Public Goods rounds, and cooperation collapsed as usual. Then they played eight consecutive rounds of Indirect Reciprocity, and cooperation built up again. Ten other groups played rounds of Indirect Reciprocity and Public Goods alternately, eight of each type. To our great surprise, players maintained cooperation in the Public Goods game at the high starting level

for 16 rounds (Milinski *et al.* 2002). We found that a player was much more likely to receive money in an Indirect Reciprocity round if she had contributed in the previous Public Goods round. As opposed to costly punishment, simply not rewarding a free-rider actually saves money for the donor in the Indirect Reciprocity round. This boosted overall efficiency; the players in the alternating treatment in fact earned a lot of money – real money, as is the rule in such experiments.

After round 16 all groups played four rounds of the Public Goods game. Cooperation remained very high in the block treatment: players obviously expected another block of Indirect Reciprocity rounds. Cooperation declined slightly in the alternating treatment: players saw a change of the previous regime. However, every second group was told that 'from now on there will be rounds only of this type of game', and cooperation collapsed immediately in both treatments. Thus, the pending risk of further rounds of a game where reputation matters forced the players to cooperate in Public Goods rounds – and had made them rich. No model had predicted this interaction effect; our experiment supported my hypothesis. The model built on our experiment came later, and proved the robustness of the interaction effect.

In another experiment, players were provided with two different pseudonyms, one that they knew was used only in some Public Goods rounds, and one that was used in other Public Goods rounds *and* in all Indirect Reciprocity rounds. Players switched immediately back and forth between cooperation and free-riding, depending on which of their two names appeared on the screen: they invested strategically in reputation, i.e. only when their good behaviour would be recognisable in the Indirect Reciprocity game.

We are obviously prepared to be selfish when unobserved, and turn altruistic as soon as others watch us. We have neurons in our amygdala that react to a pair of eyes watching us, which might switch on altruistic behaviour even when the eyes appear as symbols on a computer screen (Haley & Fessler 2005) or are just ink on paper (Bateson *et al.* 2006), a hardwired unconscious response. To save the global climate, it does not help to ask people to reduce their use of fossil energy where nobody can recognise it – they would refuse to do it. But if people can do it in public, they would like to display their altruism and collect the social reward of those watching them (Milinski *et al.* 2008). We cannot afford to lose the global climate game. This time it is not technical invention that is needed to preserve our future, but our social behaviour.

References

Bateson, M., Nettle, D. & Roberts, G. (2006) Cues of being watched enhance cooperation in a real-world setting. *Biology Letters*, **2**, 412–414.

Haley, K. J. & Fessler, D. M. T. (2005) Nobody's watching? Subtle cues affect generosity in an anonymous economic game. *Evolution and Human Behavior*, **26**, 245–256.

Hardin, G. (1968) The tragedy of the commons. *Science*, **162**, 1243–1248.

Milinski, M., Semmann, D. & Krambeck, H. J. (2002) Reputation helps solve the 'tragedy of the commons'. *Nature*, **415**, 424–426.

Milinski, M., Sommerfeld, R. D., Krambeck. H. J., Reed, F. A. & Marotzke, J. (2008) The collective-risk social dilemma and the prevention of simulated dangerous climate change. *Proceedings of the National Academy of Sciences of the USA*, **105**, 2291–2294.

Nowak, M. A. & Sigmund, K. (1998) Evolution of indirect reciprocity by image scoring. *Nature*, **393**, 573–577.

Rockenbach, B. & Milinski, M. (2006) The efficient interaction of indirect reciprocity and costly punishment. *Nature*, **444**, 718–723.

Wedekind, C. & Milinski, M. (2000) Cooperation through image scoring in humans. *Science*, **288**, 850–852.

9

Important topics in group living

Jens Krause and Graeme Ruxton

Overview

Given the vast topic of group living, this chapter highlights research areas into group living that continue to attract considerable attention or represent new developments. By these criteria, three topics stood out to us: the selfish herd, social networks and collective behaviour. The *selfish herd* is the idea that aggregation of prey animals can occur simply through the selfish actions of individuals positioning themselves so as to reduce their risk of attack. This idea is very much at the core of why animals live in groups, and the theory has been influential for a considerable period. The idea of the selfish herd is simple but subtle, and we decided to discuss it carefully, since textbook discussions on this concept often ignore four aspects of complexity: more complex and realistic geometries than are normally considered; the underlying behavioural rules that might lead to selfish herd effects; the predicted outcome of such rules in terms of properties of the group; and the interaction of selfish herd effects with other selective pressures on group size, shape and composition.

The second emerging field we choose is the application of *social network analysis* (a conceptual and statistical tool from the social sciences) to animal groups and populations. Although this topic is not completely new, recent developments represent an exponential increase in new tools for studying social networks that makes network analysis a powerful method to understand social organisation. In addition, network analysis links individual-level actions to group-level emergent properties, and can be used as a descriptive, analytic or predictive tool. We identify areas where the utility of this relatively new technique could usefully be applied, and aspects of the technique itself that are most in need of further development.

Finally, we focus on *collective behaviour*, which is another new and active area of animal grouping. Collective behaviour is a research field in which researchers investigate patterns of collective behaviour based on individuals and their interactions. Since this term (collective behaviour) is often used broadly, we begin with a discussion of what we believe collective behaviour is and is not. We then sketch out the power of individual-based simulation models to explore the link between individual-based processes and outcomes (particularly collective decision making) that emerge at the group level.

Social Behaviour: Genes, Ecology and Evolution, ed. Tamás Székely, Allen J. Moore and Jan Komdeur. Published by Cambridge University Press. © Cambridge University Press 2010.

9.1 Selfish herds

9.1.1 Introduction

The selfish herd is the idea that aggregation of prey animals can occur simply through the selfish actions of individuals positioning themselves so as to reduce their risk of attack. The term arises from W. D. Hamilton's 1971 paper. Hamilton was one of the most important evolutionary ecologists of the twentieth century, but few would regard this as his most important paper. It certainly has not had the same impact as his work on kin selection, or even that on sex ratios or the evolution of sex. It is a mark of Hamilton's greatness that one of his minor papers has still been pivotal to our understanding of animal aggregations and has amassed over 1200 citations. That this work is still relevant and important today might even have surprised Hamilton, since we suspect that he saw the main function of his paper as a correction to the erroneous viewpoint that animal aggregations evolved through benefits to the population or to the species, rather than to the individual and its genes. The paper was certainly successful in this aim, and was part of the huge shift towards a gene-centric approach which swept through evolutionary ecology in the late 1960s and early 1970s, and which has been the prevailing orthodoxy ever since. Hamilton's paper is still the centre of active research, almost 40 years after its publication. Here we will summarise past research and speculate on what the future holds for research on selfish herds.

9.1.2 What is a selfish herd?

The initial example in Hamilton's paper is so clear that we will briefly reprise it here. Imagine a population of frogs that can distribute themselves around the edge of a pond. Periodically a snake appears at a random point on the edge and captures the nearest frog to it, in either direction. The snake is equally likely to appear at any point on the edge. Where should a frog position itself so as to minimise its risk of attack? It is easy to see that each frog's probability of attack is the length of the segment of edge covering all the points that are nearer to that frog than any other edge segments (Fig. 9.1) divided by the circumference of the pond. Now the frog can do nothing to increase the circumference of the pond, so the only way to reduce its risk of attack is to reduce the size of the segment that is nearer to it than to any other frog (which is generally called the *domain of danger* – formally this could be defined as all the points in space closer to the focal animal than to any other). The way to reduce the size of the domain of danger is simply to move closer to other individuals. Indeed, the best move for an individual would be to find the smallest gap between two other individuals and then move into that gap. Of course, other individuals will want to reduce their domains of danger too, and this leads to increased aggregation driven only through the selfish attempts of individuals to decrease their own domains of danger.

This issue of domains of danger can lead to increased aggregation even when the prey are entirely immobile. Isolated individuals are most at risk from predation (they have the largest domains of danger). If we scatter frogs randomly around the edge of the pond, then by chance some will be isolated and some will be placed close to others in small aggregations. If we then allow a certain amount of predation of the type discussed above to occur, isolated individuals will be differentially attacked, and the overall level of aggregation in the population of frogs will increase because of this. This is the selfish herd; it is the formation of aggregations driven by selfish attempts to place others between yourself and danger. If it is such a simple concept, what is left for us to fill this section of the chapter with? First, the term *selfish herd* is often misused to mean other things (Box 9.1), and we will address this in the next section. Second, this simple example leaves some important questions unanswered, which we will explore in further sections:

(1) The edge of a pond was elegantly selected as a particularly simple geometry, where the universe in which prey can exist is one-dimensional and without boundaries. How does the theory generalise to more complex and realistic geometries?

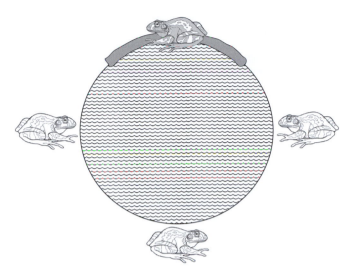

Figure 9.1 Domain of danger for a frog occupying the rim of a pond, indicated as a shaded zone for the shaded frog. A snake appears from the pond and attacks the frog that is closest (see text for details).

(2) How best should individuals move so as to take maximum advantage of the selfish-herd effect, given that the other members of the aggregation are likely to be trying to do the same?

(3) The explanation above is one that seems to lead to an aggregation that is always in flux, with individuals on the outside moving into the interior, and the density of individuals gets higher and higher as they squeeze closer together. This is not what is generally seen in nature. How can theory and observation be reconciled?

(4) There are other factors that can select for group formation. How does the selfish herd interact with them, and how important is it relative to these other factors?

Box 9.1 What the selfish herd is not

Unfortunately, if you survey a cross-section of articles citing Hamilton (1971), they often use the term *selfish herd* carelessly to describe any benefit that can arise from membership of a group. The selfish herd should properly be used to denote an aggregation that arises through the cover-seeking behaviour discussed in this chapter.

There are some important points to note about the selfish-herd mechanism. Most importantly, one individual can only decrease its own domain of danger by simultaneously increasing the domains of danger of one or more others. The overall risk across all the participants is the same regardless of whether the frogs form a tight aggregation or are spaced uniformly around the rim of the pond. The snake is successful in capturing a frog every time it appears, regardless of the spatial distribution of frogs. Thus the selfish herd affects the distribution of predation risk across a number of individuals, but it does not affect the summed overall predation risk. That is, it does not affect the likelihood of a predator's attack being successful. When seen in this light, it is clear that it is entirely inappropriate to describe processes such as

Box 9.1 Continued

collective detection of predators, or mobbing behaviour that reduce the probability that an attack will be successful, as a selfish-herd effect.

There is also the straightforward concept of dilution of risk. If, when a predator attacks a group of N individuals, it selects its victim entirely at random (with each individual being attacked with probability $1/N$); then the larger the group, the lower a given individual's probability of being targeted in any one attack. This is a clear advantage to being in a group. Indeed it can even make group membership attractive under some conditions when groups suffer higher attack rates (for example because they are easier to detect) – this is the *attack-abatement* effect (Turner & Pitcher 1986). However, dilution is conceptually separate from the selfish-herd mechanism. In dilution, all individuals within a group are assumed to have the same relative risk of predation, and individuals can only decrease their risk by joining a larger group. In the selfish herd, individuals move closer to others in order to decrease their relative risk of predation in a way that simultaneously increases the relative risk of (at least some) others. Another way to look at this is that in the case of the dilution effect the predator selects its victim entirely at random from within the attacked group, with all individuals being equally vulnerable (and spatial variation between individuals in proximity to the predator is not considered). This was not the case for the frogs and snake example, where more isolated frogs had larger domains of danger and so had a greater risk of being targeted. The only way for the frogs to be equally likely to be attacked would be if they where regularly spaced out around the rim of the pond – that is, if they were as far removed from aggregated as it is possible to be (see Bednekoff & Lima 1998 for further discussion on this point).

Interestingly, the elegant theory of attack abatement would not predict the formation of aggregations if such aggregations are much more visible to predators and so much more frequently attacked than single individuals. In contrast, the selfish-herd effect of aggregation being driven by one individual taking cover behind another pays no heed to the consequences of aggregation formation on attack rate. Thus, selfish-herd effects could actually lead to individuals aggregating even if this increases the rate at which individuals are taken by predators. Of course, if aggregated individuals were more at risk than individuals that stayed isolated, then (as pointed out by Hamilton 1971) we would expect evolutionary change over time to select against the movement behaviours that generate aggregations via the selfish-herd mechanism. Thus, only when groups do not suffer disproportionately from attacks would we expect group formation via selfish-herd effects to evolve. We can see clearly now that the selfish herd is a process driven by individuals seeking to minimise their own *relative* risk of attack; it is not a mechanism that necessarily leads to lower predation rates when prey are aggregated. In retrospect, we regret in our book *Living in Groups* (Krause & Ruxton 2002) placing our discussion on the selfish herd within a subsection on dilution of risk within a chapter on the benefits of group formation.

Thus we urge readers to be cautious when they see the phrase *selfish herd*. The selfish herd is a real and important effect (Krause & Ruxton 2002), but unfortunately the term *selfish herd* is sometimes used loosely in relation to different mechanisms and concepts. Sadly, this mixing up of concepts has a long history. Hamilton (1971) finds hints of the idea of the selfish herd in the writing of the nineteenth-century polymath Galton (1883), but – according to Hamilton – Galton 'himself presented it mixed up with another quite separate idea which he treated as if it were simply another aspect of the same thing. This was that every cow, whether marginal or interior, benefited from being part of a herd ... he mentions mutual warning and the idea that by forming at bay in outward-facing bands the cattle can present a really formidable defence against lions.'

9.1.3 Generalisation to more complex and realistic geometries

Hamilton's (1971) paper explored generalising the theory to two and three dimensions. The key issue in any geometry is that the relative risks of two individuals can be assessed by comparing their domains of danger, and an individual's domain of danger can be interpreted as containing all the points in space that are nearer to that individual than to any other. An implicit assumption of the definition of a domain of danger is that attacks are equally likely to be launched from all positions in space, and that the predator attacks the individual nearest to its launch position. The example Hamilton gives is surprise attack by a lion on a herd of cattle. He imagined that sometime before the arrival of the cattle the lion selects a position in the long grass where it crouches down and waits in ambush for prey. The herd then moves into the vicinity, and the cattle are unable to detect the lion until it attacks. The attack can therefore come from a position within the herd itself, as well as from any point outside.

One problem that Hamilton did not address with the domain of danger is the issue of domains of danger becoming infinite. For example, if all of the prey form a single aggregation in an effectively infinite space, then those individuals on the periphery of the group have infinite domains of danger (Fig. 9.2a). This is important because if one of those individuals edges closer to its neighbours but still remains on the edge of the group, then its domain of danger remains infinite and so it does not seem to benefit from aggregation. Also, the infinite domain of danger of an edge individual suggests (unrealistically) that it is infinitely more vulnerable to attack than an individual that may be very near to it but happens to be sufficiently far into the group to have a finite domain of danger. This aspect of the theory was noticed almost immediately on its publication (Vine 1971). Infinite domains of danger are an unattractive aspect of the theory in its original

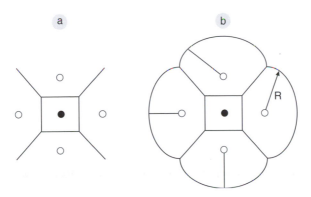

a   b

Figure 9.2 (a) Hamilton's (1971) original concept implies an infinite domain of danger (DOD) for edge individuals. (b) The limited domain of danger (LDOD) solves this problem by introducing a maximum distance R at which prey can be detected or attacked.

form, and subsequent elaborations of the theory have adopted various means to get around this problem. Morton *et al.* (1994) simply considered central individuals with finite domains of danger and ignored edge individuals. This seems unsatisfactory, given that the edge individuals do have an ecological effect on the central individuals (for example, influencing the relative sizes of their domains of danger). Further, small aggregations, with less than say 10 individuals, are likely to be dominated by edge individuals. Viscido *et al.* (2002) simply imposed finite boundaries to the space occupied by the group and so avoided any individuals having infinite domains of danger. Whilst this is more satisfactory, for many situations there is not one clear 'natural' position for these boundaries, and so the sensitivity of model predictions to different assumptions about the size and shape of the imposed finite space would certainly need very careful exploration. Reluga and Viscido (2005) avoided the problem by using a two-dimensional space with wrap-around boundaries (a torus). This avoids the problems of infinite domains of danger, but the size of the domains of peripheral individuals will still be influenced by the dimensions of the space. Finally, and most satisfactorily, James *et al.* (2004) removed the problem of infinite domains of danger (hereafter DODs) by introducing a related concept (limited domain of danger – LDOD) which cannot become infinite even for an isolated individual.

The key assumption underlying the concept of an individual's domain of danger is that an attack being initiated from anywhere in that space would be targeted on that individual. James *et al.* (2004) argue that on biological grounds this domain should never be infinite and that a further restriction should be added to the conventional DOD, since there is a maximum distance at which a predator–prey encounter can occur. Call this distance R. R might reflect the maximum distance at which a predator can detect a prey individual, or it might reflect the maximum distance over which a predator can pounce or otherwise close on a prey before the prey can make its escape. Thus the LDOD is defined as the intersection of the traditional DOD with a circle (in two dimensions) or sphere (in three dimensions) of radius R (Fig. 9.2b). Since R is

never infinite (on biological grounds) the LDOD can never be infinite.

A further pleasing aspect to the LDOD concept is that it restricts how far apart two individuals can be and still have an effect on each other. If two individuals are further than $2R$ apart, then their domains of danger are unaffected by each other, and so if one moved slightly closer to the other there would be no change in either domain of danger, and so no selection for further aggregation. However, once individuals cross this threshold, they begin to affect each other's domains of danger and so an interaction between them can occur. Thus two individuals within a distance $2R$ of each other can reasonably be thought to belong to the same loose aggregation, whereas another individual at a distance $3R$ from all other individuals would be considered to be isolated. This gives a natural way to identify the bounds of aggregations, especially attractive since R is a biological parameter and hence could potentially be evaluated empirically. The demarcation of groups of organisms has been a methodologically challenging issue, with ad hoc criteria often adopted without strong biological justification (Krause & Ruxton 2002, Stankowich 2003). It is also possible to use the LDOD concept as a way of splitting a group into central and peripheral individuals: if its LDOD is identical to the DOD then the individual is central, otherwise it is peripheral. Again, see Stankowich (2003) for discussion on the methodological issues surrounding such definitions.

It is important to remember that although oceanic fish and herbivores of the tundra and savanna may live in environments that are so open as to be effectively without boundaries from the viewpoint of predator–prey interactions; this will not be true for all ecological situations. A herd of deer that follows a path along the foot of a sheer cliff or the edge of lake may reduce its domains of danger by eliminating attacks by wolves from at least one flank. The interaction of behaviours involving attraction to habitat features that restrict predators' attacking options with selfish-herd behaviours has not been explicitly studied, but we see no reason why the two should not coexist in relatively straightforward fashion.

9.1.4 Behavioural rules underlying the selfish herd

How best should individuals move so as to take maximum advantage of the selfish-herd effect, given that the other members of the aggregation are likely to be trying to do likewise? Hamilton (1971, p. 301) acknowledged this as a challenge: 'The optimal strategy of movement for any situation is far from obvious.'

James *et al.* (2004) explored the attractiveness of different movement strategies within their LDOD framework. They considered prey that have some polarity (that is, a certain direction of movement that is 'remembered' from one moment to the next) and which must invest time in turning in order to change direction. They considered two strategies: NN (move towards your nearest neighbour in space) and NT (move towards your nearest neighbour in time; i.e. towards the individual it would take least time to reach). The nearest neighbour in space may be different from the nearest neighbour in time if changing direction takes a non-trivial amount of time. James *et al.* (2004) found that the NT strategy can invade a population playing the NN strategy but not vice versa, although full details of their evolutionary model are not provided. As they pointed out, there is empirical evidence for the use of the NT over the NN strategy from experiments with fish (Krause & Tegeder 1994).

In line with previous authors (Morton *et al.* 1994, Viscido *et al.* 2002), James *et al.* (2004) found that strategies involving movement rules based only on a single nearest neighbour lead to the formation of a number of small aggregations, rather than one large one. Morton *et al.* (1994) found greater degrees of aggregation using rules where individuals moved towards the average location of their *n*-nearest neighbours. Concerned about the biological plausibility of such a rule, they also explored a rule that they felt was less cognitively challenging. In this rule, the individual counted the numbers of individuals in the four quadrates of space centred around them and moved towards the middle of the most populous quadrate. This rule too produced a greater degree of aggregation than simply moving towards the nearest neighbour.

Viscido *et al.* (2002) also explored a more complex rule, which they called *local crowded horizon*. Here, prey move towards a point calculated as the weighted average of the positions of all other individuals, with weights declining with increasing distance from the focal individual to the individual associated with each weight. Such a rule appears to more readily produce large aggregations than some simpler rules where moves occur randomly, towards the nearest individual, or towards the gap between the nearest two neighbours. However, Viscido *et al.* (2002) were concerned to find extreme sensitivity of model predictions to the shape of the function controlling the effect of distance to an individual on its weighting factors. They were also concerned about the biological plausibility of the cognitive demands that such a rule implicitly requires of the prey. Viscido *et al.* (2001) demonstrated that the local crowded horizon rule could still lead to strong aggregation tendencies even when prey combined this rule with a tendency to increase their individual distances from a predator approaching from outside the group. Reluga and Viscido (2005) used a genetic algorithm approach to explore the evolutionary stability of the local crowded horizon rule. A parameter controlling the shape of the weighting function with distance was allowed to evolve, and generally evolved to values that caused individuals to be influenced by several other individuals, leading in turn to strong aggregation of the population.

9.1.5 The selfish-herd effect and other factors that can select for group formation

If the radius R indicates the maximum range at which a predator can detect prey, then it is reasonable to assume that attacks are only triggered when the predator is within an individual's LDOD. A model that includes this assumption inherently introduces abatement effects (Box 9.1) as well as selfish-herd effects, since the spatial distribution of prey affects the rate at which attacks occur. For example, increased overlap of LDODs might be expected to reduce the rate at which attacks occur. In order to consider selfish-herd effects in isolation, attacks would have to occur at times and positions that are unaffected by the behaviour of the prey. Indeed, the situation most commonly considered in previous models is that attacks happen at a fixed rate from random positions in the environment. This seems biologically unusual when R is defined as the detection range, since it implies that predators are assumed to launch attacks even when they can detect no prey. Hence, we suggest that in most circumstances where R represents a detection range, attacks should only occur within LDODs, and so selfish-herd effects will not be the only factor driving the overall predation risk of individuals. If R is a post-detection limit on the ability to capture prey, then attacks from outside LDODs are easier to justify biologically. It may be that the predator can detect prey nearby (and so launches an attack), but cannot gauge the distance to individuals until it has broken cover. Thus sometimes it will attack, but on launching the attack finds that the nearest prey is too far away for capture to be possible. In this case, a situation where the prey distribution does not affect the predator's attack rate can be justified, and selfish-herd effects can operate in isolation. But in most ecological circumstances the selfish-herd mechanism will not be the only factor influencing individual risks of predation, with attack-abatement effects and predator confusion being commonly experienced (Krause & Ruxton 2002).

James *et al.* (2004) argued that, for both LDOD and DOD, if there are only two individuals in the local environment, then they do not change their *relative* risk of predation by moving closer to each other; and so the selfish-herd effect alone would not lead to selection for aggregation of this pair. Thus selfish-herd effects would not drive the initial formation of a pair of individuals isolated from others, and will kick in only when some other factor (which may simply be chance) brings three or more individuals into close enough proximity to affect each other's domains of danger.

Although reduced predation risk of central individuals is a prediction of the selfish-herd mechanism, it does not follow that this mechanism is the only one that predicts lower predation risk for central individuals. For example, hover wasps *Parischnogaster alternata* nest in colonies. Centrally located nests suffer less from parasitism by ichneumon wasps

than peripheral nests (Landi *et al.* 2002). However, the hover wasps attempt to drive away parasites from the vicinity of the colony. It may be that the mechanism affording protection to central individuals is that approaches to central individuals take longer for the parasites, and so they are more likely to be detected and thwarted by the collective defence of the hover wasps.

No one suggests that the selfish-herd effect is the only or even the dominant force in the evolution of animal aggregations, or that predation will necessarily always be an evolutionary driver of aggregation. Indeed, logically and empirically, there are mechanisms by which predators can specifically target groups or even the central portions of groups (Parrish 1989, Stankowich 2003), and such behaviours would introduce counter-selection against the formation of groups. However, the simplicity, plausibility and generality of the assumptions underlying the selfish-herd mechanism suggest that it will be a widespread and potentially potent evolutionary driver.

An impressive piece of theory is the model of Beecham and Farnsworth (1999), which assumed that individuals impose attractive forces on each other through both selfish-herd and shared-vigilance effects, but also impose repulsive effects on each other as a consequence of interference competition for resources. The strengths of each of these forces vary with distance between individuals. The authors consider a static distribution of individuals (either a regular lattice arrangement or completely random) and then explore the strength and direction of the expected combination of forces (through all three mechanisms) on individuals, and thus make inferences as to how such forces would influence the shape of animal aggregations. This model is noteworthy for assuming that the probability of a predation event being successful is a declining function of the distance between the point from which the attack is launched and the position of the target individual. This means that the relative risk experienced by two individuals is related not just to the areas of their domains of danger but also to the shape of those domains. As a consequence of this, the model contains a maximum distance at which predation is possible, and thus creates a consistent methodology for determining LDOD. Further, the Beecham and Farnsworth (1999) model allows an individual's risk of predation to fall to zero if its domain of danger is entirely bordered by those of other individuals, and attacks always originate from outside the group. Such complexity likely explains why Beecham and Farnsworth did not attempt to extend their methodology to moving groups. It seems likely that dynamic change in the positioning of individuals could be simulated, and evaluation of (perhaps a simplified version of) this model could be fruitful.

9.1.6 The future of the selfish herd

An assumption of all current theory, except that of Beecham and Farnsworth, is that the relative risk of predation experienced by two individuals can be related to the ratio of the areas of their DODs or LDODs. Implicit in this is that the shape of the domain does not matter. This assumption implies that the success of attacks launched from anywhere within the domain is the same, whereas an attack launched from outside the domain is always unsuccessful. For example, using an LDOD that is affected by the interaction radius R, the success of attacks launched from a distance of $0.01\ R$ and from $0.99\ R$ are equal and non-zero, whereas an attack launched from a distance $1.01\ R$ has no chance of success. However, in many ecological scenarios, the likelihood of success might decline monotonically with the distance from which the attack is launched. Such a situation could be incorporated into selfish-herd models, although this would certainly be numerically much more demanding to evaluate since now the predation risk of an individual would be determined by the shape as well as the area of the domain of danger. A corollary of this would be that a smaller domain of danger would no longer guarantee a smaller risk of predation. The benefits of the LDOD concept could be retained in this framework by redefining R not as the distance at which predation risk falls identically to zero, but as the distance at which it falls to some specified but potentially non-zero level. The benefit that might emerge from all the extra computation involved is that of enhanced biological realism and the prospect

that the effects of the selfish-herd mechanism might be different should such a factor be introduced. There may be less selection pressure for tighter aggregation, since small domains of danger may reduce the likelihood of attacks, but those attacks that do occur will be launched over a short distance, and so are likely to be successful.

As James *et al.* (2004) suggest, the assumption that attacks are likely to be launched from anywhere within a domain is a poor representation of many ecological situations. It may be that attacks can only occur from outside the group and so individuals in central positions are immune from attack. Alternatively (or additionally) for moving groups it may be that those at the front are more vulnerable than those at the back, as these are the first to encounter waiting ambushers (Bumann *et al.* 1997). Both of these biological situations could be evaluated within the LDOD framework by shrinking the LDODs of protected individuals to zero. Evaluation of the evolutionary consequences would be valuable.

Both Morton *et al.* (1994) and Viscido *et al.* (2002) suggest that movement rules that draw on the positions of several nearest neighbours produce greater aggregation than simpler rules based on a single neighbour. It would be worthwhile exploring the robustness of this conclusion within the framework of LDODs. Modelling individuals with specific polarities that require finite time to change direction should create interest in the speed with which aggregation occurs, and interest in the evolutionary stability of rules (see Chapter 4). In addition, the authors of both these papers were understandably concerned about an individual's ability to meet the cognitive demands of these rules, so it might be stimulating to consider the robustness of strategies to the addition of error in individuals' calculated directions of movement.

More consideration should be given to the costs required to take advantage of selfish-herd effects. In the Beauchamp (2007) model, the prey respond to detection of an approaching predator by fleeing in the opposite direction. If by reacting first an individual can leap ahead of another individual, then the first individual's risk of capture decreases at the expense of the laggard. However, early detection requires high vigilance rates, which in turn reduces food gathering rates. Thus there is a cost to behaviour that shifts predation risk onto conspecifics. There is likely to be heterogeneity of risk across individuals in many situations (e.g. between edge and centre individuals), and costs too can vary between individuals. For these reasons we may see differential behavioural responses to cues of changing predator threat. For example, if a group of prey detects cues that suggest predatory attack is imminent, although they do not yet know the launch position of the attack, then we expect stronger responses from peripheral individuals with larger LDODs compared to central individuals (Krause 1994). The introduction of costs to models like that of James *et al.* (2004) would allow exploration of such heterogeneity of behavioural responses.

Empirical tests of selfish-herd theory have lagged behind theoretical developments. One of the most satisfying works is a field study of Eurasian sparrowhawk *Accipiter nisus* attacking foraging common redshanks *Tringa totanus* by Quinn and Cresswell (2006). The redshanks aggregate and are more at risk from the landward than the seaward side. The study found that redshanks were more tightly spaced on the riskier side of the flock, and further that those redshank that were attacked by sparrowhawks tended to be significantly more widely spaced than their nearest non-targeted neighbours. This comparison with neighbours is powerful, as it avoids potential confounding effects of position within the flock being associated with phenotypic or behavioural differences between individuals. Impressive as this study is, it cannot rule out the possibility that the reported effects are driven by closer aggregation of individuals inducing greater cognitive confusion in predators, rather than a selfish-herd effect. Of course, the two effects are not mutually exclusive, and the authors discuss the significant methodological challenges associated with estimating the relative importance of the two effects.

Krause (1993) took advantage of the fact that many fish respond to a chemical alarm substance called *Schreckstoff* in the water, which functions as a cue of increased predation risk. Krause observed the behaviour of groups of fish to the introduction

of *Schreckstoff* when all but one of the fish had previously been habituated to this substance. The non-habituated fish moved closer to the other fish and took up positions such that it was surrounded by others. Whilst this behaviour is strongly suggestive of the selfish-herd mechanism, note our discussion above that it is not the only mechanism that might drive such behavioural responses. However, this experimental technique (because it allows alteration of the perception of predation risk of some individuals but not others in the same arena) might prove a powerful tool for further studies.

9.2 Animal social networks: a new way of looking at animal relationships

9.2.1 Introduction

Social network theory was developed in the first half of the twentieth century by sociologists to facilitate formal description and analysis of human relationships (see Chapter 15; Scott 2000). Recently, this approach has become increasingly popular among biologists interested in social relationships of animals (Table 9.1). One of the reasons for this increased popularity is advances in statistical physics, and the availability of computer software that allows biologists to apply network theory to their study populations (Newman 2003, Croft *et al.* 2008). However, network theory is still not widely used in behavioural biology. One of the purposes of this chapter is to make this approach better known and more accessible. We strongly believe that it has great potential for enhancing our understanding of social relationships.

A network can be described as consisting of nodes (individuals) and edges (interactions between them, Fig. 9.3). Part of the appeal of the network approach is its simplicity and generality, because almost any system that comprises multiple components (whether biological or technological) can be described in the form of a network. A further strength of the network approach is that it addresses a long-standing challenge in biology, in that it provides a conceptual framework that bridges the gap between individuals

Table 9.1. Examples of animal social networks. An asterisk (*) indicates that the network approach is central to the study

Species	Authors	Research area
Fish		
Guppies *Poecilia reticulata*	Croft *et al.* 2004*, 2005*, 2006*, 2009*	Patterns of social interaction in a wild population
		Replicated networks
		Cooperation
Three-spined stickleback *Gasterosteus aculeatus*	Ward *et al.* 2002, Croft *et al.* 2005*, Pike *et al.* 2008*	Patterns of social interactions in wild populations
Insects		
Social insects	Fewell 2003*, Naug 2008*, 2009*	Modulation of foraging behaviour
Birds		
Long-tailed manakin *Chiroxiphia linearis*	McDonald 2007*, 2009*	Predicting social status
Cetaceans		
Dolphins *Tursiops* spp.	Lusseau 2003*, Lusseau & Newman 2004*, Lusseau *et al.* 2005*	Patterns of social interactions in wild populations
		Which individuals are important in tying a network together
Killer whale *Orcinus orca*	Williams & Lusseau 2006*	Social structure
Pinnipeds		
Galapagos sea lion *Zalophus wollebaeki*	Wolf *et al.* 2007*	Social structure
Primates		
Rhesus macaque *Macaca mulatta*	Chepko-Sade *et al.* 1989, de Waal 1996, Berman *et al.* 1997, Deputte & Quris 1997, Corr 2001	Social structure
		Development and perpetuation of affiliative networks
		Infant social networks
		Infant gender and socialisation process
		Changes in social networks over the lifespan of an individual
Pig-tailed macaque *Macaca nemestrina*	Flack *et al.* 2006*, Flack & Krakauer 2006*, Flack & de Waal 2007*	Policing stabilises construction of social niches in primates
Ring-tailed lemur *Lemur catta*	Nakamichi & Koyama 2000	Intra-troop affiliative relationships of females
Spider monkey *Ateles geoffroyi*	Boyer *et al.* 2006, Ramos-Fernandez *et al.* 2006*, 2009*	Foraging behaviour
Northern muriqui *Brachyteles hypoxanthus*	Strier *et al.* 2002	Male–male relationships
Emperor tamarin *Saguinus imperator*	Know & Sade 1991	Agonistic networks
Mantled howler monkey *Alouatta palliata*	Bezanson *et al.* 2002	Social structure
Western gorilla *Gorilla gorilla*	Stoinski *et al.* 2003, Bradley *et al.* 2004	Proximity patterns of female western lowland gorillas
		Extra-group, kin-biased behaviours

Table 9.1. (Continued)

Species	Authors	Research area
Chacma baboon *Papio ursinus*	Henzi *et al*. 2009*	Cyclical network structures
Primates (comparative study)	Kudo & Dunbar 2001	Network size and neocortex size
Human *Homo sapiens*	Klovdahl 1985*, Potterat *et al*. 2002*,	Disease transmission
	Eagle & Pentland 2003*, Newman	Disease transmission
	2003*, Stiller *et al*. 2003*	Mobile phone networks
		Community structure
		Social structure (Shakespeare plays)
Ungulates		
African buffalo *Syncerus caffer*	Cross *et al*. 2004*, 2005*	Modelling disease transmission, social structure
Grevy's zebra *Equus grevyi*, Onager *E. hemionus*	Sundaresan *et al*. 2007*	Comparison of social structure
Plains zebra *Equus burchelli*	Fischhoff *et al*. 2009	Social structure
Elephantidae		
African elephant *Loxodonta africana*	Wittemyer *et al*. 2005*	Multiple-tier social structure
Reptiles		
Gidgee skink *Egernia stokesii*	Godfrey *et al*. 2009*	Disease transmission
Marsupials		
Brushtail possum *Trichosurus vulpecula*	Corner *et al*. 2003*	Social-network analysis of disease transmission among captive possums
Domestic animals		
Sheep *Ovis aries*	Webb 2005	Contact structure for disease modelling
Pig *Sus scrofa* (large white landrace)	Durrell *et al*. 2004	Preferential associations

and the population. Figure 9.3 shows how one may describe the network properties of individuals, or of the entire network/population. Furthermore, it also allows the contemplation of a neglected aspect: the social (network) structure of the population can have important repercussions for the fitness of individuals (see Chapters 6, 14 and 15). The latter argument is familiar from game-theoretic models (see Chapters 4 and 18): the frequencies at which different behavioural strategies are used in a population can have fitness consequences for individuals in the population (Maynard Smith 1982). Game-theoretic models usually assume that all individuals mix freely with each other. Network theory relaxes this assumption and provides additional information because it reveals the social fine-structure of a population, thereby limiting the number of potential social contacts (see

Lieberman *et al.* 2005, using evolutionary graph theory). In many populations not everybody interacts with everybody else, but we see a structured social organisation that reflects differences between individuals in the number of social interactions, the degree to which some individuals are central or peripheral to the population network, and the tendency to interconnect different communities that form substructures within networks.

A similar point can be made about conventional epidemiological models and the modelling of socially transmitted information. The assumption of random interactions between individuals turns out to be too simplistic, and does not fit the finding that most social systems have structure that should not be neglected when studying the processes that take place in populations (Table 9.1).

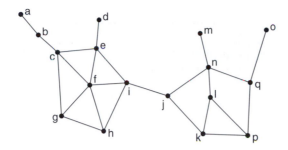

Figure 9.3 Example of a social network where nodes (filled circles) symbolise individuals and edges (lines) social connections between them. This network comprises 17 individuals (labelled a–q). See Table 9.2 for individual-based measures.

Figure 9.3 and Table 9.2 illustrate some of the features the network analysis offers. Network analysis allows us to calculate a new range of descriptive statistics that can be used to characterise the social organisation of animal populations. For example, we can calculate for each individual in the network its degree (number of immediate neighbours), cluster coefficient (the degree to which an individual's immediate neighbours are connected), path length (number of connections on the shortest path between two individuals), and node betweenness (the number of shortest paths between pairs of individuals that pass through a particular individual) (see Croft *et al.* 2008 for details). These statistics (which are just a small proportion of those available) can also be calculated for the network as a whole, which gives an idea of the local and global properties of the network. The degree can be related to the speed at which an individual might spread disease or information in a network, with highly connected individuals more likely to trigger an epidemic or a rumour. Path length and cluster coefficient might tell us something about the tendency of a pathogen to remain a local outbreak or become global in a population. Betweenness indicates how important individuals are in interconnecting different sections of the network. In the context of social learning, individuals with high betweenness that can reach into different communities are likely to be responsible for the spread of information. Many of these network statistics and others can be calculated using UCINET or similar software packages (Borgatti

et al. 2002; see also Croft *et al.* 2008) which are readily available from the internet.

Changes in the network such as the experimental removal (or addition) of individuals can potentially have a profound effect on the network, and can be measured using the above descriptive statistics. If we remove one individual (in this case *j*) from the network, this can have various effects on network structure (Fig. 9.3, Table 9.2). First of all, at the global level, the network now subdivides into two sub-networks and there is a reduction in the average path length. This subdivision into two sub-networks and the reduced path length could potentially have far-reaching consequences for the transmission of socially learnt information, for disease transmission, and for other processes in this social network. At the local (or individual) level, we can also observe important effects. Individuals *i* and *n*, which were initially central to the network, exhibit reduced betweenness after removal of *j*. This could be experimentally tested in real-life scenarios to find out whether the removal of one or more individuals does indeed produce the effect on social systems that an analysis of the network structure predicts.

In the latter example we selected an individual for removal that occupies a crucial position in the network (Fig. 9.3). Individuals could be removed from different network positions to investigate what changes the removal of single animals is likely to produce. Again, an interplay of network analysis and experimental work could be an interesting way to enhance

Table 9.2. Some individual-based measures for Figure 9.3. In brackets are the values that change after the removal of individual (or node) *j*. See text for a definition of the measures. Path lengths were calculated as distances to and from a particular node (modified after Krause *et al.* 2007)

Node/individual	Degree	Path length (to/from a node)	Clustering coefficient	Betweenness
a	1	4.75 (3)	—	0
b	2	3.875 (2.125)	0	15 (7)
c	4	3.0625 (1.5)	0.333	29 (13)
d	1	3.5625 (2.5)	—	0
e	4	2.625 (1.625)	0.333	28.5 (8.5)
f	5	2.5625 (1.5)	0.5	21.5 (5.5)
g	3	3.25 (1.875)	0.667	1.5 (1.5)
h	3	2.875 (2.125)	0.667	4.5 (0.5)
i	4 (3)	2.3125 (2)	0.333 (0.667)	65 (1)
j	3 (absent)	2.375 (absent)	0 (absent)	64 (absent)
k	3	2.9375 (2)	0.333 (1)	15
l	3	3.4375 (1.667)	0.333	2 (3)
m	1	3.6875 (2.333)	—	0 (0)
n	4 (3)	2.75 (1.5)	0	41 (6)
o	1	4.3125 (2.333)	—	0
p	3	3.4375 (1.667)	0.333	3 (3)
q	3	3.375 (1.5)	0	16 (6)
Mean	2.82 (2.625)	3.25 (1.953)	0.295 (0.403)	18.0 (3.438)

our understanding of the dynamics of social organisation in different species. Some eusocial insects show highly resilient responses to perturbations by accelerating and decelerating, or even reversing, worker development (see Chapter 1; Krause & Ruxton 2002, Naug 2009). This example shows how individual development (rather than behavioural) decisions are integrated into collective-level phenomena.

9.2.2 A brief review

Table 9.1 provides examples of species and topics that have been investigated using network theory. The table shows that non-human primates have been a focus for a long time. Social network theory was developed for analysing human relationships and therefore could be relatively easily adapted to other primate species, where similar questions were asked

and comparable sample sizes needed. From Table 9.1 the predominance of large mammalian species with complex interactions (see Chapter 14) is also apparent. Nonetheless, the social-network approach can be used with any species or population where identification of individuals is possible or where (as in the case of many social insects) interactions between particular social castes are of concern (Fewell 2003). Therefore, we predict that large areas of research where the network approach could be very useful are currently hardly touched.

The network approach has largely figured as a descriptive tool to better understand the general social organisation of a group or population (dolphins *Tursiops* spp., Lusseau 2003; fish, Croft *et al.* 2004, 2005; African buffalos *Syncerus caffer*, Cross *et al.* 2004; Galapagos sea lions *Zalophus wollebaeki*, Wolf *et al.* 2007). However, this is often just the starting point for further investigations into specific aspects of a species' behaviour and ecology. Recent work has shown how networks can be used to make predictions about changes in social systems after individuals have been removed (pig-tailed macaques *Macaca nemestrina*, Flack *et al.* 2006), when the social context has been changed (guppies *Poecilia reticulata*, Croft *et al.* 2006), or once the individuals have had time to interact and move up (or down) in the social status hierarchy (manakins *Chiroxiphia linearis*, McDonald 2007). From this work it becomes apparent that social network theory can be a descriptive, an analytic and a predictive tool to investigate animal behaviour.

9.2.3 Are we using the right terminology?

The terminology of social networks is a consequence of how the theory was first developed and used, namely to understand the relationships of humans (Scott 2000). Early applications of social network analysis among biologists also involved highly social species such as monkeys and their interaction patterns (Sade 1972, Chepko-Sade *et al.* 1989). When applying network analysis to animals, however, we may want to modify the terminology slightly since network analysis can be applied to any type of interaction between animals, for instance aggressive, sexual, cooperative or predatory behaviour. Thus it might be more appropriate to speak of animal interaction networks to express the broad use that can be made of network analysis. We would urge readers to differentiate interactions from associations. We would say that individuals A and B are *associated* if they are in close proximity at the same time, but this can occur without the behaviour or state of one individual affecting the other; such change is required for the association to count as an *interaction*.

9.2.4 What is the future of the network approach?

Here we highlight three areas that seem of particular interest, although there are potentially many more (see also Krause *et al.* 2007, Croft *et al.* 2008, Wey *et al.* 2008, Sih *et al.* 2009).

From single-species to multi-species networks

In the behavioural literature, the network approach has been largely limited to the interactions of individuals of the same species involving particular types of social interactions. This need not be the case: the network approach has been used for food webs where the basic unit is the species (Dunne *et al.* 2002, Stouffer *et al.* 2007). Also, we could envisage how the use of this approach could be extended to include disease transmission across species borders. The SARS outbreak, foot-and-mouth disease and bovine TB are just three examples in which contact patterns between individuals of different species may be analysed using network theory.

Network formation

Much of the current literature on social networks is focused on network patterns. This follows the development of many biological disciplines, in that we first categorise the different types of patterns that can be observed in nature, and then begin to address questions concerning the processes by which these patterns might have arisen. How do we get from the pattern to the process of network formation? A number of tools are available: for instance, individual-based models (IBMs) are a common tool to simulate interactions between animals (Couzin & Krause 2003). IBMs make it possible to preserve information about the order in which interactions occurred and their duration – two crucial bits of information that we need in order to better understand the dynamics of interaction patterns. A common problem with IBMs, however, is that they are sensitive to parameterisation. This means that highly specific information about the parameters of the individuals has to be available, and the same potentially applies to the interactions themselves. The model may require upfront a lot of information that we do not have, or only partially have.

Another way of looking at network formation is to consider the direct network neighbours of individuals in a network, and to allow for interactions between them that can result in positive, negative and neutral feedback (Skyrms & Permantle 2000). As a result of such interactions, existing network connections could be strengthened, or weakened. Furthermore, we could introduce a rate at which individuals also initiate new connections (and a rate at which old connections decay if no interactions take place for a while). Empirical work is just as important as modelling, because we need empirical measures for defining many of the components that are used in the development of models.

Development of network theory

The problems encountered by empiricists often create opportunities for theoreticians. The research area of social networks is full of such opportunities. Here we point out just two issues: sampling and comparability. In almost all cases when data are collected in the field or in the laboratory, we do not have a complete record of all interactions relevant to the construction of a social network. Likewise, we often cannot observe all individuals that belong to a particular group or population at each sampling interval. Currently there are estimates of how to deal with missing data points in networks, but no clear guidelines (Croft *et al.* 2008; see also D. W. Franks *et al.* 2009 for an overview of sampling methods for networks). Note that missing information when dealing with relational data (i.e. network data) can have different consequences from the situation of dealing with attribute data; the latter is the scenario most of us are familiar with.

Network comparisons pose tricky problems. Imagine we want to compare the social network structure of different populations of the same species living under different ecological conditions, to find out the influence of ecological factors on the social organisation of a particular species. There are a number of ways of making such comparisons (Croft *et al.* 2008). However, such comparisons are difficult if the networks differ in the number of individuals and the number of connections among them. This is another area in which further progress is needed to facilitate comparative studies that could potentially push the boundaries of our understanding of the social organisation of animals. Finally, we want to sound a note of caution. Much though network analysis has to offer for the behavioural sciences, it is important to keep several methodological issues in mind before this approach is used, to avoid potential 'banana skins' (James *et al.* 2009).

9.3 Collective behaviour

9.3.1 Introduction

Collective behaviour in some ways is closely related to social networks, because the individual-based models that are often used to explore collective behaviour can also provide the basis for creating interaction networks. Therefore, the interaction networks are often a sort of summary of the interactions that took place in a group or population over a certain time period.

Previously, studies of grouping had tried to explain why the strategy of group living had evolved in the first place by using a cost–benefit framework (Pulliam and Caraco 1984, Magurran 1990). However, there are now studies that address how bird flocks or fish schools manage to perform the amazing feats of synchrony and coordination that feature in virtually every natural history programme on TV. Similarly, in the insect literature, attention was firmly centred on genetic relationships to explain the evolution of eusociality, and less so on how 30 000 honey bees *Apis mellifera* manage to agree on a new nest location based on the information of 5% of scout bees that try to lead them in different directions. Collective behaviour became a new discipline in which researchers investigate how – based on individuals and their interactions – collective patterns can be explained. Individual-based models (IBMs) are a powerful tool in this context, allowing predictions to be made for collective states. In terms of methodology, the use of IBMs has brought the study of collective behaviour into close proximity with computer science, robotics and artificial intelligence. Using such IBMs has provided important insights into the process of social self-organisation and – as we will see in the following sections – has often provided simpler explanations for the social patterns that we observe in animals than the ones previously used (Hemelrijk 2000, 2005).

A concept of fundamental importance in the context of collective behaviour is that of positive (and negative) feedback. Individuals copy what others do, and the larger the numbers of individuals performing a certain behaviour the more likely it is that others will join in until negative feedback sets in (Camazine *et al.* 2001). This concept explains how large groups of animals can be coordinated in their behaviours, and provides the foundations for consensus decision making (see Chapters 6, 14 and 15; Conradt & Roper 2005). Individual interactions influence what happens at the group or population level, which in turn may select for particular behavioural strategies at the individual level (see Chapters 2 and 18; Fig. 9.4). Therefore, we have an interesting feedback loop (which is surprisingly often overlooked by humans when it comes to the cultural development of our own societies; see Chapter 15). Over time, this feedback loop may create behavioural strategies that are highly adapted to the social environment of, for example, an insect colony – and which may even allow the colony to create its own living conditions and environment, partly independent of the conditions outside the nest.

9.3.2 Simple explanations

In many cases IBMs can suggest simple explanations for seemingly complex behaviours. For example, in most animal groups, different spatial positions come with specific costs and benefits. The assumption was that individuals need to have information of the geometry of the whole group to position themselves appropriately (Krause 1994). Models of collective behaviour, however, showed that re-positioning could be achieved by changing the interaction patterns with conspecifics

within the group without information about the global geometry of the group (Couzin *et al.* 2002). Hemelrijk (2000) demonstrated in primates that aggressive behaviour of dominants is sufficient to explain their central positioning; no preference for such a position necessarily needs to be invoked. A similar argument applies to group size, which is known to affect fitness (Krause & Ruxton 2002). The ability to assess group size and to distinguish between groups of different sizes has been demonstrated in a number of different taxa (Krause & Ruxton 2002). However, when group sizes become large, this assessment may become increasingly difficult and time-consuming. Collective-behaviour models have proposed that according to the trade-off between predation risk and food competition individuals may change their aggregation tendency, which will automatically get them into groups of smaller or larger sizes with no need to constantly assess group size directly (Hoare *et al.* 2004). Similarly we can make predictions (using IBMs) for how density affects group size and number (Hensor *et al.* 2005).

9.3.3 Theory and empirical tests

A large part of the early and ongoing work on collective behaviour is on invertebrates, and in particular on eusocial insects: how they build their nests, find new nest locations, locate food or aggregate (Bonabeau *et al.* 1999, Camazine *et al.* 2001; mosquitoes, Krause *et al.* 1992; bacteria and slime moulds, Ben-Jacob *et al.* 1994, Nakagaki *et al.* 2000; honey bees, Seeley 2003; ants, Dussutour *et al.* 2004, N. R. Franks *et al.* 2009; cockroaches, Jeanson *et al.* 2005, Halloy *et al.* 2007). It took a long time before studies on vertebrates turned to collective behaviour in any major

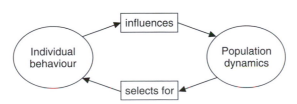

Figure 9.4. Schematic relationship between individual behaviour and population dynamics (after Kokko, unpublished; see also Chapters 4 and 18).

way, and this change is still in process. This delayed development was partly the result of a reluctance to give up on the full behavioural complexity and cognition that many vertebrates are individually capable of. Using IBMs was almost seen as a step backwards because it required a simplification of the interaction patterns of individuals to the utmost minimum. This approach has both costs and benefits: costs in terms of limiting the individual to less behavioural complexity than it is truly capable of, which may reduce the realism of the model, and benefits in the sense that this approach can propose much simpler explanations than were previously used, and thus provide an immensely powerful tool for understanding social behaviour relatively free of sociological jargon and complicated assumptions (Couzin & Krause 2003).

Because of the great potential of IBMs in exploring the relationships between individual, group and population, the field of collective behaviour is theory-driven, and empiricists have struggled to keep up with the flood of models that have emerged over the last 10–15 years. If we simply look at what is available on the model market to understand the shoaling behaviour of fish, then this is truly staggering (see introduction to Viscido *et al.* 2007). Empirical studies testing these models were missing for a long period, but this is beginning to change (Parrish & Hammer 1997, Viscido *et al.* 2004) because tracking of individual animals has become easier. Particularly interesting papers in this context are the ones on European starlings *Sturnus vulgaris* (Ballerini *et al.* 2008a, 2008b; see also Cavagna *et al.* 2008a, 2008b). A flock of over 3000 starlings was filmed during aerial manoeuvres in Rome, and video stills enabled a three-dimensional analysis of the flock structure using a sophisticated stereo photographic technique. One of the main insights from this work into the dynamics of grouping behaviour is that starlings pay attention to their 6–7 nearest neighbours regardless of their actual distance. This observation is in contrast with most models, in which a metric distance was used. The advantage of a topological distance over a metric one appears to be that the individuals are capable of maintaining strong flock cohesion even under changing densities.

Animal collective behaviour is a rapidly developing discipline, which benefits from close integration with analytic research areas such as physics and applied mathematics. Once the bottleneck of data acquisition (currently still tricky because of the need for sophisticated tracking software and time-consuming data collection) has been dealt with, we expect this field to open up to empiricists – which should enhance our understanding of the mechanisms of grouping behaviour. Recent work on decision making in vertebrate groups indicates that this is beginning to be the case (fish, Ward *et al.* 2008, Sumpter *et al.* 2008; birds, Biro *et al.* 2006; humans, Farkas *et al.* 2002, Dyer *et al.* 2008, 2009).

9.4 Conclusions and future directions

In this chapter we have discussed three topics. One, the selfish-herd effect, represents an ongoing debate, while the other two are interconnected. Network theory provides a novel method for the analysis of social relationships between animals, and collective behaviour makes use of individual-based models of animal interactions. We defined the selfish-herd effect to clarify the widespread confusion in the literature regarding the terminology. The selfish-herd effect requires a minimum of three animals and allows an individual to reduce its relative risk at the expense of others by seeking cover near or in between others. Originally proposed to explain how grouping behaviour can evolve as a result of selfish behaviour by individuals, it is arguable whether the selfish-herd effect represents an anti-predator benefit, given that it only allows for risk redistribution but not for a decrease in predation risk of most or all group members. The introduction of a limited domain of danger (LDOD) has solved the long-standing problem of quantifying the risk experienced by edge individuals in aggregations. Furthermore, it has created opportunities for empiricists to quantify the extent of the LDOD for particular predator–prey systems. The search for individual movement rules to minimise predation risk remains an interesting challenge for both theoreticians and empiricists. Likewise, little is known about how much time individuals have to follow such movement rules, because this would require information on how soon after detection by a predator a group will be attacked.

Social network theory has been around for over 50 years, although recent developments in statistical physics, graph theory and randomisation techniques provide rich tools for the analysis of animal interactions. Network theory provides a conceptual framework to link individual behaviour to the group and population level, and to understand in turn how the latter feeds back on the individual. Most applications of network theory have focused on social behaviours (cooperation, grooming etc.), but the potential is there to investigate any type of interaction among animals, be it social, aggressive, cooperative or sexual. We should therefore probably speak of *interaction networks* (rather than *social networks*), because the application of network theory is not limited to social species.

Bias in the empirical literature concerns the identification and analysis of network patterns. If we want to use network theory as a predictive tool and not just a descriptive one, we need to increase our understanding of network formation and change. Ideally an investigation of pattern and process should go hand in hand to fully utilise the potential of network theory to enhance our understanding of the social organisation of animals.

Collective behaviour is an exciting concept in the behavioural ecology of groups, although to be useful the term should not be thrown around too liberally. Great strides have been made in the last decade in using individual-based models to make predictions about the link between individual decision rules and behaviours and collective behaviours and decision making. Sadly, this modelling has tended to outstrip empirical data collection. However, as we have argued, recent technological breakthroughs provide an opportunity to close this gap. We expect more fruitful and close interaction between theory and data collection in the next few years, in ways that should greatly strengthen our understanding of collective behaviours.

Acknowledgements

JK and GDR would like to thank the editors for inviting us to contribute to this book. Discussions with Iain Couzin, Darren Croft, Christos Ioannou, Dick James, Stefan Krause, Lesley Morrell, David Sumpter, Colin Tosh and Ashley Ward on the above topics are gratefully acknowledged. Funding was provided by the EPSRC and the NERC.

Suggested readings

Selfish herd

Hamilton, W. D. (1971) Geometry for the selfish herd. *Journal of Theoretical Biology*, **31**, 295–311.

James, R., Bennett, P. G. & Krause, J. (2004) Geometry for mutualistic and selfish herds: the limited domain of danger. *Journal of Theoretical Biology*, **228**, 107–113.

Social networks

Croft, D. P., James, R. & Krause, J. (2008) *Exploring Animal Social Networks*. Princeton, NJ: Princeton University Press.

Flack, J. C., Girvan, M., de Waal, F. B. M. & Krakauer, D. C. (2006) Policing stabilizes construction of social niches in primates. *Nature*, **439**, 426–429.

McDonald, D. B. (2007) Predicting fate from early connectivity in a social network. *Proceedings of the National Academy of Sciences of the USA*, **104**, 10910–10914.

Collective behaviours

Camazine, S., Deneubourg, J., Franks, N. R. *et al.* (2001) *Self-Organization in Biological Systems*. Princeton, NJ: Princeton University Press.

Sumpter, D. J. T. (2006) The principles of collective behaviour. *Philosophical Transactions of the Royal Society B*, **361**, 5–22.

References

Ballerini, M., Cabibbo, N., Candelier, R. *et al.* (2008a) Interaction ruling animal collective behavior depends on topological rather than metric distance: Evidence from a field study. *Proceedings of the National Academy of Sciences of the USA*, **105**, 1232–1237.

Ballerini, M., Cabibbo, N., Candelier, R. *et al.* (2008b) Empirical investigation of starling flocks: a benchmark study in collective animal behaviour. *Animal Behaviour,* **76**, 201–215.

Beauchamp, G. (2007) Vigilance in a selfish herd. *Animal Behaviour,* **73**, 445–451.

Bednekoff, P. A. & Lima, S. L. (1998) Re-examining safety in numbers: interactions between risk dilution and collective detection depend upon predator targeting behaviour. *Proceedings of the Royal Society B,* **265**, 2021–2026.

Beecham, J. A. & Farnsworth, K. D. (1999) Animal group forces resulting from predator avoidance and competition minimization. *Journal of Theoretical Biology,* **198**, 533–548.

Ben-Jacob, E., Schochet, O., Tenenbaum, A. *et al.* (1994) Generic modelling of cooperative growth patterns in bacterial colonies. *Nature,* **368**, 46–49.

Berman, C. M., Rasmussen, K. L. R. & Suomi, S. J. (1997) Group size, infant development and social networks in free-ranging rhesus monkeys. *Animal Behaviour,* **53**, 405–421.

Bezanson, M., Garber, P. A., Rutherford, J. & Cleveland, A. (2002) Patterns of subgrouping, social affiliation and social networks in Nicaraguan mantled howler monkeys (*Alouatta palliata*). *American Journal of Physical Anthropology,* Suppl. 34, 44.

Biro, D., Sumpter, D. J. T., Meade, J. & Guilford, T. (2006) From compromise to leadership in pigeon homing. *Current Biology,* **16**, 2123–2128.

Bonabeau, E., Dorigo, M. & Theraulaz, G. (1999) *Swarm Intelligence: From Natural to Artificial Systems.* Oxford: Oxford University Press.

Borgatti, S. P., Everett, M. G. & Freeman, L. C. (2002) *UCINET for Windows, Version 6: Software for Social Network Analysis.* Harvard, MA: Analytic Technologies.

Boyer, D., Ramos-Fernandez, G., Miramontes, O. *et al.* (2006) Scale-free foraging by primates emerges from their interaction with a complex environment. *Proceedings of the Royal Society B,* **273**, 1743–1750.

Bradley, B. J., Doran-Sheehy, D. M., Lukas, D., Boesch, C. & Vigilant, L. (2004) Dispersed male networks in western gorillas. *Current Biology,* **14**, 510–513.

Bumann, D., Krause, J. & Rubenstein, D. I. (1997) Mortality risk of spatial positions in animal groups: the danger of being in the front. *Behaviour,* **134**, 1063–1076.

Camazine, S., Deneubourg, J. L., Franks, N. R. *et al.* (2001) *Self-Organization in Biological Systems.* Princeton, NJ: Princeton University Press.

Cavagna, A., Giardina, I., Orlandi, A. *et al.* (2008a) The STARFLAG handbook on collective animal behaviour: 1. Empirical methods. *Animal Behaviour,* **76**, 217–236.

Cavagna, A., Giardina, I., Orlandi, A., Parisi, G. & Procaccini, A. (2008b) The STARFLAG handbook on collective animal behaviour: 2. Three-dimensional analysis. *Animal Behaviour,* **76**, 237–248.

Chepko-Sade, B. D., Reitz, K. P. & Sade, D. S. (1989) Sociometrics of *Macaca mulatta* IV: network analysis of social structure of a pre-fission group. *Social Networks,* **11**, 293–314.

Conradt, L. & Roper, T. J. 2005. Consensus decision making in animals. *Trends in Ecology and Evolution,* **20**, 449–456.

Corner, L. A. L., Pfeiffer, D. U. & Morris, R. S. (2003) Social-network analysis of *Mycobacterium bovis* transmission among captive brushtail possums (*Trichosurus vulpecula*). *Preventive Veterinary Medicine,* **59**, 147–167.

Corr, J. (2001) Changes in social networks over the lifespan in male and female rhesus macaques. *American Journal of Physical Anthropology,* Suppl. 32, 54–55.

Couzin, I. D. & Krause, J. (2003) Selforganisation and collective behaviour of vertebrates. *Advances in the Study of Behavior,* **32**, 1–67.

Couzin, I. D., Krause, J., James, R., Ruxton, G. D. & Franks, N. R. (2002) Collective memory and spatial sorting in animal groups. *Journal of Theoretical Biology,* **218**, 1–11.

Croft, D. P., Krause, J. & James, R. (2004) Social networks in the guppy (*Poecilia reticulata*). *Proceedings of the Royal Society B,* **271**, 516–519.

Croft, D. P., James, R., Ward, A. J. W. *et al.* (2005) Assortative interactions and social networks in fish. *Oecologia,* **143**, 211–219.

Croft, D. P., James, R., Thomas, P. *et al.* (2006) Social structure and co-operative interactions in a wild population of guppies (*Poecilia reticulata*). *Behavioral Ecology and Sociobiology,* **59**, 644–650.

Croft, D. P., James, R. & Krause, J. (2008) *Exploring Animal Social Networks.* Princeton, NJ: Princeton University Press.

Croft, D.P., Krause, J., Darden, S.K. *et al.* (2009) Behavioural trait assortment in social networks: patterns and implications. *Behavioral Ecology and Sociobiology,* **63**, 1495–1503.

Cross, P. C., Lloyd-Smith, J. O., Bowers, J. A. *et al.* (2004) Integrating association data and disease dynamics in a social ungulate: bovine tuberculosis in African buffalo in the Kruger National Park. *Annales Zoologici Fennici,* **41**, 879–892.

Cross, P. C., Lloyd-Smith, J. O. & Getz, W. M. (2005) Disentangling association patterns in fission-fusion societies using African buffalo as an example. *Animal Behaviour*, **69**, 499–506.

Deputte, B. L. & Quris, R. (1997) Socialization processes in primates: use of multivariate analyses. 2. Influence of sex on social development of captive rhesus monkeys. *Behavioural Processes*, **40**, 85–96.

de Waal, F. B. M. (1996) Macaque social culture: development and perpetuation of affiliative networks. *Journal of Comparative Psychology*, **110**, 147–154.

Dunne, J. A., Williams, R. J. & Martinez, N. D. (2002) Food-web structure and network theory: the role of connectance and size. *Proceedings of the National Academy of Sciences of the USA*, **99**, 12917–12922.

Durrell, J. L., Sneddon, I. A., O'Connell, N. E. & Whitehead, H. (2004) Do pigs form preferential associations? *Applied Animal Behaviour Science*, **89**, 41–52.

Dussutour, A., Fourcassié, V., Helbing, D. & Deneubourg, J. L. (2004). Optimal traffic organization in ants under crowded conditions. *Nature*, **428**, 70–73.

Dyer, J. R. G., Ioannou, C. C., Morrell, L. J. *et al.* (2008) Consensus decision making in human crowds. *Animal Behaviour*, **75**, 461–470.

Dyer, J. R. G., Johansson, A., Helbing, D., Couzin, I. D. & Krause, J. (2009) Leadership, consensus decision making and collective behaviour in human crowds. *Philosophical Transactions of the Royal Society B*, **364**, 781–789.

Eagle, N. & Pentland, A. (2003) Social network computing. *Lecture Notes in Computer Science*, **2864**, 289–296.

Farkas, I., Helbing, D. & Vicsek, T. (2002) Social behaviour: Mexican waves in an excitable medium – the stimulation of this concerted motion among expectant spectators is explained. *Nature*, **419**, 132–133.

Fewell, J. H. (2003) Social insect networks. *Science*, **301**, 1867–1870.

Fischhoff, I. R., Dushoff, J., Sundaresen, S. R., Cordingly, J. E. & Rubenstein, D. I. (2009) Reproductive status influences group size and persistence of bonds in male plains zebra (*Equus burchelli*). *Behavioral Ecology and Sociobiology*, **63**, 1035–1043.

Flack, J. C. & Krakauer, D. C. (2006) Encoding power in communication networks. *American Naturalist*, **168**, 87–102.

Flack, J. C. & de Waal, F. (2007) Context modulates signal meaning in primate communication. *Proceedings of the National Academy of Sciences of the USA*, **104**, 1581–1586.

Flack, J. C., Girvan, M., de Waal, F. B. M. & Krakauer, D.C. (2006) Policing stabilizes construction of social niches in primates. *Nature*, **439**, 426–429.

Franks, D. W., James, R., Nobel, J. & Ruxton, G. D. (2009) A foundation for developing a methodology for social network sampling. *Behavioral Ecology and Sociobiology*, **63**, 1079–1088.

Franks, N. R., Dechaume-Moncharmont, F. X., Hanmore, E. & Reynolds, J. K. (2009) Speed versus accuracy in decision-making ants: expediting politics and policy implementation. *Philosophical Transactions of the Royal Society B*, **364**, 845–852.

Galton, F. (1883) *Inquiries into Human Faculty and its Development*. London: Dent.

Godfrey, S. S., Bull, C. M., James, R. & Murray, K. (2009) Network structure and parasite transmission in a group-living lizard, the gidgee skink, *Egernia stokesii*. *Behavioral Ecology and Sociobiology*, **63**, 1045–1056.

Halloy, J., Sempo, G., Caprari, G. *et al.* (2007) Social integration of robots into groups of cockroaches to control self-organized choices. *Science*, **318**, 1155–1158.

Hamilton, W. D. (1971) Geometry for the selfish herd. *Journal of Theoretical Biology*, **31**, 295–311.

Hemelrijk, C. K. (2000) Towards the integration of social dominance and spatial structure. *Animal Behaviour*, **59**, 1035–1048.

Hemelrijk, C. K. (2005) A process-oriented approach to the social behaviour of primates. In: *Self-Organisation and Evolution of Social Systems*, ed. C. K. Hemelrijk. Cambridge: Cambridge University Press, pp. 81–107.

Hensor, E. M. A., Couzin, I. D., James, R. & Krause, J. (2005) Modelling density-dependent fish shoal distributions in the laboratory and field. *Oikos*, **110**, 344–352.

Henzi, S.P., Lusseau, D., Weingrill, T., van Schaik, C. P. & Barrett, L. (2009) Cyclicity in the structure of female baboon social networks. *Behavioral Ecology and Sociobiology*, **63**, 1015–1021.

Hoare, D. J., Couzin, I. D., Godin, J.-G. J. & Krause, J. (2004) Context-dependent group-size choice in fish. *Animal Behaviour*, **67**, 155–164.

James, R., Bennett, P. G. & Krause, J. (2004) Geometry for mutualistic and selfish herds: the limited domain of danger. *Journal of Theoretical Biology*, **228**, 107–113.

James, R., Croft, D. P. & Krause, J. (2009) Potential banana skins in animal social network analysis. *Behavioral Ecology and Sociobiology*, **63**, 989–997.

Jeanson, R., Rivault, C., Deneubourg, J. L. *et al.* (2005) Self-organized aggregation in cockroaches. *Animal Behaviour*, **69**, 169–180.

Klovdahl, A. S. (1985) Social networks and the spread of infectious diseases: the AIDS example. *Social Science and Medicine*, **21**, 1203–1216.

Know, K. L. & Sade, D. S. (1991) Social behavior of the emperor tamarind in captivity: components of agonistic display and the agonistic network. *International Journal of Primatology*, **12**, 439–480.

Krause, J. (1993) The effect of 'Schreckstoff' on the shoaling behaviour of the minnow: a test of Hamilton's selfish herd theory. *Animal Behaviour*, **45**, 1019–1024.

Krause, J. (1994) Differential fitness returns in relation to spatial positions in groups. *Biological Reviews*, **69**, 187–206.

Krause, J. & Tegeder, R. W. (1994) The mechanism of aggregation behaviour in fish shoals: individuals minimise approach time to neighbours. *Animal Behaviour*, **48**, 353–359.

Krause, J. & Ruxton, G. D. (2002) *Living in Groups*. Oxford: Oxford University Press.

Krause, J., Brown, D. & Corbet, S. (1992) Spacing behaviour in resting *Culex pipiens* (Diptera, Culicidae): a computer modelling approach. *Physiological Entomology*, **17**, 241–246.

Krause, J., Croft, D. P. & James, R. (2007) Social network theory in the behavioural sciences: potential applications. *Behavioral Ecology and Sociobiology*, **62**, 15–27.

Kudo, H. & Dunbar, R. I. M. (2001) Neocortex size and social network size in primates. *Animal Behaviour*, **62**, 711–722.

Landi, M., Coster-Longman, C. & Turillazzi, S. (2002) Are the selfish herd and dilution effects important in promoting nest clustering in the hover wasp *Parischnogaster alternata* (Stenogastrinae Vespidae Hymenotypera)? *Ethology, Ecology and Evolution*, **14**, 297–305.

Lieberman, E., Hauert, C. & Nowak, M. A. (2005) Evolutionary dynamics on graphs. *Nature*, **433**, 312–316.

Lusseau, D. (2003) The emergent properties of a dolphin social network. *Proceedings of the Royal Society B*, **270**, 186–188.

Lusseau, D. & Newman, M. E. J. (2004) Identifying the role that animals play in their social networks. *Proceedings of the Royal Society B*, **271**, 477–481.

Lusseau, D., Wilson, B., Hammond, P. S. *et al.* (2005) Quantifying the influence of sociality on population structure in bottlenose dolphins. *Journal of Animal Ecology*, **75**, 14–24.

Magurran, A. E. (1990) The adaptive significance of schooling as an antipredator defense in fish. *Annales Zoologici Fennici*, **27**, 51–66.

Maynard Smith, J. (1982) *Evolution and the Theory of Games*. Cambridge: Cambridge University Press.

McDonald, D. B. (2007) Predicting fate from early connectivity in a social network. *Proceedings of the National Academy of Sciences of the USA*, **104**, 10910–10914.

McDonald, D. B. (2009) Young-boy networks without kin clusters in a lek-mating manakin. *Behavioral Ecology and Sociobiology*, **63**, 1029–1034.

Morton, T. L., Haefner, J. W., Nugala, V., Decino, R. D. & Mendes, L. (1994) The selfish herd revisited: do simple movement rules reduce predation risk. *Journal of Theoretical Biology*, **167**, 73–79.

Nakagaki, T., Yamada, H. & Tóth, Á. (2000) Maze-solving by an amoeboid organism. *Nature*, **407**, 470.

Nakamichi, M. & Koyama, N. (2000) Intra-troop affiliative relationships of females with newborn infants in wild ring-tailed lemurs (*Lemur catta*). *American Journal of Primatology*, **50**, 187–203.

Naug, D. (2008) Structure of the social network and its influence on transmission dynamics in a honeybee colony. *Behavioral Ecology and Sociobiology*, **62**, 1719–1725.

Naug, D. (2009) Structure and resilience of the social network in an insect colony as a function of colony size. *Behavioral Ecology and Sociobiology*, **63**, 1023–1028.

Newman, M. E. J. (2003) The structure and function of complex networks. *SIAM Review*, **45**, 167–256.

Parrish, J. K. (1989) Re-examining the selfish herd: are central fish safer. *Animal Behaviour*, **38**, 1048–1053.

Parrish, J. K. & Hamner, W. M. (1997) *Animal Groups in Three Dimensions*. Cambridge: Cambridge University Press.

Pike, T. W., Samanta, M., Lindstrom, J. & Royle, N. J. (2008) Behavioural phenotype affects social interactions in an animal network. *Proceedings of the Royal Society B*, **275**, 2515–2520.

Potterat, J. J., Muth, S. Q., Rothenberg, R. B. *et al.* (2002) Sexual network structure as an indicator of epidemic phase. *Sexually Transmitted Infections*, **78** (Suppl. 1), 152–15.

Pulliam, H. R. & Caraco, T. (1984) Living in groups: is there an optimal group size? In: *Behavioural Ecology: an Evolutionary Approach*, 2nd edn, ed. J. R. Krebs & N. B. Davies. Oxford: Blackwell, pp. 122–147.

Quinn, J. L. & Cresswell, W. (2006) Testing domains of danger in the selfish herd: sparrowhawks target widely spaced redshanks in flocks. *Proceedings of the Royal Society B*, **273**, 2521–2526.

Ramos-Fernández, G., Boyer, D. & Gomez, V. P. (2006) A complex social structure with fission–fusion properties can emerge from a simple foraging model. *Behavioral Ecology and Sociobiology*, **60**, 536–549.

Ramos-Fernández, G., Boyer, D., Aureli, F. & Vick, L. G. (2009) Association networks in spider monkeys (*Ateles geoffroyi*). *Behavioral Ecology and Sociobiology*, **63**, 999–1013.

Reluga, T. C. & Viscido, S. (2005) Simulated evolution of selfish herd behaviour. *Journal of Theoretical Biology*, **234**, 213–225.

Sade, D. S. (1972) Sociometrics of *Macaca mulatta*: linkages and cliques in grooming matrices. *Folia Primatologica*, **18**, 196–223.

Scott, J. (2000) *Social Network Analysis*. London: Sage.

Seeley, T. D. (2003) Consensus building during nest-site selection in honey bee swarms: the expiration of dissent. *Behavioral Ecology and Sociobiology*, **53**, 417–424.

Sih, A., Hanser, S. F. & McHugh, K. A. (2009) Social network theory: new insights and issues for behavioral ecologists. *Behavioral Ecology and Sociobiology*, **63**, 975–988.

Skyrms, B. & Permantle, R. (2000) A dynamic model of social network formation. *Proceedings of the National Academy of Sciences of the USA*, **97**, 335–339.

Stankowich, S. (2003) Marginal predation methodologies and the importance of predator preferences. *Animal Behaviour*, **66**, 589–599.

Stiller, J., Nettel, D. & Dunbar, R. I. M. (2003) The small world of Shakespeare's plays. *Human Nature*, **14**, 397–408.

Stoinski, T. S., Hoff, M. P. & Maple, T. L. (2003) Proximity patterns of female western lowland gorillas (*Gorilla gorilla gorilla*) during the six months after parturition. *American Journal of Primatology*, **61**, 61–72.

Stouffer, D. B., Camacho, J., Jiang, W. & Amaral, L. A. N. (2007) Evidence for the existence of a robust pattern of prey selection in food webs. *Proceedings of the Royal Society B*, **274**, 1931–1940.

Strier, K. B., Dib, L. T. & Figueira, J. E. C. (2002) Social dynamics of male muriquis (*Brachyteles arachnoides hypoxanthus*). *Behaviour*, **139**, 315–342.

Sumpter, D. J. T., Krause, J., James, R., Couzin, I. D. & Ward, A. J. W. (2008) Consensus decision-making by fish. *Current Biology*, **18**, 1773–1777.

Sundaresan, S. R., Fischhoff, I. R., Dushoff, J. & Rubenstein, D. I. (2007) Network metrics reveal differences in social organization between two fission-fusion species, Grevy's zebra and onager. *Oecologia*, **151**, 140–149.

Turner, G. F. & Pitcher, T. J. (1986) Attack abatement: a model for group protection by combining avoidance and dilution. *American Naturalist*, **128**, 228–240.

Vine, I. (1971) Risk of visual detection and pursuit by a predator and the selective advantage of flocking behaviour. *Journal of Theoretical Biology*, **30**, 405–422.

Viscido, S. V. (2001) The case for the selfish herd hypothesis. *Comments on Theoretical Biology*, **8**, 1–20.

Viscido, S. V., Miller, M. & Wethey, D. S. (2001) The response of a selfish herd to an attack from outside the group perimeter. *Journal of Theoretical Biology*, **208**, 315–328.

Viscido, S. V., Miller, M. & Wethey, D. S. (2002) The dilemma of the selfish herd: the search for a realistic movement rule. *Journal of Theoretical Biology*, **217**, 183–194.

Viscido, S. V., Parrish, J. K. & Grunbaum, D. (2004) Individual behavior and emergent properties of fish schools: a comparison of observation and theory. *Marine Ecology Progress Series*, **273**, 239–249.

Viscido, S. V., Parrish, J. K. & Grunbaum, D. (2007) Factors influencing the structure and maintenance of fish schools. *Ecological Modelling*, **206**, 153–165.

Ward, A. J. W., Botham, M. S., Hoare, D. J. *et al.* (2002) Association patterns and shoal fidelity in the three-spined stickleback. *Proceedings of the Royal Society B*, **269**, 2451–2455.

Ward, A. J. W., Sumpter, D. J. T., Couzin, I. D., Hart, P. J. B. & Krause, J. (2008) Quorum decision-making facilitates information transfer in fish shoals. *Proceedings of the National Academy of Sciences of the USA*, **105**, 6948–6953.

Webb, C. R. (2005) Farm animal networks: unraveling the contact structure of the British sheep population. *Preventive Veterinary Medicine*, **68**, 3–17.

Wey, T., Blumstein, D. T., Shen, W. & Jordan, F. (2008) Social network analysis of animal behaviour: a promising tool for the study of sociality. *Animal Behaviour*, **75**, 333–344.

Williams, R. & Lusseau, D. (2006) A killer whale social network is vulnerable to targeted removals. *Biology Letters*, **2**, 497–500.

Wittemyer, G., Douglas-Hamilton, I. & Getz, W. M. (2005) The socioecology of elephants: analysis of the processes creating multitiered social structures. *Animal Behaviour*, **69**, 1357–1371.

Wolf, J. B. W., Mawdsley, D., Trillmich, F. & James, R. (2007) Social structure in a colonial mammal: unravelling hidden structural layers and their foundations by network analysis. *Animal Behaviour*, **74**, 1293–1302.

A haphazard career

Ronald Noë

I was asked to explain why and how a Dutchman got to be a professor teaching animal behaviour in a French university. Someone must have thought that my story could provide some guidance for aspiring ethologists and behavioural ecologists. I am not so sure that my career path is one that should be followed, but perhaps someone can learn from my mistakes. I think I can now afford to write about them without much of a negative effect on my career. Not that I have bothered much about my 'career', but that is perhaps the core of my problem. I have never been good at preparing myself for the future, so after treading the mills of the Dutch educational system I found myself regularly confronted with steps in life that I should have prepared, if not better, then at least earlier. And so I ended up in a 'cul de sac'. But let me start from the beginning.

I can't tell you what kind of '—ist' I am exactly at this point – primatologist, behavioural ecologist or evolutionary psychologist – but I went to the university to become an ethologist. The reason was simple: I liked animals a lot, and notably the furry ones. I definitely preferred seeing them alive, healthy and doing their own thing. I understood from books by the likes of Tinbergen, Lorenz, Wickler and Eibl-Eibesfeldt that ethologists did professionally what I liked to do anyway: watch animals behave. What their books didn't say is that there are rather few positions for ethologists. Not that I wasn't warned.

During the introduction day for biology at the university we were told that about 2% of us would find jobs as biologists. That translates to about 0.1% for ethologists, I guess.

So after finishing a school in which I wasted about a third of my time learning dead languages, I enrolled in biology in Groningen. Why Groningen? I had four good reasons. Because it was not Amsterdam; it was not Leiden, where my sister studied already; it was not Utrecht, which was too close to my parents' home; and I had never been to Groningen before. As it happens Groningen was, and still is, the best place in the Netherlands for animal behaviour, but I would lie if I said that I realised that at the time. So I enjoyed highly interesting lectures in classical ethology by Gerard Baerends, Jaap Kruijt and others. The only drawback was that the ethology group of Groningen concentrated on birds and fish. Their lack of furriness forced me to look elsewhere for my master's topics, of which we did three in those days. I had my first experience with field work by following radio-collared foxes around in the night, then I watched chimpanzees in the zoo for a year, and finally did a topic in plant ecology. Fairly furry plants in fact.

The key experience was the year in the Arnhem Zoo, where I was one of Frans de Waal's first students. Perhaps the most important among Frans's many skills is that he is an incredibly keen

Social Behaviour: Genes, Ecology and Evolution, ed. Tamás Székely, Allen J. Moore and Jan Komdeur. Published by Cambridge University Press. © Cambridge University Press 2010.

observer. By analysing video tapes of complicated interactions together with him for many hours, I learned to observe the details of animal behaviour. I also learned to appreciate primates, and became interested in complicated forms of cooperation such as coalition formation. No less important was the introduction to Jan van Hooff and the animal behaviour department he was building up at the University of Utrecht.

What bothered me about the chimpanzees was that they lived in captivity. The Arnhem Zoo has a nice big enclosure, but it remains an enclosure. The foxes, the dunes in which I did my plant ecology, the nature reserve in which I lived during my chimp year, Kenya, which I toured with some friends, all reinforced my preference for working in the field. I had also become more interested in the evolutionary aspects of animal behaviour than in the mechanistic questions. I am convinced that if one wants to study the evolution of something, then one should do that in the environment that resembles the environment of origin as closely as possible. In short, I looked out for a possibility to do field work on mammals. A small problem was that I still had to do my military service and that I started the long procedure necessary to be recognised as a conscientious objector too late. In those days it was not unusual to start a PhD project with the 18 months replacement service, and I had already organised something vague on polecats at the Dutch Institute of Wildlife Research. Then one lucky day I banged my knee so badly on an iron pole during a coffee break that the damage was visible on an x-ray. That of course meant that I was not fit for military service of any kind, and free to do something else. That something else was a PhD project on baboons on Kenya's beautiful savannas.

During a primatological congress in Florence Glen Hausfater invited me to work in the Amboseli Baboon Project, led by him together with Jeanne and Stuart Altmann. With the support of Jan van Hooff and Bettie, my future wife, who made 50 copies of the proposal on a stencil machine, I obtained a four-year grant to study coalition formation in male baboons. Bettie gave up her job as a teacher and also married me, because the granting agency would otherwise not pay her airfare. I can't think of a better reason to get married.

So we were off together to Kenya to observe coalitions among male baboons, although there were none to be seen in Amboseli according to Glen, and although I knew next to nothing about the basic theories on cooperation. Luckily Glen's ignorance and my own didn't stop us from having a great time, during which I learned a lot about the organisation of a field site, about working in Africa, about primates and about the rest of wildlife. After 18 months in Amboseli I had in fact enough data to fill my thesis, but I still had money for another year of field work. We spent that in another baboon project in Kenya, which was a contrast to the Amboseli project in almost any way one could think of. Say no more.

The most important thing I learned during my PhD project was that a popular theory, in my case Trivers' idea of reciprocal altruism and related models based on the iterated Prisoner's Dilemma, can go an incredibly long way without any empirical support. It is most amazing to see that a theoretic tail can wag an empirical dog for decades and nobody cares (Noë 1990, 1992, Noë *et al.* 1991). So I spent a good deal of the rest of my career screaming out loud that theoretical models can be nice and even useful, but that once in a blue moon they need a bit of empirical support (Noë 2006).

Back in the Netherlands I spent a lot of time analysing the data and publishing the chapters of my thesis, but with my typical lack of bureaucratic talent I didn't properly organise the graduation event itself, which is quite a circus in Utrecht. Luckily enough Hans Kummer invited me to Zurich for a postdoc long before I got my doctoral title officially. I was supposed to work on captive groups of banded mongoose there, but then the university decided to construct a new building right next to their enclosure. When they proposed to build a temporary enclosure for an astronomic sum, I joked that I could work in Africa for half of that. Within weeks I found myself with exactly that sum

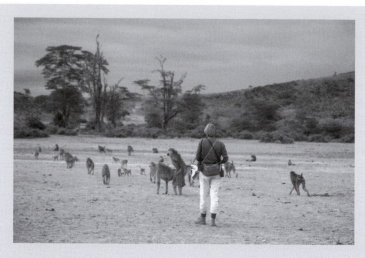

Bettie Noë-Sluijter collecting a focal animal sample in Alto's group (1982, Amboseli National Park, Kenya). Photo: Ronald Noë.

on a research account. That's what I call the opposite of bureaucracy. Perhaps we could make Zurich a kind of Lourdes for bureaucrats: a pilgrimage there could heal their morbid inclination to put spokes in the wheels of science. The pilot study I did with this unexpected grant, followed two years later by a grant from the Swiss National Research Foundation, was the start of the Taï Monkey Project in Ivory Coast – the springboard of many a career and the source of data for a long list of publications, such as Noë & Bshary (1997).

At that point in time we had salaries, an apartment, a bank account etc. in Switzerland, but no work permits. The solution came in the form of an invitation by Peter Hammerstein to work in the Max-Planck Institute in Seewiesen, Germany, supported by a grant from the Humboldt Foundation. After a little reproductive break my wife and I worked for several years in Ivory Coast in the winter and Bavaria in the summer. With Peter Hammerstein I further developed an idea that had been inspired by my work with baboons: the biological market paradigm (Noë & Hammerstein 1994, 1995, Noë 2001). The Taï Monkey Project grew into a large venture in which

we studied eight monkey species with the help of a small army of local assistants and students. All this was possible thanks to the very generous support of Wolfgang Wickler, the director of our department.

I happily lived on temporary contracts in Seewiesen until the Max-Planck Gesellschaft thought it was time to close the famous Seewiesen institute. That's when I started to worry about feeding the family. Again, the solution came from an unexpected direction: an invitation by Bernard Thierry to compete for a professorship at the Université Louis-Pasteur in Strasbourg, France. That I indeed find myself in this position today I owe to the strong support of Bernard and several other insiders who guided me through the most amazing bureaucratic procedure I have ever experienced. I don't think I beat most of the competition on merit, but more likely because I was one of the few who had the right forms filled out in time.

So, a career like mine is perhaps an idea for someone who likes a bit of adventure, enjoys living in many different countries and is willing to learn a couple of languages. It doesn't need a lot of planning, because one goes where the wind blows. However, it doesn't work without an extraordinary partner who is willing to pull up stakes about once a year and remain cheerful all the time. Such people are thin on the ground. In fact, I have only met one in my life. If you dream of a big scientific career, but are risk-adverse and worry about the economic aspects of life, you had better get organised instead. Or maybe you should avoid the study of animal behaviour altogether.

References

Noë, R. (1990) A veto game played by baboons: a challenge to the use of the Prisoner's Dilemma as a paradigm for reciprocity and cooperation. *Animal Behaviour*, **39**, 78–90.

Noë, R. (1992) Alliance formation among male baboons: shopping for profitable partners. In: *Coalitions and Alliances in Humans and Other Animals*, ed. A. H. Harcourt & F. B. M. de Waal. Oxford: Oxford University Press, pp. 282–321.

Noë, R. (2001) Biological markets: partner choice as the driving force behind the evolution of cooperation. In: *Economics in Nature. Social Dilemmas, Mate Choice and Biological Markets*, ed. R. Noë, J. A. R. A. M. van Hooff & P. Hammerstein. Cambridge: Cambridge University Press, pp. 93–118.

Noë, R. (2006) Cooperation experiments: coordination through communication versus acting apart together, *Animal Behaviour*, **71**, 1–18.

Noë, R. & Bshary R. (1997) The formation of red colobus – diana monkey associations under predation pressure from chimpanzees. *Proceedings of the Royal Society B*, **264**, 253–251.

Noë, R. & Hammerstein, P. (1994) Biological markets: supply and demand determines the effect of partner choice in cooperation, mutualism and mating. *Behavioral Ecology and Sociobiology*, **35**, 1–11.

Noë, R & Hammerstein, P. (1995). Biological markets. *Trends in Ecology and Evolution*, **10**, 336–339.

Noë, R., van Schaik, C. P. & van Hooff, J. A. R. A. M. (1991) The market effect: an explanation for pay-off asymmetries among collaborating animals. *Ethology*, **87**, 97–118.

10

Sexual behaviour: conflict, cooperation and coevolution

Tommaso Pizzari and Russell Bonduriansky

Overview

In sexually reproducing species, individual fitness is ultimately determined by social interactions over mating and fertilisation among rival members of the same sex and between prospective partners. Variation in the competitive ability to secure reproductive opportunities generates sexual selection, which promotes traits that confer a reproductive advantage in intrasexual competition through combat, scramble, courtship or manipulation, and which may benefit or harm members of the opposite sex. The ensuing intra- and intersexual coevolutionary dynamics often drag phenotypes away from naturally selected optima, producing the spectacular exaggeration that has captured the interest of generations of biologists. In this chapter, we first illustrate how the evolution of differential gametic investment by males and females (anisogamy) sets the scene for sexually dimorphic strategies and, ultimately, determines the intensity of evolutionary conflict between the sexes. In particular, we focus on intra- and interlocus sexual conflicts and their profound but poorly understood repercussions for intersexual coevolution. Second, we outline the principles of sexual selection theory, focusing on their implications for the evolution of sexual behaviour. Finally, we conclude by identifying future directions for the evolutionary analysis of sexual behaviour.

10.1 Introduction: sexual behaviour as a social trait

The lifetime reproductive success, or fitness, of an individual is measured by the representation of its genes in the gene pool of the next generation. In sexually reproducing species, individual fitness reflects the number of zygotes produced by an individual over its lifetime, and – indirectly – the ability of these zygotes to develop and reproduce. Individual variation in fitness is therefore determined by the number of reproductive partners, and the quality of their reproductive investment. In most cases, sexual reproduction is an inevitably social trait, because the reproductive behaviour of an individual will influence not only its own fitness but also the fitness of its prospective partners and that of reproductive competitors (see Chapters 2, 4, 5 and 18). Therefore, to the

Social Behaviour: Genes, Ecology and Evolution, ed. Tamás Székely, Allen J. Moore and Jan Komdeur. Published by Cambridge University Press. © Cambridge University Press 2010.

extent to which they impact reproductive success, traits that determine the outcome of inter- and intra-sexual interactions experience Darwinian selection. At the same time, these traits also function as the social environment generating the selective pressures that drive the coevolutionary response of other such reproductive traits (Moore & Pizzari 2005).

This chapter introduces the evolutionary causes underlying sex-specific selection on reproductive strategies, and explores the consequences of sexual dimorphism for the evolution of sexual behaviour. The study of sexual strategies and intersexual coevolution is vast and growing at an accelerating pace. Reviewing this field is a formidable task, and this chapter is meant only as an introduction to this topical area of social behaviour. We first introduce the concept of anisogamy and review its significance to the evolution of sexual dimorphism and sex-specific reproductive strategies. Second, we outline the fitness relationships arising over interactions within and between sexes. Third, we explain how sexual selection operates on traits that influence variation in the outcome of such sexual interactions. Fourth, we explore the consequences of social selection on sexual behaviour for the coevolution of the sexes. Finally, we conclude by outlining some promising avenues for future research.

10.2 The significance of anisogamy

Sexual reproduction generates disruptive selection on gametic investment which almost invariably leads to gametes of two different sizes, and size-disassortative fertilisation, i.e. the fusion of two gametes of unequal size, or anisogamy (Parker *et al.* 1972). The investment in large gametes (ova), which hold resources to nurture and protect the embryo, is exploited by the opposite sex, which is able to produce higher numbers of smaller and more mobile gametes (sperm) with limited cytoplasmic resources, designed to shuttle their haploid genome to the ovum. We refer to the sex producing ova as female and the sex producing sperm, and which often capitalises on female gametic investment, as male. Anisogamy

represents an evolutionarily stable strategy (ESS, see Chapter 4) relative to either size-assortative alternative. The fusion of two large gametes would provide the embryo with maximal resources, but, due to their scarcity and limited mobility, large gametes are likely to be beaten to fertilisation by small gametes. Similarly, fusion among small, resource-poor gametes would be disadvantaged due to limited parental resources and consequent impaired offspring viability (Parker 1982).

Anisogamy is the rule across multicellular sexually reproducing organisms, where ova are typically orders of magnitude larger than sperm. Even in the few species where males produce giant sperm, ova remain substantially larger. For example, the sperm of *Drosophila bifurca*, the largest sperm known, are 5.83 cm long and nearly twenty times longer than the male himself (Pitnick *et al.* 1995), yet even in this species it takes approximately six spermatozoa to equal the mass of an egg (Bjork and Pitnick 2006). Although several non-mutually exclusive hypotheses have been proposed to explain the maintenance of anisogamy (Table 10.1), a particularly relevant one invokes competition between the ejaculates of different males for fertilisation of a set of eggs (sperm competition: Parker 1970; see below). If a trade-off exists between sperm size and number, any fitness benefit from producing larger sperm (e.g. provisioning embryos with nutrients) will be marginal compared to the fitness benefits of inseminating more sperm under sperm competition (Parker 1982).

10.3 Sex-specific selection and sexual dimorphism

Darwin intuited that anisogamy has a critical impact on the evolution of sexual dimorphism. He noted that males often eagerly pursue females while females are typically coy, often 'endeavouring for a long time to escape from the male' (Darwin 1871), and drew a link between these differences in sexual behaviour and anisogamy. With special emphasis on plants and aquatic invertebrates, he wrote:

Table 10.1. Hypotheses for the evolution of numerous, small sperm. With the exception of the fertility-insurance hypothesis, the other proposed mechanisms imply some degree of sperm competition. See Pizzari & Parker (2009) for a detailed discussion

Fertility insurance	Numerous sperm are required to ensure fertilisation.	Cohen 1973
Sperm competition	Numerous sperm are selected by competition with the ejaculates of other males over fertilisation.	Parker 1982
Meiotic errors	Numerous sperm are required to compensate for deleterious mutations due to recombination errors.[a] This mechanism implies expression of sperm haplotypes and competition between the ejaculates of different males.[b] Sperm competition may also select for males that can produce many sperm without incurring high rates of recombination errors.[c]	[a] Cohen 1969, 1973 [b] Manning & Chamberlain 1994 [c] Blumenstiel 2007

We are naturally led to enquire why the male, in so many and such distinct classes, has become more eager than the female, so that he searches for her, and plays the more active part in courtship. [...] With lowly-organised aquatic animals, permanently affixed to the same spot and having their sexes separate, the male element is invariably brought to the female; and of this we can see the reason, for *even if the ova were detached before fertilisation, and did not require subsequent nourishment or protection, there would yet be greater difficulty in transporting them than the male element, because, being larger than the latter, they are produced in far smaller numbers. So that many of the lower animals are, in this respect, analogous with plants.*

Darwin 1871, p. 274, emphasis added

Darwin (1871) proposed that these sex-specific behaviours are associated with males having to compete among themselves for reproductive opportunities and females selecting reproductive partners.

10.3.1 Revisiting Bateman's principle

In 1948, Bateman experimentally tested Darwin's idea by analysing the reproductive success of individual male and female fruit flies *Drosophila melanogaster* in freely mating groups of 5–7 individuals. By assigning offspring maternity and paternity through phenotypic markers, Bateman (1948) was able to show two critical points. First, the number of offspring produced was much more variable among individual males than among individual females. Second, the number of offspring produced by a male increased sharply

with the number of females whose eggs the male had fertilised, whereas the number of offspring produced by a female did not increase as rapidly with the number of males with whom she copulated (Bateman's principle: Fig. 10.1; Wilson 1975). Bateman (1948) argued that these results demonstrated that competition over reproductive opportunities is more intense among males than among females, and that because males produce sperm at a faster rate than females produce eggs, male reproductive success is limited by the number of eggs available for fertilisation. These mechanisms were consistent with Darwin's view and provided a proximate explanation for why males are eager and females coy.

Bateman's (1948) study went largely unnoticed until Trivers (1972), Wilson (1975), Maynard Smith (1977) and, later, Clutton-Brock and Parker (1992) and Parker and Simmons (1996) discussed Bateman's principle in relation to parental investment and reproductive strategies. These models suggested that anisogamy leads to higher male potential reproductive rates. Therefore, often a male will gain more by mating with a new female (i.e. re-mating) than by investing in the current reproductive event, while the female is left with the 'cruel bind' of maternal investment, as Trivers (1972) put it. This process biases the operational sex ratio of a population (i.e. the ratio of sexually receptive males to sexually receptive females at a given point in time) towards males, thus exacerbating male–male competition over the few sexually receptive females available at any given time. In

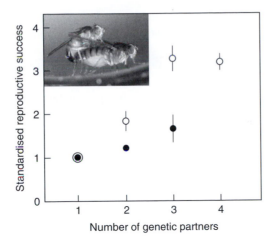

Figure 10.1 Results of Bateman's study of variation in the reproductive success of male and female *D. melanogaster* across nine different combinations of genetic markers. The graph illustrates the relationship between the number of genetic partners (i.e. partners with whom an individual has produced offspring) and the standardised individual reproductive success averaged (± SE) for each sex across the nine mating combinations conducted by Bateman (male, open data points; female, filled data points). In monogamous situations (i.e. when an individual reproduces with only one partner), male reproductive success equals that of the female (circled data point). Males can increase their reproductive success by fertilising the eggs of additional females more than females can increase their reproductive success by having their eggs fertilised by additional males. However, against this general trend two more subtle effects emerge. First, male reproductive success does not increase when mating with more than three females, indicating that sperm depletion and sperm competition may constrain optimal male re-mating frequency. Second, while not as pronounced as in males, female reproductive success shows a tendency to increase with re-mating, suggesting that females too may benefit from some degree of promiscuity. Adapted from Bateman (1948).

other words, relative parental investments by males and females dictate potential reproductive rates and the operational sex ratio of a population, explaining why intrasexual competition is often more intense in males than in females (see Chapter 11).

Recent studies have confirmed Bateman's (1948) main results of greater standardised variances in reproductive and mating success, and a stronger relationship between re-mating rates and number of offspring produced, in males than in females in many species (but see Lorch *et al.* 2008). However, the implications of these trends have come under renewed scrutiny (e.g. Dewsbury 2005, Snyder & Gowaty 2007). Sex differences in intrasexual variance in reproductive success do not necessarily explain why males compete and females choose. The sex in which intrasexual competition is less intense is not necessarily under more intense selection to select partners, because choosiness also depends on the

variability in the quality of reproductive investment among prospective partners and the costs of mating (Owens & Thompson 1994, Johnstone *et al.* 1996, Bondurianský 2001, Kokko *et al.* 2006). Similarly, it is now apparent that the operational sex ratio of a population may be decoupled from intrasexual competition. For example, males may still face more intense reproductive competition than females even when the operational sex ratio of a population is female-biased (Kokko & Monaghan 2001).

Moreover, the idea that females do not gain by re-mating, based on original interpretations of Bateman's results (Bateman 1948, Trivers 1972), has been challenged. Bateman monitored *quantitative*, not *qualitative*, changes in female reproductive success as a function of realised polyandry (number of males fertilising a set of eggs). Mounting evidence indicates that offspring viability often increases when females re-mate, especially with different partners (polyandry), indicating that females may be able to accrue qualitative benefits by re-mating. Indeed, one of Bateman's two replicate experiments indicated that the number of offspring produced by a female did increase with the degree of realised polyandry. This may be because males target the most fecund females, or because paternity is more evenly distributed across males in larger clutches. However, an alternative explanation is that *D. melanogaster* seminal fluid products, which cause females to augment their oviposition rate (Box 10.1), might have cumulative properties. Recent work has shown that, up to a point, female fecundity certainly increases with mating rate in many insects, either as a result of such chemical manipulation of female reproductive effort by males, or because males transfer nutritious nuptial gifts to their mates (Arnqvist & Nilsson 2000, Alonzo & Pizzari 2010). It appears increasingly clear, therefore, that polyandry can augment both offspring number and quality (Arnqvist & Nilsson 2000, Simmons 2005), indicating that females – like males – may be selected to mate with multiple partners (Table 10.2). Nonetheless, higher potential reproductive rates and intrasexual competition mean that optimal re-mating rates are still often likely to be lower for females than for males (Arnqvist & Nilsson 2000, Arnqvist & Rowe 2005), generating sexual conflict over re-mating decisions (see below).

Box 10.1 Are Acps potential molecular agents of intersexual cooperation, conflict or both?

Alex Wong, Laura K. Sirot and Mariana F. Wolfner

The Acps (accessory gland proteins) of *Drosophila melanogaster* may provide molecular tools to dissect the mechanisms underlying intersexual cooperation and conflict (Cordero 1995, Eberhard & Cordero 1995, Arnqvist & Rowe 2005). Acps are proteins, synthesised in the male's accessory glands, that constitute part of the seminal fluid transferred during mating. Presently, 112 putative or known *D. melanogaster* Acps have been identified (reviewed in Ravi Ram & Wolfner 2007a). Acps fall into a number of biochemical classes, including peptide hormones and their precursors, proteolytic enzymes and their regulators, sperm-binding molecules, and protective molecules such as antioxidants and antimicrobial peptides. Proteins in these classes are found in the seminal fluid of all insects and vertebrates examined to date (reviewed in Gillott 2003, Poiani 2006), and, presumably, will be found in the seminal fluid of other taxa when they are examined.

The importance of Acps in modulating reproductive phenomena associated with intersexual conflict and/or cooperation is well known in *D. melanogaster*. In female flies, Acps are essential for several post-mating effects. For example, Acp36DE facilitates sperm storage (Neubaum & Wolfner 1999), ovulin stimulates ovulation (Heifetz *et al.* 2000), sex peptide induces sexual refractoriness (i.e. unwillingness to re-mate), increased egg production and feeding, and decreased female lifespan (e.g. Chapman *et al.* 2003, Liu & Kubli 2003, Wigby & Chapman 2005, Carvalho *et al.* 2006), and CG9997 regulates the release of sperm from storage in females, and the maintenance of other post-mating effects (Ravi Ram & Wolfner 2007b). Acps have also been associated with changes in females' RNA and protein profiles that occur in response to mating (McGraw *et al.* 2004, 2008, Peng *et al.* 2005). Postcopulatory effects also require female contributions and/or functions (e.g. molecules, musculature, physiological environment: Kapelnikov *et al.* 2008), raising the interesting possibility of whether Acps are 'manipulating' the female for the male's benefit, or the female is 'exploiting' Acps for her benefit, or a combination of both. Identifying and dissecting the roles of Acps and female contributions in controlling female post-mating responses provides molecular insights into the mechanisms underlying intersexual cooperation and conflict.

For example, male–female molecular interactions involved in proteolytic cleavage (the directed splitting or degradation of proteins by enzymes) of particular Acps could underlie, or reflect, conflict or cooperation. To date, six Acps are known to be cleaved while en route to, or within, the mated female reproductive tract, including Acp36DE, ovulin, sex peptide and CG9997. Cleavage is proposed to activate sex peptide, releasing it from storage to enter the female's circulation. For ovulin, Acp36DE and CG9997, it is unknown whether cleavage is activational (e.g. liberates bioactive peptides from a precursor, or removes an inhibitory peptide) or degradational (e.g. limits how long the Acp is active in females). Cleavage of ovulin and Acp36DE appears to result from a proteolytic cascade (i.e. multiple proteolysis steps that each depend on the previous step: Ravi Ram *et al.* 2006). The Acp protease CG11864 is cleaved in the male reproductive tract en route to the female. CG11864 is, in turn, necessary for cleaving both ovulin and Acp36DE. However, this cleavage only occurs once all three proteins have entered the female, suggesting that female contributions are also necessary. Our preliminary data suggest that a female-expressed predicted protease inhibitor regulates the rate of ovulin cleavage. The processing of ovulin and Acp36DE could be a case of intersexual cooperation, in which contributions from both sexes act in concert to regulate the rate of proteolysis to maximise their reproductive output. Alternatively, the rate of proteolysis that maximises reproductive output could be different for the male and female, resulting in conflict between their contributions to bias the rate towards different optima. An interesting feature of the processing of both ovulin and Acp36DE is that the female and male contributions are exerting their effects apparently by acting within the same molecular pathway (Ravi Ram *et al.* 2006).

It is generally difficult to determine whether male–female interactions mediated by Acps are cooperative or conflicting. The rapid rate of molecular evolution of some Acps is consistent with sexual selection (Haerty *et al.* 2007, Panhuis *et al.* 2006), but conflict and cooperation cannot be distinguished using sequence data alone. Complementary approaches, which attempt to associate variation in fitness components with allelic variation at Acp loci, have yielded tantalising results (Fiumera *et al.* 2005, 2006, 2007). In one case, an Acp allele associated with decreased female longevity was also associated with sperm competitive ability, and a different Acp that has been shown to decrease female longevity (sex peptide) also appears to increase male reproductive success (increased egg production and mating-refractoriness by their mates: see Fiumera *et al.* 2006 and references therein). While it is tempting to interpret these longevity effects in the light of sexual conflict, it is important to note that lifespan reduction may be a tolerated negative side effect of positive effects on female fitness. Interestingly, one recent study has found evidence that Acps affect offspring fitness (Priest *et al.* 2007). Ultimately, then, more comprehensive fitness measures are required to determine the contributions of specific Acps to male and female fitness.

In conclusion, the identification of male-derived molecules that affect female post-mating reproductive behaviours, physiology and output provides a class of

Box 10.1 Continued

molecular probes with which to tease apart the 'male side' of molecular interactions between the sexes. Recent studies identifying genes regulated by Acps, or whose products interact with Acps (such as a recently reported receptor for sex peptide: Yapici *et al.* 2008) provide molecular probes for the 'female side'. Studies that integrate the activities of these gene sets into molecular pathways, and identify each gene's effect on male and female fitness, have the potential to address the mechanisms underlying conflict or cooperation. For example, identification of female molecules that interact with Acps (e.g. Yapici *et al.* 2008) will allow tests for coevolution of the male and female molecules, which would support certain models of sexual selection.

Table 10.2. Some direct and indirect mechanisms that may favour the maintenance of female polyandry. Direct selection on female fecundity or fertility would result in a positive relationship between female re-mating rate and the number of offspring produced, tested by Bateman (1948). However, the Bateman approach would not detect positive effects of re-mating on female longevity, and offspring fitness. See Simmons (2005), Cornell & Tregenza (2007) and Kempenaers (2007) for recent discussions of female re-mating

Selection mechanism	Fitness payoff	Hypothesis
Direct selection	Female fertility	Pursuit of sufficient sperm supplies. Bet-hedging against the risk of partner infertility.
	Female fecundity, longevity	Mating is associated with commodities such as nutrients with cumulative effects on female fitness.
	Female fertility	Bet-hedging against the risk of infertility determined by genetic incompatibility between gametes.
	Female longevity	Resisting re-mating is more costly to a female than accepting re-mating (convenience polyandry).
	Female longevity	Paternal care from multiple males reduces maternal investment.
Indirect selection	Offspring viability	Increased offspring heterozygosity, genome-wide or at candidate loci.
	Offspring viability	Avoidance of inbreeding depression.
	Offspring viability	Increased probability that some young will survive (genetic bet-hedging).
	Offspring viability	Increased offspring viability fostered by sperm competition and genetic covariance between ejaculate quality and viability (good sperm).
	Sons' reproductive success	Increased fertilising efficiency of sons (sexy sperm).
	Offspring viability and reproductive success	Females re-mate with partners of better genetic quality than previous partners (trading up).
	Offspring reproductive success and grand-offspring viability.	Reduced risk of offspring inbreeding in species where breeding occurs within family groups, due to the fact that the offspring of polyandrous females may have different fathers.

In addition, the original interpretation of Bateman's (1948) results does not take into account the effect of the competition between the ejaculates of different males to fertilise a set of eggs (sperm competition), which often occurs when females mate multiply. Sperm competition weakens the relationship between male copulation success and fertilisation success. In the absence of sperm competition, an average ejaculate is often sufficient to fertilise all the female's eggs, and variation in fertilisation success is mostly determined by female fecundity. Under sperm competition, however, fertilisation success is determined by the outcome of the competition with ejaculates of competing males, and copulation may not necessarily result in fertilisation. Bateman, however, equated mating success with fertilisation success and concluded that males with higher re-mating rates produced more offspring. Bateman was aware of potential problems associated with female promiscuity, but the evolutionary significance of sperm competition would only be recognised 22 years after Bateman's study by Parker (1970). Dewsbury (2005) pointed out that Bateman's principle has been translated into: 'males that copulate with more females produce more offspring than males that copulate with fewer females', but this is not necessarily true under sperm competition.

The correct interpretation of Bateman's results is more circular: males that fertilised the eggs of more females fertilised more eggs overall. Sperm competition therefore limits selection on male re-mating (Shuster & Wade 2003, 2005). Sperm competition can also promote increased ejaculate expenditure by the male, and sperm production may weaken the relationship between copulation success and fertilisation success (Dewsbury 2005). Similarly, males may face a trade-off between seeking additional partners and protecting paternity in current partners. Thus, by copulating with more females, a male may reduce the number of offspring that he fathers with each of these females (Shuster & Wade 2005). Some evidence of sperm depletion emerged from one of Bateman's replicate experiments, where males that fertilised the eggs of three females produced more offspring than males that fertilised the eggs of four females. In

addition, under some conditions (see Parker & Begon 1993), sperm competition may promote the production of fewer but larger sperm. This strategy appears paradoxical because it pushes males towards female-like patterns of gametic investment and might relax sexual selection on male re-mating rates (Pizzari 2006). Finally, sperm competition reduces male confidence in paternity, and this is expected to reduce paternal investment (Queller 1997).

10.3.2 Implications of Bateman's principle

A new picture is beginning to emerge in which anisogamy influences intrasexual competition and the evolution of sex roles in a more complex way than originally believed. First, anisogamy often means that the most successful males will have much higher reproductive success than the most successful females in a population. Second, under sperm competition, confidence in paternity is reduced. These mechanisms explain why males often tend to invest more than females in the pursuit of new reproductive opportunities, and consequently why sexual selection is typically more intense on males (Queller 1997, Kokko *et al.* 2006). To a degree these mechanisms may also help explain why females may be more intensely selected to discriminate among prospective partners.

This does not mean, however, that reproductive competition is unimportant in females and sexual preference unimportant in males. Even the very nature of traditional sex roles is being revisited (Bondurianksy 2001, Clutton-Brock 2007). That sex roles may be reversed under some exceptional ecological circumstances has long been recognised. Until recently, however, sex-role-reversed species were considered the exception that confirms the rule. We are now beginning to realise that female–female competition and male selection of partners also occur in species with traditional sex roles (Bondurianksy 2001), and that sex-role-reversed species may represent one end of a continuous gradient, along which the relative intensity of reproductive competition and selection to re-mate varies within each sex. For example, in a population of two-spotted gobies *Gobiusculus flavescens* a gradual decline in males over the breeding season shifts the operational sex ratio from male-biased at the beginning of the season to female-biased towards the end of the season (Forsgren *et al.* 2004; see Chapter 11). Sex roles shift accordingly, with male–male competition and male courtship early in the season replaced by female–female competition and female courtship later on (Forsgren *et al.* 2004). The ecological plasticity of sex roles was neatly demonstrated in the bushcricket *Metaballus* sp. (Gwynne & Simmons 1990). The ejaculate of male bushcrickets contains a nutrient-rich component (the spermatophylax) that is readily consumed by the female. When females were fed a poor diet, spermatophylaxes became a particularly valuable resource, and females competed fiercely with one another over access to males and their spermatophylaxes.

In conclusion, Bateman's (1948) study crystallised the traditional view that anisogamy results in males competing more intensely for access to reproductive opportunities than females. However, new empirical and theoretical research suggests that sex differences in reproductive competition and sexual preference arise through a more complex network of underlying mechanisms than previously appreciated. In the next section, we discuss how asymmetries in reproductive competition between sexes influence the potential for evolutionary cooperation and conflict within and between sexes.

10.4 Sexual cooperation and conflict

With a clearer view of sex roles and sex-specific selective pressures acting on sexual behaviour, we now briefly explore the fitness implications of social interactions within and between sexes, and discuss the different social mechanisms arising from such interactions. We consider interactions within sexes first, and then between sexes.

As we have seen, under most circumstances, males compete to fertilise the eggs of a female, and thus are in evolutionary conflict with each other. Eggs often represent a fitness-related resource whose consumption (i.e. fertilisation) by a male excludes consumption by other males and simultaneously diminishes the

number of eggs available to other males. Intrasexual competition therefore favours behaviours that enable the acquisition of a larger share of reproductive resources. Often, however, the reproductive investment of a male in a female may 'unintentionally' benefit competing males mating with the same female. For example, a male can increase the quantity and/or the viability of the offspring produced by a female through a number of mechanisms, including the provision of nuptial gifts, the stimulation of maternal investment or oviposition rate, or parental care. Similarly, the ejaculate of a male may neutralise immunological barriers and render the female reproductive tract less hostile to subsequent, rival inseminations (Hodgson & Hosken 2006). In these cases, information on whether a female has already mated with another male or will do so in the near future might enable a male to benefit from the reproductive investment of rival males inseminating the same female. For example, a male may fertilise the eggs that will have been produced through the investment of another male, or father offspring that will benefit from the care of another male (Alonzo & Pizzari 2010). One possible outcome of such parasitic coevolutionary dynamics among competing males is for a male to reduce reproductive investment in a female, and thus the overall amount and/or quality of reproductive resources available to the males mating with her. Similarly, competition among males over access to receptive females can lead to male sexual harassment of females which ultimately reduces the availability of receptive females in such populations (Le Galliard *et al.* 2005). Situations in which intrasexual competition reduces the resources available to competitors have been interpreted as a reproductive tragedy of the commons (see Chapter 6; Rankin *et al.* 2007).

In principle, it is even possible that a male may spitefully pay a net fitness cost to actively reduce the availability or quality of reproductive resources for rival males (see Chapter 5). Several studies have claimed that intrasexual competition may lead to spiteful behaviours (e.g. Baker 1983, Foster 1983, Greenfield 1994). However, often seemingly spiteful behaviours result – on average – in a net fitness benefit (rather than a cost) to the actor, indicating that, rather than being spiteful, such behaviours are often self-ish (Foster *et al.* 2001, West *et al.* 2007). Situations in which males benefit by cooperating to reproduce with the same female are scarcer and less intuitive. Such situations may arise when individual males have a higher probability of mating by cooperating with other males. In addition, it has been recently shown that in species where male reproductive investment has a relatively strong and cumulative impact on reproductive success (due for example to different mechanisms that stimulate female fecundity), the reproductive success of each of two individual males can be higher when they both mate with the same female rather than when each mates with a different female (Alonzo & Pizzari 2010).

At a mechanistic level, successful reproduction also requires a degree of coordination and cooperation between partners. However, from an evolutionary perspective, the fitness interests of two prospective partners may either converge or diverge. When a male and a female meet, both may gain – or both may lose by mating with each other. In such situations mating will be sought or avoided by mutual interest. Convergence of fitness interests over mating decisions mostly occurs when two individuals can only reproduce with each other – in other words, when both partners maximise fitness through lifetime genetic monogamy. The advent of molecular tools to assign paternity in the 1980s and 1990s, combined with studies of sexual behaviour, has dispelled the myth that most species are genetically monogamous, showing instead that some members of at least one sex typically mate with multiple partners.

So does true genetic monogamy ever exist, or is it simply a useful theoretical abstraction? The answer is that it does exist, but it is rare. Strict genetic monogamy is expected to evolve when the pursuit of multiple partners is a less profitable strategy than investing in reproduction with a single partner. This may arise under ecological and life-history conditions in which reproductive partners are scarce or difficult to access, biparental care is a prerequisite for reproductive success, and reproductive success increases with the experience and coordination of reproductive pairs (see Chapter 11). Even under strict genetic monogamy,

however, males and females are still likely to experience different selection pressures on some genes (sex-specific selection generating intralocus sexual conflict: see below). Some form of evolutionary conflict between the sexes (sexual conflict) thus appears to be an unavoidable feature of sex itself.

Sexual conflict arises whenever females and males cannot maximise their fitness simultaneously and in exactly the same way. There are two mechanisms through which this can happen. First, sexual conflict over reproductive decisions occurs whenever parental investment is costly and alternative reproductive opportunities are available to at least one of the partners. If multiple reproductive opportunities are available to an individual, sexual conflict arises with members of the opposite sex over the partitioning of its reproductive investment across reproductive events (Lessells 2006). Such conflict between actual or prospective partners over reproductive decisions is mediated by conflict between different sexually antagonistic loci (interlocus sexual conflict). In addition, independently of social interactions between reproductive partners, conflict can also arise over the evolution of genetic loci subject to sex-specific selection (intralocus sexual conflict).

10.4.1 Interlocus sexual conflict

At the genetic level, conflict between reproductive partners over reproductive decisions is manifested in the evolution of separate loci that function to further the interests of one sex at the expense of the other, such as loci that enhance males' ability to coerce females into mating, and other loci that enhance females' ability to resist male advances. These sexually antagonistic genes at different (and perhaps often sex-limited) loci convey a competitive advantage to the carrier but impose a fitness cost on its partners. This results in *interlocus* sexual conflict. We adopt an example used by Parker (2006) to illustrate this. Imagine two sex-limited loci: M is expressed in males and F in females. M prescribes 'in situation X, attempt to mate', and F prescribes 'in situation X, attempt to avoid mating', where mating and not mating are respectively the optimal responses of males and females in situation X. Mutant alleles at M (or F) that help male (female) carriers reach their own reproductive optimum will be at a selective advantage despite the costs imposed on reproductive partners, creating an evolutionary conflict between the two loci (Parker 2006).

Consider the case of the blue-headed wrasse *Thalassoma bifasciatum*. The males of this reef fish defend territories where females convene to spawn their eggs, but some of the more colourful males are able to attract more eggs than they can fertilise. On average, 7% of the eggs shed by a female visiting one of these attractive males will not be fertilised, because males economise their sperm allocation across multiple females (Warner *et al.* 1995). From the perspective of a sperm-depleted male this makes sense: by attracting more spawning females he can father more offspring even if a small proportion of the eggs of each female will not be fertilised. However, an individual female visiting an attractive male will produce 7% fewer offspring than a female visiting a less successful male. The harm inflicted by attractive male wrasse appears a collateral by-product of male reproductive strategies: within the limited resources available to a male, strategies that maximise his reproductive success also happen to reduce female fitness. Several cases of sexual conflict are likely to be mediated by such collateral damage of the other sex (e.g. Morrow *et al.* 2003). Even when both sexes gain by mating, sexual conflict may arise over subsequent reproductive decisions such as how much each partner should invest in the current reproductive event, and whether each should re-mate with other partners, and the frequency at which they should do so.

An individual can coerce reproductive partners into reproductive decisions that increase its own reproductive success. Sexual coercion often occurs through sexual harassment (Clutton-Brock & Parker 1995). However, an individual may also coerce partners through sexual intimidation or punishment (Clutton-Brock & Parker 1995). Here, the actor enforces cooperation by imposing or threatening to impose fitness costs on the recipient. For example, if a male punishes a female every time that she refuses to mate with him (or that she mates with a competitor),

the female is expected to learn to mate with him (or not mate with others), provided that the cumulative harm of punishment has the potential to outweigh the costs associated with mating with this male (Clutton-Brock & Parker 1995). However, despite some anecdotal evidence consistent with sexual punishment (Clutton-Brock & Parker 1995, Valera *et al.* 2003), the experimental demonstration of these social mechanisms remains elusive. A similarly sinister scenario may occur where males may actually gain *directly* by damaging their partners. First, by harming females, a male might cause them to forgo re-mating with other males in order to avoid even greater harm (Johnstone & Keller 2000). Second, by reducing females' life expectancy, a male might be able to induce them to elevate their short-term reproductive effort as a terminal investment strategy (Lessells 2005).

An additional factor that may exacerbate sexual conflict is that typically partners are not related to each other genetically, therefore eliminating kin-selected mechanisms of altruism. As Dawkins (1976) pointed out in *The Selfish Gene*, if evolutionary conflict occurs even between a parent and its own offspring, the potential for conflict will be that much greater among partners who are not usually genetically related. The role of kin selection in sexual conflict has been investigated by Parker (1979) and Kokko and Ots (2006) with respect to inbreeding decisions. Inbreeding is the mating between close relatives, and, by increasing the reproductive success of a related partner, inbreeding would in principle enable an individual to increase its own inclusive fitness, in the absence of inbreeding costs. However, inbreeding can severely depress offspring fitness through two mechanisms: (1) increased probability that deleterious recessive alleles will be expressed, and (2) loss of fitness advantages associated with heterozygosity (overdominance). Selection on inbreeding is therefore determined by the relative magnitude of inbreeding depression. Because of asymmetries in male and female reproductive investment, selection on inbreeding is sex-specific. In general, theory predicts that males should be more inbreeding-tolerant than females (Parker 1979, 2006, Kokko & Ots 2006). If investment in a given reproductive event (e.g. parental and mating investment) is lower for males than for females we expect that – with intermediate levels of inbreeding depression – males gain but females lose fitness by reproducing with a relative. Consistent with this prediction, male red junglefowl *Gallus gallus* are just as likely to inseminate a full-sib sister as an unrelated female when experimentally exposed to either type of female, and may even inseminate more sperm in their sisters (Pizzari *et al.* 2004). Female junglefowl, on the other hand, appear to select against the sperm of full-sib brothers following insemination, suggesting that sexual conflict over inbreeding promotes counteracting strategies. With increasing male reproductive investment or with reduced female availability, male inbreeding tolerance is expected to decline and converge towards female levels (Parker 1979, 2006, Kokko & Ots 2006).

In principle, interlocus conflict might give rise to sexually antagonistic coevolution, where antagonistic alleles accumulate at different sex-limited loci as each sex evolves counter-adaptations to retain control over reproduction. A popular way to visualise this process is to picture the two sexes as locked in an intimate dance in which each step by one dancer is matched by the steps of the other on the dance floor of evolutionary time. Demonstrating such an intimate coevolutionary process is challenging, and experimental studies have provided ambiguous results.

Work by Rice and colleagues on *D. melanogaster* has produced tantalising glances of sexually antagonistic coevolution. When females were prevented from coevolving with males, they evolved to be less able to resist the costs of mating, and suffered higher mortality rates (Rice 1996). Holland and Rice (1999) experimentally evolved male and female lines under different mating systems. In one treatment, three males competed to fertilise the eggs of a single female (enforced male competition). In a second treatment, each female was paired with a single randomly assigned male (enforced monogamy). By crossing these lines, experimentally evolved for 47 generations, with partners from the stock population with intermediate levels of male competition, Holland and Rice (1999) showed that males from the enforced-monogamy lines had evolved to be more benign to their partners than males from

the enforced-male-competition lines. Subsequent work showed that enforced monogamy had resulted in smaller males with proportionally smaller and less efficient testes (Pitnick *et al.* 2001). However, asymmetries in effective population size, density and inbreeding between experimental treatments may have confounded the effect of sexual selection in Holland and Rice's experiment (e.g. Snook 2001).

Follow-up experiments by Wigby and Chapman (2004) exposed *D. melanogaster* populations to three different treatments of experimental evolution which manipulated the sex ratio of a population, while maintaining population size constant: (a) male-biased (intense male competition and high potential for sexual conflict), (b) female-biased (relaxed male competition and reduced potential for sexual conflict), and (c) equal sex ratios as control. This elegant design enabled the authors to demonstrate that, consistent with previous findings, female-biased regimes led to the evolution of less male-resistant females that suffered greater harm when exposed to males than the more male-resistant females from the male-biased lines. However, contrary to predictions, males did not differ in their ability to harm females across treatments, suggesting that differential male harm was likely determined by differences in mating frequencies rather than by specific sexually antagonistic male traits. A similar experimental design was used by Crudgington *et al.* (2005) to study sexual conflict in *D. pseudoobscura*. Crudgington *et al.* (2005) quantified the effect of selection treatments on reproductive fitness payoffs under different male density treatments, thus disentangling the effects of an evolutionary response to sexual selection from the proximate effects of population density. Males evolved under elevated male competition intensity displayed an increased ability to inhibit female re-mating propensity. However, contrary to expectations, male selection history did not affect female fitness, but – consistent with Wigby and Chapman's (2004) findings – male density did. In addition, females evolved under elevated sexual selection were relatively more fecund and enjoyed relatively high reproductive success. Further research is clearly needed to disentangle these perplexing results.

10.4.2 Intralocus sexual conflict

We have seen in the previous sections that anisogamy leads to sex-specific selection on numerous traits. However, because the sexes share much of the genome, many genes underlying the expression of such traits will be expressed in both males and females. This means that adult males and females are expected to experience contrasting patterns of selection on many shared loci, and on the phenotypic traits whose expression is influenced by such loci. As a result, an allele might have sexually antagonistic effects on fitness, enhancing fitness when expressed in one sex but reducing fitness when expressed in the other sex. Evolutionary conflict might therefore arise between different alleles segregating at the same locus, with opposite fitness effects (i.e. male-beneficial/female-detrimental versus male-detrimental/female-beneficial). Such *intralocus* sexual conflict may impede the evolution of traits that are homologous in males and females towards their sex-specific phenotypic optima, because such traits tend to be affected by the same genes in both sexes (Lande 1980, Rice 1984).

The key distinction between interlocus and intralocus forms of sexual conflict is that the former reflects sexually antagonistic coevolution between different loci (male-benefit and female-benefit loci) in the genome, whereas the latter reflects sexually antagonistic coevolution between different alleles (male-benefit and female-benefit alleles) within a single locus. Note, however, that male- or female-benefit loci involved in interlocus sexual conflict may also be prime epicentres of intralocus sexual conflict, since alleles segregating at such loci will tend to enhance fitness when expressed in one sex, but may reduce fitness when expressed in the other sex, unless such loci are fully sex-limited in their expression. The evolutionary resolution of intralocus sexual conflict lies in restricting the inheritance or expression of sexually antagonistic alleles to the sex in which these alleles are beneficial, thus reducing the intersexual genetic correlation and permitting a closer approach to optimal sexual dimorphism (Bonduriansky & Chenoweth 2009). This can be achieved by reducing

trait heritability through opposite-sex parents via genomic imprinting (Day & Bonduriansky 2004, Bonduriansky & Rowe 2005). Similarly, the evolution of sex-linkage (Rice 1984), sex-limited trait expression (Rhen 2000), or even more complex facultative mechanisms (Bonduriansky & Chenoweth 2009), could mitigate intralocus sexual conflict.

The puzzle of intralocus sexual conflict centres on three related questions. First, how widespread and important are such conflicts, both taxonomically and in relation to particular traits? Second, are such conflicts transient, with the evolution of genomic modifications rapidly mitigating their severity (see above), or are they a long-term (even permanent) impediment to the evolution of optimal sexual dimorphism? With regard to the first question, although evidence is still very limited, laboratory and field studies have provided direct evidence of such conflict in taxa ranging from insects to mammals and birds (Chippindale *et al.* 2001, Fedorka & Mousseau 2004, Brommer *et al.* 2007, Foerster *et al.* 2007). Influence of intersexual genetic correlations on sexual behaviour provides additional, indirect evidence (see below). A much broader taxonomic survey is, of course, needed before firm conclusions can be reached. The second question is more difficult to answer, and will require a better empirical and theoretical understanding of the genetic basis of sexually dimorphic traits. Bedhomme and Chippindale (2007) have argued that intralocus sexual conflicts may be intractable. Moreover, novel conflicts may arise as a by-product of sexual coevolution, including interlocus sexual conflict (see below). The mitigating evolution of genetic architecture is unlikely to keep pace (see Bonduriansky and Chenoweth 2009). The third question is the most difficult of all: what are the long-term implications of intralocus sexual conflict for intersexual coevolution? This form of sexual conflict has generally been viewed as a break on intersexual coevolution and the evolution of sexual dimorphism (e.g. Lande 1980, Pischedda & Chippindale 2006). However, theory also suggests the intriguing possibility that intralocus sexual conflict could play a role in adaptive evolution and speciation (Lande & Kirkpatrick 1989, Bonduriansky & Chenoweth 2009).

In the next sections, we outline sexual selection theory and discuss how asymmetries in reproductive competition between sexes influence the operation of sexual selection.

10.5 Sexual selection

Competition over reproductive opportunities generates individual variation in the number and quality of reproductive partners among members of the same sex. Sexual selection is the evolutionary process that arises from this variation to promote traits that confer an advantage in competition for mates. Variance in relative number and quality of reproductive partners among same-sex individuals represents the opportunity for sexual selection. Traits whose expression

covaries with the number and quality of reproductive partners are the targets of sexual selection. An evolutionary response to sexual selection occurs when there is sufficient additive genetic variance underlying the sexually selected trait or combination of traits under sexual selection.

Darwin (1859, 1871) proposed the idea of sexual selection to explain why in many species males but not females display exaggerated traits that could not be explained by viability selection, and why such male traits displayed more divergence between closely related species than did female traits. Darwin identified two mechanisms, often called intra- and intersexual selection, through which a trait can influence reproductive competition (Fig. 10.2). We discuss each of these mechanisms below.

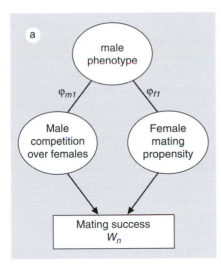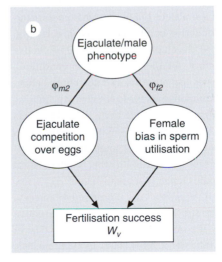

Figure 10.2 Episodes of sexual selection on males. (a) At a pre-insemination stage, sexual selection operates on male phenotypic traits that covary with mating success (W_n). Such covariance may arise through a direct effect of a trait on intrasexual competition over access to partners (φ_{m1}), or through an effect on female behaviour that influences mating success (φ_{f1}). (b) When the ejaculates of multiple males compete for fertilisation, sexual selection continues to operate after insemination on the subset of the male population that managed to mate with at least one female. Here, sexual selection operates on phenotypic traits of the male and/or of the ejaculate that covary with fertilisation success (W_v) through a direct effect on sperm competition (φ_{m2}) or through an effect on female responses in sperm utilisation that bias fertilisation success (φ_{f2}). Overall male reproductive success is therefore determined by the product of $W_n \times W_v$. Interactions between male and female phenotypes/genotypes pre- and post-insemination create additional sources of variance in male reproductive success with non-transitive effects (see text).

10.5.1 Intrasexual selection: alternative tactics, cross-dressing and sexual coalitions

Members of the same sex interact in various ways in competition over access to reproductive partners. Competition often occurs through scrambles in which competitors independently search for partners. Often, the access to mating opportunities is determined through direct ritualised contests between males. In social species, the outcome of these pair-wise contests can lead to dominance hierarchies, in which socially dominant individuals consistently outcompete subordinates, and the distribution in mating success is heavily skewed towards a dominant minority. In some cases, male–male competition occurs without direct interactions – a male may outcompete others by retaining reproductive condition and resources over a prolonged period of time, displaying at more suitable times, etc. (Murphy 1998). Intrasexual selection in males is thought to underlie the evolution of traits enabling males to reach reproductive territories and reproductive condition relatively early (e.g. protandry: the development of male reproductive condition before female reproductive condition), seek out females (e.g. motility and searching behaviours), and monopolise access to females (e.g. fighting behaviours, armaments, large body size, high levels of plasma testosterone). Intrasexual selection also encompasses aspects of sperm competition (i.e. variation in sperm competitive ability that is independent of cryptic female choice, discussed below).

When high variance in reproductive success occurs within the predominant tactic, alternative tactics within the same sex can invade and persist in a population (Shuster & Wade 2003). In many species, males have evolved alternative sexual tactics, often associated with drastically different phenotypes and behaviours (Oliveira *et al.* 2008, Gross 1996). Male alternative tactics often reflect different ways to optimise a trade-off between investments in different episodes of sexual selection. Tactics focused on monopolising females or territories face relatively low risk of cuckolding by other males (see below), while tactics that do not involve defence of females or territories (such as sneaking, discussed below) face higher

risk of losing paternity and invest preferentially in ejaculate traits associated with fertilising efficiency, as in the bluegill sunfish *Lepomis macrochirus* (Fig. 10.3). Alternative tactics are also common in insects. In many scarabeid beetles (e.g. *Onthophagus taurus*), large, 'major' males express horns that they use in combat with rivals, whereas small, 'minor' males lack horns and resemble females. A male's status as 'major' or 'minor' is condition-dependent, being determined by the quality of diet that he encounters as a larva (Emlen 1994). 'Majors' defeat 'minors' in combat, but 'minors' are more agile in scramble competition within narrow underground tunnels where females lay eggs (Moczek & Emlen 2000). Interestingly, only the 'major' males help females to provision larvae with dung, thus producing larger offspring and sons that are more likely to be 'majors' (Hunt & Simmons 2000). The bluegill sunfish and dung beetle examples illustrate conditional polymorphisms, but some polymorphisms have a strictly genetic basis (Shuster & Wade 2003). For example, in the Gouldian finch *Erythrura gouldiae* both sexes exhibit black-, red- and yellow-headed morphs, with red-headed males dominating other morphs and both reds and blacks preferring mating partners of their own colour (Pryke & Griffith 2006, 2007). Similarly, genetically based alternative female tactics may evolve, possibly in response to reproductive costs imposed by males. Sexually antagonistic coevolution may in principle lead to the evolution of alternative female phenotypes, which may be followed by the evolution of male polymorphism (Gavrilets & Waxman 2002), particularly when mating is non-random with respect to male and female forms (Härdling & Bergsten 2006).

The maintenance of genetically based polymorphisms is often interpreted in terms of frequency-dependent selection on different tactics, whilst conditional polymorphisms are thought to be maintained in the same way as other condition-dependent secondary sexual traits: alternative tactics convert condition into fitness at different rates, and individuals are expected to switch to the tactic that provides the highest fitness payoff given their current condition (or status: Gross 1996). However, a more realistic approach may be to consider the evolution of

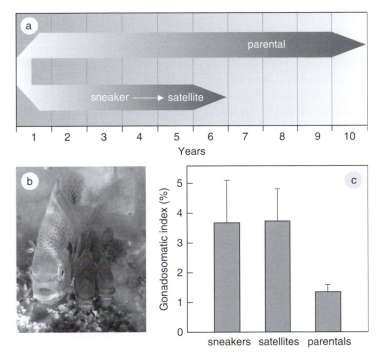

Figure 10.3 Alternative tactics in the bluegill sunfish *Lepomis macrochirus*. (a) Developmental pathways of alternative tactics. Early in their ontogeny males encounter a switch which can turn them into either parentals – which are large, reach sexual maturity late in life, build nests, court females and guard their eggs – or into cuckolding males. These males are smaller, reach sexual maturity earlier than parentals and encounter another developmental switch. When they are young and relatively small, they act as sneakers, darting into nests and ejaculating rapidly between the 'guard' male and female. When they grow bigger, sneakers turn into satellites (adapted from http://publish.uwo.ca/~bneff/research_beea.htm). (b) Satellites can enter nests by mimicking females (from http://publish.uwo.ca/~bneff/research_beea.htm). (c) Both sneakers and satellites invest more somatic tissue into gonads to produce larger ejaculates (adapted from Stoltz & Neff 2006). In addition, because satellites can reach the eggs undisturbed, and proximity to eggs favours fertilisation in external fertilisers, satellites do not need to release nearly as many sperm as a parental to have an equal share of paternity. Similarly, sneakers produce ejaculates of higher quality that outcompete those of parentals even after controlling for number of sperm ejaculated (Fu *et al.* 2001, Neff & Stoltz 2006).

conditional polymorphisms in terms of genetically based switchpoints that determine the environmental (i.e. conditional) threshold at which a given genotype switches from one phenotype (tactic) to another (Tompkins & Hazel 2007). Below we discuss two of the most striking examples of alternative tactics: 'cross-dressing' (i.e. sexual mimicry) and sexual coalitions.

In a phylogenetically diverse set of species, alternative sexual tactics occur in which some members of one sex develop a phenotype and behaviour strikingly similar to the opposite sex (Oliveira *et al.* 2008). Males

which mimic females and readily copulate with other males are not exclusive to the bluegill sunfish encountered above, but occur in several taxa, including insects, cephalopods, crustaceans, fishes, amphibians, snakes and birds (Forsyth & Alcock 1990, Field & Keller 1993, Laufer & Ahl, 1995, Willmott & Foster 1995, Howard *et al.* 1997, Shine *et al.* 2001, Hanlon *et al.* 2005, Gonçalves *et al.* 2005, Jukema & Piersma 2006). Female mimicry appears to serve two functions. First, it enables mimics to approach females defended by other males undisturbed and copulate opportunistically. Second, by copulating with other males, female mimics may in principle be able to deplete the sperm reserves of rival males, and by so doing gain an advantage in sperm competition (see below). Females too may adopt alternative sexual tactics based on male mimicry. Male mimicry by females often appears to be maintained in part by male sexual harassment. For example, in several butterflies and damselflies, male-mimics (andromorphs) receive less male attention and, as a result, less harassment than females that do not resemble males (e.g. Robertson 1985, van Gossum & Sherrat 2008), although recent studies suggest differences in mating rates between andromorph and gynomorph (female-like) females may be rather weak and short-lived (Sirot *et al.* 2003). It would appear that male mimicry is associated with a frequency-dependent selective advantage. However, the selective mechanisms are unclear. One possibility is that andromorphs can persist at low levels because when they are rarer than males they are mistaken for males. An alternative, non-mutually exclusive hypothesis is that when andromorphs are scarcer than gynomorphs, males may specialise in seeking gynomorphs (van Gossum & Sherrat 2008). However, mimicking males which are more conspicuous may also expose females to higher costs, including higher predation risk (Robertson 1985).

In another frequently observed tactic, members of the same sex cooperate in groups (coalitions) to access reproductive opportunities. This behaviour often occurs among males and was already noted by Darwin (1871), who discussed the anecdotal account of two young feral bulls *Bos taurus domesticus* cooperating (unsuccessfully, as it turned out) to evict the dominant older bull. At first, the evolutionary significance of this tactic seems paradoxical. Why should an individual help competitors? There are three possible answers to this question. The simplest answer is that under some circumstances each member of a coalition will on average increase his own chances of reproductive success by cooperating rather than acting individually. The second explanation is that a male may give up some of his own mating opportunities to other males to win their support in conflict or in exchange for other direct benefits such as

food (Duffy *et al.* 2007). The third answer is kin selection. Even when a male that joins a coalition is likely to reduce his own reproductive success, by helping individuals that are more genetically related to him than the population average, he may obtain inclusive fitness benefits that outweigh the direct costs (see Chapters 6 and 13; Kokko & Lindström 1996). There is some evidence indicating that males may cooperate preferentially with individuals that are more genetically related to them than the average male in the population (e.g. Packer *et al.* 1991, Höglund *et al.* 1999, Petrie *et al.* 1999, Shorey *et al.* 2000, Höglund 2003, Krakauer 2005; but see Loiselle *et al.* 2007). Because the skew in reproductive success among males of a coalition tends to increase with coalition size (Packer *et al.* 1991, Alatalo *et al.* 1992, Widemo & Owens 1995), it has been suggested that kin-selection mechanisms may contribute to determine optimal coalition size (Kokko & Lindström 1996). For example, male African lions *Panthera leo* form coalitions in which males cooperate to monopolise females, and the per capita rate of male reproductive success increases with coalition size (Packer *et al.* 1991). However, as coalitions become larger, male reproductive success becomes progressively more skewed and, simultaneously, males become more likely to join the coalitions of genetically related individuals (Packer *et al.* 1991). These results have been interpreted as evidence that males that join large coalitions do so to help relatives reproduce rather than to increase their own reproductive success (Packer *et al.* 1991). This may be the case if reproductive success is consistently skewed against certain individuals and these individuals have information about their disadvantaged role when they decide to join a coalition. In this way, low-quality males may make the best of a bad situation, gaining at least some fitness by helping their relatives to reproduce. Alternatively, if all coalition members share the same probability of high dividends, the decision of joining a coalition may simply be directly selected. While the evolution of male sexual coalitions remains to be fully understood, it appears likely that in most cases a combination of direct and kin selection may explain this tactic. To fully understand the functional significance of sexual coalitions we must therefore measure the intensity of local reproductive competition, the degree of genetic relatedness among coalition members relative to the population average, and the fitness payoffs experienced by individual coalition members.

10.5.2 Intersexual selection

Reproductive competition among members of the same sex is often mediated by the response of prospective partners, whose propensity to copulate can be consistently biased towards certain phenotypes and/or genotypes. Such intersexual selection promotes traits that are more effective at attracting (or coercing) prospective mating partners. Intersexual selection on males has driven the evolution of spectacularly exaggerated secondary sexual characters displayed to females in courtship. Females may prefer (i.e. be more predisposed to mate with) males possessing exaggerated sexual ornaments (e.g. certain pheromone profiles, complex song, large or elaborate ornaments, bright pigmentation), although we know relatively little about how female response changes over a male phenotypic gradient (e.g. from low to high song complexity). This response pattern, called preference function, describes the behavioural rules underpinning mating decisions, and measures the form, direction and intensity of intersexual selection on male phenotypes. Females sometimes sample several males and resist their advances before mating. In fact, a cryptic form of female mate choice can even occur after copulation, when females discriminate among sperm from different partners (see below). In general, however, the more restrictive the preference criteria and the higher the female choosiness (i.e. investment in sampling before mating), the higher the costs of choice for females. In some taxa (e.g. some insects, birds, fish), females too can be ornamentated, although usually less so than males (Kraaijeveld *et al.* 2007). While female ornaments have long been considered by-products of sexual selection for male ornaments, recent evidence suggests that female ornaments can in fact have independent genetic determination (Wright *et al.* 2008)

and play an important role in male sexual preferences and sperm allocation.

A number of proximate mechanisms can lead to mating preferences. In some cases, the sensory system of the receiver may be predisposed to detect and respond to certain stimuli for reasons that are independent of male signals, and that might pre-date the evolution of such signals. Signals that more closely match this sensory predisposition (bias) will therefore have a competitive advantage. When sensory bias is maintained by natural selection, males may evolve to exploit such sensory predispositions of the female nervous system (Basolo 1990, Ryan 1998, Rodd *et al.* 2002), and this may enable males to manipulate females into mating even when mating harms females (Holland & Rice 1998). Cultural transmission may also play an important role in the development of mating preferences. In species with biparental care, sexual preferences can develop through sexual imprinting, where young develop a preference template based on the phenotype of their opposite-sex parent. Neat experimental studies in zebra finches *Taeniopygia guttata* indicate that sexual imprinting may develop through a peak shift, whereby a male develops a preference for female types that are less similar to his father (i.e. more feminine) than his mother (ten Cate *et al.* 2006).

Sexual preferences may be learnt from peers, too. There is evidence that females may learn to copy the preferences of other females in the population. Mate-choice copying can drastically intensify intersexual selection on the preferred trait, particularly when costs of sampling and selecting partners are high (Pruett-Jones 1992). However, provided that the culturally transmitted preference is for partners with the highest lifetime fitness, indirect selection (see below) may promote this behaviour even when associated with moderate net fitness costs (Servedio & Kirkpartick 1996).

The coevolution of signallers (typically males) and receivers (typically females) poses a number of puzzles (see Chapter 8). One question concerns the functions of multiple male display signals within the same species (Møller & Pomiankowski 1993), and the existence of independent female preferences for such signals (Brooks & Couldridge 1999). Optimality models predict that, when signals and preferences are costly, less effective signals and less beneficial preferences will be lost until only the most efficient signal and preference remain (Iwasa & Pomiankowski 1994). So how can we account for the multiple signals and preferences observed in real animals? Several hypotheses have been developed. For example, multiple signals may provide information on different aspects of mate quality, may convey information about the same aspect of quality more reliably, or may be maintained if costs are low (Møller *et al.* 1993), and empirical studies have provided a range of different answers (Andersson *et al.* 2002, Omland 1996). More work is needed to assess the generality of these patterns.

Another interesting question concerns the evolution of signal honesty: do male sexual displays tend to reveal male mate quality accurately and, if so, what keeps low-quality males from cheating by expressing misleading signals? An early answer was provided by Zahavi (1975; see also Amotz Zahavi's profile), who argued that the high costs of display-trait expression ensure that only high-quality males are able to produce attractive displays and, furthermore, that displays function as handicaps that showcase males' ability to bear them. Subsequent theoretical analyses showed that costly displays can indeed evolve, although the viability costs of such displays are likely to decrease, not increase, with male quality or condition (Getty 1998). It has also become clear that condition dependence plays a key role in secondary sexual trait expression and the maintenance of honesty. Condition represents the quantity of metabolic resources available to an individual, and the efficiency with which it is able to convert those resources into fitness (Rowe & Houle 1996). Secondary sexual trait expression is typically strongly condition-dependent: only males in the highest condition express large, costly displays (Bondurianksy 2007, Cotton *et al.* 2004). Condition dependence thus enables individual males to optimise the trade-off between secondary sexual trait expression and viability, with each male expressing its signal and weapon traits to the greatest degree that it can afford, given its condition. Females selecting males with the most attractive displays thus typically obtain partners in high condition, which may carry fewer parasites, transfer more or better sperm, and perhaps provide genetic benefits (see below).

10.5.3 Post-insemination sexual selection

Sexual selection theory was revolutionised in the 1980s and 1990s when the advent of molecular tools to assign paternity, combined with careful studies of sexual behaviour, revealed that in many species females can mate with multiple males so as to expose their eggs to multiple ejaculates simultaneously (Birkhead & Møller 1998, Simmons 2001, Pizzari & Parker 2009; see also Tim Birkhead's profile). That some degree of female promiscuity occurred in some species was already known. Aristotle (*c.*350 BCE) had already pointed out that hens sometimes mate with two roosters, and some chicks resemble one male and others his rival. Darwin, too, recognised female promiscuity in some taxa. However, female promiscuity was considered an exception, and further discussion of this prurient subject was avoided until Parker (1970) explored the evolutionary implications of female re-mating in insects. Parker recognised that female re-mating can extend intrasexual selection to a post-insemination stage by forcing the ejaculates of different males to compete for fertilisation, a process that he called sperm competition. At approximately the same time, entomologists also realised that when a female obtains sperm from multiple males, she can bias fertilisation success in favour of the sperm of certain partners (e.g. Childress & Hartl 1972). These observations led to the hypothesis that polyandrous females can extend intersexual selection to a post-insemination stage via differential sperm uptake, storage and utilisation mechanisms. Females' ability to discriminate against sperm from certain males *during and after copulation* was called cryptic female mate choice (Thornhill 1983, Eberhard 1996).

Mounting evidence suggests that sperm competition drives the evolution of a whole set of male traits that increase fertilising efficiency under a competitive scenario (Pizzari & Parker 2009). A typical macroevolutionary response to sperm competition is an increase in the rate of sperm production through larger and – sometimes – more efficient testes, which enable males to outcompete rivals by inseminating more sperm (Simmons 2001, Pizzari & Parker 2009). Species evolving under higher levels of sperm competition often also evolve more competitive sperm morphologies (Pizzari & Parker 2009), seminal fluid products that increase the number of eggs fertilised by an ejaculate at the expense of the fitness of competing ejaculates (see Box 10.1), and complex male genitalic morphology enabling males to inseminate sperm further into the female reproductive tract, remove sperm inseminated into the same female by previous rivals (Rivera et al. 2004), or even to pierce the female body wall and deposit sperm directly into the female's body cavity (Stutt & Siva-Jothy 2001, Tatarnic et al. 2006)!

Sperm competition also underlies the evolution of phenotypic plasticity in male sexual behaviour. At a microevolutionary scale sperm competition presents individual males with three challenges. First, a trade-off may occur between guarding a female to prevent her from re-mating, and mating with new females. In socially monogamous birds, a male guards his social partner in the days leading to egg laying, when an insemination is most likely to result in fertilisation, and will seek extra-pair copulations when his social partner has laid her eggs and is busy incubating (Beecher & Beecher 1979). In other species, males have evolved mechanisms to minimise this trade-off by defending paternity vicariously. This can be done through seminal-fluid peptides that inhibit female re-mating propensity (Box 10.1), while in some birds inhibition of female re-mating is achieved through stimuli associated with mounting (Løvlie et al. 2005). In other species males leave antiaphrodisiac compounds that render females unattractive to males (Scott 1986, Andersson et al. 2000), or block the female genital tract through highly derived seminal-fluid products that appear to prevent future inseminations by functioning as chastity belts, although the evidence that such male plugs prevent re-mating is ambiguous (Simmons 2001, Moreira et al. 2007).

Second, trade-offs occur between the resources allocated to securing mating opportunities and those invested in ejaculates, and among expenditures in different ejaculates. Experimental work has shown that, in a wide range of taxa (e.g. insects, crustaceans, reptiles, amphibians, birds and mammals), males allocate sperm differentially according to the reproductive value of a copulation, as determined by the level of sperm competition associated with a female, in a way that is often generally consistent with the predictions of game-theoretic models of ejaculate expenditure (Wedell et al. 2002, Pizzari et al. 2003). Interestingly, males from monogamous species with little or no sperm competition appear incapable of strategic sperm allocation (Pound 1999). Recent studies have also demonstrated potential for cryptic male mate choice, whereby males allocate sperm or ejaculate components differentially based on female mate quality (Bonduriansky 2001, Wedell et al. 2002, Pizzari et al. 2003, 2004).

Third, female ability to bias sperm utilisation is also a potentially potent evolutionary agent. Several sperm and male genitalic traits have been interpreted as male adaptations to manipulate females' uptake and storage of sperm, and its use in fertilisation (Eberhard 1996, Pitnick et al. 2009). The copulatory and postcopulatory behaviour of a male is also expected to promote the preferential utilisation of his sperm by the female. As in pre-insemination intersexual selection, male stimulation may occur through the exploitation of pre-existing biases. For example, cuticular plates in the female reproductive tract of the damselfly *Calopteryx haemorrhoidalis asturica* possess mechanoreceptive sensilla (sensory organs sensitive to mechanical pressure or distortion) which influence female oviposition behaviour. The male intromittent organ (aedeagus) stimulates female sensilla, inducing the female to eject previously stored sperm, and wider male organs are more effective at inducing this female behaviour (Córdoba-Aguilar 1999).

10.5.4 Interactions between episodes of sexual selection

While they are often studied in isolation, different episodes (or mechanisms) of sexual selection, such as pre- and post-insemination selection, may interact, generating either synergistic or conflicting selection on male phenotypes (Hunt et al. 2009).

For example, in feral populations of Soay sheep *Ovis aries* dominant rams enjoy privileged access to sexually receptive females, but, over the breeding season, these males produce increasingly less competitive ejaculates, allowing subdominant males to gain some paternity (Preston *et al*. 2001). Similarly, intersexual selection may either reinforce or conflict with intrasexual selection (Hunt *et al*. 2009). For example, female guppies *Poecilia reticulata* have long been known to prefer males with extensive carotenoid-based orange pigmentation (particularly in populations where predators do not target brightly coloured males: Endler 1986). A recent study based on artificial inseminations of ejaculates from different males has neatly shown that after controlling for the number of sperm inseminated, the ejaculates of brightly coloured males have a fertilising advantage in sperm competition (Evans *et al*. 2003), suggesting that this male phenotype is also advantaged in post-insemination sexual selection through sperm competition (e.g. males with more carotenoids produce sperm that are more resistant to oxidative stress and thus of higher fertilising efficiency). In feral populations of domestic fowl *Gallus gallus domesticus*, male access to females is strongly influenced by social status, and females display a preference for socially dominant males (Pizzari & Birkhead 2000). When female ability to mate exclusively with preferred males is curtailed through sexual coercion by subordinate males, female fowl are able to manipulate reproductive success in favour of dominant males through two behavioural mechanisms. First, they attract the attention of dominant males when approached by subdominants, which increases the likelihood that such approaches will fail and dominant males will inseminate females instead (Pizzari 2001). Second, female fowl may bias sperm retention following insemination, and appear to be more likely to eject the ejaculates inseminated by subdominant males through forced matings (Pizzari & Birkhead 2000).

In other cases, intra- and intersexual selection episodes generate opposing selection on the male phenotype. For example, in the cockroach *Nauphoeta cinerea*, the male pheromone blend that confers intrasexual dominance is relatively unattractive to females (Moore & Moore 1999). Similarly, in the carrion fly *Prochyliza xanthostoma*, males with relatively elongated heads are more attractive to females, but tend to lose fights against males with less elongated heads (Bonduriansky & Rowe 2003). Finally, in the house mouse *Mus musculus domesticus*, males induce female sperm utilisation through prolonged copulatory stimulation (e.g. slower penile thrusts), but, in the presence of a competitor, sexual behaviour changes drastically and males reduce stimulation (e.g. more vigorous, more frequent thrusts) to ejaculate sooner (Preston & Stockley 2006). Opposing sexual selection vectors may either weaken net sexual selection, or result in the evolution of alternative phenotypic optima and alternative reproductive strategies (see above). In part, the outcome of such interactions is dictated by whether different selective episodes operate simultaneously on the same population (as may be the case for male–male competition and female preference: Hunt *et al*. 2009) or sequentially, whereby one operates on the subset selected by the previous episode (as may be the case for female selection of partners and cryptic female choice).

10.6 The evolution of sexual preferences

Sexual preferences – reflecting the target, direction and form of intersexual selection – can influence the fitness of the choosing individual, the fitness of its chosen partners, and the fitness of the resulting offspring. The evolution of sexual preferences has been a topic of intense interest and controversy among evolutionary biologists since this mechanism was proposed by Darwin (1871). Here, we explore the mechanisms of direct and indirect selection on sexual preferences, with special emphasis on the evolution of female sexual preferences.

10.6.1 Direct selection: fitness benefits and the chase-away hypothesis

Female preference is under direct natural selection whenever male phenotypes vary in their effects on female reproductive success and/or longevity. Natural selection will promote female preference for male types that maximise female fitness. For example, males of several insect species provide females with nutritious gifts in the form of prey or highly specialised seminal products in the ejaculate (spermatophylax) which are digested by the female. In some butterflies and bushcrickets the nutrients delivered by the spermatophylax can increase female fecundity and longevity (e.g. Gwynne 1984, Wiklund *et al.* 1993, Wedell 1994). Natural selection is therefore expected to promote preference for male types associated with larger direct fitness benefits to the female.

Holland and Rice (1998) proposed a verbal model to provide an alternative explanation for the evolution of female preference, based on the avoidance of fitness costs imposed by manipulative males rather than the pursuit of fitness benefits: the *chase-away* hypothesis. Under sexual conflict, males can obtain a reproductive advantage over their rivals while reducing the fitness of their partners (see above). Here, natural selection is expected to promote female preferences that minimise these direct costs by discriminating against the most harmful males. As females run away from antagonistic male manipulation, males are selected to escalate or modulate their manipulation of female reproductive decisions. Holland and Rice (1998) argue that exaggerated male sexual ornaments evolve because they enable males to manipulate female reproductive decisions by exploiting latent sensory bias.

10.6.2 Indirect selection: Fisherian runaway and good genes

Additive genetic variance (see Chapters 1 and 2) in female preference and male attractiveness also sets the scene for indirect selection on female preference. Female mate choice results in the build-up of positive genetic covariance through linkage disequilibrium between female preference and male attractiveness – that is, if females tend to mate with the males that they find most attractive, offspring will tend to inherit (and pass on to their own offspring) both alleles for attractiveness-enhancing male traits, and alleles for female preference for the attractive traits. When

this happens, female preference will be indirectly selected as a result of intersexual selection on male attractiveness. This original verbal argument, developed by Fisher (1930), was formally explored through progressively more realistic and complex genetic models (Lande 1981, Kirkpatrick 1982, Pomiankowski *et al.* 1991, Kokko *et al.* 2006). Imagine for simplicity a species where female preference is coded by one locus with two alleles: P, coding for preference for male trait T, and p, coding for random mating. Imagine also that the male trait T is coded by one locus segregating for two alleles: T, producing a large trait, and t, producing a small trait. To the extent to which P-females mate with preferred T-males, P and T alleles will become progressively genetically associated within individual genomes through linkage disequilibrium. This genetic association between P and T means that, as T is sexually selected over t, P will also be indirectly selected because of its association with T. In this positive feedback mechanism, female preference determines intersexual selection for a male trait, which in turn generates indirect selection on female preference for that trait. P and T are therefore expected to spread in a population at ever faster rates. In reality, however, both preference and ornament traits are likely to be controlled by multiple genes (i.e. they are quantitative traits). The coevolutionary trajectories of quantitative preference and ornament traits are complex and depend on three main factors: (1) the intensity of net selection (i.e. sexual and natural selection) on the ornament, (2) the degree of additive genetic variance in the ornament, and (3) the degree of additive genetic covariance between the ornament and the preference. Several studies have also considered costs of mate choice and thus natural selection on preference.

In general, quantitative genetic models of Fisherian runaway consistently identify scenarios of two types. In the first type, preference and ornament approach at ever-decreasing speed a stable equilibrium line or point in which sexual selection for further ornament exaggeration is balanced by natural selection of similar intensity but opposite direction; net selection on the ornament is thereby reduced to zero. In the second type of scenario, ornament and preference 'run away' from equilibrium at ever-increasing speed (i.e. the equilibrium is unstable). Whether a population will 'walk towards' or 'run away' from equilibrium depends on the relative magnitude of the ratio of the additive genetic covariance between ornament and preference to the additive genetic variance in the ornament (Andersson 1994, Mead & Arnold 2004). Both scenarios have the potential to lead to an exaggeration of the average ornament and preference in a population across successive generations (Mead & Arnold 2004).

Fisherian runaway models rest on the assumptions that male attractiveness is heritable, and that it covaries genetically with female preference. There is some empirical support for these assumptions. A positive genetic correlation between male attractiveness and female preference has been observed in some species (e.g. Bakker & Pomiankowski 1995). In addition, evidence for the heritability of male attractiveness and reproductive success has been detected in a number of species (e.g. Hedrick 1988, Moore 1990, Wedell & Tregenza 1999, Head *et al.* 2005, Taylor *et al.* 2007). These father–son relationships should be interpreted with caution, however, because they may arise through environmental rather than genetic effects (see below). For example, females may invest more resources in offspring fathered by more attractive males, thus enhancing their sons' attractiveness (e.g. Sheldon 2001).

Below, we review two related outstanding issues associated with the evolution of sexual preferences: (1) the lek paradox, and (2) genetic compatibility.

What (if anything) is the lek paradox?

Some of the most striking examples of social behaviour in the context of mating occur in the 'lek' aggregations of certain birds, mammals, insects and other animals. Here, females choose among several displaying males, but seem to get nothing but sperm for their efforts, since males seem to provide no resources to the female or her offspring. In a seminal paper, Borgia (1979) drew attention to an apparent contradiction in theoretical predictions that he dubbed the *paradox of the lek* (see also Marion Petrie's profile): persistent

directional selection from female preferences should deplete genetic variation in fitness-related traits, eliminating any heritable difference between attractive and unattractive males. If attractive fathers are no more likely to produce high-fitness offspring than unattractive fathers, then what do females gain by being choosy? The lek paradox highlighted a general difficulty with the good-genes model for the evolution of female preferences (see above), discussed earlier by Williams (1975) and Maynard-Smith (1978). The lek paradox has motivated a great deal of theoretical and empirical work, and continues to do so. We argue, however, that the lek paradox is due for a conceptual re-evaluation in light of recent theoretical and empirical advances.

As noted above, the lek paradox originally focused on the maintenance of female preferences despite the presumed lack of additive genetic variation for fitness-related traits in stable (equilibrium) populations (Borgia 1979, Taylor & Williams 1982, Bradbury & Gibson 1983). Later, Kirkpatrick (1986) showed that additive genetic variation in secondary sexual traits such as male displays could, in general, be maintained by opposing vectors of sexual and viability selection. In other words, any sexual advantage from enhanced attractiveness would be negated by an equivalent disadvantage from reduced viability, resulting in net stabilising (balancing) selection on sexual display. Population-genetic theory shows that, if male displays are under net stabilising (not directional) selection, then additive genetic variation can be maintained. However, stabilising selection on male display traits could not in itself maintain additive genetic variance for *fitness* (i.e. good genes) – since fitness is always under directional selection – and, therefore, could not account for the persistence of female preferences.

Curiously, empirical surveys soon showed that populations in fact exhibit considerable levels of additive genetic variation in traits closely associated with fitness (Mousseau & Roff 1987, Pomiankowski & Møller 1995). This evidence seemed to solve one aspect of the paradox while deepening another. If substantial genetic variation for fitness exists in populations, then female choice for good genes is possible after all. But how is genetic variation for fitness maintained? How can good genes persist despite persistent directional selection via female preferences?

An early solution to the problem of how additive genetic variation for fitness could be maintained was suggested by Hamilton and Zuk (1982), based on continual coevolution between hosts and parasites. The host allele conferring greatest resistance to infection at present would soon be rendered ineffectual by pathogen evolution, which would select for a new, more resistant host allele, and so forth. If the most attractive displays are produced by the healthiest males, then choosy females will benefit because their offspring will inherit good genes for resistance to parasites. Current theory suggests that continual coevolution between males and females could maintain additive genetic variation in fitness in much the same way as host–parasite coevolution (Gavrilets *et al.* 2001, Gavrilets & Hayashi 2006; see also Iwasa & Pomiankowski 1995). Several other mechanisms have also been proposed (Pomiankowski & Moller 1995, Rowe & Houle 1996, Miller & Moore 2007). Most influential was Rowe and Houle's (1996) *genic capture* model, which proposed that secondary sexual traits evolve condition-dependent expression through the 'capture' of genetic variation at numerous loci that affect condition. They suggested that genic capture could provide a large enough mutational target to maintain genetic variation in condition despite directional selection.

Thus, at the turn of the twenty-first century, several models appeared to account for the maintenance of additive genetic variation for fitness, and empirical studies suggested that this variation was in fact sufficient to account for female preferences. The lek paradox was resolved! Or so it seemed, until recent studies on Australian *Drosophila* suggested that the maintenance of additive genetic variation is illusory: although abundant genetic variation may segregate for any one trait, this is negated by the covariance structure among traits, such that multivariate additive genetic variation *in the direction of sexual selection* is virtually nil (Blows *et al.* 2004, Hine *et al.* 2004, van Homrigh *et al.* 2007). To put it another way, sexual selection acts on trait combinations reflecting the effects of multiple loci, and there is little or no genetic variation for

more attractive combinations. These findings appear to reinstate the lek paradox in something close to its original form, with the added complication of challenging well-established models.

While the good-genes controversy has raged on, however, several alternative explanations for the maintenance of female preferences were available that did not depend on good genes at all, and could thus circumvent the lek paradox. These explanations may now provide the best way forward.

First, whereas the lek paradox assumes that female preferences are maintained by indirect selection (i.e. enhanced offspring fitness), it has been recognised from the start that direct selection could, in principle, also account for female preferences (Borgia 1979, Taylor & Williams 1982, Reynolds & Gross 1990, Kirkpatrick & Ryan 1991). In other words, if females can obtain greater direct benefits (e.g. receive more resources) or pay lower direct costs (e.g. suffer lower risk of infection) by choosing certain males, then female preference can be maintained even in the absence of additive genetic variation in fitness. Given that sexual ornaments tend to be strongly condition-dependent (Rowe & Houle 1996), perhaps the most attractive males are generally also the healthiest (i.e. least parasite-ridden), and best-endowed with resources (such as nutrients) that can be transferred to females. The potential role of direct selection is also supported by theoretical analyses suggesting that indirect selection is generally too weak to account for the evolution of elaborate displays and preferences (Kirkpatrick 1996, Kirkpatrick & Barton 1997; but see Houle & Kondrashov 2002). Since males make no obvious contributions to females or offspring in lekking species, direct selection on female preferences must be subtle or cryptic, but it remains a possibility worth exploring.

Second, whereas the lek paradox reflects the assumption that indirect selection is generated by 'good genes', it is becoming increasingly apparent that paternally heritable variation (in the broad sense) can be mediated by non-genetic inheritance mechanisms in a wide variety of taxa, including taxa lacking obvious forms of paternal investment (reviewed in Bonduriansky & Day 2009; Chapters 1 and 2). If such mechanisms allow for the transfer of paternal condition to offspring, they can generate indirect selection on female preferences. Moreover, unlike additive genetic variation, indirect selection generated by environmental heterogeneity cannot be depleted by directional selection. Consider the example of the fly *Telostylinus angusticollis*, in which females appear to receive nothing but tiny ejaculates from males. Bonduriansky and Head (2007) showed that male condition and body size are strongly affected by larval diet quality, and males reared on rich larval diet produce larger offspring. Females may thus benefit indirectly by mating with large males, even if variation in body size is purely phenotypic. Such effects are well known in species where males provide nutrients or other forms of paternal investment (Dussourd *et al.* 1988, Gwynne 1988, Smedley & Eisner 1996, Griffith *et al.* 1999, Hunt & Simmons 2000), but few studies have investigated this possibility in species lacking obvious forms of paternal investment.

Finally, whereas the lek paradox reflects the assumption that female preferences confer benefits for females, theory suggests that preference need not confer any benefits at all, and can even be deleterious. Such models include the Fisher runaway process, and the evolution of maladaptive female preferences via male exploitation of female sensory bias, or other forms of sexual conflict (see above). As we have already noted, intralocus sexual conflict in particular poses a considerable dilemma for classic 'good genes' models of sexual selection and the evolution of mate preferences. Intralocus sexual conflict represents a fundamental challenge for such genetic models of mating preference because sexually antagonistic alleles may cause high-fitness males to sire low-quality daughters (Chippindale *et al.* 2001, Rice & Chippindale 2001). If males are merely advertising genes whose benefits in sons are balanced by costs in daughters, there will be no net benefit of mate choice to females. But the situation may be even worse than that in XX/XY sex-determination systems. Male-attractiveness genes are predicted to accumulate disproportionately on the X-chromosome (Rice 1984; although the empirical evidence remains equivocal: e.g. see Fitzpatrick 2004), which fathers pass only to their daughters. High-quality males may therefore not even pass their attractiveness on to their sons. Intralocus sexual conflict may thus negate the benefits of mate choice for females, posing a severe challenge to our understanding of the evolution of mate choice (Pischedda & Chippindale 2006). Intralocus sexual conflict turns the lek paradox on its head: how can female preferences for attractive males be maintained if such preferences are *opposed* by indirect selection?

So where are we, three decades after Borgia (1979) first drew attention to the lek paradox? In our view, four key questions remain to be answered: (1) How much heritable variation for fitness is maintained, and by what mechanisms? (2) What are the magnitude and sign of indirect selection on female preferences? (3) What is the relative importance of direct and indirect selection in maintaining female preferences in lekking species? (4) How much do these parameters vary among taxonomic groups? Seemingly, despite the tremendous conceptual and empirical advances of recent years, the lek paradox continues to haunt us.

Non-transitive preferences: genetic compatibility

An additional mechanism that may contribute to the evolution of sexual preferences (and to explaining the lek paradox) is the possibility that offspring fitness is influenced by the interaction of paternal and maternal genotypes. Such interactions between parental genotypes mean that while one individual will maximise the fitness of its offspring by reproducing with partner *A*, another individual may do best by mating with partner *B* – and, if so, there will be no directional selection on male traits. Inbreeding avoidance provides a classic example (see above), but non-transitive mechanisms may be more general. It has been suggested that genome-wide heterozygosity may be an important predictor of viability (Brown 1997, Kempenaers 2007). With the exception of inbreeding avoidance, evidence of sexual preference based on genome-wide genetic compatibility is presently scarce. However, heterozygosity at specific candidate loci may be an important factor in modulating sexual preferences. In vertebrates, one such candidate region is the major histocompatibility complex (MHC), a group of linked genes which are critically involved in the recognition and presentation of foreign antigens to T-lymphocytes, a group of white blood cells involved in cell-mediated immunity (Hughes & Yeager 1998).

Studies in humans and domestic fowl have produced evidence for MHC heterozygote advantage with respect to resistance to several pathogens (e.g. Nevo & Beiles 1992, Thursz *et al.* 1997, Carrington *et al.* 1999, Jeffery *et al.* 2000, Senseney *et al.* 2000). Together, these studies suggest that MHC heterozyotes recognise a wider range of antigens and/or have more efficient recognition of the same antigens (Hughes & Nei 1992), and that disassortative mating among MHC haplotypes should be favoured because it increases MHC heterozygosity and diversity of offspring. However, only a few studies have been able to distinguish between genome-wide heterozygosity and MHC heterozygosity (e.g. Arkush *et al.* 2002, Penn *et al.* 2002). Other studies investigating the relationship between MHC heterozygosity and immune resistance have produced more ambiguous results (e.g. Paterson *et al.* 1998, Langefors *et al.* 2001, Lohm *et al.* 2002, Ilmomen *et al.* 2007). In addition, it is possible that an optimal degree of heterozygosity may occur beyond which an organism risks autoimmunity problems (Milinski 2006). This appears to be the case in three-spined sticklebacks *Gasterosteus aculeatus*, in which pathogen resistance peaks at intermediate MHC heterozyogsity and females prefer males with intermediate numbers of different MHC genes (Reusch *et al.* 2001).

Genetic compatibility therefore promotes sexual preferences that are non-transitive, i.e. not shared by the majority of the population, and such preferences are expected to maintain variation in traits affecting male reproductive success.

10.7 Intersexual coevolution

We pointed out above that, while sexual selection can benefit both males and females, it also can create evolutionary conflict between the sexes. Sexual selection on male traits can result in the displacement of females from their optimal phenotypes for sexually homologous traits (intralocus sexual conflict). Furthermore, phenotypes that are advantaged in sexual selection may impose direct fitness costs on their partners, for example through reduced fertility or reduced longevity (interlocus sexual conflict), suggesting that mating preference for more successful partners may be particularly costly. However, we have also shown that indirect selection might in principle promote preference for successful partner types when additive genetic variance available to intersexual selection underlies attractiveness and viability, and high genetic covariance occurs between attractiveness and sexual preference.

Understanding the coevolutionary trajectories of the sexes hinges, in part, upon establishing the relative magnitude of direct and indirect selection on mating preference. Under what conditions do we expect females to evolve a preference for male types successful in reproductive competition through indirect selection, and under what conditions do we expect natural selection to prevail and promote female resistance against these males? When the spread of sexually selected traits in one sex reinforces selection on preference for such traits in the other and vice versa, intersexual coevolution is a mutualistic process. However, when the spread of sexually selected traits in one sex generates natural selection to resist or avoid these traits in the opposite sex, intersexual coevolution will be antagonistic, mediated by evolutionary arms races between different loci of the same genome (interlocus sexual conflict).

In 1979 Parker formulated the question as follows (see also Parker 2006). Suppose a male mutation that enables its bearers to outcompete rival males over access to females spreads in a population, and that this mutation also imposes a fitness cost on females such that, all else being equal, the fitness of females mating with the mutant male type is lower than the fitness of females mating with the common male type. Females mating with mutant males would produce sons who will inherit a competitive advantage from their fathers. Would we expect females to evolve resistance against, or preference for, the male mutant? In the former case, direct costs outweigh indirect benefits and females pay a net cost, in the latter the opposite is true (Pizzari & Snook 2003).

Stewart *et al.* (2005) tested this idea by experimentally creating genetic polymorphism for female resistance in *D. melanogaster*. Wild-type females interacted with multiple males which exposed them to male-induced harm but simultaneously provided them with the possibility of producing offspring that would inherit high-male-fitness genes from their fathers. In contrast, females of the red-eye genotype were mated singly by a randomly selected male. The red-eye allele thus protected these females from male harassment but also excluded indirect benefits of sexual selection. In other words, eye colour was used as a genetic marker for female resistance. The study monitored the evolutionary fate of the two genotypes and found that the red-eye genotype increased in frequency over successive generations, a result which was interpreted as evidence that female resistance evolves through natural selection favouring avoidance of direct fitness costs. However, this interpretation warrants caution for several reasons. First, rather than engineering a female genotype that is truly resistant to male harm, the study provided red-eye females with cost-free resistance. Second, the fitness advantage conferred by the red-eye protection allele may have resulted simply from the reduced number of flies in the environment where red-eyed females mated (i.e. a density effect), rather than from reduced exposure to males per se. Third, Stewart *et al.* (2005) assumed that elimination of direct harm reduced the potential for indirect benefits to exactly the same degree, but many forms of direct harm involve males' *incidental* interference with female foraging or reproduction (e.g. via males' use or obstruction of resources, production of waste, physical interactions unrelated to mating, etc). Such harm is unlikely to depend strongly on female mating behaviour or associated morphological and physiological traits, and thus cannot be traded off against indirect benefits – it forms no part of the optimisation equation that shapes the evolution of female mating strategy. For all three reasons, this experiment is likely to overestimate the advantage of a 'protection' allele that reduces or eliminates direct

harm that females experience as a result of their sexual interactions with males. More recent studies have produced an ambiguous picture (Fig. 10.4).

Intralocus sexual conflict also poses fascinating questions about intersexual coevolution. Above, we outlined the challenges it poses for understanding the coevolution of male secondary sexual traits and female preferences. Because the sexes share much of the genome, sexual selection on a locus in males can displace females from their phenotypic optimum, as well as negate the indirect benefits of mate choice. From this perspective, intralocus sexual conflict represents a brake on sexual coevolution. However, because intralocus sexual conflict can cause both sexes to evolve in response to sexual selection on one sex, it could also carry populations across valleys in the fitness landscape, facilitate niche shifts, and even promote speciation (Lande & Kirkpatrick 1989). Imagine a secondary sexual trait (such as leg length in a fly) exaggerated by sexual selection in males and, to a lesser extent, in females. Increased leg length may at first be costly for females but, once mean leg length attains a certain threshold, it could allow for the exploitation of a new niche (such as rough tree bark). Viability selection might then promote further evolution of leg length in both sexes, and favour reproductive isolation mechanisms. Intralocus sexual conflict could thus have a broad range of important implications for evolution, and we have barely begun to scratch the surface of this problem (Bondurianksy & Chenoweth 2009).

What do these results tell us collectively? Sexual selection can promote male types that are harmful to females, and this harm can translate into net female costs which set the scene for female resistance and antagonistic coevolution. However, differential mating costs do not always translate into antagonistic coevolution between the sexes. Indirect benefits can potentially be sufficiently high to outweigh direct costs, setting the scene for mutualistic intersexual coevolution. It is likely that the relative magnitude of direct and indirect effects is highly labile, and future research should focus on the ecological and life-history mechanisms that predispose populations to antagonistic intersexual coevolution.

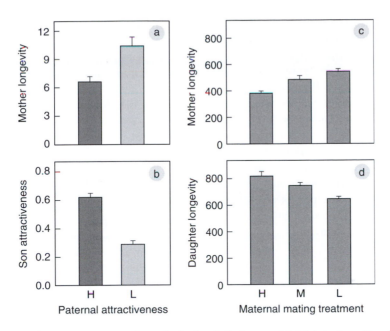

Figure 10.4 Direct and indirect consequences of sexual selection. In the house cricket *Acheta domesticus*, (a) females experimentally mated to more attractive males suffered reduced longevity (± SE), but (b) these costs were offset by indirect benefits determined by superior reproductive performance of sons (adapted from Head *et al.* 2005). Female *D. melanogaster* (c) experimentally exposed to higher re-mating rates (H) suffered higher mortality and accelerated reproductive senescence which resulted in an overall cost in lifetime reproductive success (LRS) compared to females exposed to medium (M) and low (L) re-mating rates, but (d) H females produced daughters that enjoyed on average higher lifetime reproductive success compared to the daughters of both M and L females, suggesting that the inclusive fitness of females mating at a high rate may not be lower than the inclusive fitness of more resistant females (adapted from Priest *et al.* 2008). These indirect benefits appear to be particularly important in the initial stages of the demographic expansion of a population (Priest *et al.* 2008).

10.8 Conclusions and future directions

Sex permeates and motivates many aspects of social behaviour, and over the past 30 years we have seen an explosion of research interest in the amazing diversity of sexual behaviour and associated morphological, physiological and life-history traits. This work has demonstrated that Darwin's intuition of sexual selection as the evolutionary force driving such diversity was generally correct, revealing sexual selection as a pervasive and potent agent of evolutionary change. However, we are also beginning to realise that sexual behaviour is subject to far more complex evolutionary dynamics than originally anticipated. We face a number of exciting challenges. We need a deeper understanding of the evolutionary implications of

anisogamy, and a more comprehensive theoretical framework for understanding the operation of sexual selection, integrating its pre- and post-insemination episodes. We must also resolve the coevolutionary trajectories of the sexes, and understand the way socio-environmental conditions modulate the 'virulence' of intersexual conflict and its evolutionary consequences.

Four emerging approaches promise to catalyse future research. First, key to these challenges will be to determine the genetic basis of sexual behaviour and sexually selected traits. Functional genomics and post-genomic tools provide an unprecedented opportunity to explore the genetic architecture of sexual traits and their molecular evolution under sexual selection and intersexual coevolution (Andersson & Simmons 2006). Second, adaptive dynamic modelling can be used to complement game theory and quantitative genetic models to investigate evolutionary dynamics within and between sexes (Gavrilets & Hayashi 2006). Third, quantitative tools based on multivariate analyses can be successfully applied to the study of the operation of sexual selection on suites of traits (Blows 2007), and finally, social network analysis can be similarly used to study the dynamics of sexual networks (see Chapter 9; Krause *et al.* 2007). We are on the brink of a new era in the study of sexual behaviour, and if the past 30 years are anything to go by, we very much look forward to it!

Acknowledgements

We are grateful to Margo Adler, Laura Sirot, Nina Wedell, Mariana Wolfner, Alex Wong and an anonymous reviewer for detailed and constructive suggestions on a draft of this chapter. We are also grateful to the editors for inviting us to contribute this chapter, and for their continued support.

Suggested readings

Andersson, M. (1994) *Sexual Selection*. Princeton, NJ: Princeton University Press.

Arnqvist, G & Rowe, L. (2005) *Sexual Conflict*. Princeton, NJ: Princeton University Press.

Bateman, A. J. (1948) Intra-sexual selection in *Drosophila*. *Heredity*, **2**, 349–368.

Eberhard, W. G. (1996) *Female Control: Sexual Selection by Cryptic Female Choice*. Princeton, NJ: Princeton University Press.

Holland, B. & Rice, W. R. (1998) Perspective. Chase-away sexual selection: antagonistic seduction versus resistance. *Evolution*, **52**, 1–7.

Parker, G. A. (1970) Sperm competition and its evolutionary consequences in the insects. *Biological Reviews*, **45**, 525–567.

Parker, G. A. (2006) Sexual conflict over mating and fertilization: an overview. *Philosophical Transactions of the Royal Society B*, **361**, 235–259.

Rice, W. R. (1984) Sex chromosomes and the evolution of sexual dimorphism. *Evolution*, **38**, 735–742.

References

Alatalo, R. V., Höglund, J., Lundberg, A. & Sutherland, W. J. (1992) Evolution of black grouse leks: female preferences benefit males in larger leks. *Behavioral Ecology*, **3**, 53–59.

Alonzo, S. H. & Pizzari, T. (2010) Male fecundity stimulation: conflict and cooperation within and between the sexes. *American Naturalist*, **175**, 174–185.

Andersson, J., Borg-Karlson, A.-K. & Wiklund, C. (2000) Sexual cooperation and conflict in butterflies: a male-transferred anti-aphrodisiac reduces harassment of recently mated females. *Proceedings of the Royal Society B*, **267**, 1271–1275.

Andersson, M. (1994) *Sexual Selection*. Princeton, NJ: Princeton University Press.

Andersson, M. & Simmons, L. W. (2006) Sexual selection and mate choice. *Trends in Ecology and Evolution*, **21**, 296–302.

Andersson, S., Pryke, S., Ornborg, J., Lawes, M. J. & Andersson, M. (2002) Multiple receivers, multiple ornaments, and a trade-off between agonistic and epigamic signaling in a widowbird. *American Naturalist*, **160**, 683–691.

Aristotle (350 BCE) *History of Animals*. Books IV–VI. Loeb Classical Library 438. London: Heinemann, 1970.

Arkush, K. D., Giese, A. R., Mendonca, H. L. *et al.* (2002) Resistance to three pathogens in the endangered winter-run chinook salmon (*Oncorhynchus tshawytscha*): effects of inbreeding and major histocompatibility complex genotypes. *Canadian Journal of Fisheries and Aquatic Sciences*, **59**, 966–975.

Arnqvist, G. & Nilsson, T. (2000) The evolution of polyandry: multiple mating and female fitness in insects. *Animal Behaviour*, **60**, 145–164.

Arnqvist, G. & Rowe, L. (2005) *Sexual Conflict*. Princeton, NJ: Princeton University Press.

Baker, R. R. (1983) Insect territoriality. *Annual Review of Entomology*, **28**, 65–89.

Bakker, T. C. M. & Pomiankowski, A. (1995) The genetic basis of female mate preferences. *Journal of Evolutionary Biology*, **8**, 129–171.

Basolo, A. L. (1990) Female preference predates the evolution of the sword in swordtail fish. *Science*, **250**, 808–810.

Bateman, A. J. (1948) Intra-sexual selection in *Drosophila*. *Heredity*, **2**, 349–368.

Bedhomme, S. & Chippindale, A. K. (2007) Irreconcilable differences: when sexual dimorphism fails to resolve sexual conflict. In: *Sex, Size and Gender Roles: Evolutionary Studies of Sexual Size Dimorphism*, ed. D. J. Fairbairn, W. U.

Blanckenhorn & T. Székely. Oxford: Oxford University Press, pp. 185–194.

Beecher, M. & Beecher, I. (1979) Sociobiology of bank swallows: reproductive strategy of the male. *Science*, **205**, 1282–1285.

Birkhead, T. R. & Møller A. P., eds. (1998) *Sperm Competition and Sexual Selection*. London: Academic Press.

Bjork, A. & Pitnick, S. (2006) Intensity of sexual selection along the anisogamy-isogamy continuum. *Nature*, **441**, 742–745.

Blows, M. W. (2007) A tale of two matrices: multivariate approaches in evolutionary biology. *Journal of Evolutionary Biology*, **20**, 1–8.

Blows, M. W., Chenoweth, S. F. & Hine, E. (2004) Orientation of the genetic variance-covariance matrix and the fitness surface for multiple male sexually selected traits. *American Naturalist*, **163**, 329–340.

Blumenstiel, J. P. (2007) Sperm competition can drive a male-biased mutation rate. *Journal of Theoretical Biology*, **249**, 624–632.

Bonduriansky, R. (2001) The evoluton of male mate choice in insects: a synthesis of ideas and evidence. *Biological Reviews of the Cambridge Philosophical Society*, **76**, 305–339.

Bonduriansky, R. (2007) The evolution of condition dependent sexual dimorphism. *American Naturalist*, **169**, 9–19.

Bonduriansky, R. & Chenoweth, S. F. (2009) Intralocus sexual conflict. *Trends in Ecology and Evolution*, **24**, 280–288.

Bonduriansky, R. & Day, T. (2009) Nongenetic inheritance and its evolutionary implications. *Annual Review of Ecology, Evolution, and Systematics*, **40**, 103–125.

Bonduriansky, R. & Head, M. (2007) Maternal and paternal condition effects on offspring phenotype in *Telostylinus angusticollis* (Diptera: Neriidae). *Journal of Evolutionary Biology*, **20**, 2379–2388.

Bonduriansky, R. & Rowe, L. (2003) Interactions among mechanisms of sexual selection on male body size and head shape in a sexually dimorphic fly. *Evolution*, **57**, 2046–2053.

Bonduriansky, R. & Rowe, L. (2005) Intralocus sexual conflict and the genetic architecture of sexually dimorphic traits in *Prochyliza xanthostoma* (Diptera: Piophilidae). *Evolution*, **59**, 1965–1975.

Borgia, G. (1979) Sexual selection and the evolution of mating systems. In: *Sexual Selection and Reproductive Competition in Insects*, ed. M. S. Blum & N. A. Blum. New York, NY: Academic Press, pp. 19–80

Bradbury, J. W. & Gibson, R. M. (1983) Leks and mate choice. In: *Mate Choice*, ed. P. Bateson. Cambridge: Cambridge University Press, pp. 109–138.

Brommer, J. E., Kirkpatrick, M., Qvarnström, A. & Gustafsson, L. (2007) The intersexual genetic correlation for lifetime fitness in the wild and its implications for sexual selection. *PLoS ONE*, **2** (1), e744.

Brooks, R. & Couldridge, V. (1999) Multiple sexual ornaments coevolve with multiple mating preferences. *American Naturalist*, **154**, 37–45.

Brown, J. L. (1997) A theory of mate choice based on heterozygosity. *Behavioral Ecology*, **8**, 60–65.

Carrington, M., Nelson, G. W., Martin, M. P. *et al.* (1999) HLA and HIV-1: heterozygote advantage and B*35-Cw*04 disadvantage. *Science*, **283**, 1748–1752.

Carvalho, G. B., Kapahi, P., Anderson, D. J. & Benzer, S. (2006) Allocrine modulation of appetite by the sex peptide of *Drosophila*. *Current Biology*, **16**, 692–696.

Chapman, T., Bangham, J., Vinti, G. *et al.* (2003) The sex peptide of *Drosophila melanogaster*: female post-mating responses analyzed by using RNA interference. *Proceedings of the National Academy of Sciences of the USA*, **100**, 9923–9928.

Childress, D. & Hartl, D. L. (1972) Sperm preference in *Drosophila melanogaster*. *Genetics* **71**, 417–427.

Chippindale, A. K., Gibson, J. R. & Rice, W. R. (2001) Negative genetic correlation for adult fitness between the sexes reveals ontogenetic conflict in *Drosophila*. *Proceedings of the National Academy of Sciences of the USA*, **98**, 1671–1675.

Clutton-Brock, T. (2007) Sexual selection in males and females. *Science*, **318**, 1882–1885.

Clutton-Brock, T. H. & Parker, G. A. (1992) Potential reproductive rates and the operation of sexual selection. *Quarterly Review of Biology*, **67**, 437–456.

Clutton-Brock, T. H. & Parker, G. A. (1995) Sexual coercion in animal societies. *Animal Behaviour*, **49**, 1345–1365.

Cohen, J. (1969) Why so many sperms? An essay on the arithmetic of reproduction. *Science Progress*, **57**, 23–41.

Cohen, J. (1973) Cross-overs, sperm redundancy and their close association. *Heredity*, **31**, 408–413.

Cordero, A. (1995) Ejaculate substances that affect female insect reproductive physiology and behavior: honest or arbitrary? *Journal of Theoretical Biology*, **192**, 453–461.

Córdoba-Aguilar, A. (1999) Male copulatory sensory stimulation induces female ejection of rival sperm in a damselfly. *Proceedings of the Royal Society B*, **266**, 779–784.

Cornell, S. J. & Tregenza, T. (2007) A new theory for the evolution of polyandry as a means of inbreeding avoidance. *Proceedings of the Royal Society B*, **274**, 2873–2879.

Cotton, S., Fowler, K. & Pomiankowski, A. (2004) Do sexual ornaments demonstrate heightened condition-dependent expression as predicted by the handicap hypothesis? *Proceedings of the Royal Society B*, **271**, 771–783.

Crudgington, H. S., Beckerman, A. P., Brüstle, L., Green, K. & Snook, R. R. (2005) Experimental removal and elevation of sexual selection: does sexual selection generate manipulative males and resistant females? *American Naturalist*, **165**, S72–87.

Darwin, C. (1859) *On the Origin of Species by Means of Natural Selection*. London: John Murray.

Darwin, C. (1871) *The Descent of Man, and Selection in Relation to Sex*. London: John Murray.

Dawkins, R. (1976) *The Selfish Gene*. Oxford: Oxford University Press.

Day, T. & Bondurianksy, R. (2004) Intralocus sexual conflict can drive the evolution of genomic imprinting. *Genetics*, **167**, 1537–1546.

Dewsbury, D. A. (2005) The Darwin–Bateman paradigm in historical context. *Integrative and Comparative Biology*, **45**, 831–837.

Duffy, K. G., Wrangham, R. W. & Silk, J. B. (2007) Male chimpanzees exchange political support for mating opportunities. *Current Biology*, **17**, R586–587.

Dussourd, D. E., Ubik, K., Harvis, C. *et al.* (1988) Biparental defensive endowment of eggs with acquired plant alkaloid in the moth Utetheisa ornatrix. *Proceedings of the National Academy of Sciences of the USA*, **85**, 5992–5996.

Eberhard, W. G. (1996) *Female Control: Sexual Selection by Cryptic Female Choice*. Princeton, NJ: Princeton University Press.

Eberhard, W. G. & Cordero, C. (1995) Sexual selection by cryptic female choice on male seminal products: a new bridge between sexual selection and reproductive physiology. *Trends in Ecology and Evolution*, **10**, 493–496.

Emlen, D. J. (1994) Environmental control of horn length dimorphism in the beetle Onthophagus acuminatus (Coleoptera: Scarabaeidae). *Proceedings of the Royal Society B*, **256**, 131–136.

Endler, J. A. (1986) *Natural Selection in the Wild*. Princeton, NJ: Princeton University Press.

Evans, J. P., Zane, L., Francescato, S. & Pilastro, A. (2003) Directional postcopulatory sexual selection revealed by artificial insemination. *Nature*, **421**, 360–363.

Fedorka, K. M. & Mousseau, T. A. (2004) Female mating bias results in conflicting sex-specific offspring fitness. *Nature*, **429**, 65–67.

Field, S. A. & Keller, M. A. (1993) Alternative mating tactics and female mimicry as post-copulatory mate-guarding behaviour in the parasitic wasp Cotesia rubecula. *Animal Behaviour*, **46**, 1183–1189.

Fisher, R. A. (1930) *The Genetical Theory of Natural Selection*. Oxford: Clarendon Press.

Fitzpatrick, M. J. (2004) Pleiotropy and the genomic location of sexually selected genes. *American Naturalist*, **163**, 800–808.

Fiumera, A. C., Dumont, B. L. & Clark, A. G. (2005) Sperm competitive ability in *Drosophila melanogaster* associated with variation in male reproductive proteins. *Genetics*, **169**, 243–257.

Fiumera, A. C., Dumont, B. L. & Clark, A. G. (2006) Natural variation in male-induced 'cost-of-mating' and allele-specific association with male reproductive genes in *Drosophila melanogaster*. *Philosophical Transactions of the Royal Society B*, **361**, 355–361.

Fiumera, A. C., Dumont, B. L. & Clark, A. G. (2007) Associations between sperm competition and natural variation in male reproductive genes on the third chromosome of *Drosophila melanogaster*. *Genetics*, **176**, 1245–1260.

Foerster, K., Coulson, T., Sheldon, B.C. *et al.* (2007) Sexually antagonistic genetic variation for fitness in red deer. *Nature*, **447**, 1107–1109.

Forsgren, E., Amundsen, T., Borg, A. A. & Bjelvenmark, J. (2004) Unusually dynamic sex roles in a fish. *Nature*, **429**, 551–554.

Forsyth, A. & Alcock, J. (1990) Female mimicry and resource defense polygyny by males of a tropical rove beetle, *Leistrophus versicolor* (Coleoptera: Staphylinidae). *Behavioral Ecology and Sociobiology*, **26**, 325–330.

Foster, K. R., Wenseleers, T. & Ratnieks, F. L. W. (2001) Spite: Hamilton's unproven theory. *Annales Zoologici Fennici*, **38**, 229–238.

Foster, M. S. (1983) Disruption, dispersion, and dominance in lek-breeding birds. *American Naturalist*, **122**, 53–72.

Fu, P., Neff, B.D. & Gross, M.R. (2001) Tactic-specific success in sperm competition. *Proceedings of the Royal Society B*, **268**, 1105–1112.

Gavrilets, S. & Hayashi, T. I. (2006) The dynamics of two- and three-way sexual conflicts over mating. *Philosophical Transactions of the Royal Society B*, **361**, 345–354.

Gavrilets, S. & Waxman, D. (2002) Sympatric speciation by sexual conflict. *Proceedings of the National Academy of Sciences of the USA*, **99**, 10533–10538.

Gavrilets, S., Arnqvist, G. & Friberg, U. (2001) The evolution of female mate choice by sexual conflict. *Proceedings of the Royal Society B*, **268**, 531–539.

Getty, T. (1998) Handicap signalling: when fecundity and viability do not add up. *Animal Behaviour*, **56**, 127–130.

Gillott, C. (2003) Male accessory gland secretions: modulators of female reproductive physiology and behavior. *Annual Review of Entomology*, **48**, 163–184.

Gonçalves, D., Matos, R., Fagundes, T. & Oliveira, R. (2005) Bourgeois males of the peacock blenny, *Salaria pavo*, discriminate female mimics from females? *Ethology*, **111**, 559–572.

Greenfield, M. D. (1994) Synchronous and alternating choruses in insects and anurans: common mechanisms and diverse functions. *American Zoologist*, **34**, 605–615.

Griffith, S. C., Owens, I. P. F. & Burke, T. (1999) Environmental determination of a sexually selected trait. *Nature*, **400**, 358–360.

Gross, M. R. (1996) Alternative reproductive strategies and tactics: diversity within sexes. *Trends in Ecology and Evolution*, **11**, A92–98.

Gwynne, D. T. (1984) Courtship feeding increases female reproductive success in bushcrickets. *Nature*, **307**, 361–363.

Gwynne, D. T. (1988) Courtship feeding in katydids benefits the mating male's offspring. *Behavioral Ecology and Sociobiology*, **23**, 373–377.

Gwynne, D. T. & Simmons, L. W. (1990) Experimental reversal of courtship roles in an insect. *Nature*, **346**, 172–174.

Haerty, W., Jagadeeshan, S., Kulathinal, R. J. *et al.* (2007) Evolution in the fast lane: rapidly evolving sex- and reproduction-related genes in *Drosophila* species. *Genetics*, **177**, 1321–1335.

Hamilton, W. D. & Zuk, M. (1982) Heritable true fitness and bright birds: a role for parasites? *Science*, **218**, 384–387.

Hanlon, R. T., Naud, M.-J., Shaw, P. W. & Havenhand, J. N. (2005) Transient sexual mimicry leads to fertilization. *Nature*, **433**, 212.

Härdling, R. & Bergsten, J. (2006) Nonrandom mating preserves intrasexual polymorphism and stops population differentiation in sexual conflict. *American Naturalist*, **167**, 401–409.

Head, M. L., Hunt, J., Jennions, M. D. & Brooks, R. (2005) The indirect benefits of mating with attractive males outweigh the direct costs. *PLoS Biology*, **3** (2), e33.

Hedrick, A. V. (1988) Female choice and the heritability of attractive male traits: an empirical study. *American Naturalist*, **132**, 267–276.

Heifetz Y., Lung, O., Frongillo, E. A. & Wolfner, M. F. (2000) The Drosophila seminal fluid protein Acp26Aa stimulates release of oocytes by the ovary. *Current Biology*, **10**, 99–102.

Hine, E., Chenoweth, S. F. & Blows, M. W. (2004) Multivariate quantitative genetics and the lek paradox: genetic variance male sexually selected traits of *Drosophila serrata* under field conditions. *Evolution*, **58**, 2754–2762.

Hodgson, D. J. & Hosken, D. J. (2006) Sperm competition promotes the exploitation of rival ejaculates. *Journal of Theoretical Biology*, **243**, 230–234.

Höglund, J. (2003) Lek-kin in birds: provoking theory and surprising new results. *Annales Zoologici Fennici*, **40**, 249–253.

Höglund, J., Alatalo, R. V., Lundberg, A., Rintamäki, P. T. & Lindell, J. (1999) Microsatellite markers reveal the potential for kin selection on black grouse leks. *Proceedings of the Royal Society B*, **266**, 813–816.

Holland, B. & Rice, W. R. (1998) Perspective. Chase-away sexual selection: antagonistic seduction versus resistance. *Evolution*, **52**, 1–7.

Holland, B. & Rice, W. R. (1999) Experimental removal of sexual selection reverses intersexual antagonistic coevolution and removes a reproductive load. *Proceedings of the National Academy of Sciences of the USA*, **96**, 5083–5088.

Houle, D. & Kondrashov, A. S. (2002) Coevolution of costly mate choice and condition-dependent display of good genes. *Proceedings of the Royal Society B*, **269**, 97–104.

Howard, R. D., Moorman, R. S. & Whiteman, H. H. (1997) Differential effects of mate competition and mate choice on eastern tiger salamanders. *Animal Behaviour*, **53**, 1345–1356.

Hughes, A. L. & Nei, M. (1992) Maintenance of Mhc polymorphism. *Nature*, **355**, 402–403.

Hughes, A. L. & Yeager, M. (1998) Natural selection at Major Compatibility Complex loci of vertebrates. *Annual Review of Genetics*, **32**, 415–435.

Hunt, J. & Simmons, L. W. (2000) Maternal and paternal effects on offspring phenotype in the dung beetle *Onthophagus taurus*. *Evolution*, **54**, 936–941.

Hunt, J., Breuker, C. J., Sadowski, J. A. & Moore, A. J. (2009) Male–male competition, female mate choice and their interaction: determining total sexual selection. *Journal of Evolutionary Biology*, **22**, 13–26.

Ilmonen, P., Penn, D. J., Damjanovich, K. *et al.* (2007) Major histocompatibility complex heterozygosity reduces fitness in experimentally infected mice. *Genetics*, **176**, 2501–2508

Iwasa, Y. & Pomiankowski, A. (1994) The evolution of mate preferences for multiple sexual ornaments. *Evolution*, **48**, 853–867.

Iwasa, Y. & Pomiankowski, A. (1995) Continual change in mate preferences. *Nature*, **377**, 420–422.

Jeffery, K. J. M., Siddiqui, A. A., Bunce, M. *et al.* (2000) The influence of HLA class I alleles and heterozygosity on the outcome of human T cell lymphotropic virus type T infection. *Journal of Immunology*, **165**, 7278–7284.

Johnstone, R. A. & Keller, L. (2000) How males can gain by harming their mates: sexual conflict, seminal toxins, and the cost of mating. *American Naturalist*, **156**, 368–377.

Johnstone, R. A., Reynolds, J. D. & Deutsch, J. C. (1996) Mutual mate choice and sex differences in choosiness. *Evolution*, **50**, 1382–1391.

Jukema, J. & Piersma, T. (2006) Permanent female mimics in a lekking shorebird. *Biology Letters*, **2**, 161–164.

Kapelinikov, A., Rivlin, P. K., Hoy, R. R. & Heifetz, Y. (2008) Tissue remodeling: a mating-induced differentiation program for the *Drosophila* oviduct. *BMC Developmental Biology*, **8**, 114.

Kempenaers, B. (2007) Mate choice and genetic quality: a review of the heterozygosity theory. *Advances in the Study of Behavior*, **37**, 189–278.

Kirkpatrick, M. (1982) Sexual selection and the evolution of female choice. *Evolution*, **36**, 1–12.

Kirkpatrick, M. (1986) The handical mechanism of sexual selection does not work. *American Naturalist*, **127**, 222–240.

Kirkpatrick, M. (1996) Good genes and direct selection in the evolution of mating preferences. *Evolution*, **50**, 2125–2140.

Kirkpatrick, M. & Barton, N. H. (1997) The strength of indirect selection on female mating preferences. *Proceedings of the National Academy of Sciences of the USA*, **94**, 1282–1286.

Kirkpatrick, M. & Ryan, M. J. (1991) The evolution of mating preferences and the paradox of the lek. *Nature*, **350**, 33–38.

Kokko, H. & Lindström, J. (1996) Kin selection and the evolution of leks: whose success do young males maximize? *Proceedings of the Royal Society B*, **263**, 919–923.

Kokko, H. & Monaghan, P. (2001) Predicting the direction of sexual selection. *Ecology Letters*, **4**, 159–165.

Kokko, H. & Ots, I. (2006) When not to avoid inbreeding. *Evolution*, **60**, 467–475.

Kokko, H., Jennions, M. D. & Brooks, R. (2006) Unifying and testing models of sexual selection. *Annual Review of Ecology, Evolution and Systematics*, **37**, 43–66.

Kraaijeveld, K., Kraaijeveld-Smit, F. J. L. & Komdeur, J. (2007) The evolution of mutual ornamentation. *Animal Behaviour*, **74**, 657–677.

Krause, J., Croft, D. P. & James, R. (2007) Social network theory in the behavioural sciences: potential applications. *Behavioral Ecology and Sociobiology*, **62**, 15–27.

Krakauer, A. H. (2005) Kin selection and cooperative courtship in wild turkeys. *Nature*, **434**, 69–72.

Lande, R. (1980) Sexual dimorphism, sexual selection, and adaptation in polygenic characters. *Evolution*, **34**, 292–305.

Lande, R. (1981) Models of speciation by sexual selection on polygenic traits. *Proceedings of the National Academy of Sciences of the USA*, **78**, 3721–3725.

Lande, R. & Kirkpatrick, M. (1989) Ecological speciation by sexual selection. *Journal of Theoretical Biology*, **133**, 85–98.

Langefors, A., Lohm, J., Grahn, M., Andersen, O. & von Schantz, T. (2001) Association between major histocompatibility complex class IIB alleles and resistance to *Aeromonas salmonicida* in Atlantic salmon. *Proceedings of the Royal Society B*, **268**, 479–485.

Laufer, H. & Ahl, J. S. B. (1995) Mating behavior and methyl farnesoate levels in male morphotypes of the spider crab, *Libinia emarginata* (Leach). *Journal of Experimental Marine Biology and Ecology*, **193**, 15–20.

Le Galliard, J. F., Fitze, P. S., Ferriere, R. & Clobert, J. (2005) Sex ratio bias, male aggression, and population collapse in lizards. *Proceedings of the National Academy of Sciences of the USA*, **102**, 18231–18236.

Lessells, C. M. (2005) Why are males bad for females? Models for the evolution of damaging male behavior. *American Naturalist*, **165**, 546–563.

Lessells C. M. (2006) The evolutionary outcome of sexual conflict. *Philosophical Transactions of the Royal Society B*, **361**, 301–317.

Liu, H. & Kubli, E. (2003) Sex peptide is the molecular basis of the sperm effect in *Drosophila melanogaster*. *Proceedings of the National Academy of Sciences of the USA*, **100**, 9929–9933.

Lohm, J., Grahn, M., Langefors, A. *et al.* (2002) Experimental evidence for major histocompatibility complex-allele-specific resistance to a bacterial infection. *Proceedings of the Royal Society B*, **269**, 2029–2033.

Loiselle, B. A., Ryder, T. B., Durães, R. *et al.* (2007) Kin selection does not explain male aggregation at leks of 4 manakin species. *Behavioral Ecology*, **18**, 287–291.

Lorch, P. D., Bussiére, L. & Gwynne, D. T. (2008) Quantifying the potential for sexual dimorphism using upper limits on Bateman gradients. *Behaviour*, **145**, 1–24.

Løvlie, H., Cornwallis, C. K. & Pizzari, T. (2005) Male mounting alone reduces female promiscuity in the fowl. *Current Biology*, **15**, 1222–1227.

Manning, J. T. & Chamberlain, A. T. (1994) Sib competition and sperm competitiveness: an answer to 'why so many sperms?' and the recombination/sperm number correlation. *Proceedings of the Royal Society B*, **256**, 177–182.

Maynard-Smith, J. (1977) Parental investment: a prospective analysis. *Animal Behaviour*, **25**, 1–9.

Maynard-Smith, J. (1978) *The Evolution of Sex*. Cambridge: Cambridge University Press.

McGraw, L. A., Gibson, G., Clark, A. G. & Wolfner, M. F. (2004) Genes regulated by mating, sperm, or seminal proteins in mated female *Drosophila melanogaster*. *Current Biology*, **14**: 1509–1514.

McGraw, L. A., Clark, A. G. & Wolfner, M. F. (2008) Post-mating gene expression profiles of female *Drosophila melanogaster* in response to time and to four male accessory gland proteins. *Genetics*, **179**, 1395–408.

Mead, L. S. & Arnold, S. J. (2004) Quantitative genetic models of sexual selection. *Trends in Ecology and Evolution*, **19**, 264–271.

Milinski, M. (2006) The major histocompatibility complex, sexual selection, and mate choice. *Annual Review of Ecology, Evolution, and Systematics*, **37**, 159–186.

Miller, C. W. & Moore, A. J. (2007) A potential resolution of the lek paradox through indirect genetic effects. *Proceedings of the Royal Society B*, **274**, 1279–1286.

Moczek, A. P. & Emlen, D. J. (2000) Male horn dimorphism in the scarab beetle, *Onthophagus taurus*: do alternative reproductive tactics favour alternative phenotypes? *Animal Behaviour*, **59**, 459–466.

Møller, A. P. & Pomiankowski, A. (1993) Why have birds got multiple sexual ornaments? *Behavioral Ecology and Sociobiology*, **32**, 167–176.

Moore, A. J. (1990) The inheritance of social dominance, mating behaviour, and attractiveness to mates in *Nauphoeta cinerea*. *Animal Behaviour*, **39**, 388–397.

Moore, A. J. & Moore, P. J. (1999) Balancing sexual selection through opposing mate choice and male competition. *Proceedings of the Royal Society B*, **266**, 711–716.

Moore, A. J. & Pizzari, T. (2005) Quantitative genetic models of sexual conflict based on interacting phenotypes. *American Naturalist*, **165**, S88–97.

Moreira, P. L., Nunes, V. L., Martín, J. & Paulo, O. S. (2007) Copulatory plugs do not assure high first male fertilisation success: sperm displacement in a lizard. *Behavioral Ecology and Sociobiology*, **62**, 281–288.

Morrow, E. H., Arnqvist, G. & Pitnick, S. (2003) Adaptation versus pleiotropy: why do males harm their mates? *Behavioral Ecology*, **14**, 802–806.

Mousseau, T. A. & Roff, D. A. (1987) Natural selection and the heritability of fitness components. *Heredity*, **59**, 181–197.

Murphy, C. G. (1998) Interaction-independent sexual selection and the mechanisms of sexual selection. *Evolution*, **52**, 8–18.

Neff, B. D. & Stoltz, J. A. (2006) Sperm competition in a fish with external fertilization: the contribution of sperm number, speed, and length. *Journal of Evolutionary Biology*, **19**, 1873–1881.

Neubaum, D. M. & Wolfner, M. F. (1999) Mated *Drosophila melanogaster* females require a seminal fluid protein, Acp36DE, to store sperm efficiently. *Genetics*, **153**, 845–847.

Nevo, E. & Beiles, A. (1992) Selection for class-Ii Mhc heterozygosity by parasites in subterranean mole rats. *Experientia*, **48**, 512–515.

Oliveira, R., Taborski, M. & Brockman, J. H. (2008) *Alternative Reproductive Tactics*. Cambridge: Cambridge University Press.

Omland, K. E. (1996) Female mallard mating preferences for multiple male ornaments. *Behavioral Ecology and Sociobiology*, **39**, 353–360.

Owens, I. P. F. & Thompson, D. B. A. (1994) Sex differences, sex ratios and sex roles. *Proceedings of the Royal Society B*, **258**, 93–99.

Packer, C., Gilbert, D. A., Pusey, A. E. & O'Brien, S. J. (1991) A molecular genetic analysis of kinship and cooperation in African lions. *Nature*, **351**, 562–565.

Panhuis, T. M., Clark, N. L. & Swanson, W. J. (2006) Rapid evolution of reproductive proteins in abalone and *Drosophila*. *Philosophical Transactions of the Royal Society B*, **361**, 261–268.

Parker, G. A. (1970) Sperm competition and its evolutionary consequences in the insects. *Biological Reviews*, **45**, 525–567.

Parker, G. A. (1979) Sexual selection and sexual conflict. In: *Sexual Selection and Reproductive Competition in Insects*, ed. M. S. Blum & N. A. Blum. New York, NY: Academic Press, pp. 123–166.

Parker, G. A. (1982) Why are there so many tiny sperm? Sperm competition and the maintenance of two sexes. *Journal of Theoretical Biology*, **96**, 281–294.

Parker, G. A. (2006) Sexual conflict over mating and fertilization: an overview. *Philosophical Transactions of the Royal Society B*, **361**, 235–259.

Parker, G. A. & Begon, M. E. (1993) Sperm competition games: sperm size and sperm number under gametic control. *Proceedings of the Royal Society B*, **253**, 255–262.

Parker, G. A. & Simmons, L. W. (1996) Parental investment and the control of sexual selection: predicting the direction of sexual competition. *Proceedings of the Royal Society B*, **263**, 315–321.

Parker, G. A., Smith, V. G. F. & Baker, R. R. (1972) Origin and evolution of gamete dimorphism and male-female phenomenon. *Journal of Theoretical Biology*, **36**, 529–553.

Paterson, S., Wilson, K. & Pemberton, J. M. (1998) Major histocompatibility complex variation associated with juvenile survival and parasite resistance in a large unmanaged ungulate population (*Ovis aries* L.). *Proceedings of the National Academy of Sciences of the USA*, **95**, 3714–3719.

Peng, J., Zipperlen, P. & Kubli, E. (2005) Drosophila sex-peptide stimulates female innate immune system after mating via the Toll and Imd pathways. *Current Biology*, **15**, 1690–1694.

Penn, D. J., Damjanovich, K. & Potts, W. K. (2002) MHC heterozygosity confers a selective advantage against multiple-strain infections. *Proceedings of the National Academy of Sciences of the USA*, **99**, 11260–11264.

Petrie, M., Krupa, A. & Burke, T. (1999) Peacocks lek with relatives even in the absence of social and environmental cues. *Nature*, **401**, 155–157.

Pischedda, A. & Chippindale, A.K. (2006) Intralocus sexual conflict diminishes the benefits of sexual selection. *PLoS Biology* 4 (11), e356.

Pitnick, S., Spicer, G. S. & Markow, T. A. (1995) How long is a giant sperm? *Nature*, **375**, 109.

Pitnick, S. Miller, G. T., Reagan, J. & Holland, B. (2001) Males' evolutionary responses to experimental removal of sexual selection. *Proceedings of the Royal Society B*, **268**, 1071–1080.

Pitnick, S., Wolfner, M. F. & Suarez, S. S. (2009) Ejaculate-female and sperm-female interactions. In: *Sperm Biology: an Evolutionary Perspective*, ed. T. R. Birkhead, D. J. Hosken & S. Pitnick. London: Academic Press, pp. 247–304.

Pizzari, T. (2001) Indirect female choice through manipulation of male behaviour by female fowl, Gallus g. domesticus. *Proceedings of the Royal Society B*, **268**, 181–186.

Pizzari, T. (2006) Evolution: the paradox of sperm leviathans. *Current Biology*, **16**, R462–464.

Pizzari, T. & Birkhead, T. R. (2000) Female feral fowl eject sperm of subdominant males. *Nature*, **405**, 787–789.

Pizzari, T. & Parker, G. A. (2009) Sperm competition and sperm phenotype. In: *Sperm Biology: an Evolutionary Perspective*, ed. T. R. Birkhead, D. J. Hosken & S. Pitnick. London: Academic Press, pp. 207–245.

Pizzari, T. & Snook, R. R. (2003) Perspective. Sexual conflict and sexual selection: chasing away paradigm shifts. *Evolution*, **57**, 1223–1236.

Pizzari, T., Cornwallis, C. K., Løvlie, H., Jakobsson, S. & Birkhead, T. R. (2003) Sophisticated sperm allocation in a bird. *Nature*, **426**, 70–74.

Pizzari, T., Løvlie, H. & Cornwallis, C. K. (2004) Sex-specific, counteracting responses to inbreeding in a bird. *Proceedings of the Royal Society B*, **271**, 2115–2121.

Poiani A., 2006. Complexity of seminal fluid: a review. *Behavioral Ecology and Sociobiology*, **60**, 289–310.

Pomiankowski, A. & Møller, A. P. (1995) A resolution of the lek paradox. *Proceedings of the Royal Society B*, **260**, 21–29.

Pomiankowski, A., Iwasa, Y. & Nee, S. (1991) The evolution of costly mate preferences I. Fisher and biased mutation. *Evolution*, **45**, 1422–1430.

Pound, N. (1999) Effects of morphine on electrically evoked contractions of the vas deferens in two congeneric rodent species differing in sperm competition intensity. *Proceedings of the Royal Society B*, **266**, 1755–1758.

Preston, B. T. & Stockley, P. (2006) The prospect of sexual competition stimulates premature and repeated ejaculation in a mammal. *Current Biology*, **16**, R239–241.

Preston, B. T., Stevenson, I. R., Pemberton, J. M. & Wilson K. (2001) Dominant rams lose out by sperm depletion. *Nature*, **409**, 681–682.

Priest, N. K., Roach, D. A. & Galloway, L. F. (2007) Cross-generational fitness benefits of mating and seminal fluid. *Biology Letters*, **4**, 6–8.

Priest, N. K., Galloway, L. F. & Roach, D. A. (2008) Mating frequency and inclusive fitness in *Drosophila melanogaster*. *American Naturalist*, **171**, 10–21.

Pruett-Jones, S. (1992) Independent versus nonindependent mate choice: do females copy each other? *American Naturalist*, **140**, 1000–1009.

Pryke, S. R. & Griffith, S. C. (2006) Red dominates black: agonistic signalling among head morphs in the colour polymorphic Gouldian finch. *Proceedings of the Royal Society B*, **273**, 949–957.

Pryke, S. R. & Griffith, S. C. (2007) The relative role of male vs. female mate choice in maintaining assortative pairing among discrete colour morphs. *Journal of Evolutionary Biology*, **20**, 1512–1521.

Queller, D. C. (1997) Why do females care more than males? *Proceedings of the Royal Society B*, **264**, 1555–1557.

Rankin, D. J., Bargum, K. & Kokko, H. (2007) The tragedy of the commons in evolutionary biology. *Trends in Ecology and Evolution*, **22**, 643–651.

Ravi Ram, K. & Wolfner, M. F. (2007a) Seminal influences: *Drosophila* Acps and the molecular interplay between males and females during reproduction. *Integrative and Comparative Biology*, **47**, 1–19.

Ravi Ram, K. & Wolfner, M. F. (2007b) Sustained post-mating response in *Drosophila melanogaster* requires multiple seminal fluid proteins. *PLoS Genetics*, **3** (12), e238.

Ravi Ram, K., Sirot, L. K. & Wolfner, M. F. (2006) A predicted seminal astacin-like protease is required for the processing of reproductive proteins in *Drosophila melanogaster*. *Proceedings of the National Academy of Sciences of the USA*, **103**, 10674–10679.

Reusch, T. B. H., Haberli, M. A., Aeschlimann, P. B. & Milinski, M. (2001) Female sticklebacks count alleles in a strategy of sexual selection explaining MHC polymorphism. *Nature*, **414**, 300–302.

Reynolds, J. D. & Gross, M. R. (1990) Costs and benefits of female mate choice: is there a lek paradox? *American Naturalist*, **136**, 230–243.

Rhen, T. (2000) Sex-limited mutations and the evolution of sexual dimorphism. *Evolution*, **54**, 37–43.

Rice, W. R. (1984) Sex chromosomes and the evolution of sexual dimorphism. *Evolution*, **38**, 735–742.

Rice, W. R. (1996) Sexually antagonistic male adaptation triggered by experimental arrest of female evolution. *Nature*, **381**, 232–234.

Rice, W. R. & Chippindale, A. K. (2001) Intersexual ontogenetic conflict. *Journal of Evolutionary Biology*, **14**, 685–693.

Rivera, A. C., Andres, J. A., Córdoba-Aguilar, A. & Utzeri, C. (2004) Postmating sexual selection: allopatric evolution of sperm competition mechanisms and genital morphology in calopterygid damselflies (Insecta: Odonata). *Evolution*, **58**, 349–359.

Robertson, H. M. (1985) Female dimorphism and mating behaviour in a damselfly, *Ischnura ramburi*: females mimicking males. *Animal Behaviour*, **33**, 805–809.

Rodd, F. H., Hughes, K. A., Grether, G. & Baril, C. T. (2002) A possible non-sexual origin of a mate preference: are male guppies mimicking fruit? *Proceedings of the Royal Society B*, **269**, 475–481.

Rowe, L. & Houle, D. (1996) The lek paradox and the capture of genetic variance by condition dependent traits. *Proceedings of the Royal Society B*, **263**, 1415–1421.

Ryan, M.J. (1998) Sexual selection, receiver biases, and the evolution of sex differences. *Science*, **281**, 1999–2002.

Scott, D. (1986) Sexual mimicry regulates the attractiveness of mated *Drosophila melanogaster* females. *Proceedings of the National Academy of Sciences of the USA*, **83**, 8429–8433.

Senseney, H. L., Briles, W. E., Abplanalp, H. & Taylor, R. L. (2000) Allelic complementation between MHC haplotypes B-Q and B-17 increases regression of Rous sarcomas. *Poultry Science*, **79**, 1736–1740.

Servedio, M. R. & Kirkpatrick, M. (1996) The evolution of mate choice copying by indirect selection. *American Naturalist*, **148**, 848–867.

Sheldon, B. C. (2001) Differential allocation: tests, mechanisms and implications. *Trends in Ecology and Evolution*, **15**, 397–402.

Shine, R., Phillips, B., Waye, H., LeMaster, M. & Mason, R. T. (2001) Benefits of female mimicry in snakes. *Nature*, **414**, 267.

Shorey, L., Piertney, S., Stone, J. & Höglund, J. (2000) Fine-scale genetic structuring on *Manacus manacus* leks. *Nature*, **408**, 352–353.

Shuster, S. M. & Wade, M. J. (2003) *Mating Systems and Strategies*. Princeton, NJ: Princeton University Press.

Shuster, S. M. & Wade, M. J. (2005) Don't throw Bateman out with the bathwater! *Integrative and Comparative Biology*, **45**, 945–951.

Simmons, L. W. (2001) *Sperm Competition and its Evolutionary Consequences in the Insects*. Princeton, NJ: Princeton University Press.

Simmons, L. W. (2005) The evolution of polyandry: sperm competition, sperm selection, and offspring viability. *Annual Review of Ecology, Evolution, and Systematics*, **36**, 125–146.

Sirot, L. K., Brockmann, H. J., Marinis, C. & Muschett, G. (2003) Maintenance of a female-limited polymorphism in *Ischnura ramburi* (Zygoptera: Coenagrionidae). *Animal Behaviour*, **66**, 763–775.

Smedley, S. R. & Eisner, T. (1996) Sodium: a male moth's gift to its offspring. *Proceedings of the National Academy of Sciences of the USA*, **93**, 809–813.

Snook, R. (2001) Sexual selection: conflict, kindness and chicanery. *Current Biology*, **11**, R337–341.

Snyder, B. F. & Gowaty, P. A. (2007) A reappraisal of Bateman's classic study of intrasexual selection. *Evolution*, **61**, 2457–2468.

Stewart, A. D., Morrow, E. H. & Rice, W. R. (2005) Assessing putative interlocus sexual conflict in *Drosophila melanogaster* using experimental evolution. *Proceedings of the Royal Society B*, **272**, 2029–2035.

Stoltz, J. A. & Neff, B. D. (2006) Male size and mating tactic influence proximity to females during sperm competition in bluegill sunfish. *Behavioral Ecology and Sociobiology*, **59**, 811–818.

Stutt, A. D. & Siva-Jothy, M. T. (2001) Traumatic insemination and sexual conflict in the bed bug *Cimex lectularius*. *Proceedings of the National Academy of Sciences of the USA*, **98**, 5683–5687.

Tatarnic, N. J., Cassis, G. & Hochuli, D. F. (2006) Traumatic insemination in the plant bug genus *Coridromius* Signoret (Heteroptera: Miridae). *Biology Letters*, **2**, 58–61.

Taylor, M., Wedell, N. & Hosken, D. (2007) The heritability of attractiveness. *Current Biology*, **17**, R959–960.

Taylor, P. D. & Williams, G. C. (1982) The lek paradox is not resolved. *Theoretical Population Biology*, **22**, 392–409.

ten Cate, C., Verzijden, M. & Etman, E. (2006) Sexual imprinting can induce sexual preferences for exaggerated parental traits. *Current Biology*, **16**, 1128–1132.

Thornhill, R. (1983) Cryptic female choice and its implications in the scorpionfly Harpobittacus nigriceps. *American Naturalist*, **122**, 765.

Thursz, M. R., Thomas, H. C., Greenwood, B. M. & Hill, A. V. S. (1997) Heterozygote advantage for HLA class-II type in hepatitis B virus infection. *Nature Genetics*, **17**, 11–12.

Tomkins, J. L. & Hazel, W. (2007) The status of the conditional evolutionarily stable strategy. *Trends in Ecology and Evolution*, **22**, 522–528.

Trivers, R. L. (1972) Parental investment and sexual selection. In: *Sexual Selection and the Descent of Man, 1871–1971*, ed. B. Campbell. Chicago, IL: Aldine, pp. 136–179.

Valera, F., Hoi, H. & Kristin, A. (2003) Male shrikes punish unfaithful females. *Behavioral Ecology and Sociobiology*, **14**, 403–408.

van Gossum, H. & Sherratt, T. M. (2008) A dynamical model of sexual harassment and its implications for female-limited polymorphism. *Ecological Modelling*, **210**, 212–220.

van Homrigh, A., Higgie, M., McGuigan, K. & Blows, M. W. (2007) The depletion of genetic variance by sexual selection. *Current Biology*, **17**, 528–532.

Warner, R. R., Shapiro, D. Y., Marcanato, A. & Petersen, C. W. (1995) Sexual conflict – males with the highest mating success convey the lowest fertilization benefits to females. *Proceedings of the Royal Society B*, **262**, 135–139.

Wedell, N. (1994) Dual function of the bushcricket spermatophore. *Proceedings of the Royal Society B*, **258**, 181–185.

Wedell, N. & Tregenza, T. (1999) Successful fathers sire successful sons. *Evolution*, **53**, 620–625.

Wedell, N., Gage, M. J. G. & Parker, G. A. (2002) Sperm competition, male prudence and sperm-limited females. *Trends in Ecology and Evolution*, **17**, 313–320.

West, S. A., Griffin, A. S. & Gardner, A. (2007) Social semantics: altruism, cooperation, mutualism, strong reciprocity and group selection. *Journal of Evolutionary Biology*, **20**, 415–432.

Widemo, F. & Owens, I. P. F. (1995) Lek size, male mating skew and the evolution of lekking. *Nature*, **373**, 148–151.

Wigby, S. & Chapman, T. (2004) Female resistance to male harm evolves in response to manipulation of sexual conflict. *Evolution*, **58**, 1028–1037.

Wigby, S. & Chapman, T. (2005) Sex peptide causes mating costs in female *Drosophila melanogaster*. *Current Biology*, **15**, 316–321.

Wiklund, C., Kaitala, A., Lindfors, V. & Abenius, J. (1993) Polyandry and its effect on female reproduction in the green-veined white butterfly (*Pieris napi* L.). *Behavioral Ecology and Sociobiology*, **33**, 25–33.

Williams, G. C. (1975) *Sex and Evolution*. Princeton, NJ: Princeton University Press.

Willmott, H. E. & Foster, S. A. (1995) The effects of rival male interaction on courtship and parental care in the four-spine stickleback, *Apeltes quadracus*. *Behaviour*, **132**, 997–1010.

Wilson, E. O. (1975) *Sociobiology: the New Synthesis*. Cambridge, MA: Harvard University Press.

Wright, D., Kerje, S., Brändström, H. *et al.* (2008) The genetic architecture of a female sexual ornament. *Evolution*, **62**, 86–98.

Yapici, N., Kim, Y. J., Ribeiro, C. & Dickson, B. J. (2008) A receptor that mediates the post-mating switch in *Drosophila* reproductive behaviour. *Nature*, **451**, 33–37.

Zahavi, A. (1975) Mate selection: selection for a handicap. *Journal of Theoretical Biology*, **53**, 205–214.

In celebration of questions, past, present and future

Geoff A. Parker

But I now see that the whole problem is so intricate that it is safer to leave its solution for the future.

Darwin (1874) on the evolution of the unity sex ratio; later solved by Fisher (1930)

A vital part of science is the compulsion to ask questions, even if, like Darwin, we cannot always find an answer. I admit to being surprised, almost offended, when people claim not to be interested in animals, what animals do, and why they do it. I don't care at all if someone isn't interested in my other preoccupations – jazz, exhibition poultry – why should they be? But somehow I can't accept that it is possible not to have an interest in the evolution of behaviour – the evolution of our own behaviour, and ultimately why we are what we are. Indeed, it seems impossible to gain insight about ourselves without considering the diversity of animal life, and our place in it all.

Maybe that, and my fascination for natural history, was why I changed almost immediately from medicine to zoology as a student at Bristol University in 1962. Medicine would have offered affluence and security, but when 'push came to shove', I opted for the risk and adventure of following my obsession. Biology – indeed science itself – offers a philosophy and insight into the nature of life that applied science and technology does not. So when I began my PhD, staring hard at the intense melee of dungflies

swarming on a cowpat, I was utterly fascinated, and never thought that what I was doing was odd. An occupation such as trying to find a better way to sell baked beans was odd: that merely provided a living. It was an immense privilege to be paid to do my hobby.

The most amazing thing about dungflies at cattle droppings in their seasonal population peaks is the sheer number of them, the swirling chaos of activity, with males leaping around searching for females as they arrive, and locked in struggles with other males for possession of females (Parker 2001). Original photos from my thesis have been published several times over the years, but help to show what happens. Once a male has found a gravid female, he copulates and then guards the female while she oviposits in the dung. Particularly during oviposition, searching males repeatedly attack the pair, and the guarding male (whose genitalia are now free from the female) shows an elaborate series of behavioural responses to deflect an attacking male away from the female. Most attacks are deflected with minimal disturbance, but should the attacker manage to touch the female with his front tarsi (e.g. when two males attack simultaneously), he attempts to insert himself between the female and the guarding male. An intense and protracted struggle then develops, and larger males have an advantage. If there is a take-over, the new

Social Behaviour: Genes, Ecology and Evolution, ed. Tamás Székely, Allen J. Moore and Jan Komdeur. Published by Cambridge University Press. © Cambridge University Press 2010.

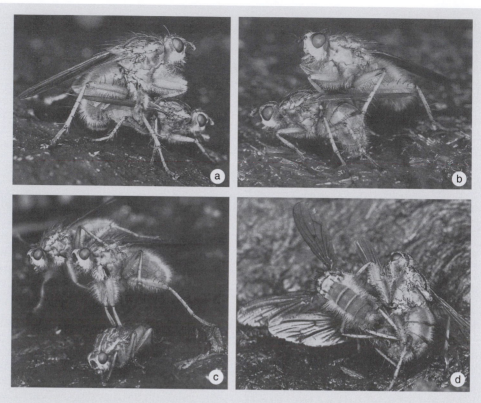

Some of the original dungfly photographs from my PhD thesis (Parker 1968). (a) Pair copulating on a cattle dropping. (b) After copulation: male guarding and female ovipositing. (c) A guarding male deflecting an attacking male. (d) A struggle between two males for the possession of a female.

male copulates with the female – the last male to mate gains on average over 80% of the eggs, which is why he guards his female during oviposition.

The dungfly mating system is a wonderful one to study. I like to believe that my PhD provided much-needed quantitative evidence for fine-grained adaptation arising through the male–male competition, at a time when Darwin's theory of sexual selection was not a favoured interpretation (Parker 1978, 2006a). I think there were also other benefits. A good model system should make one ask wider questions (Parker 2001), and I owe to the dung-flies the fact that I became interested in a range of general problems, such as sperm competition, the evolution of two sexes, animal contests, animal

distributions and sexual conflict (Parker 2009). In fact, much of my time in the last four decades has been dedicated to extending ideas arising from that early empirical study. Mostly, I have been involved in studying antisocial behaviour, and in particular how conflicts of interest between individuals are resolved.

The behavioural-ecology explosion of the 1970s was an amazing time for our subject area (Parker 2006a, 2009). If I were to try to summarise its impact, I would opt for three key aspects: (1) a shift from interpretations based on group selection or 'survival value for the species' to explanations based on advantages to genes or individuals, (2) the rapid development of optimality models for understanding adaptation, based on maximisation of individual or inclusive fitness, and (3) the appreciation of underlying evolutionary conflicts of interest between individuals. 'Maximisation of fitness' certainly doesn't mean a local maximum for the fitness of the population, though this might occur. Maynard Smith & Price (1973) proposed that we seek a competitive optimum or an evolutionarily stable strategy (ESS), i.e. a strategy such that when played by most of the population, all mutants deviating from the population strategy achieve lower fitness than an individual playing the population strategy (see Chapter 4). Thus fitness is maximised in a competitive sense: in game-theory terms, we seek a strategy that is a best reply to itself. Even that is not sufficient; we also require that the ESS is 'continuously stable', i.e. that selection will drive towards it. Observations are compared with model predictions, not to test whether adaptation has occurred (which is an assumption), but rather to gain evidence that the selective forces that have moulded the adaptation have been correctly identified (Parker & Maynard Smith 1990).

The behavioural-ecology explosion had a downside: the 'sociobiology debate' (Segerstråle 2000). Following the publication of Wilson's (1975) *Sociobiology* book, the approach suffered controversy and attack, because sociobiologists discussed the nature of human behaviour. I was horrified that 'the baby might be thrown out with the bath water'. It would have been a tragedy if the new and exciting science that was developing had become consigned to the dustbin for political reasons. I was personally reluctant to speculate in print about human behaviour. As a behavioural ecologist, I of course had great faith in the approach. But human behaviour is a complex mix of nature and nurture, and a theoretical basis for the evolutionary rules underlying learning and motivation was underdeveloped (and probably still is). It is easier to make progress with flies. And newsreels of the Nazi death camps that had haunted me so much as a child made me worry about the political consequences of hypotheses about human biology. Nowadays, human behavioural ecology (renamed evolutionary psychology; see Chapter 15) is a thriving discipline; it is hard to believe it had so divisive a birth.

Much has changed since the 1970s – the advances are huge. We now have much better techniques for comparative analysis, molecular biology has generated amazing possibilities for evolutionary biology, and our computing power is immense. Models based on the underlying mechanisms are replacing the early 'black box' approach, in which one constructed a model without any knowledge of the mechanistic constraints. Since an optimality model is a device for maximising against a set of trade-offs and other physiological constraints, the more we know about the true nature of those constraints the better the model is likely to be. There are two modelling extremes (Parker & Maynard Smith 1990): the most general models are mainly heuristic, aiming to emphasise the question and the sorts of answers that may be possible; the most specific models are tailored for given systems and have empirically determined parameters, and aim to make exact predictions for that system.

My current interests are rather diverse. Since 1990, I have been modelling sperm allocation under postcopulatory sexual selection, and although my collaborators and I have spent much time on this, we still need more theory, and many more empirical studies to determine the mechanisms involved. In particular, we need to ask how the resolution of precopulatory and postcopulatory sexual conflicts are linked, since the payoffs for precopulatory strategies depend on what happens at the postcopulatory levels (Parker 2006b).

Much of my time since 2000 has been spent investigating the evolution of complex life cycles in helminth parasites. There are so many questions to answer about parasite evolution, and though a start has been made, it is remarkable that so little was achieved until the past two decades. I should like to understand more about such things as the mechanisms by which parasites add new hosts, why complex migrations are made in intermediate hosts, how some helminths evade their host's responses, why there is asexual reproduction in trematodes but not acanthocephalans or nematodes, and so on.

What about future studies of social behaviour? My interests have mainly concerned conflicts in biology and their resolution; these are usually relevant to social behaviour, particularly conflicts within the family, and questions about the simultaneous resolution of the three linked games, sib competition, parent–offspring conflict, and sexual conflict over parental investment or mating decisions. I should love to know more about the balance between scramble competition between sibs and signalling true need to parents in the evolution and maintenance of begging signals. There is also room for further theory about sexual conflicts, concerning both parental investment and mating/fertilisation.

We still have plenty of questions to answer, and each answer throws up several more questions. Since its early controversies, and the exhilaration of its originality and creativity, behavioural ecology has by now matured into a flourishing research area in biology. It is an exciting time for our discipline.

References

Darwin, C. (1874) *The Descent of Man and Selection in Relation to Sex*, 2nd edn. London: John Murray.

Fisher, R. A. (1930) *The Genetical Theory of Natural Selection*. Oxford: Clarendon Press.

Maynard Smith, J. & Price, G. R. (1973) The logic of animal conflicts. *Nature*, **246**, 15–18.

Parker, G. A. (1968) The reproductive behaviour and the nature of sexual selection in *Scatophaga stercoraria* L. Unpublished PhD thesis, University of Bristol.

Parker, G. A. (1978) Selfish genes, evolutionary games, and the adaptiveness of behaviour. *Nature*, **274**, 849–855.

Parker, G. A. (2001) Golden flies, sunlit meadows: a tribute to the yellow dungfly. In: *Model Systems in Behavioural Ecology: Integrating Conceptual, Theoretical, and Empirical Approaches*, ed. L. A. Dugatkin. Princeton, NJ: Princeton University Press, pp. 3–26.

Parker, G. A. (2006a) Behavioural ecology: the science of natural history. In: *Essays on Animal Behaviour: Celebrating 50 years of Animal Behaviour*, ed. J. R. Lucas & L. W. Simmons, Burlington MA: Elsevier, pp. 23–56.

Parker, G. A. (2006b) Sexual conflict over mating and fertilization: an overview. *Philosophical Transactions of the Royal Society B*, **361**, 235–259.

Parker, G. A. (2009) Reflections before dusk. In: *Leaders in Animal Behavior: the Second Generation*, ed. L. Drickamer & D. A. Dewsbury. Cambridge: Cambridge University Press, pp. 429–464.

Parker, G. A. & Maynard Smith, J. (1990) Optimality theory in evolutionary biology. *Nature*, **348**, 27–33.

Segerstråle, U. (2000) *Defenders of the Truth: the Battle for Science in the Sociobiology Debate and Beyond*. Oxford: Oxford University Press.

Wilson, E. O. (1975) *Sociobiology: the New Synthesis*. Cambridge, MA: Harvard University Press.

11

Pair bonds and parental behaviour

Lisa McGraw, Tamás Székely and Larry J. Young

Overview

Pair bonds and parental behaviour are among the most variable social traits. To understand *how* and *why* these traits are so variable, we investigate three issues in this chapter. First, we present an overview of recent work on molecular and neural aspects of pair bonds and parental care using microtine rodents as model organisms. We focus on two neuropeptides, oxytocin and vasopressin, and show that although both molecules are found in both sexes, oxytocin plays a more prominent role in regulating parenting and pair bonding in females, whereas vasopressin serves this role in males. Variation in the expression of oxytocin and vasopressin receptors appears to contribute to species and individual differences in social behaviour. These studies also show that although oxytocin and vasopressin function in distinct brain regions, they act within the same neural circuit. Therefore, females and males appear to accomplish behavioural changes in pair bonding and parental care by altering the responsiveness of the same neural circuit. Second, studies of pair bonds and parental care in natural populations have revealed that these traits are often tied together. Cost–benefit analyses of both traits in a game-theoretic framework provide novel insights into how diverse pair bonding and parental care may have evolved. Recent work emphasises the role of social environment in influencing pair bonding and care. Finally, we point out that currently there is a schism between proximate and ultimate approaches to understanding pair bonding and parental care. We propose to bridge this gap by using a bottom-up approach that builds upon the vole research paradigm, and a top-down approach that seeks to establish molecular and neural bases of behavioural variation in taxa that exhibit highly diverse pair bonds and care.

11.1 Introduction

Historically, many biologists idealised the monogamous family life in terms of sexual and parental commitment, perhaps because fidelity and cooperation between parents reflected the cultural values of Western society. For example, Lack (1968) suggested that over 90% of all bird species were genetically monogamous, possessed strong social bonds between partners and exhibited biparental care of offspring. However, several years later, Trivers (1972, 1974) recognised that, on the contrary, family life is

Social Behaviour: Genes, Ecology and Evolution, ed. Tamás Székely, Allen J. Moore and Jan Komdeur. Published by Cambridge University Press. © Cambridge University Press 2010.

often rife with conflicts, and the interests of males and females of a breeding pair often differ (sexual conflict). Trivers, based on the groundbreaking work by Bateman (1948; see Chapter 10), predicted that males should behave in ways that maximise their lifetime reproductive success by engaging in opportunistic extra-pair matings, and that females should be choosy and select mates that increase the genetic quality of their offspring. More recent studies further suggest that females may also gain indirect benefits by mating with multiple males (Jennions & Petrie 2000, Tregenza & Wedell 2000, Zeh & Zeh 2001). In the past decades, advances in genetic techniques to assess relatedness of offspring, coupled with field studies of natural populations, have revealed that, as Trivers (1972, 1974) predicted, genetic monogamy is rarely the norm. Instead, many species that were previously thought to be genetically monogamous are now considered to be socially monogamous, and sexual fidelity by all individuals in a population is exceedingly uncommon (reviewed in Westneat & Stewart 2003, Wolff & MacDonald 2004, Solomon & Keane 2007). While, in most cases, sexual fidelity can no longer be considered a useful measure for defining monogamy, two other attributes of many socially monogamous species, the pair bond and biparental care of offspring, often accompany this mating strategy (Møller 2007, Reichard 2007).

As pair bonds and biparental care of offspring are often (though not always) a characteristic feature of monogamous mating systems, they have long been the subject of investigation for scientists from a variety of disciplines. While we have learned a tremendous amount about pair bonding and parental care over the past few decades, scientists from distinct and non-overlapping fields of biology have performed much of this research with little communication between them. At one extreme, geneticists, endocrinologists and neurobiologists have primarily been interested in understanding the proximate mechanisms that underlie pair bond formation and parental care (see Chapter 3). These investigators use a mechanistic approach to identify the genes, hormones and neural circuits that regulate these processes (reviewed by Numan & Insel 2003, Young &

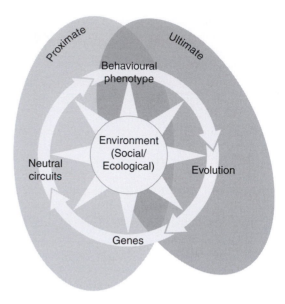

Figure 11.1 A conceptual framework of the dynamic processes influencing behavioural phenotypes such as pair bonding and/or parental care. In this chapter, we emphasise the importance of considering comprehensively how genes, neural circuits and selection pressures work together to generate the behavioural phenotype, and how both the social and ecological environment may further influence each of these individual components. Whereas proximate research approaches have linked genes and neural circuits to behaviours (left) and ultimate research approaches have considered how selection pressures may drive the evolution of behaviours (right), few studies have integrated the two approaches to derive a comprehensive understanding of the complex dynamics that generate pair bonds and parental care.

Wang 2004, Adkins-Regan 2005). These researchers are often limited to working on inbred strains of laboratory animals with limited behavioural repertoires that may not accurately reflect the diversity of natural populations. In contrast, evolutionary biologists and behavioural ecologists have focused on understanding the ultimate questions that lead to diversity in parenting styles or mating tactics, and focus on how life-history strategies, ecology and cooperation and/ or conflict between individuals shape the evolution of pair bonding and parental care (reviewed by Clutton-Brock 1989, Black 1996, Balshine-Earn *et al.* 2002,

Bennett & Owens 2002, Houston *et al.* 2005). These researchers typically study animals in their natural environments, and many of these organisms are not amenable to laboratory, genetic or neural studies.

The integration of proximate and ultimate research approaches and perspectives is imperative for gaining a comprehensive understanding of how genes, hormones, neural circuitry, the environment and evolutionary pressures work together to generate diversity in pair-bonding and parental behaviours (Fig. 11.1). In this chapter, we present an overview of the proximate biological mechanisms that shape pair bonding and parental care, and then review how ultimate approaches have led us to a greater understanding of how natural selection shapes these behaviours. Finally, we suggest areas in which scientists from different disciplines can interact to facilitate an integrated understanding of these processes.

11.2 The prairie vole model

Much of our basic understanding of the genes, hormones and neural circuits that ultimately regulate social behaviours has been derived from experiments using traditional laboratory animals such as Norway rats *Rattus norvegicus* and house mice *Mus musculus* (reviewed in Insel & Young 2000, Meaney 2001, Young & Insel 2002, Numan & Insel 2003, Bielsky & Young 2004, Curley & Keverne 2005, Hammock & Young 2007a). Although these laboratory-bred species have proven valuable for this purpose, they provide little insight into how variation in the proximate mechanisms that regulate social behaviour leads to diversity in these traits, or how these mechanisms are shaped by selective forces to drive the evolution of social behaviour. Furthermore, as these species do not form pair bonds, they cannot be used to reveal the mechanisms underlying attachment between mates. However, arvicoline rodents, or voles, have provided enormous insight into both proximate and ultimate aspects of pair bonding and parental care (Young & Wang 2004, Carter *et al.* 1995).

Prairie voles *Microtus ochrogaster* are cooperatively breeding, socially monogamous rodents that have been extensively studied both within their natural environments and in the laboratory for over two decades. Early field studies led to the initial classification of the social structure of prairie voles as being primarily monogamous (Getz *et al.* 1981, 1990). In nature, most adult prairie voles form long-lived pair bonds with their mates (Getz *et al.* 1981, 1993, Getz & Hofmann 1986, Getz & Carter 1996), and, as predicted by their mating system, both females and males participate in important aspects of parental care (McGuire & Novak 1984a, Oliveras & Novak 1986, Solomon 1993, Wang & Insel 1996, Lonstein & DeVries 1999). In the laboratory, mated pairs develop a partner preference, preferring the company of their partner over that of a novel stimulus animal (Williams *et al.* 1992), and if one sexual partner dies, the remaining animal of the pair will typically not establish a pair bond with a new partner (Pizzuto & Getz 1998). Furthermore, in the laboratory removal of the partner leads to behaviours reminiscent of depression (Bosch *et al.* 2009). While the early classification of prairie voles as a monogamous species remains valid in some sense, recent studies using molecular markers to determine relatedness among individuals in natural or semi-natural populations have determined that a striking number of offspring are the result of extra-pair matings (Solomon *et al.* 2004, Ophir *et al.* 2008a). Thus, like most species that were initially thought to be genetically monogamous, prairie voles are now classified as socially monogamous. Furthermore, there is considerable variation, both within and across prairie vole populations, in the percentage of individuals who display pair bonds and biparental care (Getz *et al.* 1990, 1992, Roberts *et al.* 1998, Cochran & Solomon 2000, Cushing *et al.* 2001, Lucia *et al.* 2008, Solomon & Crist 2008).

11.2.1 From genes to brains to behaviour: laboratory studies of pair bonding and parental care in voles

While the social behaviour of prairie voles has been extensively studied in their natural environment, they are also easily maintained in a laboratory setting where animals are systematically outbred so that, like animals observed in their natural environments,

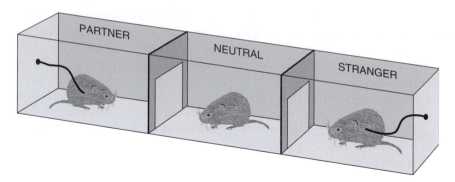

Figure 11.2 The partner preference test is a simple laboratory assay to measure pair bonding in rodents. In this test, males and females are paired for a given amount of time (usually eight hours or longer), during which they are free to interact and mate. After a brief separation, they are then subjected to the partner preference test. To test for a male's partner preference, his female mate is tethered in one chamber of a three-chambered apparatus and a second, unrelated, mated stranger female is tethered in another chamber. The male is then placed in the middle chamber, and he is free to roam throughout the arena for three hours. A partner preference is measured by quantifying the total time he spends in contact with his mate compared to the time spent with the stranger. A female's partner preference can be examined by tethering males instead of females.

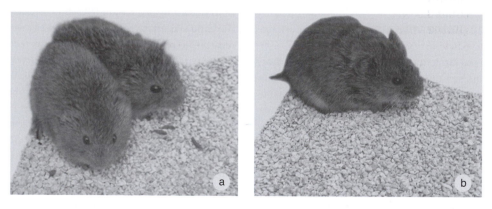

Figure 11.3 Comparative studies of (a) socially monogamous prairie voles *Microtus ochrogaster* and (b) promiscuous meadow voles *M. pennsylvanicus* have provided enormous insight into the molecular and neurobiological basis of sociobehavioural traits.

they display tremendous individual variation in social behaviours. Within the controlled laboratory setting, it is possible to measure social behaviours that can typically only be inferred from field studies. For example, the partner preference test is commonly used to assess the formation of the pair bond between sexual partners (Fig. 11.2; Williams *et al.* 1992), and parental behaviour can be easily quantified in controlled environments (Wang *et al.* 1994). These qualities make

prairie voles an ideal model organism for identifying individual differences in the proximate mechanisms underlying social behaviour. In addition, comparative studies between socially monogamous prairie voles and two closely related, non-monogamous and uniparental vole species, meadow *M. pennsylvanicus* and montane *M. montanus* voles, have provided invaluable insights into the mechanisms that underlie species differences in social behaviour (Fig. 11.3).

Although many genes and molecular events influence pair bonds and parental care (for review, see Young & Insel 2002), in this section we focus on two behavioural modulators, oxytocin and vasopressin, that exemplify how the prairie vole model has helped bridge some of the gaps between genes, the brain and behaviour.

11.2.2 Oxytocin: a molecule of female social behaviour

In voles, like many rodents, maternal behaviour begins at parturition as mothers begin to lick and pull the emerging fetuses from the vagina. Females continue to clean the pups, removing the amniotic sac, amniotic fluid, umbilical cord and placenta. After birth, females continue to provide maternal care through typical behaviours such as retrieving displaced pups, licking and grooming pups, constructing and maintaining the nest, hovering over the pups and nursing (McGuire & Novak 1984b). There is considerable species diversity in the development of maternal nurturing behaviour among mammals. Many species only exhibit maternal responsiveness towards pups after exposure to the hormonal changes that accompany pregnancy and birth (Young & Insel 2002). However, in some species, juveniles and/or virgin adults display maternal-like behaviour. For example, most sexually naive, juvenile (20 days of age) prairie voles exhibit spontaneous maternal behaviour, or alloparental behaviour if they are exposed to novel pups, perhaps an adaptation important in communal nests in which older offspring stay in their natal nest (Solomon 1991, Roberts *et al.* 1998, Olazábal & Young 2005). In contrast, juvenile meadow voles and house mice rarely display alloparental care. As female prairie voles mature, approximately half of the individuals lose maternal responsiveness and will either ignore pups or, often, will attack and kill the pups (Solomon 1991, Roberts *et al.* 1998, Olazábal & Young 2005). The tremendous species and individual variation in vole maternal care provides an excellent opportunity to study the mechanisms underlying the diversity and regulation of maternal behaviour.

The hormones associated with pregnancy and lactation, including oestrogen, progesterone, prolactin and oxytocin, all synchronise the peripheral physiology associated with pregnancy, delivery and lactation with the onset of maternal behaviour (see Chapter 3; Young & Insel 2002). Here we will limit our discussion to the neuropeptide oxytocin, as it has been shown to contribute to variation in parenting styles both within and across species (Young & Insel 2002). Vaginocervical stimulation during parturition, along with suckling during nursing, stimulates the release of oxytocin from the posterior pituitary into the general circulation, where it stimulates uterine contractions during labour and milk ejection during lactation (Burbach *et al.* 2006). Oxytocin is also released from neurons concentrated in the hypothalamus, where it modulates maternal behaviour (Numan & Insel 2003). The initial studies implicating oxytocin in the regulation of maternal care came from observations of virgin female rats. Rats that were hormone-primed to simulate pregnancy became maternal one hour following an injection of oxytocin into the brain (Pedersen & Prange 1979). Likewise, when female rats were given an antagonist that blocked oxytocin's receptor, they exhibited delayed onset of maternal behaviour (Leengoed *et al.* 1987). Oxytocin appears to trigger the onset of maternal behaviour through stimulating several brain regions involved in olfactory processing, emotionality, and reward and reinforcement (Insel & Young 2000). Studies in domestic sheep *Ovis aries* have revealed that oxytocin facilitates the selective bond between the ewe and her lamb within minutes after birth (Kendrick *et al.* 1987, 1997).

Oxytocin's actions in both the periphery and the brain are mediated by a G-protein-coupled oxytocin receptor (OTR). OTRs are localised in several brain regions that have been implicated in the regulation of maternal care. Interestingly, there is remarkable individual and between-species variation in OTR distribution in the brain that appears to contribute to diversity in parenting styles (Olazábal & Young 2006a). Prairie voles have high densities of OTR in the nucleus accumbens, a region of the brain associated with reward and reinforcement, compared to montane and meadow voles, which do not exhibit spontaneous parental care (Fig. 11.4; Insel & Shapiro 1992, Young

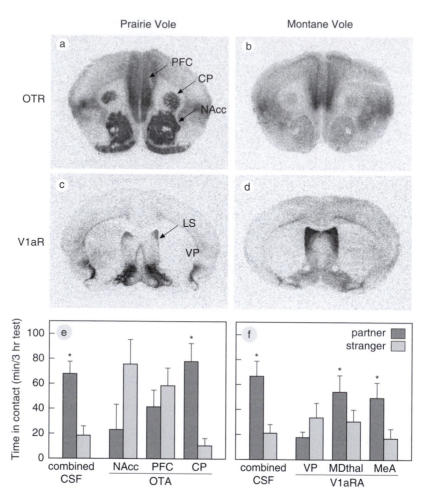

Figure 11.4 (a) Socially monogamous prairie voles have higher densities of oxytocin receptor (OTR) in brain regions such as the nucleus accumbens (NAcc) and caudate putamen (CP), but not the prefrontal cortex (PFC), than do (b) non-monogamous montane voles. (c) Prairie voles also have higher densities of vasopressin 1a receptor (V1aR) in the ventral pallidum (VP), but lower density of receptors in the lateral septum (LS) than do (d) montane voles. (e) If a selective OTR antagonist (OTA) is infused into the NAcc (but not the CP) of female prairie voles, partner preference formation, measured as the amount of time spent in social contact during a 3-hour partner preference test, is diminished compared to control females that were injected with cerebrospinal fluid (CSF). (f) Likewise, if a selective V1aR antagonist (V1aRA) is infused into the VP (but not the medial dorsal thalamus (Mdthal) or medial amygdala (MeA)) in prairie vole males, mating-induced partner preference is blocked compared to controls. Figure modified from Young & Wang (2004).

& Wang 2004, Olazábal & Young 2006b). OTR density in the nucleus accumbens also appears to drive individual differences in maternal care in prairie voles, as both juvenile and adult females that provide a greater degree of spontaneous maternal care (assessed by the amount of time they spent huddling over pups) have higher densities of OTR in the nucleus accumbens (Fig. 11.5; Olazábal & Young 2006a, 2006b). Further, when antagonists that block the OTR are injected into the nucleus accumbens of adult female prairie voles,

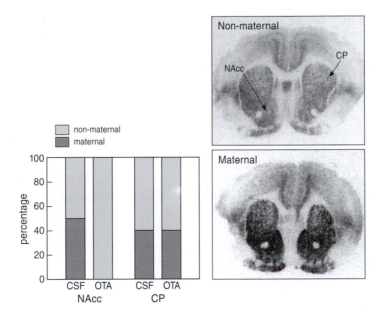

Figure 11.5 Female prairie voles exhibit considerable variation in the density of oxytocin receptor (OTR) in both the nucleus accumbens (NAcc) and the caudate putamen (CP); females that display maternal behaviour when presented with pups have much higher densities of OTR in these regions than females that ignore or attack pups. When a selective OTR antagonist (OTA) is injected into the NAcc, females spend significantly less time hovering over pups compared to females injected with a cerebrospinal fluid (CSF) control. However, when a selective OTR antagonist is injected into the CP, no difference in maternal behaviour is observed between experimental and control animals. Bars show the percentage of maternal and non-maternal animals.

they fail to display spontaneous maternal behaviour (Fig. 11.5; Olazábal & Young 2006b). Thus, in voles, the presence of OTRs in the nucleus accumbens plays a role in the display of spontaneous maternal behaviour. The activation of OTRs in the olfactory bulb and the preoptic area has also been implicated in the regulation of maternal behaviour in rats (Yu *et al.* 1996, Pedersen *et al.* 1994).

In female voles, in addition to its role in eliciting maternal behaviour, oxytocin also plays a prominent role in regulating the formation of a partner preference with her mate. A partner preference is a laboratory proxy for the pair bond and is assessed by quantifying the amount of time spent in contact with the partner versus a novel stranger of the same stimulus value (Fig. 11.2). Female prairie voles display a partner preference following at least six hours cohabitation and mating with a male (Williams *et al.*

1992). Longer periods of cohabitation are required for partner preference formation if mating is prevented. During copulation, vaginocervical stimulation is thought to cause the release of oxytocin within the female's brain. In the absence of mating, an infusion of oxytocin into the brain during cohabitation with a male accelerates the development of a partner preference (Williams *et al.* 1994). Similarly, when females are given an antagonist that blocks OTRs, pair bonding does not occur even after extensive mating bouts (Insel & Hulihan 1995, Young 1999). Interestingly, as with the case for maternal responsiveness, it is the OTRs in the nucleus accumbens that are critical for the development of the pair bond. Selectively infusing an OTR antagonist into the nucleus accumbens prior to mating prevents the development of the pair bond (Young *et al.* 2001). As mentioned above, females in non-monogamous vole species have few

OTRs in the nucleus accumbens, suggesting that species differences in the formation of pair bonds may be attributed, in part, to species differences in the location of the receptors for oxytocin (Young & Wang 2004).

The involvement of OTRs in the nucleus accumbens in partner preference formation suggests a potential neural mechanism by which a simple peptide and its receptor can stimulate social bonding. Studies in transgenic mice suggest that oxytocin is involved in the neural processing of social information, given that oxytocin-deficient mice display social amnesia (Ferguson et al. 2000). The nucleus accumbens is part of the mesolimbic dopamine reward and reinforcement regions of the brain, and has been implicated in drug abuse and addiction (see Chapter 17; Wise 2002). Oxytocin and dopamine interact within the nucleus accumbens to stimulate partner preference formation, as dopamine is also released within the nucleus accumbens during mating (Young & Wang 2004). In the nucleus accumbens, simultaneous activation of OTRs and dopamine receptors may result in the establishment of an association between the social olfactory cues of the partner, and the rewarding or reinforcing aspects of copulation, reminiscent of classical conditioning, and thus promoting the selective affiliation of the female with her mate.

These studies of the role that oxytocin plays in parenting and pair bonding demonstrate several interesting points. First, diversity in OTR expression patterns in the brain seems to lead to diversity in parenting styles and pair-bonding behaviour, suggesting that selection on genomic elements that regulate OTR expression may be an important force that shapes social behaviour. Second, the brain regions involved in maternal care and pair bonding are also critical components of reward and reinforcement circuitry. The intriguing overlap between these systems suggests that attachment in prairie vole partners is akin to an addiction to one another through a process of sexual imprinting, or learning, mediated by odour (Lim et al. 2004a). Finally, there is considerable overlap between the mechanisms that modulate maternal care for the offspring and those that modulate pair

bonding between mates. The latter observation raises the intriguing possibility that, at least in rodents, pair bonding may actually evolve through the tweaking of the neurochemistry and neural circuitry that has evolved to promote the mother–infant relationships that is present in all mammalian species.

11.2.3 Vasopressin: a molecule of male social behaviour

Paternal behaviour, although common in fishes and birds, is only observed in a handful of mammals, and most of these are socially monogamous. Since paternal care is absent in both house mice and rats, the majority of our understanding of the proximate mechanisms underlying paternal care comes from studies of socially monogamous species such as prairie voles. Male prairie voles obviously cannot nurse their offspring, although they participate in all other aspects of pup care including licking, grooming, retrieving, nest maintenance and huddling. Sexually naive adult male prairie voles also exhibit spontaneous paternal behaviour, thus making them an excellent model for understanding the regulation of paternal care.

Much of the work investigating the mechanisms underlying paternal behaviour in prairie voles has focused on arginine vasopressin rather than oxytocin. Vasopressin is structurally similar to oxytocin, and the genes for these two peptides appear to have emerged through a gene duplication (Ivell & Dietmar 1985). Like oxytocin, vasopressin is also synthesised in the hypothalamus and secreted into the general circulation, where it regulates water retention and blood pressure. However, vasopressin released in the brain also modulates other social behaviours such as territoriality and aggression in Syrian hamsters *Mesocricetus auratus* (Albers & Bamshad 1998), social recognition in mice (Bielsky et al. 2004), and pair bonding and paternal care in prairie voles (Young & Wang 2004). Vasopressin distribution is highly sexually dimorphic in the brain, with males having much higher levels of vasopressin in some regions than females (Bamshad et al. 1993, Wang et al. 1996).

Early comparative studies of the socially monogamous prairie vole and the non-monogamous meadow vole revealed surprising differences in vasopressin dynamics in a region of the brain called the lateral septum as a function of sexual experience (Wang *et al.* 1996). In promiscuous meadow voles, vasopressin levels in the lateral septum did not differ between fathers and sexually inexperienced males. However, in the biparental prairie voles, sexual experience resulted in a decrease in vasopressin content in the septum, which was coincident with an increase in paternal responsiveness. This decrease in content may reflect a release of vasopressin from neuronal fibres in the region. This comparison suggested that species differences in vasopressin release in this brain region following pairing with a female might account for differences in social behaviours. To test the hypothesis that vasopressin modulates paternal care, the lateral septum of sexually naive prairie vole males was infused with either vasopressin, an antagonist to the vasopressin receptor (V1aR), or a saline control. Males that were treated with vasopressin showed an increase in paternal behaviours such as grooming, crouching over and retrieving pups, while males that were treated with the vasopressin receptor antagonist spent less time tending the pups in comparison to control males (Wang *et al.* 1994).

Like oxytocin in females, vasopressin in males is not only associated with paternal behaviour, but is a key component in regulating pair-bond formation. When male prairie voles are given infusions of vasopressin, they form partner preferences with a female partner even in the absence of mating, while infusion of V1aR antagonists diminishes partner preference formation (Winslow *et al.* 1993). Like oxytocin in females, vasopressin may also trigger partner preference formation in males through promoting recognition of his mate through olfactory cues. For example, in rats, antagonists against V1aR in certain regions of the brain (see below) inhibit social recognition abilities, but infusion of vasopressin in these same brain regions facilitates social recognition (Landgraf *et al.* 1995, 2003, Everts & Koolhaas 1999). Also similarly to oxytocin in females, vasopressin appears to act via

dopamine pathways in the brain that trigger reward responses (Young & Wang 2004).

As with the OTR, there are remarkable species differences in V1aR distribution in the brain between monogamous and non-monogamous vole species (Fig. 11.4). Specifically, socially monogamous male prairie voles have high densities of V1aR in the ventral pallidum, while non-monogamous vole species do not (Insel *et al.* 1994). Males in other monogamous species, such as common marmosets *Callithrix jacchus* (Young *et al.* 1999) and the California mouse *Peromyscus californicus* (Bester-Meredith *et al.* 1999), have similarly high levels of V1aR in this ventral forebrain region compared to related non-monogamous species (Fig. 11.6). In prairie voles, when V1aR antagonists are injected directly into the ventral pallidum or the lateral septum, partner preference formation is inhibited (Liu *et al.* 2001, Lim *et al.* 2004b). To test whether species differences in V1aR densities in the ventral pallidum truly contribute to monogamous versus non-monogamous behaviours, Lim *et al.* (2004b) used viral vector-mediated gene transfer to over-express *avpr1a*, the gene that encodes V1aR, in the ventral pallidum of male meadow voles (Fig. 11.7). When the manipulated males of this non-monogamous species were allowed to cohabitate and mate with a female, they displayed pair-bond behaviours as measured by the partner preference test.

In these voles, a highly repetitive DNA sequence, or microsatellite, upstream of *avpr1a* appears to play an important role in generating diversity in V1aR expression patterns and in social behaviour (Fig. 11.8). In the socially monogamous prairie vole this microsatellite element spans over 430 base pairs, but it is shorter than 50 base pairs in the promiscuous meadow and montane voles. Initial comparative DNA studies focused attention on the instability of this microsatellite and its potential for contributing to variation in V1aR patterns in the brain. Microsatellite elements are by nature highly unstable, and therefore variation in the length or composition of this element could conceivably alter V1aR expression patterns. To further test the hypothesis that variation in this microsatellite might alter gene expression, rat cell culture lines were constructed in which a luciferase reporter

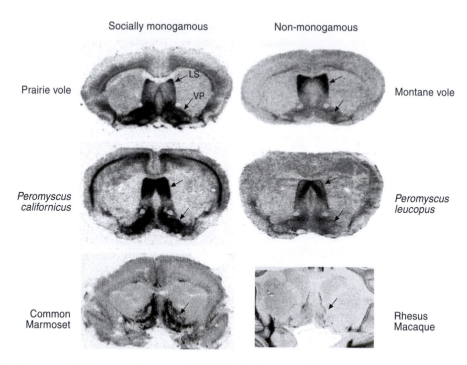

Figure 11.6 Comparison of vasopressin 1a receptor (V1aR) distribution in socially monogamous versus non-monogamous mammals. Arrows indicate the lateral septum (LS) and the ventral pallidum (VP).

gene, which allows one to visualise and quantify gene expression, was placed downstream of the prairie vole *avpr1a* promoter region (Hammock & Young 2004). By varying only the microsatellite sequence, it was possible to demonstrate that variation in the length of the microsatellite significantly affects gene expression in cell culture, further supporting the hypothesis that even subtle length variations in the microsatellite found within prairie voles may contribute to variation in gene expression patterns and social behaviour.

The microsatellite element in the promoter of the *avpr1a* gene is highly variable among individual prairie voles, and this variation has been associated with individual variation in V1aR density in the brain. Hammock and Young (2005) genotyped the *avpr1a* microsatellite locus in individual laboratory-reared prairie voles, and selectively bred animals to produce offspring that were homozygous for either short or long microsatellite elements. When these male offspring were tested for typical paternal behaviours, males with longer microsatellite alleles had higher

V1aR expression in the lateral septum, and exhibited increased paternal behaviour and an increased propensity to form a partner preference for their mates (Hammock & Young 2005). A subsequent study in another prairie vole population also found a correlation between microsatellite length and V1aR density, although the specific brain regions affected were different between the two studies (Ophir *et al.* 2008b). The unstable nature of the microsatellite element may function as an evolutionary tuning knob to create diversity in sociobehavioural traits that selective pressures can act upon (Hammock & Young 2007b). While this microsatellite element appears to play an important role in generating differences in social behaviour between prairie and meadow voles, other promiscuous vole species have microsatellites similar in size to prairie voles, suggesting that this region was deleted in a common ancestor of the montane and meadow voles. Thus, the microsatellite element itself is not a universal genetic feature that controls monogamy in all vole species (Fink *et al.* 2006), but

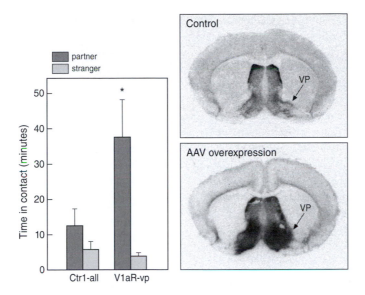

Figure 11.7 Lim *et al.* (2004a, 2004b) used adeno-associated viral vector-mediated gene transfer (AAV) to over-express the gene that encodes vasopressin 1a receptor (V1aR) in the ventral pallidum (VP) of non-monogamous male meadow voles. Compared to control males, AAV-injected males spent significantly more time with their partner than with a strange female in the partner preference test.

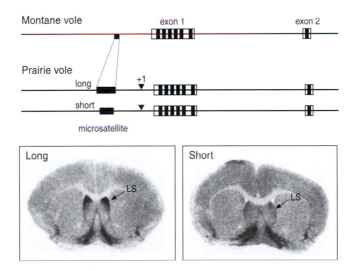

Figure 11.8 The length of a microsatellite element approximately 700 bp upstream of the transcription start site of *avpr1a* is less than 50 bp long in non-monogamous montane voles, but is greater than 430 bp long in the socially monogamous prairie vole. This microsatellite element is highly variable among prairie vole individuals. Prairie vole males that were bred to be homozygous for long microsatellite alleles have higher densities of V1aR in the lateral septum (LS) compared to prairie vole males that were bred to be homozygous for short microsatellite alleles.

illustrates how subtle variations in genetic elements can generate extensive variations in the expression of genes involved in pair bonding and parental care. Whether variation in microsatellite length is a factor contributing to natural variation in mating strategy in nature remains to be confirmed (see below).

As with oxytocin in females, vasopressin appears to facilitate pair-bond formation in males by acting via dopamine reward and reinforcement centres in the brain, and dopamine itself plays an important role in regulating pair-bond formation (see Chapter 17). Interestingly, dopamine may also serve to maintain the pair bond by preventing males from bonding with other females during extra-pair matings. D2 dopamine receptor activation facilitates partner preferences, while D1 dopamine receptor activation prevents partner preference formation (Aragona *et al.* 2006). Thus, the D1 and D2 dopamine receptors have antagonistic influences on initial pair bond formation. However, once a pair bond has been established and maintained for two weeks, males show a significant increase in the density of D1, but not D2, receptors in the nucleus accumbens. This increase in D1 receptors following the initial pair-bond formation may serve to prevent subsequent pair-bond formation. Interestingly, non-monogamous meadow voles have high levels of D1 receptors in the nucleus accumbens even prior to mating.

11.2.4 Similarities between the OTR and V1aR systems

A comparison of the mechanisms underlying female and male pair bonding and parental behaviours reveals distinct yet complementary mechanisms. First, while oxytocin and vasopressin are different neuropeptides, they share a common structure (differing by only two amino acids) and originated evolutionarily from a common ancestral gene (Ivell & Dietmar 1985). Second, although these molecules are found in both sexes, oxytocin plays a more prominent role in regulating parenting and pair-bonding behaviours in females, while vasopressin serves this role in males. Third, in both females and males, variation in the expression of oxytocin and vasopressin

receptors appears to contribute to both species and individual differences in social behaviour. Finally, although oxytocin and vasopressin function in distinct brain regions to facilitate pair bonding, they act within the same neural circuit, since the ventral pallidum is a major output of neurons within the nucleus accumbens. Therefore, females and males have evolved independent mechanisms to regulate pair bonding and parental care, but both sexes accomplish this behaviour change by altering the responsiveness of the same neural circuit.

11.2.5 Can these laboratory studies be translated to animals in their natural environments?

Although laboratory studies of vasopressin, oxytocin and their receptors in voles have contributed immensely to our understanding of the genes, hormones and neural circuits that underlie pair-bond formation and parental care, only a few researchers have begun to examine these systems in the context of what is known about voles in natural or semi-natural populations. Although resident, territorial male–female prairie vole pairs comprise the majority of social units during breeding months, other social units are also commonly observed in this species. Within a prairie vole population, it is common to find male–female pairs with philopatric young, single females living alone, wanderer males that have large home ranges overlapping with multiple territories, extended families where offspring remain to take care of subsequent litters, as well as extended social groups that can consist of up to six breeding females that participate in cooperative care of offspring (Getz *et al.* 1990).

The prevalence of monogamous behavioural strategies in prairie vole populations appears to have a strong ecological component. Within a single population, social structure varies temporally in relation to breeding season. During the primary breeding season (spring–autumn), approximately 73% of social units consist of either male–female pairs or singly breeding females (Getz *et al.* 1990, 1992). During non-breeding winter months, a larger percentage of social units are groups rather than pairs or single animals (Cochran & Solomon 2000, Lucia *et al.* 2008, Solomon & Crist 2008). Interestingly, the composition of social structures as well as social behaviours may vary considerably between prairie vole populations from different geographical ranges. For example, compared to populations of prairie voles from Illinois, prairie voles from a Kansas population appear to be less social, display lower levels of physical contact between adults, have lower levels of alloparental and parental behaviour, and are more aggressive (Roberts *et al.* 1998, Cushing *et al.* 2001; but see Ophir *et al.* 2007). Thus, like genes and brain circuitry, components of the ecological environment such as climate, vegetation or predators (see below) may play an important role in generating the diversity in social behaviours in this species.

A few researchers have begun to relate what is known about prairie voles in their natural environments to what has been learned in the laboratory. As mentioned above, during the breeding season the majority of male prairie voles are socially monogamous and display a resident strategy where they form a pair bond with a female, defend a territory and assist the female in the rearing of offspring. A few males, however, assume a wandering tactic where they acquire large home ranges that overlap territories of one or more resident pairs. Wanderer males typically only sire offspring via extra-pair fertilisations and provide no care for their young (Getz *et al.* 1993). To determine how these two distinct male reproductive tactics relate to V1aR expression patterns in the lateral septum and ventral pallidum, Ophir *et al.* (2008c) observed sexually naive adult prairie voles within semi-natural, outdoor enclosures and used radio telemetry to track patterns of each vole's spatial use. After approximately three weeks, they assessed paternity by genotyping developing embryos and then examined the distribution of V1aR in adult male forebrains. After three weeks, most males (74%) were classified as a member of a bonded pair, while the remaining males assumed the wandering tactic. Interestingly, neither male mating tactic, male mating success, nor the male's propensity to engage in extra-pair copulations was correlated with V1aR densities in either the ventral pallidum or the lateral septum. Instead, V1aR density in the posterior cingulate/retrosplenial cortex, a region of the brain involved in spatial learning and memory, predicted reproductive success in wanderers. Among wanderer males, those with lower densities of V1aR in this brain region assumed larger home territories and sired more offspring. Further, among all successfully breeding males, those with lower densities of V1aR in the posterior cingulate/retrosplenial cortex were more likely to engage in extra-pair matings (Fig. 11.9). In a second study, Ophir *et al.* (2008b) explored the relationship between the microsatellite polymorphism upstream of *avpr1a*, V1aR distribution within the brain and field measures of monogamy and fitness. Although microsatellite length corresponded to the density of V1aR receptors within the brain, as has been shown in laboratory experiments (described above), these differences did not correspond to male mating tactic or reproductive success as measured by resident versus wanderer strategy and rates of extra-pair fertilisations. It should be noted that this finding does not preclude a role of this microsatellite element in population-wide variation in behaviour and evolution, but rather suggests that in this small study other factors (e.g. variation in mating frequency or environmental influences) may have had more significant impact in behavioural variability.

Although only a few studies in voles have sought to link mechanistic laboratory studies to animals in their natural settings, the results from these studies exemplify the complexity underlying social behaviours such as pair bonding and parental care and the clear need for more studies that link laboratory and field research. In voles, ecological correlates appear to have profound effects on the social behaviours of prairie voles, and laboratory studies do not necessarily predict what occurs in natural populations. It will continue to be of great importance to discover how a complex environment contributes to the expression of genes relevant to pair bonding and parental care, as well as to determine other genes and brain regions that play a prominent role in these behaviours, both in the laboratory and in the field (see Chapters 1 and 21).

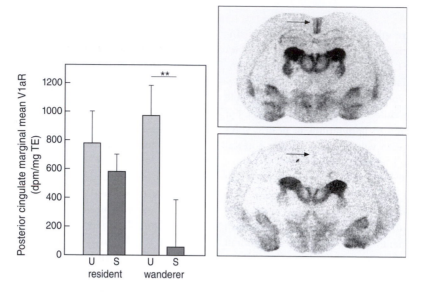

Figure 11.9 Variation in vasopressin 1a receptor (V1aR) expression (demonstrated by top and bottom images) in the posterior cingulate/retrosplenial cortex (arrow) predicts space use and mating success (U, unsuccessful; S, successful) in male prairie voles that have adopted the 'wandering' strategy in semi-natural environments. Unsuccessful males display higher densities of V1aR in this region. (V1aR expression measured as ^{125}I-linear-AVP-specific binding disintegrations per minute (dpm) in tissue equivalence (TE)).

11.3 The evolution and diversity of pair bonds and parental behaviour

11.3.1 From pair bonds to parental care

Studies described above in voles demonstrate genetic and neurobiological links between monogamy and biparental care, since the same genes and neural circuits are involved in regulating both pair bonding and parental behaviour. These behaviours are also tied from an ecological perspective, since prolonged pair bonds often (but not always) invoke social monogamy and extensive care of the young, usually by both parents. Note however, that these terms (pair bond, parental care: Box 11.1) combine behaviourally and phylogenetically different traits under a single label. For instance, pair bonding and social monogamy may be of different intensity and duration, and the type of pair bond may range from a short exclusive association between a male and female lasting only for a few minutes (or days) to a lifetime mutual partnership between a pair of animals over many years (see below; Black 1996, Reichard 2007).

Box 11.1 The terminology of pair bonds and parental care

The terminology in studies of pair bonds and parental care is often confusing, and researchers use terms interchangeably. This is not correct, because the meanings and implications of these terms are different (Clutton-Brock 1991):

Pair bond – a long-term selective social attachment between a mating pair. The existence of a pair bond does not imply sexual fidelity. A pair bond is typically associated with a shared territory and nest.

Parental care – any form of parental behaviour that appears to increase the fitness of an offspring. This is a descriptive term, and has no implication about costs such as time, energy or reduced future reproductive success that the parent may incur. In the broad sense it may include any activity that increases offspring fitness, for instance depositing a large egg-yolk. In the narrow sense it refers only to the care of the eggs and young when they are detached from the parent's body (Clutton-Brock 1991).

Parental effort – the expenditure of parental resource on the offspring. It does not necessarily imply that the expenditure has implications for the parents' future fitness.

Parental investment – defined by Trivers (1972) as 'any investment by the parent in an individual offspring that increases the offspring's chance of surviving (and hence reproductive success) at the cost of parent's ability to invest in other offspring'. An often overlooked component of Trivers' definition is that investment is not measured at the time when the parent provides care for the young, but rather in the long term, by how much it takes away from the parent's future success. Few studies have ever quantified parental investment *sensu* Trivers (1972). Mock and Parker (1997) correctly pointed out that measuring parental investment is the empiricists' nightmare, because it requires that both the benefit (to offspring survival) and cost (to parent's future success) be demonstrated before any parental behaviour can qualify as parental investment.

Partner preference – a laboratory measure of the preference to associate with a partner or novel opposite-sex conspecific. Pair-bonded individuals typically spend more time in close proximity to their partner than to a novel stimulus animal. The presence of a partner preference does not, however, imply the establishment of a pair bond.

11.3.2 Costs, benefits and conflict

One of the fundamental circumstances that is thought to generate prolonged pair bonds and biparental care of the young in natural populations is when both the male and the female benefit from such an association (Lack 1968, Clutton-Brock 1991, Black 1996). Since females typically (with a few exceptions such as sex-role-reversed species) invest more in production of gametes and offspring than males (see Chapter 10; Bateman 1948, Trivers 1972), the costs of rearing offspring subsequent to parturition (or hatching) can be a substantial burden for them. Thus, long-term pair bonds and biparental care are likely to emerge when females are unable to raise their offspring alone.

Male attendance and participation in offspring care can provide direct benefits to both the female and the young such as additional food, enhanced thermoregulation of eggs and young, and protection from predators and infanticide (e.g. Trivers 1972, Wilson 1975, Dunbar & Dunbar 1980, McKinney *et al.* 1984, Wingfield *et al.* 1990, Clutton-Brock 1991, Lott 1991, Fuentes 1999, Reichard 2007). In humans, paternal involvement in childhood has a positive association with offspring IQ at the age of 11 (Nettle 2008).

Experimental removal of one parent (usually the male) supports the hypothesis that biparental care of offspring provides direct benefits, as it often enhances the survival of the young and/or puts less strain on the female (Clutton-Brock 1991, Liker 1995, Gubernick & Teferi 2000, McGuire & Bemis 2007). Parents that are deserted by their mate increase their workload (Osorno & Székely 2004), and removing or handicapping the mate (for instance by attaching small weights or clipping feathers) usually produces a response in the remaining (or non-handicapped) mate's behaviour, usually elevated care, in mammals (Cantoni & Brown

1997), birds (Wright & Cuthill 1990, Sanz *et al.* 2000, Whittingham *et al.* 1994, Griggio *et al.* 2005), fishes (Raadik *et al.* 1990, Itzkowitz *et al.* 2001) and insects (Hunt & Simmons 2002, Rauter & Moore 2004, Smiseth *et al.* 2005). However, the parents appear to have a limited capacity to compensate for the missing (or reduced) contribution of their mate, so compensation is usually partial (Harrison *et al.* 2009). Biparental care can also influence fecundity by decreasing the inter-birth interval, presumably by decreasing the energy load on the female. For example, female California mice assisted by their mate had shorter inter-birth intervals than unassisted females (Cantoni & Brown 1997).

In addition to the numerous benefits, monogamy and biparental care can be considerably costly, since caring for the young takes substantial time and energy, leaving the caring parent vulnerable to predation, lowered immune response, decreased metabolism and malnutrition (Clutton-Brock 1991, Balshine-Earn *et al.* 2002, Bonneaud *et al.* 2003, Cheney & Cote 2003, Houston *et al.* 2005, Tieleman *et al.* 2008). In addition, monogamy can be costly for the individual as one's entire reproductive investment is dependent on the fitness and fidelity of one's mate.

The preceding cost–benefit analyses suggest that pair-bond formation and biparental care of young often do benefit both sexes, although these traits may also emerge for a variety of other reasons. First, if the behavioural options of males or females are limited, so that they cannot easily establish new pair bonds, remaining with one's current mate is often the best strategy for maximising reproductive success. For instance, in territorial birds and primates, the mate of a would-be-polygynous male can behave aggressively towards females that intrude upon the territory, often succeeding in evicting intruders and thus reinforcing the pair bond by curbing the opportunity for her mate to find a new partner (Dietz 1993, Slagsvold & Lifjeld 1994, Liker & Székely 1997). Similarly, males may also coerce females to be monogamous if guarding the female from being promiscuous is the male's best option (Getz *et al.* 1987, Gowaty 1996, Williams 1996). Even in humans, direct or indirect coercing of females has occurred throughout history, in spite of polyandry conferring various advantages to females (Kempenaers 2007, Zeh & Zeh 2001).

Monogamy may also prevail if the male is only able to defend a single breeding site (Davies 1989, Veiga 1992, Gowaty 1996). Harsh physical environment (extreme cold or hot, humid or dry) may also select for the emergence of pair bonds and biparental care (Wilson 1975, Clutton-Brock 1991), although convincing evidence is scarce because adaptations to these extreme environments may also involve changes in life-history strategies, population density and a suite of other traits, making it difficult to disentangle what is cause and what is consequence (see section 11.3.3 and Chapter 18).

To distinguish between competing hypotheses as to how pair bonds and biparental care of offspring arose, one needs to manipulate these traits and measure the effects separately for males and females, ideally throughout their lifetime. For example, as mentioned above, many researchers experimentally remove one parent and then examine the reproductive success of the remaining parent and of the offspring. These types of experimental studies of monogamy, however, are typically focused on short-term measures (e.g. examining changes in breeding success immediately following manipulation). Observational studies nonetheless suggest that in species that form pair bonds lasting several years, reproductive success typically drops after mate change (Ens *et al.* 1996, McNamara & Forslund 1996). Therefore mate change, at least in those species that exhibit prolonged pair bonds, reduces reproductive performance, perhaps because the newly formed pair members need to learn to cooperate with each other (Black 1996).

Because the benefits of care (producing viable offspring) are shared between the biological parents, whereas each parent pays the cost of parental care individually, there is often a conflict between parents concerning who should provide the care (Lessells 1999, Houston *et al.* 2005). For example, both males and females may seek out and engage in extra-pair copulations, shirk their parental care obligations or manipulate their partners to invest more effort into offspring care. Thus a conflict of interest emerges when each parent prefers the other to do the hard work of raising offspring (Lessells 1999, Arnqvist & Rowe 2005, Houston *et al.* 2005).

Conflict between parents has been well described in a small passerine bird, the Eurasian penduline tit

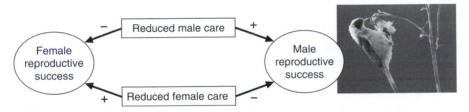

Figure 11.10 Sexual conflict between parents in penduline tits *Remiz pendulinus*. By reducing care provisioning, male penduline tits seek new females and thus increase their own reproductive success, consistent with the Bateman rule (see Chapter 10). Male desertion, however, harms the female's interest, because in response she either spends time and energy on raising the young unassisted, or abandons the clutch. Conversely, reduced care by the female increases her reproductive success by allowing her to re-mate and re-nest, although it harms her mate's reproductive interest. The arrows and the positive and negative signs indicate correlation coefficients or standardised path coefficients. After Szentirmai *et al.* (2007). Photo by Csaba Daróczi.

Remiz pendulinus, which exhibits short pair bonds, lasting up to a week, and sequential polygamy by both sexes. Both males and females may have up to six mates in a single breeding season. In this species, only one parent incubates the eggs and rears the young, but about one-third of clutches are abandoned by both parents before incubation starts (Persson & Öhrström 1989). Sexual conflict between parents appears to drive these unusual breeding behaviours. By deserting their mate and their eggs, male penduline tits increase their annual reproductive success, since many deserting males breed with new females (Fig. 11.10; Szentirmai *et al.* 2007). Desertion by the female, however, is costly to males, because the male either stays with the eggs and cares for them, which takes substantial time, or he also deserts the eggs so that the eggs are left to die. In either case, the male pays a cost of being deserted by his mate.

Interestingly, the reproductive interest of the female penduline tit is the same, but opposes that of the male. By deserting her mate, she usually produces a new clutch, whereas when her mate deserts her, she has decreased reproductive success. Therefore, in the penduline tit, short pair bond, polygamy and offspring desertion improve the reproductive success of the deserting parent, but reduce the reproductive success of the mate of the deserter (Fig. 11.10)

In most cases, leaving a partner is only a good strategy if there are unmated individuals in the population willing to engage in new pair bonds (see Chapter 4). In nature, unlike most laboratory environments, the parents interact with other individuals, and these interactions can influence whether they keep their partner and cooperate with them to rear their young, or whether they divorce and seek a new mate. For example, in populations where the adult sex ratio is skewed, one sex may increase their reproductive success more than the other sex by breaking the pair bond and deserting their mate, or by keeping their social mate but engaging in extra-pair copulations (Székely *et al.* 1999, Pilastro *et al.* 2001, Balshine-Earn *et al.* 2002).

Game-theoretic models (see Chapter 4) have been used to identify conditions when parental behaviours (e.g. staying with the partner or divorcing, caring for the brood or deserting, or the amount of parental effort invested) are evolutionarily stable strategies. Using these types of models, Houston and Davies (1985) sought to establish the joint optimum parental effort for both parents, and showed that for stable biparental care to exist each parent should respond to its mate's effort. For instance, if one partner reduces its effort to care for offspring, the other partner should increase the amount of care it provides, but not fully compensate. One assumption of this model is that parents had only a single interaction to decide how much effort they should put into raising their young. In reality, however, one parent may make up its mind before the other, or the parents may repeatedly interact to arrive at a shared workload (Box 11.2).

Box 11.2 Models of parental effort

Alasdair I. Houston

Houston and Davies (1985) modelled the interaction between parents over care as an evolutionary game (see Chapter 4). Each parent chooses a level of parental care (i.e. a parental effort) independently of the effort of its mate (this is sometimes referred to as a game based on sealed bids). The success of the current breeding attempt increases as the total parental care increases. Thus each parent benefits from a large total amount of care. Each parent pays a cost, in terms of future reproductive success, that increases with its own level of parental care. For any level of care by the male, we can calculate the level of care by the female that gives her the highest total reproductive success (current plus future reproductive success). This is the female's best response to the male's effort. Repeating this procedure for a range of male efforts gives us the female's best response curve. Using the same procedure, we can find the male's best response curve. The evolutionarily stable levels of care satisfy the following condition: the female adopts her best effort given the male's effort, and the male adopts his best effort given the female's effort. In other words, each parent adopts its best response to the effort of the other, so neither has any reason to change its behaviour. The best-response functions show under-compensation, i.e. a decrease in effort by one parent is not fully compensated for by the increase in effort by the other parent.

Although the derivation of the evolutionarily stable efforts is based on the concept of a best response, the approach does not involve any interaction between the parents. The best response is the response that would be expected to occur over evolutionary time, not during a breeding attempt. The resulting evolutionarily stable levels of care are the levels that should be seen if each parent makes its decision independently of the decision of the other. The model implicitly assumes that all males are the same and all females are the same, so all individuals of a given sex use the same effort. This means that a partner's effort provides no information and hence there is no point in responding to it.

But the assumption that a parent does not respond to the behaviour of its mate is not realistic. Many experiments have induced a change in the behaviour of one parent and have found that the other parent changed its behaviour in response (Harrison *et al.* 2009). Why shouldn't we represent this responsiveness by assuming that animals adopt the Houston–Davies best-response function as a way of responding to the effort of their mate during a breeding attempt? This will be called the Houston–Davies rule. McNamara *et al.* (1999) establish that such a way of responding is not evolutionarily stable. Assume that parents use the Houston–Davies rule. Now consider a mutant female that adopts a fixed level of care, regardless of the behaviour of her mate. Such a female can select her effort so as to maximise her total reproductive success given the rule adopted by the male. Her resulting total reproductive success is higher than that of females that use the Houston–Davies best response to determine their behaviour. The mutant female exploits her mate by being lazy.

If members of a sex differ in quality then it is advantageous for an individual to adjust its effort in response to the effort of its partner. This leads us to consider the evolution of rules for negotiating with the other parent about the level of care that will be adopted. McNamara *et al.* (1999) assume that there is a period of negotiation that decides the behaviour that parents will adopt to raise their young. No costs or benefits are incurred during this period. Once negotiation is over, the cost that a parent incurs depends on its quality and its effort. A rule specifies the level of care adopted by a parent during negotiation as a function of its quality and its partner's most recent level of care. At evolutionary stability the female's rule is the best rule to use against the male's rule, and the male's rule is the best rule to use against the female's rule, i.e. the rules are best responses to each other. In contrast, the resulting efforts are not evolutionary best responses to each other. The evolutionarily stable negotiation rule does not increase effort by as much as the Houston–Davies rule when the partner reduces its effort (i.e. it does not compensate as much) and young receive less care than if parents adopted the Houston–Davies efforts.

Johnstone and Hinde (2006) show how models involving negotiation can predict that one parent should increase its effort in response to an increase by its mate. As in the model of McNamara *et al.* (1999), negotiation is costless and the cost to a parent of the negotiated effort depends on this effort and the parent's quality. The crucial feature of the model of Johnstone and Hinde is that parents do not have perfect knowledge about the condition of their young. A rule now specifies how effort during the negotiation phase depends on a parent's state, its perception of the condition of the young, and the partner's most recent effort. An increase in the effort of one parent then has two effects on its partner. The first decreases the value of further care, and hence makes it advantageous to decrease the level of parental care. This is the standard effect seen in previous models. The novel effect is that the increase in effort provides information that it is important to feed the young. This makes it advantageous to increase the level of parental care. The predicted outcome depends on the magnitude of these effects. If one parent is better informed about the condition of the young, it should devote more effort to the young, respond more strongly to changes in the condition of the young, and compensate more strongly for a decrease in the effort of its partner.

Relaxing the assumption of a single interaction between parents provided two new insights (McNamara *et al.* 2002, Johnstone & Hinde 2006). First, the negotiated parental effort is typically less than one achieved by a single decision. Second, there are situations when the young fare better with one parent than with two. Supporting the latter counterintuitive theoretical argument, Royle *et al.* (2002) showed using an aviary experiment that offspring received greater per capita investment from single female zebra finches *Taeniopygia guttata* than from both parents working together, and the sons of single mothers were more attractive as adults than their biparentally reared male siblings. They argued that the difference between single and biparental offspring was due to the reduction in care provided by the female when she shared care responsibilities with her mate. Royle *et al.* (2002), however, measured parental investment as the amount of seed consumed by the parents, and one may argue that food intake does not directly correspond to parental investment (Box 11.1).

11.3.3 The significance of ecological and social environment

Pair bonds and parental care are plastic social behaviours that can be readily moulded by selection pressures emerging from the environment. In the laboratory, experimental animals are sheltered from environmental fluctuations, have permanent access to food and drinking water and are typically housed in enclosures where they are isolated from other individuals in the population. Theoretical and field studies, however, suggest that the interactions between individuals and the environment, and between parents and other individuals in the population, can greatly influence the strength of the pair bond, and affect how much each parent invests in offspring care (Ens *et al.* 1996, McNamara & Forslund 1996, Houston *et al.* 2005, Kokko & Jennions 2008).

Social behaviour is often different between low- versus high-food habitats (Davies 1991, Getz *et al.* 2003). For instance, experimental supplementation of food in natural habitats of voles and passerine birds induced a decrease in the size of female ranges, and female ranges in the resource-rich areas were more aggregated and overlapped (Davies & Lundberg 1984, Ostfeld 1986, Ims 1987). Since male ranges were not affected by the supplementary food, the breeding systems shifted towards higher incidences of polygamy (Davies 1991). Short-term manipulation of food resources in natural habitats, however, is not fully satisfactory, because resources, carrying capacities and population densities may fluctuate many-fold in nature, with complex interactions between density-dependent mortalities and social behaviour (see Chapter 18).

The social environment (e.g. competitors, peers and potential mates) likely generates selection on pair bonds and parental care (social selection, see Chapters 2, 5 and 10). Thus, how the parents perceive mating opportunities may influence whether or not they stay with the mate and provide care. For instance, with a male-biased sex ratio in the breeding population, females reduced their care and the incidence of polyandry increased (Davies 1992, Pilastro *et al.* 2001). In the past, parental behaviour was considered largely an input trait that gives rise to variations in mating system, mate choice and sexual selection (Trivers 1974, Emlen & Oring 1977). However, more recent studies have emphasised the dynamic nature of parental behaviour, pair bonds, mate choice and sexual selection (Alonzo & Warner 2000, Székely *et al.* 2000, Kokko & Jennions 2003). For example, Forsgren *et al.* (2004) showed a striking temporal plasticity in mating competition of two-spotted gobies *Gobiusculus flavescens*. Over the breeding season, fierce male–male competition and intensive male courtship behaviours were replaced by female–female competition and actively courting females. In this species, the males provide uniparental care of the eggs, and the shift, Forsgren *et al.* (2004) argued, was due to a decline in sexually

active males that skewed the sex ratio towards females as the breeding season proceeded.

The complex interactions between the physical and social environments and their effects on behaviour are only beginning to be understood. For instance, food availability may affect both pair bonding and parental care indirectly by generating density-dependent effects. The Kentish plover *Charadrius alexandrinus* is a small shorebird with a polygamous breeding system whereby one parent typically deserts the brood so that only a single parent attends and defends the precocial chicks. Kosztolányi *et al.* (2006) postulated that in resource-rich habitat brood desertion should be more common than in resource-poor habitat, because the young are expected to develop faster and thus require less care. However, resource-rich habitats attracted plovers from the surrounding areas, and as a response to the increased plover density, vicious fights for feeding territories ensued that sometimes ended by killing the neighbours' chicks. Therefore, in contrast to the postulated relationship, in the resource-rich habitat the young required more care, especially in the form of defence, and pair bonds lasted longer than in the resource-poor habitat.

11.3.4 Insights from phylogenetic studies

Behavioural ecologists typically explore the evolution of diversity in social behaviour by observing behavioural patterns in the context of natural history and phylogenetic relationships. Throughout the animal kingdom there are many forms of pair bonds and parental care, and their frequencies vary not only among phylogenetically distinct taxa, but also among closely related taxa (Fig. 11.11, Box 11.3). Although parental care is not found in all organisms (e.g. many oysters (Ostreidae) simply cast their eggs and sperm into the seawater: Ó Foighil & Taylor 2000), many invertebrates have sophisticated nurturing systems where parental care is essential for the survival of the offspring (e.g. Wilson 1975, Tallamy 1999, Walling *et al.* 2008). Parental care, in its simplest form, may consist only of guarding eggs and young from predators, or providing them with a safe environment to develop, or providing nutrients for growth (Clutton-

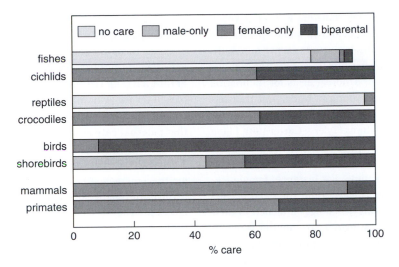

Figure 11.11 Frequencies of the care provider in teleost fishes (422 families), cichlid fishes (182 genera), squamate reptiles (938 genera), crocodilians (21 species), birds (9600 species), shorebirds (203 species), mammals (1117 genera) and primates (203 species) (after Reynolds *et al.* 2002). The percentages of fish species do not add up to 100 because they are based on numbers of families that show exclusively one form of care (393 families).

Box 11.3 Variation in parental care among tropical frogs

Tropical frogs exhibit unusually diverse parental care systems (Crump 1996, Summers *et al.* 2006): egg attendance, egg transport, tadpole attendance, tadpole transport, tadpole feeding or internal gestation have been observed in approximately 20% of frog species (Lehtinen & Nussbaum 2003). The male, the female or both parents may provide parental care. Most members of microhylid frogs in Papua New Guinea have terrestrial eggs that are deposited in small holes in the ground or in epiphytes, and these eggs develop directly into free-living froglets. For instance, *Oreophryne anthonyi* deposits its eggs in moist cavities of epiphytic plants, and both parents take care of the eggs and froglets (Gunther 2005). In other microhylid frogs the male – rarely the female – broods the terrestrial eggs. Adult females guard the terrestrial eggs in the Jamaican frog *Eleutherodactylus cundalli*, and the fully metamorphosed froglets are transported on the back of the female (Diesel *et al.* 1995). Froglets may be transported by the male in microhylid frogs (Bickford 2002, Gunther 2005): they jump off at different points, reducing the competition for food and the opportunities for inbreeding between froglets. In Taiwan, male *Chirixalus eiffingeri* attend the clutches during embryonic development, and the female provides the oophagous (egg-eating) tadpoles by laying unfertilised eggs (Chen *et al.* 2005). In the Amazonian poison frog *Dendrobates ventrimaculatus* the male transports the oophagous tadpoles between water bodies to assist their development (Poelman & Dicke 2007).

Brock 1991, Tallamy 1999, Balshine-Earn *et al.* 2002). Elaborate parental behaviour in some species can be quite bizarre: examples include gastric or mouth-brooding of young in fish and frogs, building massive terrestrial mounds or arboreal nests for incubating the eggs and rearing young in birds, and transferring nutrients to young through secretion from specialised skin in caecilians (Tyler & Carter 1981, Ligon 1999, Hansell 2000, Kupfer *et al.* 2006).

Parenting in its most intense form may last for extended periods of time. For instance, female ice-fish *Chionobathyscus dewitti* from the deep oceans around Antarctica carry their eggs attached to their pelvic fins for an estimated six months (Kock & Pshenichnov 2006), and care provisioning in primates, elephants and whales may extend for years so that the parent–offspring relationship gradually becomes a social network of parents and their adult offspring (see Chapter 14). Likewise, the relationships between sexual partners can range from short exclusive associations between a male and female that may last only for a few minutes or days to life-long mutual partnerships between the pair (see below; Black 1996, Reichard 2007).

This small sampling of the range of parental care and pair bonds demonstrates how the terms used to describe these traits (parental care, pair bond, monogamy) combine behaviourally and phylogenetically different traits under a single label. By examining the continuum of variation in these traits across taxa and using phylogenetic methods, we can ask fundamental questions that experimental studies cannot address (see Chapter 5). Data on natural diversity of mating strategies and on parental care are rapidly accumulating not only from temperate regions, where natural history and field research have a long tradition, but also from the tropics, thanks to the emergence of biodiversity-driven research. These data, coupled with powerful statistical approaches and robust phylogenetic hypotheses, are producing major advances in understanding of the natural diversity in social behaviour.

First, phylogenetic analyses can infer historic patterns in behavioural evolution. Approximately 20% of bony fish families harbour at least some species in which the adults provide post-zygotic care, ranging from internal gestation by females (or males in

pipefishes and seahorses) to external brooding or nest defence by either or both parents. The evolution of care can be conceptually divided into two pathways depending on the mode of fertilisation: external or internal (Fig. 11.12). In externally fertilising fishes parental care is mainly (or exclusively) provided by males, and phylogenetic reconstruction suggests that paternal care evolved repeatedly in lineages in which males build and defend spawning sites (Mank & Avise 2006). The most parsimonious explanation for the emergence of maternal care in these taxa involves the change in fertilisation mode from external to internal, whereas biparental care most likely evolved independently from maternal and paternal care in species exhibiting external fertilisation (Mank & Avise 2006).

Recent phylogenetic studies (see Chapter 5) have also examined the relationship between the emergence of parental care and monogamy. It has been hypothesised that biparental care evolved in response to more demanding young, and that pair bonding evolved as a consequence of selection for biparental care. Critical examinations of these hypotheses have provided mixed results. On the one hand, demanding young constrain the parents to monogamy and biparental care as predicted (i.e. monogamy and biparental care are tightly coupled in shorebirds: Thomas & Székely 2005), although unexpectedly, whether changes in pair bonds pre-dated the changes in parental care or vice versa is ambiguous. On the other hand, contrary to the traditional view, evolutionary changes in parental care type appear to be dependent on the intensity of sexual selection in cichlid fishes (Gonzales-Voyeur *et al.* 2008) where female-only care emerged as a consequence of intense sexual selection among males. The latter result turns a famous dictum, 'What governs the operation of sexual selection is the relative parental investment of the sexes in their offspring' (Trivers 1972), on its head, and suggests that in some instances sexual selection is more likely to drive parental care than vice versa.

Although the selective forces that lead to pair bonds and parental care may differ, these traits typically coevolve. For instance, the incidence of polygamy increases with female-biased parental care in passerines and shorebirds (Searcy & Yasukawa

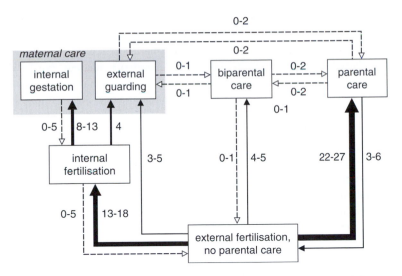

Figure 11.12 Maximum-parsimony inferences of parental care modes in actinopterygian fishes (Mank & Avise 2006). Arrow sizes reflect relative numbers of evolutionary transitions; numerals adjacent to the arrows are minimum and maximum estimated numbers of evolutionary transitions. Broken arrows indicate transitions that might or might not have occurred.

1995, Thomas & Székely 2005). In mammals, however, Komers and Brotherton (1997) argued that monogamy is decoupled from paternal care since there are many examples where pair bonding occurs without paternal care. Re-analysis of the latter study in an appropriate phylogenetic framework, however, is warranted because inspection of Komers and Brotherton's (1997) Table 1 reveals a highly significant relationship between the incidence of monogamy and paternal care (Spearman rank correlation, $r_s = 0.352$, $n = 159$ species, $p < 0.001$).

Comparative analyses can predict the ecological and life-history traits that lead to the evolution of pair bonds and biparental care. Large eggs and long lifespans are often (but not always, e.g. in cichlid fishes: Kolm *et al.* 2006) associated with long-term pair bonds and elaborate parental care. For instance frogs with large eggs exhibit elaborate caring behaviour (Summers *et al.* 2006). However, it is not clear whether large egg size resulted in selection of biparental care, or whether the development of biparental care led to the evolution of large eggs. Similarly, the existence of parental-care bias (i.e. the difference in care between males and females) is often associated

with non-monogamous mating systems where the sex providing less care tends to have more flashy sexual ornaments than the more parental sex. Again, it is not clear whether this relationship is driven by natural selection acting on the caring parent, sexual selection influencing pair bonds, or both (Bennett & Owens 2002, Kokko & Jennions 2003).

Finally, phylogenetic studies can test the consequences of pair bonds and parental strategies for macroevolution, speciation and extinction (see Chapter 5). For instance, live-bearing lineages in bony fishes appear to exhibit significantly higher rates of cladogenesis than externally brooding sister clades (Mank & Avise 2006), and shorebird clades with less demanding young have accelerated phenotypic evolution compared to those with demanding offspring (Thomas *et al.* 2006).

11.4 Conclusions and future directions

Our current understanding of pair bonds and parental care is largely subdivided into two distinct research fields with very little overlap. Conceptual and historical divides continue to segregate both the experimental questions and the researchers in the field. However, a dialogue between researchers from different perspectives is sorely needed, to unify the field and to produce a holistic and integrated understanding of diversity in social organisation in nature. In this chapter we have described how laboratory studies of voles have made a large impact in beginning to understand the genetic and neurological basis of these behaviours. We then described how theoretical models and field studies in a variety of organisms have generated a broad understanding of how these traits may have evolved, and the ecological factors that likely play a significant role in the expression of these traits in nature.

We envisage that a three-pronged approach is needed for new insights into the evolution of pair bonds, mating systems and parental care. First, researchers are attempting to bridge the gap between proximate and ultimate understanding of pair bonds and parental care. The few studies that have tried to incorporate both proximate and ultimate approaches towards the study of these traits (i.e. the vole studies described above: Ophir *et al.* 2008a, 2008b, 2008c) illustrate the complex nature of these behaviours and underscore the necessity of integrating the two research methodologies. Collaborations between researchers from different disciplines and parallel studies of organisms in the field and in the laboratory are an essential progression towards gaining a comprehensive understanding of proximate and ultimate aspects of pair bonds and parental care.

The experiments described above in voles, in which laboratory discoveries were extended by observing the animals' behaviours within semi-natural enclosures, are an important step, and provide an example of integrating laboratory and field studies. In this context, animals are free to choose their mates, establish and defend territories and develop social structures that are not feasible in the constrained confines of the laboratory. Further, behaviours and reproductive success can be monitored in the field, and at least some ecological components that may influence social behaviours are in place. Since some of the most detailed examples of pair bonding and parental care have been best described through field

studies of birds, a natural extension of this research is to perform complementary studies in aviaries, where the genetic and neural architecture of pair bonding and parental behaviour can be directly tested by manipulating animals using technologies developed in the laboratory. For example, genetic manipulations of genes in particular brain regions can be performed in animals that are reared in semi-natural environments, allowing for a clearer perspective of how gene-by-environment interactions contribute to the complexity of these traits (see Chapters 1 and 2). Further, DNA samples that are routinely collected in many field studies can be used to investigate the contribution of genetic diversity of specific genes to variation in behaviour. Examination of gene expression profiles and genomic analysis should be combined with field-collected data to identify genetic mechanisms contributing to pair bonding and parental care in natural populations. As the vole studies have demonstrated, the seemingly straightforward genetic and neural mechanisms that appear to drive these complex behaviours in the laboratory are often confounded when animals are allowed to interact with their ecological and social environments. As molecular and genetic tools become more widely available for non-model species, and more researchers begin to integrate proximate and ultimate approaches towards understanding pair bonding and parental care in a variety of species, many of the seemingly complex variables that lead to variation and evolution of pair bonding and parental care will become apparent.

Second, phylogenetic studies have identified a number of taxa with large variation in pair bonds, mating systems and parental care. Laboratory methodologies, such as have been performed in a few species of voles, can be applied across numerous taxa to identify the evolutionary history of the genes and brain regions that give rise to the diversity of pair bonds and parental care in species beyond rodents. For example, the phylogenetic plasticity in the expression of the genes encoding vole oxytocin and vasopressin receptors likely contributes to the diversity in pair bonding and parental care, and is a potential target for natural selection. However, our understanding of the roles of these systems is limited to a few mammalian species, and studies that extend this line of research to other model systems are greatly needed. Homologues of both oxytocin and vasopressin occur in most vertebrates and influence a variety of social behaviours in taxa ranging from fish to birds to mammals (Goodson & Bass 2001, Goodson *et al.* 2005, Soma 2006). Thus, these molecules and their receptors are potential candidates for regulating pair bonding and parental care in other species that display these traits, although few studies have investigated this. Pair bonding and parental care behaviours have perhaps been most extensively studied in birds, where most species are socially monogamous and males typically help care for offspring, yet it is still unknown whether mesotocin and vasotocin (non-mammalian vertebrate homologues of oxytocin and vasopressin, respectively) play a central role in these behaviours. Only with increased dialogue and collaboration between researchers in diverse fields will we gain a truly integrative understanding of the diversity in social structure in the animal kingdom.

Finally, the vast majority of animal species have not been named, let alone had their breeding systems studied in detail. Insects, fish and frogs that live in challenging environments have developed specific adaptations to cope with their environments, and these may involve adaptations in social traits, pair bonds and parenting styles. Discovering the breeding systems of tropical, deep-sea and alpine species is one of the fundamental tasks in biodiversity research, and will expand the frontiers of our understanding. New data on natural history, coupled with powerful phylogenetic analyses, behavioural experiments and detailed analyses using genetic and neuroscience tools, will likely reveal novel functions and mechanisms that may not only advance evolutionary biology but that are also relevant to human health and biomedical research (Chivian & Bernstein 2008).

Acknowledgements

We are grateful for the comments of Bart Kempenaers, Geoff Parker, Alex Ophir, Allen Moore and Jan Komdeur. TS was supported by NERC (NE/C004167/1), FP6/2002–2006 (GEBACO, 28696) and FP6–2005-NEST-Path (INCORE, 043318).

Suggested readings

Balshine-Earn, S., Kempenaers, B. & Székely, T. (2002) Conflict and co-operation in parental care. *Philosophical Transactions of the Royal Society B*, **357**, 237–404.

Hammock, E. A. D. & Young, L. J. (2005) Microsatellite instability generates diversity in brain and sociobehavioural traits. *Science*, **308**, 1630–1634.

Houston, A. I., Székely, T. & McNamara, J. M. (2005) Conflict over parental care. *Trends in Ecology and Evolution*, **20**, 33–38.

Reichard, U. H. (2007) Monogamy: past and present. In: *Monogamy: Mating Strategies and Partnerships in Birds, Humans and Other Mammals*, ed. U. H. Reichard & C. Boesch. Cambridge: Cambridge University Press, pp. 3–26.

Young, L. J. & Insel, T. R. (2002) Hormones and parental behaviour. In: *Behavioural Endocrinology*, 2nd edn, ed. J. B. Becker, S. M. Breedlove, D. Crews & M. M. McCarthy. Cambridge, MA: MIT Press, pp. 331–369.

References

Adkins-Regan, E. (2005) *Hormones and Animal Social Behavior.* Princeton, NJ: Princeton University Press.

Albers, H. E. & Bamshad, M. (1998) Role of vasopressin and oxytocin in the control of social behavior in Syrian hamsters (*Mesocricetus auratus*). *Progress in Brain Research*, **119**, 395–408.

Alonzo, S. & Warner, R. (2000) Dynamic games and field experiments examining intra- and inter-sexual conflict: explaining counter-intuitive mating behavior in a Mediterranean wrasse, *Symphodus ocellatus*. *Behavioral Ecology*, **11**, 56–70.

Aragona, B. J., Liu, Y., Yu, Y. J. *et al.* (2006) Nucleus accumbens dopamine differentially mediates the formation and maintenance of monogamous pair bonds. *Nature Neuroscience*, **9**, 133–139.

Arnqvist, G. & Rowe, L. (2005) *Sexual Conflict.* Princeton, NJ: Princeton University Press.

Balshine-Earn, S., Kempenaers, B. & Székely, T. (2002) Conflict and co-operation in parental care. *Philosophical Transactions of the Royal Society*, **357**, 237–404.

Bamshad, M., Novak, M. A. & Devries, G. J. (1993) Sex and species differences in the vasopressin innervation of sexually naive and parental prairie voles, *Microtus ochrogaster* and meadow voles, *M. pennsylvanicus. Journal of Neuroendocrinology*, **5**, 247–255.

Bateman, A. J. (1948) Intra-sexual selection in *Drosophila. Heredity*, **2**, 349–368.

Bennett, P. M. & Owens, I. P. F. (2002) *Evolutionary Ecology of Birds*. Oxford: Oxford University Press.

Bester-Meredith, J. K., Young, L. J. & Marler, C. A. (1999) Species differences in paternal behavior and aggression in *Peromyscus* and their associations with vasopressin immunoreactivity and receptors. *Hormones and Behavior*, **36**, 25–38.

Bickford, D. (2002) Male parenting of New Guinea froglets. *Nature*, **418**, 601–602.

Bielsky, I. F. & Young, L. J. (2004) Oxytocin, vasopressin and social recognition in mammals. *Peptides*, **25**, 1564–1574.

Bielsky, I. F., Hu, S.-B., Szegda, K. L., Westphal, H. & Young, L. J. (2004) Profound impairment in social recognition and reduction in anxiety in vasopressin V1a receptor knockout mice. *Neuropsychopharmacology*, **29**, 483–493.

Black, J. M., ed. (1996) *Partnerships in Birds*. Oxford: Oxford University Press.

Bonneaud, C., Mazuc, J., Gonzalez, G. *et al.* (2003) Assessing the cost of mounting an immune response. *American Naturalist*, **161**, 367–379.

Bosch, O. J., Nair, H. P., Ahern, T., Neumann, I. D. & Young, L. J. (2009) The CRF system mediates increased passive stress-coping behavior following the loss of a bonded partner in a monogamous rodent. *Neuropsychopharmacology*, **34**, 1406–1415.

Burbach, P., Young, L. J. & Russell, J. (2006) Oxytocin: synthesis, secretion and reproductive functions. In: *Knobil and Neill's Physiology of Reproduction*, 3rd edn, ed. J. D. Neill. St Louis, MO: Elsevier, pp. 3055–3128.

Cantoni, D. & Brown, R. (1997) Paternal investment and reproductive success in the California mouse, *Peromyscus californicus. Animal Behaviour*, **54**, 377–386.

Carter, C. S., Devries, A. C. & Getz, L. L. (1995) Physiological substrates of mammalian monogamy: the prairie vole model. *Neuroscience and Biobehavioral Reviews*, **19**, 303–14.

Cheney, K. & Cote, I. (2003) Indirect consequences of parental care: sex differences in ectoparasite burden and cleaner-seeking activity in longfin damselfish. *Marine Ecology Progress Series*, **262**, 267–275.

Chivian, E. & Bernstein, A. (2008) *Sustaining Life*. Oxford: Oxford University Press.

Clutton-Brock, T. H. (1989) Mammalian mating systems. *Proceedings of the Royal Society B*, **236**, 339–372.

Clutton-Brock, T. H. (1991) *The Evolution of Parental Care*. Princeton, NJ: Princeton University Press.

Cochran, G. & Solomon, N. (2000) Effects of food supplementation on the social organization of prairie voles (*Microtus ochrogaster*). *Journal of Mammalogy*, **81**, 746–757.

Crump, M. (1996) Parental care among the amphibia. *Advances in the Study of Behavior*, **25**, 109–144.

Curley, J. P. & Keverne, E. B. (2005) Genes, brains and mammalian social bonds. *Trends in Ecology and Evolution*, **20**, 561–567.

Cushing, B. S., Martin, J., Young, L. J. & Carter, C. S. (2001) The effects of peptides on partner preference formation are predicted by habitat in prairie voles. *Hormones and Behavior*, **39**, 48–58.

Davies, N. B. (1989) Sexual conflict and the polygamy threshold. *Animal Behavior*, **38**, 226–234.

Davies, N. B. (1991) Mating systems. In: *Behavioural Ecology*, 3rd edn, ed. J. R. Krebs & N. B. Davies. Oxford: Blackwell, pp. 263–294.

Davies, N. B. (1992) *Dunnock Behaviour and Social Evolution*. Oxford: Oxford University Press.

Davies, N. B. & Lundberg, A. (1984) Food distribution and a variable mating system in the dunnock (*Prunella modularis). Journal of Animal Ecology*, **53**, 895–912.

Diesel, R., Baurle, G. & Vogel, P. (1995) Cave breeding and froglet transport: a novel pattern of anuran brood care in the Jamaican frog, *Eleutherodactylus cundalli. Copeia*, **1995**, 354–360.

Dietz, J. (1993) Polygyny and female reproductive success in golden lion tamarins, *Leontopithecus rosalia. Animal Behaviour*, **46**, 1067–1078.

Dunbar, R. & Dunbar, E. (1980) The pairbond in klipspringer. *Animal Behaviour*, **28**, 219–229.

Emlen, S. T. & Oring, L. W. (1977) Ecology, sexual selection, and the evolution of mating systems. *Science*, **197**, 215–223.

Ens, B., Choudhury, S. & Black, J. M. (1996) Mate fidelity in monogamous birds. In: *Partnerships in Birds*, ed. J. M. Black. Oxford: Oxford University Press, pp. 344–401.

Everts, H. G. & Koolhaas, J. M. (1999) Differential modulation of lateral septal vasopressin receptor blockade in spatial learning, social recognition, and anxiety-related behaviors in rats. *Behavioural Brain Research*, **99**, 7–16.

Ferguson, J. N., Young, L. J., Hearn, E. F., Insel., T. R. & Winslow, J. T. (2000) Social amnesia in mice lacking the oxytocin gene. *Nature Genetics*, **25**, 284–288.

Fink, S., Excoffier, L. & Heckel, G. (2006) Mammalian monogamy is not controlled by a single gene. *Proceedings of the National Academy of Sciences of the USA*, **103**, 10956–10960.

Forsgren, E., Amundsen, T., Borg, A. & Bjelvenmark, J. (2004) Unusually dynamic sex roles in a fish. *Nature*, **429**, 551–554.

Fuentes, A. (1999) Reevaluating primate monogamy. *American Anthropologist*, **100**, 890–907.

Getz, L. L. & Carter, C. S. (1996) Prairie-vole partnerships. *American Scientist*, **84**, 56–62.

Getz, L. L. & Hofmann, J. E. (1986) Social-organization in free-living prairie voles, *Microtus ochrogaster*. *Behavioral Ecology and Sociobiology*, **18**, 275–282.

Getz, L. L., Carter, C. S. & Gavish, L. (1981) The mating system of the prairie vole Microtus ochrogaster: field and laboratory evidence for pair bonding. *Behavioral Ecology and Sociobiology*, **8**, 189–194.

Getz, L. L., Hofmann, J. E., Klatt, B., Verner, L., Cole, F. & Lindroth, R. (1987) Fourteen years of population fluctuations of *Microtus ochrogaster* and *M. pennsylvanicus* in east-central Illinois. *Canadian Journal of Zoology*, **65**, 1317–1325.

Getz, L. L., McGuire, B., Hofmann, J. E., Pizzuto, T. & Frase, B. (1990) Social organization and mating system of the prairie vole, *Microtus ochrogaster*. In: *Social Systems and Population Cycles in Voles*, ed. T. Tamarin, R. Ostfeld, S. Pugh & G. Bujalska. Basel: Birkhauser, pp. 69–80.

Getz, L. L., Gudermuth, D. & Benson, S. (1992) Pattern of nest occupancy of the prairie vole, *Microtus ochrogaster*, in different habitats. *American Midland Naturalist*, **128**, 197–202.

Getz, L. L., McGuire, B., Hofmann, J. E., Pizzuto, T. & Frase, B. (1993) Social organization of the prairie vole (*Microtus ochrogaster*). *Journal of Mammalogy*, **74**, 44–58.

Getz, L. L., McGuire, B. & Carter, C. (2003) Social behavior, reproduction and demography of the prairie vole, *Microtus ochrogaster*. *Ethology, Ecology and Evolution*, **15**, 105–118.

Gonzales-Voyeur, A., Fitzpatrick, J. & Kolm, N. (2008) Sexual selection determines parental care in cichlid fishes. *Evolution*, **62**, 2015–2026.

Goodson, J. L. & Bass, A. H. (2001) Social behavior functions and related anatomical characteristics of vasotocin/vasopressin system in vertebrates. *Brain Research Reviews*, **35**, 246–265.

Goodson, J. L., Saldanha, C., Hahn, T. & Soma, K. (2005) Recent advances in behavioral neuroendocrinology: insights from studies on birds. *Hormones and Behavior*, **48**, 461–473.

Gowaty, P. (1996) Battles of the sexes and origins of monogamy. In: *Partnerships in Birds*, ed. J. M. Black. Oxford: Oxford University Press, pp. 21–52.

Griggio, M., Matessi, G. & Pilastro, A. (2005) Should I stay or should I go? Female brood desertion and male counter-strategy in rock sparrows. *Behavioral Ecology*, **16**, 435–441.

Gubernick, D. & Teferi, T. (2000) Adaptive significance of male parental care in a monogamous mammal. *Proceedings of the Royal Society B*, **267**, 147–150.

Gunther, R. (2005) Derived reproductive modes in New Guinean anuran amphibians and description of a new species with paternal care in the genus *Callulops* (Microhylidae). *Journal of Zoology*, **268**, 153–170.

Hammock, E. A. D. & Young, L. J. (2004) Functional microsatellite polymorphisms associated with divergent social structure in vole species. *Molecular Biology and Evolution*, **21**, 1057–1063.

Hammock, E. A. D. & Young, L. J. (2005) Microsatellite instability generates diversity in brain and sociobehavioral traits. *Science*, **308**, 1630–1634.

Hammock, E. A. D. & Young, L. J., eds. (2007a) *Neuroendocrinology, Neurochemistry, and Molecular Neurobiology of Affiliative Behavior*. New York, NY: Springer-Verlag.

Hammock, E. A. D. & Young, L. J. (2007b) On switches and knobs, microsatellites and monogamy. *Trends in Genetics*, **23**, 209–212.

Hansell, M. (2000) *Bird Nests and Construction Behaviour*. Cambridge: Cambridge University Press.

Harrison, F., Barta, Z., Cuthill, I. & Székely, T. (2009) How is sexual conflict over parental care resolved: a meta-analysis. *Journal of Evolutionary Biology*, **22**, 1800–1812.

Houston, A. I. & Davies, N. B. (1985) Evolution of cooperation and life history in dunnocks. In: *Behavioural Ecology: the Ecological Consequences of Adaptive Behaviour*, ed. R. Sibly & R. H. Smith. Oxford: Blackwell, pp. 471–487.

Houston, A. I., Székely, T. & McNamara, J. (2005) Conflict over parental care. *Trends in Ecology and Evolution*, **20**, 33–38.

Hunt, J. & Simmons, L. (2002) Behavioural dynamics of biparental care in the dung beetle *Onthophagus taurus*. *Animal Behaviour*, **64**, 65–75.

Ims, R. (1987) Responses in spatial organisation and behaviour to manipulations of the food resource in the vole *Clethrionomys rufocanus*. *Journal of Animal Ecology*, **56**, 585–596.

Insel, T. R. & Hulihan, T. (1995) A gender-specific mechanism for pair bonding: oxytocin and partner preference formation in monogamous voles. *Behavioral Neuroscience*, **109**, 782–789.

Insel, T. R. & Shapiro, L. E. (1992) Oxytocin receptor distribution reflects social organization in monogamous and polygamous voles. *Proceedings of the National Academy of Sciences of the USA*, **89**, 5981–5985.

Insel, T. R. & Young, L. J. (2000) Neuropeptides and the evolution of social behavior. *Current Opinion in Neurobiology*, **10**, 784–789.

Insel, T. R., Wang, Z. & Ferris, C. F. (1994) Patterns of vasopressin receptor distribution associated with social organization in microtine rodents. *Journal of Neuroscience*, **14**, 5381–5392.

Itzkowitz, M., Santangelo, N. & Richter, M. (2001) Parental division of labour and the shift from minimal to maximal role specializations: an examination using a biparental fish. *Animal Behaviour*, **61**, 1237–1245.

Ivell, R. & Dietmar, R. (1985) Structure and comparison of the oxytocin and vasopressin genes from rat. *Proceedings of the National Academy of Sciences of the USA*, **81**, 2006–2010.

Jennions, M. & Petrie, M. (2000) Why do females mate multiply? A review of the genetic benefits. *Biological Reviews*, **59**, 677–688.

Johnstone, R. A. & Hinde, C. A. (2006) Negotiation over offspring care: how should parents respond to each other's efforts? *Behavioral Ecology*, **17**, 818–827.

Kempenaers, B. (2007) Mate choice and genetic quality: a review of the heterozygosity theory. *Advances in the Study of Behavior*, **37**, 189–278.

Kendrick, K. M., Keverne, E. B. & Baldwin, B. A. (1987) Intracerebroventricular oxytocin stimulates maternal behaviour in the sheep. *Neuroendocrinology*, **46**, 56–61.

Kendrick, K. M., Costa, A. P. C. D., Broad, K. D. *et al.* (1997) Neural control of maternal behavior and olfactory recognition of offspring. *Brain Research Bulletin*, **44**, 383–395.

Kock, K. & Pshenichnov (2006) Evidence for egg brooding and parental care in icefish and other nototheniods in the Southern Ocean. *Antarctic Science*, **18**, 223–227.

Kokko, H. & Jennions, M. (2003) It takes two to tango. *Trends in Ecology and Evolution*, **18**, 103–104.

Kokko, H. & Jennions, M. (2008) Parental investment, sexual selection and sex ratios. *Journal of Evolutionary Biology*, **21**, 919–948.

Kolm, N., Goodwin, N., Balshine, S. & Reynolds, J. (2006) Life history evolution in cichlids 1: revisiting the evolution of life histories in relation to parental care. *Journal of Evolutionary Biology*, **19**, 66–75.

Komers, P. & Brotherton, P. (1997) Female space use is the best predictor of monogamy in mammals. *Proceedings of the Royal Society B*, **264**, 1261–1270.

Kosztolányi, A., Székely, T., Cuthill, I., Yilmaz, K. & Berberoglu, S. (2006) The influence of habitat on brood-rearing behaviour in the Kentish plover. *Journal of Animal Ecology*, **75**, 257–265.

Kupfer, A., Muller, H., Antoniazzi, M. *et al.* (2006) Parental investment by skin feeding in a caecilian amphibian. *Nature*, **440**, 926–929.

Lack, D. (1968) *Ecological Adaptations for Breeding in Birds*, London: Methuen.

Landgraf, R., Gerstberger, R., Montkowski, A. *et al.* (1995) V1 vasopressin receptor antisense oligodeoxynucleotide into septum reduces vasopressin binding, social discrimination abilities, and anxiety-related behavior in rats. *Journal of Neuroscience*, **6**, 4250–4258.

Landgraf, R., Frank, E., Aldag, J. M. *et al.* (2003) Viral vector-mediated gene transfer of the vole V1a vasopressin receptor in the rat septum: improved social discrimination and active social behaviour. *European Journal of Neuroscience*, **18**, 403–411.

Leengoed, E. V., Kerker, E. & Swanson, H. H. (1987) Inhibition of postpartum maternal behaviour in the rat by injecting an oxytocin antagonist into the cerebral ventricles. *Journal of Endocrinology*, **112**, 275–282.

Lehtinen, R. & Nussbaum, R. (2003) Parental care: a phylogenetic perspective. In: *Reproductive Biology and Phylogeny of Anura*, ed. B. G. M. Jamieson. Enfield, NH: Science Publishers, pp. 343–386.

Lessells, C. M. (1999) Sexual conflict in animals. In: *Levels of Selection in Evolution*, ed. L. Keller. Princeton, NJ: Princeton University Press, pp. 75–99.

Ligon, J. (1999) *Evolution of Avian Breeding Systems*. New York, NY: Oxford University Press.

Liker, A. (1995) Monogamy in precocial birds: a review. *Ornis Hungarica*, **5**, 1–14.

Liker, A. & Székely, T. (1997) Aggression among female lapwings, *Vanellus vanellus*. *Animal Behaviour*, **54**, 797–802.

Lim, M. M., Murphy, A. & Young, L. J. (2004a) Ventral striatopallidal oxytocin and vasopressin V1a receptors in the monogamous prairie vole (*Microtus ochrogaster*). *Journal of Comparative Neurology*, **468**, 555–570.

Lim, M. M., Wang, Z., Olazábal, D. E., Ren, X., Terwillger, E. F. & Young, L. J. (2004b) Enhanced partner preference in a promiscuous species by manipulating the expression of a single gene. *Nature*, **429**, 754–757.

Liu, Y., Curtis, J. T. & Wang, Z. (2001) Vasopressin in the lateral septum regulates pair bond formation in male prairie voles (*Microtus ochrogaster*). *Behavioral Neuroscience*, **115**, 910–919.

Lonstein, J. & De Vries, G. (1999) Comparison of the parental behavior of pairbonded female and male prairie voles (*Microtus ochrogaster*). *Physiology and Behavior*, **66**, 33–40.

Lott, D. (1991) *Intraspecific Variation in the Social Systems of Wild Vertebrates*. Cambridge: Cambridge University Press.

Lucia, K., Keane, B., Hayes, L. *et al.* (2008) Philopatry in prairie voles: an evaluation of the habitat saturation hypothesis. *Behavioral Ecology*, **19**, 774–783.

Mank, J. & Avise, J. (2006) The evolution of reproductive and genomic diversity in ray-finned fishes: insights from phylogeny and comparative analysis. *Journal of Fish Biology*, **69**, 1–27.

McGuire, B. & Bemis, W. E. (2007) Parental care. In: *Rodent Societies: an Ecological and Evolutionary Perspective*, ed. J. O. Wolff & P. W. Sherman. Chicago, IL: University of Chicago Press, pp. 231–242.

McGuire, B. & Novak, M. (1984a) A comparison of maternal behaviour in the meadow vole (*Microtus pennsylvanicus*), prairie vole (*M. ochrogaster*) and pine vole (*M. pinetorum*). *Animal Behaviour*, **32**, 1132–1141.

McGuire, B. & Novak, M. (1984b) A comparison of maternal behaviors in the meadow vole, prairie vole and pine vole. *Animal Behaviour*, **32**, 1132–1141.

McKinney, F., Cheng, K. & Bruggers, D. (1984) Sperm competition in apparently monogamous birds. In: *Sperm Competition and the Evolution of Animal Mating Systems*, ed. R. L. Smith. New York, NY: Academic Press, pp. 523–545.

McNamara, J. M. & Forslund, P. (1996) Divorce rates in birds: predictions from an optimization model. *American Naturalist*, **147**, 609–640.

McNamara, J. M., Gasson, C. & Houston, A. (1999) Incorporating rules for responding into evolutionary games. *Nature*, **401**, 368–371.

McNamara, J. M., Houston, A., Barta, Y. & Osorno, J.-L. (2002) Should young ever be better off with one parent than two? *Behavioral Ecology*, **14**, 301–310.

Meaney, M. J. (2001) Maternal care, gene expression, and the transmission of individual differences in stress reactivity across generations. *Annual Review of Neuroscience*, **24**, 1161–1192.

Mock, D. W. & Parker, G. A. (1997) *The Evolution of Sibling Rivalry*. Oxford: Oxford University Press.

Møller, A. (2007) The evolution of monogamy: mating relationships, parental care and sexual selection. In: *Monogamy: Mating Strategies and Partnerships in Birds, Humans and Other Mammals*, ed. U. H. Reichard & C. Boesch. Cambridge: Cambridge University Press, pp. 29–41.

Nettle, D. (2008) Why do some dads get more involved than others? Evidence from a large British cohort. *Evolution and Human Behavior*, **29**, 416–423.

Numan, M. & Insel, T. R. (2003) *The Neurobiology of Parental Behavior*. New York, NY: Springer-Verlag.

Ó Foighil, D. & Taylor, D. (2000) Evolution of parental care and ovulation behavior in oysters. *Phylogenetics and Evolution*, **15**, 301–313.

Olazábal, D. E. & Young, L. J. (2005) Variability in 'spontaneous' maternal behavior is associated with anxiety-like behavior and affiliation in naive juvenile and adult female prairie voles (*Microtus ochrogaster*). *Developmental Psychobiology*, **47**, 166–178.

Olazábal, D. E. & Young, L. J. (2006a) Species and individual differences in juvenile female alloparental care are associated with oxytocin receptor density in the striatum and the lateral septum. *Hormones and Behavior*, **49**, 681–687.

Olazábal, D. E. & Young, L. J. (2006b) Oxytocin receptors in the nucleus accumbens facilitate 'spontaneous' maternal behavior in adult female prairie voles. *Neuroscience*, **141**, 559–568.

Oliveras, D. & Novak, M. (1986) A comparison of paternal behavior in the meadow vole *Microtus pennsylvanicus*, the pine vole *M. pinetorum* and the prairie vole *M. ochrogaster*. *Animal Behaviour*, **34**, 519–526.

Ophir, A.G., Phelps, S.M., Sorin, A.B. & Wolff, J.O. (2007) Morphological, genetic, and behavioural comparisons of two prairie vole populations in the field and laboratory. *Journal of Mammalogy*, **88**, 989–999.

Ophir, A. G., Phelps, S. M., Sorin, A. B. & Wolff, J. O. (2008a) Social but not genetic monogamy is associated with greater breeding success in prairie voles. *Animal Behaviour*, **75**, 1143–1154.

Ophir, A. G., Campbell, P., Hanna, K. & Phelps, S. M. (2008b) Field tests of cis-regulatory variation at the prairie vole avpr1a locus: Association with V1aR abundance but not sexual or social fidelity. *Hormones and Behavior*, **54**, 694–702.

Ophir, A., Wolff, J. & Phelps, S. (2008c) Variation in neural V1aR predicts sexual fidelity and space use among male prairie voles in semi-natural settings. *Proceedings of the National Academy of Sciences of the USA*, **105**, 1249–1254.

Osorno, J. & Székely, T. (2004) Sexual conflict and parental care in magnificent frigatebirds: full compensation by deserted females. *Animal Behaviour*, **68**, 337–342.

Ostfeld, R. (1986) Territoriality and mating systems of California voles. *Journal of Animal Ecology*, **55**, 691–706.

Pedersen, C. A. & Prange, A. J. (1979) Induction of maternal behavior in virgin rats after intracerebroventricular administration of oxytocin. *Proceedings of the National Academy of Sciences of the USA*, **76**, 6661–6665.

Pedersen, C. A., Caldwell, J., Walker, C., Ayers, G. & Mason, G. (1994) Oxytocin activates the postpartum onset of rat maternal behavior in the ventral tegmental and medial preoptic areas. *Behavioral Neuroscience*, **108**, 1163–1171.

Persson, O. & Öhrström, P. (1989) A new avian mating system: ambisexual polygamy in the penduline tit *Remiz pendulinus*. *Ornis Scandinavica*, **20**, 105–111.

Pilastro, A., Biddau, T., Marin, G. & Mingozzi, T. (2001) Female brood desertion increases with number of available mates in the rock sparrow. *Journal of Avian Biology*, **32**, 68–72.

Pizzuto, T. & Getz, L. L. (1998) Female prairie voles (*Microtus ochrogaster*) fail to form a new pair after loss of mate. *Behavioural Processes*, **43**, 79–86.

Poelman, E. & Dicke, M. (2007) Offering offspring as food to cannibals: oviposition strategies of Amazonian poison frogs (*Dendrobates ventrimaculatus*). *Evolutionary Ecology*, **21**, 215–227.

Raadik, T., Bourke, D., Clarke, M. & Martin, A. (1990) Behaviour and reproductive success of pairs and lone parents in the convict cichlid *Heros nigrofasciatus*. *Animal Behaviour*, **39**, 594–596.

Rauter, C. M. & Moore, A. J. (2004) Time constraints and trade-offs among parental care behaviours: effects of brood size, sex and loss of mate. *Animal Behaviour*, **68**, 695–702.

Reichard, U. H. (2007) Monogamy: past and present. In: *Monogamy: Mating Strategies and Partnerships in Birds, Humans and Other Mammals*, ed. U. H. Reichard & C. Boesch. Cambridge: Cambridge University Press, pp. 3–26.

Reynolds, J. D., Goodwin, N. B. & Freckleton, R. P. (2002) Evolutionary transitions in parental care and live-bearing in vertebrates. *Philosophical Transactions of the Royal Society B*, **357**: 269–281.

Roberts, R. L., Miller, A. K., Taymans, S. E. & Carter, C. S. (1998) Role of social and endocrine factors in alloparental behavior of prairie voles (*Microtus ochrogaster*). *Canadian Journal of Zoology*, **76**, 1862–1868.

Royle, N., Hartley, I. & Parker, G. (2002) Sexual conflict reduces offspring fitness in zebra finches. *Nature*, **416**, 733–736.

Sanz, J., Kranenbarg, S. & Tinbergen, J. (2000) Differential response by males and females to manipulation of partner contribution in the great tit (*Parus major*). *Journal of Animal Ecology*, **69**, 74–84.

Searcy, W. & Yasukawa, K. (1995) *Polygyny and Sexual Selection in Red-Winged Blackbirds*. Princeton, NJ: Princeton University Press.

Slagsvold, T. & Lifjeld, J. T. (1994) Polygyny in birds: the role of competition between females for male parental care. *American Naturalist*, **143**, 59–94.

Smiseth, P. T., Dawson, C., Varley, E. & Moore, A. J. (2005) How do caring parents respond to mate loss? Differential response by males and females. *Animal Behaviour*, **69**, 551–559.

Solomon, N. G. (1991) Current indirect fitness benefits associated with philopatry in juvenile prairie voles. *Behavioral Ecology and Sociobiology*, **29**, 277–282.

Solomon, N. G. (1993) Comparison of parental behavior in male and female prairie voles (*Microtus ochrogaster*). *Canadian Journal of Zoology*, **71**, 434–437.

Solomon, N. G. & Crist, T. (2008) Estimates of reproductive success for group-living prairie voles, *Microtus ochrogaster*, in high-density populations. *Animal Behaviour*, **76**, 881–892.

Solomon, N. G. & Keane, B. (2007) Reproductive strategies in female rodents. In: *Rodent Societies: an Ecological and Evolutionary Perspective*, ed. J. O. Wolff & P. W. Sherman. Chicago, IL: University of Chicago Press, pp. 42–56.

Solomon, N. G., Keane, B., Knoch, L. & Hogan, P. (2004) Multiple paternity in socially monogamous prairie voles (*Microtus ochrogaster*). *Canadian Journal of Zoology*, **82**, 1667–1671.

Soma, K. (2006) Testosterone and aggression: Berthold, birds and beyond. *Journal of Neuroendocrinology*, **18**, 543–551.

Summers, K., Mckeon, C. & Heying, H. (2006) The evolution of parental care and egg size: a comparative analysis in frogs. *Proceedings of the Royal Society B*, **273**, 687–692.

Székely, T., Cuthill, I. & Kis, J. (1999) Brood desertion in Kentish plover: sex differences in remating opportunities. *Behavioral Ecology*, **10**, 983–993.

Székely, T., Webb, J. & Cuthill, I. (2000) Mating patterns, sexual selection and parental care: an integrative approach. In: *Vertebrate Mating Systems*, ed. M. Apollonio, M. Festa-Bianchet & D. Mainardi. London: World Science Press, pp. 194–223.

Szentirmai, I., Székely, T. & Komdeur, J. (2007) Sexual conflict over care: antagonistic effects of clutch desertion on reproductive success of male and female penduline tits. *Journal of Evolutionary Biology*, **20**, 1739–1744.

Tallamy, D. (1999) Semelparity and the evolution of maternal care in insects. *Animal Behavior*, **57**, 2373–2383.

Thomas, G. & Székely, T. (2005) Evolutionary pathways in shorebird breeding systems: sexual conflict, parental care, and chick development. *Evolution*, **59**, 2222–2230.

Thomas, G., Freckleton, R. & Székely, T. (2006) Comparative analyses of the influence of developmental mode on phenotypic diversification rates in shorebirds. *Proceedings of the Royal Society B*, **273**, 1619–1624.

Tieleman, B. I., Dijkstra, T., Klasing, K., Visser, G. & Williams, J. (2008) Effects of experimentally increased costs of activity during reproduction on parental investment and self-maintenance in tropical house wrens *Behavioral Ecology*, **19**, 949–959.

Tregenza, T. & Wedell, N. (2000) Genetic compatibility, mate choice and patterns of parentage. *Molecular Ecology*, **9**, 1013–1027.

Trivers, R. L. (1972) Parental investment and sexual selection. In: *Sexual Selection and the Descent of Man, 1871–1971*, ed. B. Campbell. Chicago, IL: Aldine, pp. 136–179.

Trivers, R. L. (1974) Parent–offspring conflict. *American Zoologist*, **14**, 249–264.

Tyler, M. & Carter, D. (1981) Oral birth of the young of the gastric brooding frog *Rheobatrachus silus*. *Animal Behaviour*, **29**, 280–282.

Veiga, J. (1992) Why are house sparrows predominantly monogamous: a test of hypotheses. *Animal Behaviour*, **43**, 361–370.

Walling, C. A., Stamper, C. E., Smiseth, P. T. & Moore, A. J. (2008) Genetic architecture of sex differences in parental care. *Proceedings of the National Academy of Sciences of the USA*, **105**, 18430–18435.

Wang, Z., Ferris, C. F. & De Vries, G. J. (1994) Role of septal vasopressin innervation in paternal behavior in prairie voles (*Microtus ochrogaster*). *Proceedings of the National Academy of Sciences of the USA*, **91**, 400–4.

Wang, Z., Zhou, L., Hulihan, T. J. & Insel, T. R. (1996) Immunoreactivity of central vasopressin and oxytocin pathways in microtine rodents: a quantitative comparative study. *Journal of Comparative Neurology*, **366**, 726–737.

Wang, Z. X. & Insel, T. R. (1996) Parental behavior in voles. *Advances in the Study of Behavior*, **25**, 361–384.

Westneat, D. F. & Stewart, I. R. K. (2003) Extra-pair paternity in birds: causes, correlates and conflict. *Annual Review of Ecology, Evolution and Systematics*, **34**, 365–396.

Whittingham, L., Dunn, P. & Robertson, R. (1994) Female response to reduced male parental care in birds: an experiment in tree swallows. *Ethology, Ecology and Evolution*, **96**, 260–269.

Williams, J. R., Catania, K. & Carter, C. (1992) Development of partner preferences in female prairie voles (*Microtus ochrogaster*): the role of social and sexual experience. *Hormones and Behavior*, **26**, 339–349.

Williams, J. R., Insel, T. R., Harbaugh, C. R. & Carter, C. S. (1994) Oxytocin administered centrally facilitates formation of a partner preference in prairie voles (*Microtus ochrogaster*). *Journal of Neuroendocrinology*, **6**, 247–250.

Williams, T. (1996) Mate fidelity in penguins. In: *Partnerships in Birds*, ed. J. M. Black. Oxford: Oxford University Press, pp. 268–285.

Wilson, E. O. (1975) *Sociobiology: the New Synthesis*, Cambridge, MA: Harvard University Press.

Wingfield, J., Hegner, R.-E., Dufty Jr., A. & Ball, G. (1990) The 'challenge hypothesis': theoretical implications for patterns of testosterone secretion, mating systems and breeding strategies. *American Naturalist*, **136**, 829–846.

Winslow, J., Hastings, N., Carter, C. S., Harbaugh, C. & Insel, T. (1993) A role for central vasopressin in pair bonding in monogamous prairie voles. *Nature*, **365**, 545–548.

Wise, R. A. (2002) Brain reward circuitry: insights from unsensed incentives. *Neuron*, **36**, 229–240.

Wolff, J. O. & MacDonald, D. W. (2004) Promiscuous females protect their offspring. *Trends in Ecology and Evolution*, **19**, 127–134.

Wright, J. & Cuthill, I. (1990) Biparental care: short-term manipulations of partner contribution and brood size in the starling. *Behavioral Ecology*, **1**, 116–124.

Young, L. J. (1999) Frank A. Beach Award. Oxytocin and vasopressin receptors and species-typical social behaviors. *Hormones and Behavior*, **36**, 212–221.

Young, L. J. & Insel, T. R. (2002) Hormones and parental behaviour. In: *Behavioral Endocrinology*, 2nd edn, ed. J. B. Becker, S. M. Breedlove, D. Crews & M. M. McCarthy. Cambridge, MA: MIT Press, pp. 331–369.

Young, L. J. & Wang, Z. (2004) The neurobiology of pair bonding. *Nature Neuroscience*, **7**, 1048–1054.

Young, L. J., Wang, Z. & Insel, T. R. (1999) Neuroendocrine bases of monogamy. *Trends in Neuroscience*, **21**, 71–75.

Young, L. J., Lim, M. M., Gingrich, B. & Insel, T. R. (2001) Cellular mechanisms of social attachment. *Hormones and Behavior*, **40**, 133–138.

Yu, G.-Z., Kaba, H., Okutani, F. & Higuchi, T. (1996) The olfactory bulb: a critical site of action for oxytocin in the induction of maternal behaviour in the rat. *Neuroscience*, **72**, 1083–1088.

Zeh, J. & Zeh, D. (2001) Reproductive mode and the genetic benefits of polyandry. *Animal Behaviour*, **61**, 1051–1063.

Mating systems and genetic variation

Marion Petrie

I can't remember a time when I wasn't interested in social behaviour, and I chose a biology degree course where animal behaviour was a key component. Sussex University was an exciting place to be as an undergraduate in the early 1970s when sociobiology was coming to the fore, and I was lucky enough to have John Maynard Smith as my personal tutor. John's enthusiasm for applying evolutionary principles to animal behaviour was an inspiration that I still value today. When I started doing a PhD on moorhens *Gallinula chloropus* the working title for my thesis was 'the function of winter flocking in moorhens' – why animals live in groups was a key issue in the 1970s. It was whilst watching flocks that I noticed birds fighting in front of potential mates. Moorhens cannot be sexed in the field so it was not immediately clear whether it was males fighting for females or vice versa, and I can remember still my surprise and delight when I came back home and looked up the birds' numbers and sizes to discover that it was the smaller females fighting in front of males. It became clear that they were fighting for access to a particular male, and I started to wonder what it was about this male that was worth fighting for.

At this time there was virtually no work on female choice, and my first paper, published in *Science* in 1983, provided some of the first evidence that females can show strong mate preference. It was entitled 'Female moorhens compete for small fat males' (Petrie 1983), which has had the unexpected consequence of endearing me to small fat males everywhere! Fat males were able to expend more effort on parental care, were thus capable of incubating more clutches in the season, and were thus highly prized as mates. It was during that time that I realised that no one had studied the quintessential sexually selected species, the peafowl *Pavo cristatus*, and that, whilst Darwin had suggested that the peacock's train had evolved through female choice, no one had experimentally tested this idea. For my first postdoc with Tim Halliday at the Open University I established a field study at Whipsnade Park on a free-ranging population of peafowl. I showed that females did prefer males with elaborate trains (Petrie *et al.* 1991), and that experimental removal of eye-spots from the train resulted in a decline in mating success (Petrie & Halliday 1994). After establishing that female preferences occur, I then asked, 'why would evolution have favoured choosy females in a species where, unlike the moorhen, males perform no parental care'? What sort of selective benefits do females gain from their choice of an attractive male, and do they gain obvious direct reproductive benefits or indirect genetic benefits for their offspring? I considered these questions during a fellowship at Oxford. I found no evidence

Social Behaviour: Genes, Ecology and Evolution, ed. Tamás Székely, Allen J. Moore and Jan Komdeur. Published by Cambridge University Press. © Cambridge University Press 2010.

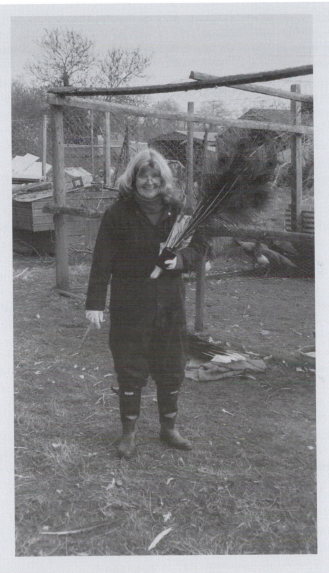

Dressed for action. Photo: Tom Pike.

that females gain direct benefits (e.g. Birkhead & Petrie 1995), but I did find that females gain viability advantages for their offspring from matings with attractive males. Even when obvious maternal effects and environmental differences were controlled for, I found that the offspring of attractive males survive better (Petrie 1994).

The discovery that females gain genetic benefits for offspring poses a major problem, sometimes known as the 'lek paradox' (see Chapter 10). Simply stated, this is: why is there any heritable variation left in the fitness indicator traits that females base their choice on? Theoretically, strong directional selection as a result of female choice and natural selection should remove any genetic variation in fitness. However, despite these theoretical expectations there clearly is genetic variation in sexually selected ornaments (Petrie *et al.* 2009), and indeed, some indication that there is more genetic variation in sexually selected species with higher variance in mating success (Petrie *et al.* 1998).

How can this be? I have recently developed a new idea that may provide the first self-sustaining solution to the lek paradox. Using a simulation modelling approach with my colleague Gilbert Roberts at Newcastle, we have shown that female choice can sustain a higher mutation rate when compared with random mating. An increase in mutation rate can sustain genetic variability among males, which can promote female choice, and a greater level of choice can promote a higher mutation rate (Petrie & Roberts 2007). This is counterintuitive but, essentially, the higher mating success that accrues to an individual with any beneficial mutation can lead to the maintenance of the associated higher mutation rate. I am intrigued by the possibility that sexual selection can maintain genetic variation, and feel that this area is ripe for empirical testing. In general, the role of selection on the heritable genetic mechanisms for generating variation (such as recombination) is something that needs to be incorporated more into our evolutionary models. At the moment we tend to think only in terms of selection removing variation, but its role in generating variation could result in major changes in our evolutionary thinking.

It also appears that, regardless of mechanism, there could be a strong link between levels of genetic variation in a population and the observed mating system. Whether or not males can attract multiple mates is critical in determining whether they expend their reproductive effort on displaying or caring for offspring. Theoretically, I have argued that caring males cannot invade a population of displaying males when there are strong genetic benefits to females (Petrie & Lipsitch 1994). There can only be strong genetic benefits to females when there is a lot of variance in the genetic quality of males. Although so far I have only developed this idea in relation to female choice for male partners, I also feel that relatively high variation in female genetic quality may explain the evolution of male-only care. It may only pay males to look after the offspring of females that don't help with parental care when the offspring of these females inherit their mother's high genetic quality. The relative degree of genetic variation among males and females could be critical in determining the future benefits that accrue from display or parental care. This factor is often overlooked in explaining the evolution of sex roles, but I believe this could change as we understand more about the maintenance of genetic variation in populations.

The following are the principles that have guided my research (in no particular order):

- Watching animals and questioning their behaviour, or entering or plotting data and looking at variation, is the best way to discover new research questions.
- Focusing on one question that has associated alternative but testable hypotheses leads to citable publications. *Question, hypothesis, prediction, test* is my mantra to my students.
- One of John Maynard Smith's guiding principles, which has always stayed with me, was 'if you can't write it on the back of a matchbox then you haven't understood it.'

References

Birkhead, T. R. & Petrie, M. (1995) Ejaculate features and sperm utilisation in the peafowl *Pavo cristatus*. *Proceedings of the Royal Society B*, **261**, 153–158.

Petrie, M. (1983) Female moorhens compete for small fat males. *Science*, **220**, 413–415.

Petrie, M. (1994) Improved growth and survival of offspring of peacocks with more elaborate trains. *Nature*, **371**, 598–599.

Petrie, M. & Halliday, T. (1994) Experimental and natural changes in the peacock's (*Pavo cristatus*) train can affect mating success. *Behavioral Ecology and Sociobiology*, **35**, 213–217.

Petrie, M. & Lipsitch, M. (1994) Avian polygyny is most likely in populations with high variability in heritable male fitness. *Proceedings of the Royal Society B*, **256**, 275–280.

Petrie, M. & Roberts, G. (2007) Sexual selection and the evolution of evolvability. *Heredity*, **98**, 198–205.

Petrie, M., Halliday, T. R. & Sanders, C. (1991) Peahens prefer peacocks with elaborate trains. *Animal Behaviour*, **41**, 323–331.

Petrie, M., Doums, C. & Møller, A. P. (1998) The degree of extra-pair paternity increases with genetic variability. *Proceedings of the National Academy of Sciences of the USA*, **95**, 9390–9395.

Petrie, M., Cotgreave, P. & Pike, T. W. (2009) Variation in the peacock's train shows a genetic component. *Genetica*, **135**, 7–11.

12

Adaptations and constraints in the evolution of delayed dispersal: implications for cooperation

Jan Komdeur and Jan Ekman

Overview

Cooperation is a ubiquitous feature of life. While many instances of cooperation are explicable as the selfish motives of individuals, other forms of cooperation, such as cooperative breeding in which individuals live and breed in mixed-sex groups of three or more adults and share in providing care at a single breeding attempt, are difficult to explain. Given that the majority of cooperative breeders exhibit delayed dispersal, it would appear that delayed dispersal plays a role in the evolution of cooperative breeding. However, there are several species that, despite the absence of cooperative breeding, live in family units. Thus it is important to understand the specific fitness consequences of delayed dispersal independently of the confounding fitness consequences of helping behaviour.

In this chapter we focus on how delayed dispersal has evolved or can be maintained in the absence of cooperative breeding. We do this by exploring the proximate and ultimate factors involved in the evolution of delayed dispersal in species which exhibit delayed dispersal but do not cooperate by helping to raise non-descendant relatives. We show that the benefits of delaying dispersal and being philopatric to maintain a family association can come either as direct fitness gained through enhanced survival in family groups (e.g. better predator defence or food access) and/or enhanced future reproduction. Survival benefits from cooperation among group-living kin are likely to be a more general candidate of a fitness component selecting for family cohesion than the inclusive fitness gains from alloparental care. Therefore, parental tolerance of retained offspring, coupled with territoriality, is likely to be a cornerstone of family cohesion in territorial species by providing the offspring benefits (e.g. safe haven) until they disperse. The potential for group-living effects to select for delayed dispersal is evident from the variety of family groups that exist in the absence of cooperative breeding.

Directing attention to these general group-living effects, in both cooperatively and non-cooperatively breeding species, has the potential to account for the large unexplained variation in the length of time the offspring stay, and the variation in sociality among many vertebrate species. A more inclusive approach to family cohesion would incorporate the short- and long-term fitness consequences of delayed dispersal of offspring both for the offspring and for their parents, and should be the focus of future research. This research should include species with and without cooperative breeding.

Social Behaviour: Genes, Ecology and Evolution, ed. Tamás Székely, Allen J. Moore and Jan Komdeur. Published by Cambridge University Press. © Cambridge University Press 2010.

12.1 Introduction

Cooperation is a ubiquitous feature of life. Individuals cooperate in hunting, feeding, fending off enemies and migrating from one site to another (Wilson 1975, Dugatkin 1997). Many insects, fish, birds and mammals live and breed in colonies, and males and females cooperate in mating and/or care provisioning (Chapters 10 and 11). Behaviour that provides a benefit to another individual and, importantly, has evolved at least partly because of this benefit, can be defined as cooperative (West *et al.* 2007). But why do animals cooperate? Behavioural ecologists traditionally addressed this question by studying adaptation and the effects of environment on behaviour and reproductive success (see Paul Sherman's profile). Individuals may cooperate with their relatives to enhance the reproductive output of their kin (e.g. Koenig *et al.* 1992, Mumme 1992, Emlen 1995, 1997, Russell & Hatchwell 2001, Richardson *et al.* 2003), and males and females cooperate to raise young in many insect, fish and bird species (Smiseth & Moore 2004, Houston *et al.* 2005). Furthermore, if the environment is harsh (e.g. extremely cold or hot) and there is high predation risk, then cooperation among conspecifics is expected in order to cope with the environment, food and enemies. Emperor penguins *Aptenodytes forsteri* have developed a social behaviour for when it gets cold. During extremely low temperatures, they huddle together in groups that may comprise several thousand penguins. That way, most individuals of the group have a part of their body protected and warmed by the other penguins. However, is this cooperation? There is a continual movement of penguins from the outside of the group to the centre, thereby displacing the warmer and more protected penguins to the outside where they will take their turn in the worst places against the wind and raw cold (Ancel *et al.* 1997).

There are, however, differences between individuals, populations and species in the extent of cooperation. These differences are explained in the context of evolutionary theory (Chapter 6), which states that individuals are selected for their ability to efficiently translate resources into survival and reproductive success, maximising their genetic contribution to future generations (Hamilton 1964a, 1964b, Maynard Smith 1964). Individuals are thus expected to employ a strategy that maximises their own fitness, even if it leads to a decrease in fitness of their partner or of other group or family members. This would appear to lead to a world dominated by selfish behaviour. As a consequence, the evolution of investment should be driven by the relative costs and benefits of this investment (e.g. Maynard Smith 1977, Clutton-Brock 1991). For example, the amount of paternal care to offspring may be adjusted in line with confidence of genetic parentage (Westneat & Sherman 1993).

Many instances of apparent cooperation are, after detailed investigation, explicable as the selfish motives of individuals; however, other forms of cooperation have proved more difficult to explain. For example, in some species individuals live and breed in mixed-sex groups of three or more adults and share in providing parental care at a single breeding attempt (Brown 1987, Stacey & Koenig 1990). Systems may include a breeding pair assisted by non-breeding helpers, as in the grey wolf *Canis lupus* (Derix *et al.* 1993) and the naked mole-rat *Heterocephalus glaber* (O'Riain *et al.* 2000). Alternatively a dominant pair may be accompanied by subordinates, of one or both sexes, that share reproduction with the dominant of the opposite sex, as in the Lake Tanganyika cichlid *Neolamprologus pulcher* (Dierkes *et al.* 1999), dwarf mongoose *Helogale parvula* (Rood 1990), meerkat *Suricata suricatta* (Griffin *et al.* 2003), superb fairy-wren *Malurus cyaneus* (Double & Cockburn 2003) and the Seychelles warbler *Acrocephalus sechellensis* (Richardson *et al.* 2002). Among vertebrates, cooperative breeding is found in at least 9% of birds (Cockburn 2006), 3% of mammals (Brown 1987) and in some fish species (Taborsky 1994), with a particularly high frequency of 19% in oscine passerine species, i.e. the true songbird species (Cockburn 2003), as well as in Australian birds (Russell 1989, Arnold & Owens 1998) and primates (Kappeler 2008). Whatever the structure of the system, the fact that the majority of cooperative breeders exhibit delayed dispersal of offspring that do not breed independently but instead remain on their natal territories and care for young that are not their own genetic offspring (*alloparental care*), provides an intriguing evolutionary paradox. The key issue in understanding the evolution of alloparental care is to understand the formation of family units. Although in such family units helping may occur, the role of helping for the evolution of delayed dispersal remains unknown.

Traditionally, the evolution of vertebrate cooperative breeding systems has been viewed as a two-step process: first, there is a decision by mature individuals to join a group and forgo independent breeding, and second, there is a decision by subordinates in a group to become helpers (Emlen 1982). The first step should be the key to the formation of family units, and is usually attributed to the existence of ecological or life-history constraints on independent breeding (Emlen 1982, Arnold & Owens 1998, 1999, Hatchwell & Komdeur 2000). The second step envisages that individuals that become helpers within a group must gain a net fitness benefit (Emlen 1982). Non-breeding subordinates can increase their fitness indirectly by enhancing the reproductive success of close relatives (who carry the same genes). However, in most species the indirect genetic fitness benefit gained from helping is likely to be considerably less than the potential direct genetic gain from immediate independent breeding (Brown 1987). Indeed, in some systems where subordinates are unrelated to the dominant breeders such indirect benefits are not possible at all. Therefore, understanding why mature individuals do not, or cannot, breed independently is the key to understanding the evolution of cooperative breeding.

One of the inherent difficulties in studies of 'why stay?' and 'why help?' questions is that the two behaviours are inevitably closely coupled. This is because most studies investigating the fitness consequences of helping have considered the decisions to remain on the natal territory into the breeding season as the switch point. However, Brown (1987) suggests that the greatest insights into cooperative breeding will come from comparisons of species in which delaying dispersal and delaying breeding on the one hand and helping on the other are uncoupled. In a typical cooperative breeder, at least some individuals engage in both of these behaviours by becoming

non-breeding helpers on their natal territory, but it is important to note that some individuals and some species can be characterised by any combination of the two. For example, individuals may delay breeding and delay dispersal by remaining in their natal social group but provide no assistance in raising offspring. The two questions, 'why stay?' and 'why help?', represent two independent behavioural decisions, although the costs and benefits of one decision may affect the potential fitness consequences of the other decision. Studying species exhibiting delayed dispersal that do not help allows analyses of the specific fitness consequences of delayed dispersal without obfuscation by the confounding fitness consequences of helping behaviour. This approach has been put to effective use in a few intraspecific comparisons where such uncoupling is feasible (e.g. Reyer 1984, Emlen & Wrege 1988, Komdeur 1996, Khan & Walters 1997).

In general, however, species that exhibit delayed dispersal of offspring but do not help have attracted little attention until recently (Ekman et al. 2004, Ekman 2006), although a number of studies have revealed that the offspring forgo personal reproduction, remain associated with their parents and yet do not provide alloparental care (Table 12.1). The absence of alloparental care in such species is not an artefact stemming from lack of observations. Parents sometimes actively prevent offspring from approaching the nest (Verbeek & Butler 1981, Strickland 1991, Burt & Peterson 1993, Ekman et al. 1994). One reason for the lack of attention to such species is that the young do not exhibit the apparent altruism that has been the focus of research into cooperative breeding in the past decades. Any inclusive fitness benefits of helping would certainly augment benefits of delayed dispersal, but they appear to be neither necessary nor sufficient to explain why dispersal should be delayed. In the past, explanations for delayed dispersal have mainly focused on constraints rather than adaptation, and both have been regarded as mutually exclusive explanations of delayed dispersal (Ekman et al. 2004). This is because the duality of explanations for kin-structured groups could be highlighted with, on the one hand, explanations representing constraints on dispersal and, on the other hand, explanations

Table 12.1. Species with offspring delaying dispersal beyond the first breeding season. The off-spring do not breed independently and do not provide alloparental care while in the family groups

Species	Reference
Mammals	
Tamarisk gerbil *Meriones tamariscinus*	Tchabovsky & Bazykin 2004
Wolverine *Gulo gulo*	Vangen *et al.* 2001
Brown bear *Ursus arctos*	Støen *et al.* 2006
Birds	
Red kite *Milvus milvus*	Newton *et al.* 1994
Common buzzard *Buteo buteo*	Walls & Kenward 1996
Siberian jay *Perisoreus infaustus*	Ekman *et al.* 1994
Grey (Canadian) jay *Perisoreus canadensis*	Strickland 1991
Steller's jay *Cyanocitta stelleri*	Brown 1963
Green (Texas) jay *Cyanocorax yncas*	Gayou 1986
Western (California) scrub jay *Aphelocoma californica*	Carmen 2004
Eurasian magpie *Pica pica*	Eden 1987, Birkhead 1991
Northwestern crow *Corvus caurinus*	Verbeek & Butler 1981
Song wren *Cyphorhinus phaeocephalus*	Robinson 2000
Western bluebird *Sialia mexicana*	Dickinson *et al.* 1996
Chinspot batis *Batis molitor*	Hockey *et al.* 2005
Chowchilla *Orthonyx spaldingii*	Jansen 1999, Frith *et al.* 1997
Speckled warbler *Chthonicola sagittata*	Gardner *et al.* 2003
Brown thornbill *Acanthiza pusilla*	Green & Cockburn 2001
Australian magpie *Gymnorhina tibicen*	Veltman 1989
Reptiles	
Squamate reptile *Egernia* sp.	Chapple 2003

representing adaptations to handle these constraints, such as improved fitness.

In this chapter we focus on the evolution of delayed dispersal and living in kin groups rather than cooperation as such. We do this by discussing the emerging evidence for an adaptive response to constraints in access to breeding and the importance of factors influencing survival value (referred to as ultimate factors) in the control of timing of dispersal. First, we discuss the constraints on access to breeding and the causal (proximate) factors involved in the formation of family groups. Second, we discuss the emerging evidence for adaptive responses, other than helping behaviour, to these constraints in access to breeding. We focus on fitness benefits achieved from forms of cooperation other than helping behaviour, because the latter has been intensively explored (e.g. MacDonald & Moehlman

1982, Stacey & Koenig 1990, Koenig & Dickinson 2004, Cezilly 2007), whereas species with delayed dispersal of non-helping offspring have attracted little attention (Ekman *et al.* 2004). We argue that constraints and adaptation of delayed dispersal should not be seen as mutually exclusive explanations of delayed dispersal, rather as complementary explanations. We do this by uncoupling delayed dispersal and cooperative breeding in vertebrate species, which allows us to investigate the proximate and ultimate factors involved in the evolution of delayed dispersal.

12.2 Delayed dispersal and its significance

Delayed dispersal is a loosely defined concept only relating independence to time. The moment of independence can vary, and there are no fixed time limits defining when dispersal is considered delayed. But delayed dispersal, whatever its timing, represents a challenge to evolutionary theory when there are costs from a postponement of independence. A fitness cost is manifested in loss of lifetime reproduction, and the most obvious such cost is incurred when sexually mature offspring forgo reproductive opportunities and remain non-breeding on their birth site. Conflict over reproduction (Chapters 10 and 11) can be rife, with mechanisms of incest avoidance helping prevent mating within families and suppressing offspring reproduction (Koenig & Haydock 2004), in particular when reproduction requires a territory (Cockburn 2004). Conflict over reproduction may also prevent the offspring from acquiring breeding status through inheritance of the birth site, although this is not universal (Brown 1978a, Fitzpatrick & Woolfenden 1984, Zahavi 1990). Ascending to breeding status after the death of a same-sex parent confers the risk of an incestuous relationship with the remaining parent. This conflict seems generally to be resolved to the advantage of the parent. The inherent sexual conflict that stems from close relatedness in families will therefore select for natal dispersal, i.e. dispersal of young from birth place to place of first breeding attempt (Perrin & Mazalov 1999, Perrin & Lehmann 2001), and this raises the question of how a delay in natal dispersal can be maintained despite its costs. Delayed dispersal could impinge on the ability to find a breeding vacancy of high quality, with repercussions for future reproduction (Nilsson & Smith 1988). The challenge posed by delayed dispersal is to define the precise costs, and to determine to what extent the offspring response can be reconciled with adaptive behaviour.

12.3 Access to reproduction: constraints and adaptive responses

Constraints on access to resources required for reproduction, such as territories, nesting sites or partners have been seen as a unifying phenomenon of family living (Brown 1969, Emlen 1982, Pruett-Jones & Lewis

1990). Family groups form when offspring remain non-breeding and can wait for a breeding opportunity at the natal site (Keller & Waller 2002, Perrin & Lehmann 2001). As a response to incest taboos and reproductive conflict offspring reproduction is often suppressed in families (Koenig & Haydock 2004). The offspring will eventually have to leave their birth site to reproduce, given that inbreeding costs and incest avoidance block inheritance of the birth site as a main route to acquire breeding status. In what appears to be a response to lack of breeding opportunities elsewhere in the form of shortage of territories (Selander 1964), nesting sites (Walters et al. 1992) or breeding partners (Faaborg 1986, Pruett-Jones & Lewis 1990), natal philopatry is seemingly behaviourally imposed by external conditions.

The idea that environmental conditions, and habitat saturation in particular, limits breeding populations in territorial animals has a long history with its roots in population ecology. A process describing how habitats become saturated in crowded populations was termed the *buffer effect* by Kluyver and Tinbergen (1953). Their model was designed to explain the regulation of population numbers in a habitat of varying quality. As a basic premise it assumes that habitats are filled in order of quality. First optimal habitats becomes filled, and then suboptimal habitats, until there is no suitable habitat available for reproduction (Brown 1969). As habitats of better quality are gradually filled up, remaining vacant space eventually becomes of such poor quality that would-be breeders deem it unsuitable as breeding habitat. The fraction of the population without a territory will become floaters until a breeding vacancy becomes available.

The observation that non-breeding offspring formed the additional members (supernumeraries) in family groups suggested that the buffer effect might also account for why territorial animals associate in families (Selander 1964). It becomes relevant for explaining the occurrence of natal philopatry in that it provides an answer to why individuals remain non-breeding, which then serves as a premise for postponed dispersal and family living. The buffer effect could easily be adapted to family living by assuming that constraints on access to critical resources prevent non-breeding offspring from breeding. Families should then build up in saturated environments as a direct corollary of the fact that offspring remain on their birth site rather than become floaters leaving the birth site (Brown 1969). Testing for the role of the buffer effect in population regulation requires that the presence of floaters is demonstrated, which is now well supported by breeder-removal experiments. Removal of breeders from a territory resulted in floaters of the same sex rapidly moving in to fill the breeding opportunity, which demonstrates that they were previously precluded from settling by established territory owners (Newton 1998). In family-living species the presence of non-breeding supernumeraries may in any case be obvious, with no need to resort to removal experiments.

However, the question at the heart of family living concerns the lifetime implications arising from a postponed reproductive debut. The buffer effect tells us little about what makes a habitat suitable. It is a strict population model limited to describing the proximate control of how populations are distributed over habitats. It does not make any connections between behaviour and life-history trade-offs or lifetime reproductive success, but habitats are considered unsuitable simply because they are not used. It was only with a formulation of the fitness consequences of delayed dispersal in terms of reproductive success by Brown (1978b) that a comparison of the costs and benefits of dispersal alternatives in fitness terms became possible. Emlen (1982) developed this idea, seeing adaptive delayed dispersal from the perspective of a long-term life-history trade-off in what has become known as the *ecological constraints model*.

12.4 Delayed dispersal: ecological constraints or trade-off decision?

Although ecological constraints seemingly focus on the role of limited access to resources, it is essentially an adaptive explanation in which delayed dispersal is portrayed as the outcome of a lifetime trade-off. The constraint is essentially the cost in an adaptive trade-off. Life history accounts for delayed reproductive

debut as a response to excessive reproductive costs from breeding at an early age. Such costs could come in the form of developmental investments or physiological expenditures for sexual maturation. The ecological constraints model differs from general life-history models only insofar as it specifically identifies environmental conditions as the source of a cost. Emlen (1982) envisioned a lifetime trade-off where reproduction was postponed under environmental conditions that limit access to resources and make their acquisition risky. Although not technically incorporating a trade-off mechanism, the model is built on the assumption that dispersal and independent reproduction should be delayed only when it carries compensating fitness gains over the individual's lifetime. Individuals can only be expected to delay dispersal if the benefits they receive – due to increased survival or increased reproductive benefits, including indirect and future benefits – exceed the benefits they would receive if they were not in the group. While 'ecological constraints' have generally been associated with proximate mechanisms limiting immediate dispersal, the ultimate motives of staying in the group (Macedo & Bianchi 1997, Baglione *et al.* 2005) have largely gone unnoticed. Yet, the adaptive basis of the ecological constraints model was explicitly stated by Emlen (1982): 'Thus we must consider the long-term trade-offs of early dispersal against the postponement of dispersal with its possible compensating benefits for later reproduction.' What is seemingly a contradiction between the facts that a postponement of dispersal is constrained by environmental conditions while it should simultaneously be an adaptive choice is reconciled by the difference in perspective. Constraints on access to resources, such as a lack of mates and/or breeding territories, address the proximate mechanism controlling immediate dispersal, while a trade-off decision portrays the effects of constraints from a lifetime perspective. It should then be kept in mind that an adaptive value of delayed dispersal does not exclude simultaneous selection for an early start of breeding, even though overall lifetime reproductive output in absolute terms may very well be limited by constraints on access to resources early in life. Immediate dispersal and an early reproductive debut can indeed confer higher reproductive output over the lifetime, given the availability of adequate resources (Eikenaar *et al.* 2008). Fitness is a relative measure, based on how the reproductive success from different options compare. Individuals make choices under all kinds of constraints (Kokko & Ekman 2002, Kokko 2007), and the adaptive value of delayed dispersal depends on how behaviour translates constraints into reproductive success.

Several models have elaborated on mechanisms by which natal dispersal could be an adaptive response. These models differ in time perspective. One set of models focuses on the period of family coherence, including mechanisms such as *safe haven*, in which the natal territory functions as a safe place where young have a higher chance of surviving (Brown 1987, Ekman & Rosander 1992, Kokko & Ekman 2002), and *group augmentation*, in which natal philopatry leads to an increase in overall group size which, because larger groups are better at competing with other groups or deterring predators, increases the survival of all group members, including those that delay dispersal (Wiley & Rabenold 1984, Green & Cockburn 2001, Kokko *et al.* 2001, Griesser *et al.* 2006). Another approach focuses on the benefits the offspring can gain from delaying dispersal from acquiring better territories as independent breeders after having left the family (Stacey & Ligon 1987, 1991, Kokko & Lundberg 2001).

A number of field studies have correlated postponement of dispersal to environmental conditions (Koford *et al.* 1986, Emlen 1991). Cogent support for a causal role of ecological constraints in delay of the reproductive debut was found in several studies. For example, removal of a breeder from a territory resulted in philopatric offspring of the same sex rapidly moving in from other groups to fill the breeding opportunity in the acorn woodpecker *Melanerpes formicivorus* (Hannon *et al.* 1985), the red-cockaded woodpecker *Picoides borealis* (Walters *et al.* 1992), the superb fairy-wren (Pruett-Jones & Lewis 1990, Ligon *et al.* 1991) and the Seychelles warbler (Komdeur 1992). Dispersal not only requires a territory of a suitable quality, which could include resources such as access to partners, but more generally dispersal also requires other resources such as access to food.

Evidence for a role of food in the offspring decision to postpone independence comes from experimental manipulations of food levels, which have been shown to induce both dispersal and natal philopatry. In a unique experiment the natural food resources were depleted in family territories of the western bluebird (Fig. 12.1; Dickinson & McGowan 2005). In winter, the bluebird is dependent mainly on berries of the oak mistletoe *Phoradendron villosum* for food. Dickinson and McGowan removed half of the mistletoe by volume, and in response sons (the philopatric sex) left the depleted territory. Likewise offspring in a Spanish population of the carrion crow *Corvus corone* that were given additional food (dog food) in their birth territory were more likely to delay dispersal (Baglione *et al.* 2006). These experiments show that offspring are more likely to stay when territories are of higher quality in terms of food levels.

Evolutionary transitions during the expansion of passerines over the northern hemisphere during the latter half of the Tertiary (Neogene period, starting around 35 MYA) likewise suggest that energy shortage and food competition could limit the possibilities for family living, and strong seasonality may actually be a factor shaping large-scale global patterns. The oscine passerines stem from the southern hemisphere supercontinent Gondwanaland. The Corvida (corvids, shrikes and allies) branch is of Australopapuan origin (Ericson *et al.* 2002) while according to the most recent analyses the Passerida (finches, sparrows, tits and allies) clade arrived into the northern hemisphere through Africa (Fuchs *et al.* 2006). Family living seems to have been the ancestral trait in both these branches (Holmes *et al.* 2002, Cockburn 2003). Family groups among the oscine passerines are still found primarily in tropical and subtropical areas in the southern hemisphere, mainly in Australia and Africa (Russell 1989, Cockburn 2003, Ligon & Burt 2004), while the behaviour is rare in the northern hemisphere. With a Gondwanan origin and with family living being ancestral, the most parsimonious explanation for the absence of family living among the oscine passerines in the northern hemisphere is a loss of the ancestral behaviour. One possible reason for this loss could be selection driven

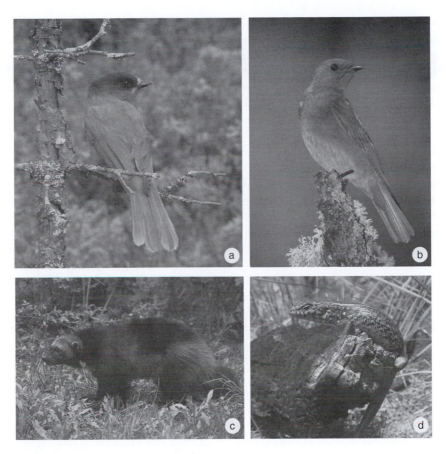

Figure 12.1 Four species with delayed dispersal of offspring that do not breed independently and do not provide allopa-rental care. (a) Siberian jay *Perisoreus infaustus* (photo: Jan Ekman); (b) Western bluebird *Sialia mexicana* (photo: Peter LaTourrette); (c) Wolverine *Gulo gulo* (photo: Dave Watts); (d) Squamate reptile *Egernia* sp. (photo: Geoff White).

by within-family competition for energy following the exposure to low temperatures, few hours of daylight and non-renewing food resources. These are all factors that would put a strain on the energy budget (Ekman & Ericson 2006).

Comparative analyses (Chapter 5) are consistent with experimental results on the role of food for family living, and indicate that local food competition may have shaped regional and continental patterns in family living. Such comparisons represent a different level of analysis, and are able to address the origin of traits, in contrast to their current utility, which is all that an analysis based on fitness estimates can examine (see Paul Sherman's profile). Family living among

passerines in Africa and Australia is more common in open and more productive bush land, whereas it is rare under desert-like conditions with lower food levels (Ford *et al.* 1988, Duplessis *et al.* 1995). The absence of family living in desert areas not only shows that natal philopatry is sensitive to food resource levels, but it also suggests that family living may no longer be permissive when resource levels become low. A phylogenetically controlled study of the acrocephaline warblers, using information on the evolutionary relationships of organisms to compare the warbler species, has indicated a similar role of food levels (Leisler *et al.* 2002). Given that resources are rare and thinly distributed, there may be no possibility for natal philopatry or family living. Just as related-ness can confer inclusive fitness gains from cooperation, promoting family living, relatedness can turn local competition into a disruptive force driving the offspring to leave and resulting in family dissolution. Competition should not be imposed on relatives under severe conditions, for the same inclusive-fitness reasons that drive cooperation among relatives.

There is also substantial support for the view that the delay in dispersal is a trade-off decision under individual control. Natal dispersal can be postponed despite the seeming availability of suitable habitat (Komdeur et al. 1995, Macedo & Bianchi 1997). Likewise, dispersal is not always delayed in crowded populations (Baglione et al. 2006, Doerr & Doerr 2006). Such observations are at odds with a notion that the offspring should disperse as soon as constraints are lifted. One way of strengthening such assessments is to see to what extent they coincide with the preferences as seen through the offspring's eyes. Such supporting evidence has in some cases been obtained by studying offspring preferences for dispersal and settlement (Komdeur 1992, Ekman et al. 2001a). For instance, in the Seychelles warbler the benefits, in terms of future breeding success and survival, of remaining on high-quality territories as non-breeders outweigh the benefits of independent breeding on lower-quality territories. Consequently, non-breeding Seychelles warblers dispersed to take up a breeding vacancy only in territories classified as of high quality, and conversely non-breeding individuals from high-quality territories rarely dispersed to fill vacancies in territories classified as of low quality (Komdeur 1992). Another line of evidence comes from comparing the timing of dispersal among siblings, which reveals that delaying dispersal can be the preferred option. Priority access to resources does not necessarily translate into early dispersal, and dominant brood or litter mates sometimes postpone dispersal and leave later than their subordinate siblings (Black & Owen 1987, Ekman et al. 2002, Pasinelli & Walters 2002, Dahle & Swenson 2003). The lesson from this dominance-related behaviour is that the implications of constraints go beyond environmental conditions, and that they also depend on individual

properties. Thus identification of a constraint is insufficient to explain variation in natal philopatry. These studies indicate that natal dispersal is a trade-off decision under individual control.

Comparisons of lifetime reproductive success of individuals delaying dispersal with that of individuals that do not delay dispersal provides the strongest evidence for an adaptive delayed dispersal, supporting Emlen's (1982) assumption of compensating benefits later in life arising from postponement of dispersal. An understanding of the role of ecological constraints for natal philopatry has been severely hampered, however, by the fact that the consequences of behaviour have rarely been assessed over a lifetime (Komdeur & Richardson 2007). This is because in most studies individual survival and reproductive estimates, and thus calculations of total lifetime reproductive success, are confounded by dispersal outside the study population and the complex patterns of shared parentage of broods and extra-pair parentage. However, those studies capable of addressing fitness values through the relative difference in lifetime reproductive success rather than the proximate control of immediate dispersal show that the prospects from delaying dispersal may indeed not be bleak at all, which is in line with Emlen's (1982) assumption. The offspring can actually do better over a lifetime by delaying dispersal (Ekman et al. 1999, Robbins & Robbins 2005, Hawn et al. 2007).

12.5 Role of design and life history

The behavioural responses and reproductive data over an entire lifetime show that environmental constraints are but one component shaping natal dispersal. Not only is access to resources a function of their abundance, but there can also be social constraints on the acquisition of resources. Likewise, the options for trade-offs over a lifetime will depend on the individual's life history (Kokko & Lundberg 2001, Hardling & Kokko 2003, Covas & Griesser 2007). The central idea underlying the role of environmental constraints (and the buffer effect) for family living is that the offspring should only disperse when there is a suitable vacancy. Yet what is suitable is meaningful only from a lifetime-fitness perspective. Short-lived species have little leeway to forgo any vacancy. Their lifetime reproduction is metered out over only a few reproductive events, and selection against philopatry will be high. It is in line with life-history theory that long-lived species have more scope to trade in a delay in reproductive debut for later gains (Goodman 1974, Schaffer 1974).

Delayed dispersal can be a strategy to wait for a breeding vacancy of better quality (Komdeur 1992, Ekman et al. 2001a), to enhance the probability that an individual ascends to the dominant breeding position (e.g. Emlen 1982, MacDonald & Moehlman 1982, Brown 1987, Stacey & Koenig 1990, Solomon & French 1997), or to allow individuals to gain resources through 'budding off' of a portion of the territory (Woolfenden & Fitzpatrick 1984, Komdeur & Edelaar 2001). An adaptive delayed dispersal should represent a trade-off where there is some waiting period after which further gains in quality of the vacancy from

further delay do not justify the cost in lost breeding opportunities. Yet the possibility of such gains will have to be within the limits of life history. Habitat properties that are crucial to survival and reproduction have been identified in two long-lived species with delayed dispersal, the Eurasian oystercatcher *Haematopus ostralegus* (Ens et al. 1992) and the Siberian jay *Perisoreus infaustus* (Box 12.1; Ekman et al. 2001a). Offspring that postpone their reproductive debut for longer also obtain better territories in both species. Such possibilities for a long-term lifetime trade-off have largely been overlooked in studies of family-living species in which the main interest has been on the inclusive fitness consequences of cooperation during breeding (Brown 1987). While such data may explain the existence of alloparental care, they have less to say about family living in the first place as an arena allowing the expression of alloparental care (Emlen 1982, 1997, Ekman 2006).

Box 12.1 The adaptive significance of delayed dispersal in the Siberian jay

The Siberian jay (Fig. 12.1) inhabits northern-hemisphere boreal taiga forest. Breeding success is poor due to high predation, mainly by other corvids that hunt using visual cues (Eggers et al. 2005a). Thus dense forest forms prime breeding habitat with higher reproductive success (Griesser et al. 2007). The Siberian jay lives in small territorial family groups of up to around half a dozen members formed around a breeding pair (Ekman et al. 1994). About one offspring in three delays independence, and may stay with its family for up to three years. Behaviourally dominant offspring initially choose to forgo dispersal to take up territories in vacant habitat with open forest where breeding success is low, whereas their dispersing siblings settle as immigrants in groups of unrelated birds (Ekman et al. 2001a). Dominant offspring disperse later than their siblings, which they evict (Ekman et al. 2002). Once the dominant offspring become breeders they obtain better territories, and they enjoy higher lifetime reproductive success, than their subordinate siblings (Ekman et al. 1999). While in company with their parents, retained offspring further enjoy survival benefits from a preferential (nepotistic) treatment (Griesser et al. 2006) where parents provide protection against predators and tolerance in sharing of food (Ekman et al. 1994), while these benefits are withheld from immigrants joining family groups. Unlike in most species where the offspring postpone dispersal, Siberian jays do not gain any indirect fitness or take part in the care of younger siblings hatched from subsequent broods (Ekman et al. 1994). Given the high risk of nest predation, activity around the nest is one of the main threats to reproductive success, and retained offspring are actively prevented from approaching the nest (Eggers et al. 2005b, 2006, Ekman et al. 1994).

Although trade-offs are a general principle in the evolution of life-history traits, they have rarely been invoked as explanations for the timing of natal dispersal (Brown 1987). Yet the potential for reproduction/survival trade-offs over a lifetime should be substantial among long-lived species living in family groups. Several mechanisms could provide an opportunity to sacrifice reproduction early in life, allowing it to be traded in for a higher lifetime reproductive success. The costs involved in such a trade-off may explain why philopatric green woodhoopoe *Phoeniculus purpureus* females enjoy a long breeding career and high lifetime reproductive success by remaining non-breeding on the birth site for 2–3 years, whereas dispersal does not seem to bear on territory quality (Hawn *et al.* 2007). We may expect selection promoting a delay in the debut when reproduction at an early age is counteracted by an excessive penalty in high mortality risk.

Despite the possibility that adaptive adjustment in timing of dispersal should be open primarily to long-lived species, this relationship remains an open question. Phylogenetically controlled comparisons have sometimes identified long lifespan as a unifying trait for family living (Arnold & Owens 1998). Yet results are conflicting, which may reflect different approaches to biases in datasets of uneven quality, rather than any absence of a role for life history (Cockburn 2003). One problem with this comparison is that it is based on a grouping differing in more than one respect. The difference could therefore be an effect of migratory habits rather than life history. The material currently available is biased, with philopatry represented mainly by species from tropical and subtropical environments in the southern hemisphere, and lack of philopatry mainly by migratory species from temperate and boreal environments in the northern hemisphere. Hence sociality is compounded by migratory habits. Further, the role of longevity has so far been explained from a population build-up and habitat saturation, which leaves out the effects of adaptive life-history trade-offs (Arnold & Owens 1998). The potential of explaining variation in dispersal between species in terms of trade-offs associated with life-history traits remains to be explored (Covas & Griesser 2007).

12.6 Staying at home: adaptive variation in length of parental behaviour

Parents need to provision their dependent offspring. Yet there is no time limit on how long they should continue to provide care, although the offspring's needs change as they mature. Even if inexperienced offspring may no longer need provisioning after becoming nutritionally independent, they could still benefit from other forms of parental behaviour that could boost survival prospects, such as providing predator alerts or protection against conspecific aggression. Adaptive gains from such parental behaviours depend on offspring demand and parental capacity to provide care, and parents should provide these forms of protection as long as there is a payoff (Chapter 11). Thus the duration of parental investments is not fixed in time, and plasticity in the duration of parental behaviour should be treated as an adaptive response. Furthermore, this variation should affect the value to offspring from remaining in the family group, and the incentive to delay dispersal could thus be a response to adaptive variation in parental behaviour.

Kin selection theory states that individuals are only expected to behave altruistically if the fitness benefits they gain via their relatives are greater than the costs of such behaviour (Chapter 5; Hamilton 1964a, 1964b, Maynard Smith 1964). Kin cooperation will be favoured by selection only if $rb - c > 0$, where r is the genetic relatedness between the helper and the offspring helped, b is the fitness benefit to the offspring helped, and c is the fitness cost of helping (Hamilton 1964a, 1964b). Hamilton's rule therefore predicts higher payoff of cooperation when the benefits (b) or relatedness (r) are higher, and lower levels when the costs (c) are high. However, the case for kin selection is not as strong as was once considered, especially for vertebrates (Cockburn 1998, Clutton-Brock 2002). This, together with a change of emphasis towards ecological constraints, has resulted in a trend shifting the focus in studies of family living (and communal breeding) away from relatedness (r) and towards the effects of costs (c) and benefits (b). This shift overlooks the fact that cooperation in family flocks is not confined to the provision of care by mature offspring to younger siblings (alloparental care). Mature offspring may themselves be the beneficiaries of parental behaviour. There could be selection for parental investments in offspring beyond their nutritional independence, provided Hamilton's rule is fulfilled while the offspring are an evolutionary asset to their parents. The prolonged parental care may be pivotal in explaining why non-breeding offspring choose to wait in their birth site until they can disperse and become breeders elsewhere (Ekman *et al.* 2001b). Offspring that cannot acquire a territory or other resources to allow independent breeding face the choice of where to spend the waiting time until their reproductive debut. Remaining non-breeding paves the way for family living is one, but not their only, option. Offspring in many species disperse without becoming breeders, to remain floaters or to settle as immigrants together with unrelated group members (Brown 1969, Newton 1998). In species where the offspring delay dispersal but do not cooperate in breeding, the birth site must offer something the offspring cannot gain elsewhere, and parental investments in mature offspring could provide this unique benefit. Brown and Brown (1984) attributed the involvement of parents in the dispersal decision of their offspring, which they called *parental facilitation*, to a role in enhancing survival and the prospects of obtaining reproductive status. There are few data that can be used to evaluate the effects of parental facilitation, while any consideration of fitness effects due to family living has so far been largely confined to studying the effects of alloparental care. The emphasis on cooperative breeding is evident from the fact that Cockburn (1998) and Hatchwell (1999) could find enough data to review the fitness effects of alloparental care, whereas there is as yet not enough field data to review whether the higher survival of philopatric Siberian jays (Griesser *et al.* 2006) is a general phenomenon.

Although philopatric offspring as a rule seem to gain inclusive fitness by assisting in providing care to siblings in subsequent broods, their first challenge is generally to survive a non-breeding season in the family group. Most species where the offspring postpone dispersal are single-brooded (Brown 1978b). It is only in a few multi-brooded species where the offspring

have an opportunity to gain fitness by providing care to younger siblings in the same breeding season they were born. To what extent can the parents' behaviour enhance first-year survival of the offspring and be an incentive to delay dispersal? Conflicts over resources in social groups often take the form of contests, and parental tolerance could then hold a key role in giving their offspring access to resources, thus providing an incentive to remain on the birth site. A number of studies of parental behaviour in family groups have been able to document that parents are more tolerant towards offspring than towards non-kin group members (Scott 1980, Barkan *et al.* 1986, Black & Owen 1989, Ekman *et al.* 1994, Pravosudova & Grubb 2000, Dickinson & McGowan 2005). Dominants that are unrelated to the group are more likely to evict young. This is most obvious when territories get taken over by new dominants, as for example in African lions *Panthera leo* (Pusey & Packer 1987) and white-faced capuchins *Cebus capucinus* (Jack & Fedigan 2004a, 2004b), where takeovers result in the immediate killing or eviction of unrelated young.

This is not to say that parent–offspring relations are without conflict, or that related dominant individuals are always tolerant. For example, in the superb fairywren any female offspring still in the natal territory at the start of the next breeding season are forced by the mother to disperse (Mulder 1995). Overall it is clear that in cooperative breeding systems those individuals that remain on natal territories may only be able to do so because the dominant group members allow them to. Yet data on parental tolerance and its implications for family living are still limited in comparison to the effort devoted to communal breeding. The reasons for this paucity of data could be that such tolerance is taken for granted as a part of parental care, and is therefore overlooked in the field.

12.7 Fitness implications of parental tolerance

One implication of parental tolerance is reduced foraging interference. Relaxed social interference carries over in several effects. Parental tolerance implies that the offspring are less likely to have their feeding interrupted, which lifts or at least mitigates a time constraint on offspring feeding. Facing less interference, the offspring are freer to allocate time to predator protection without compromising their food intake. Group members that do not enjoy a similar tolerance risk being displaced at any time, and give priority to feeding at the expense of vigilance (Griesser 2003). The role of parental tolerance in reducing interference at foraging would be valuable if access to food is critical for the decision to sit out the waiting time to become breeder at the natal site. Indeed, such a critical role of food in the offspring's decision to leave or stay is exactly what was shown independently by the manipulation of food, as described above for the western bluebird (Dickinson & McGowan 2005) and the carrion crow (Baglione et al. 2006).

Anti-predator behaviour has rarely been invoked as a reason for offspring delaying independence and staying in a family group. Reduced foraging interference relieves offspring of time constraints during feeding and allows them to invest in predator defence, but the involvement of parents and other relatives in predator protection can be more direct, alerting the offspring to presence and attacks from predators. A variety of anti-predator behaviours, including alarm calling (Griesser & Ekman 2004), vigilance (Rasa 1986, 1989, Griesser 2003) and mobbing and sentinels (Rasa 1979, Horrocks & Hunte 1986, McGowan & Woolfenden 1989, Clutton-Brock et al. 1999, Wright et al. 2001a, 2001b), have been associated with living in family groups. The look-out behaviour of sentinels in social mammals and birds has been described as cooperative behaviour (Clutton-Brock et al. 1999, Wright et al. 2001b), but it is not obvious if predator responses such as alarm calling (Sherman 1985) or mobbing (Ostreiher 2003) always have a function of warning or protecting relatives even in family units. The existence of the anti-predator behaviour is in itself not a sufficient incentive for delaying dispersal. The anti-predator behaviour should also specifically benefit relatives. Otherwise the offspring could gain benefits elsewhere, and the parental behaviour would be no incentive to stay. Relatives are the main beneficiaries of behaviours alerting to the presence of predators when family groups are composed exclusively or largely of family members. However, the relevance of anti-predator behaviour to family living becomes obvious from observations showing that it is specifically directed towards alerting relatives. Relatedness made the difference to behaviours such as alarm calling and predator mobbing in the Siberian jay (Griesser & Ekman 2004, 2005), since parents give alarm calls primarily when in company with a related offspring. The value of such parental investments in offspring survival becomes obvious when the extent of predation risk is considered. By attaching radio transmitters it was possible to retrieve first-year birds that disappeared in winter, and they had all been killed by predators, primarily hawks (Griesser et al. 2006).

A preferential treatment of offspring by parents would provide little incentive to delay dispersal unless it entails survival benefits. And indeed, first-year Siberian jays survive better due to lower predation risk in the role of retained offspring than if they disperse in their first summer of life to settle with unrelated group members (Griesser et al. 2006). Given that predators pose such a threat to survival, the parental behaviour of providing protection should be a strong incentive to wait in the natal territory for a breeding vacancy. On the other hand, if the parents disappear there would be little reason for the offspring to remain at their birth site – and indeed, this is what happens. In several species retained offspring do disperse when their parents disappear or are removed (Balcombe 1989, Ekman & Griesser 2002, Eikenaar et al. 2007), which strongly supports Brown and Brown's (1984) suggestion that parental facilitation can be pivotal to delayed dispersal. Once the parents are gone the benefits of waiting at the birth site will have vanished, and the offspring would be equally well off in the company of unrelated individuals elsewhere. This would hold in particular in the event of losing one parent, as incest taboos would generally prevent ascending to reproductive status by mating with the remaining parent. When a dominant individual dies or disappears, group young of the same sex may attempt to occupy the vacant breeding position. If the parent of the opposite sex is still alive and dominant, this pattern of inheritance would result in incestuous mating. To avoid this, young should be selective when it comes to territory inheritance. In the Florida scrub-jay *Aphelocoma coerulescens*, territory inheritance occurs more often when the surviving breeder is a step-parent of the potential heir rather than its natural parent (Woolfenden & Fitzpatrick 1986, Balcombe 1989). Similarly, males of *Antechinus agilis*, a small dimorphic carnivorous marsupial, are more likely to remain philopatric if the mother is removed at the time of weaning (Cockburn *et al.* 1985). In the acorn woodpecker (Koenig *et al.* 1998), the red-cockaded woodpecker (Daniels & Walters 2000) and the superb fairy-wren (Cockburn *et al.* 2003), dominants have even been observed to give up their breeder positions when all the opposite-sex members of the group are closely related to them. These results show that incest avoidance can lead to individuals giving up breeding opportunities and, therefore, to increased dispersal. An alternative way that females can avoid incestuous matings with related group members is through extra-group paternity with unrelated males from outside the territory. Once the parents are gone the kin benefits of allowing young to remain are reduced, or absent, for dominant individuals less related to the young, whereas the costs of group living remain. Consequently, dominants that are unrelated to the group young are more likely to evict young (as discussed above).

12.8 Long-term benefits of philopatry

The life of offspring in species with family living goes through two phases. First they spend a period as family members on their birth site, and then they either inherit the birth site or, as seems more common, spend the rest of their lives as independent breeders after having dispersed. The fitness consequences of family living have been linked to cooperation within the family group, but the fitness consequences for the period after dispersal may be an important consequence of delaying dispersal, and even its main fitness benefit. The time spent as an independent breeder can be a large portion of the lifetime, with the consequence that lifespan or length of reproductive career becomes the most important determinant of lifetime reproductive success (Fitzpatrick *et al.* 1989, Rowley & Russell 1989, Ekman *et al.* 1999, Hawn *et al.* 2007).

Given the focus on within-group dynamics among social animals, there is as yet little information on how life as an independent breeder depends on the timing of dispersal. In the green woodhoopoe, females but not males fare better if they delay dispersal. This difference among females is linked to a higher mortality of females that started to reproduce early. The difference between the sexes could reflect a survival (or fecundity) trade-off where starting to breed early carries excessive mortality costs (Hawn *et al.* 2007). Habitat quality seems to be the key factor to long-term benefits of delayed dispersal in the Siberian jay (Ekman *et al.* 2001a) and the oystercatcher (Ens *et al.* 1992). Breeders seem to obtain better-quality territories when they delay dispersal in these species. Furthermore, living and cooperating in groups will affect how a species interacts with other species. Cooperating animals may benefit in that they have an advantage of numbers in intraspecific resource competition. They may also be better able to defend themselves or their young from predators (e.g. Griesser & Ekman 2004, 2005), or they may themselves be better at preying on other species (e.g. Nudds 1978, Safi & Kerth 2007). Nest predation is high among Siberian jays, and philopatric offspring settled in territories with better protection. Nest predation can be so extensive that annual variation in breeding numbers is not buffered by non-breeding survival, with the change in breeding numbers to the ensuing year showing a negative correlation with the extent of nest predation in the previous year (Eggers *et al.* 2005a, 2005b). The selection from nest predation seems so strong that parents adjust nest sites and reproductive investments to the perceived risk of predation (Eggers *et al.* 2006).

Delayed dispersal and sociality may affect interactions with other species, but it is also important to realise that these behaviours may be the consequence of such interactions. For example, individuals may initially delay dispersal and form groups to avoid predation, either because of safety in numbers or because they group around an 'umbrella' species that helps protect them from predators (Chapter 9). Therefore, understanding how delayed dispersal and sociality

Table 12.2. Social systems with delayed offspring dispersal

System	Examples	Reference
Dispersal delayed beyond 1st breeding		
Territorial		
With alloparental care	Most cooperative breeders	Brown 1987
Without alloparental care	See Table 12.1	
Colonial	White-fronted bee-eater *Merops bullockoides*	Emlen & Wrege 1988
Lekking [a]	Black grouse *Tetrao tetrix*	Hoglund *et al.* 1999
Brood merging (brood parasitism)	White-bearded manakin *Manacus manacus*	Shorey *et al.* 2000
	Goldeneye *Bucephala clangula*	Andersson & Ahlund 2000
	Eider *Somateria mollissima*	Andersson & Waldeck 2007
Dispersal delayed into 1st non-breeding (winter) season		
Territorial	Varied tit *Sittiparus varius*	Harrap & Quinn 1995
Migratory	Geese *Anser* sp.	Weiss & Kotrschal 2004
	Swans *Cygnus* sp.	Scott 1980
	Common crane *Grus grus*	Alonso *et al.* 2004
Non-territorial		
Alloparenting	Partridge *Perdix perdix*	Dahlgren 1990

[a] Lekking: a gathering of males for the purposes of competitive mating display to attract females.

affects both intraspecific and interspecific interactions is an extremely complicated concept, one that has been the focus of relatively little research.

12.9 Conclusions and future directions

Association in family groups arises as the offspring delay dispersal, and in doing so they are often assumed to incur an evolutionary cost in lost personal reproduction. This applies to cooperatively breeding species with only one breeding pair in the group (singular breeders), which appears to be the predominant mating pattern among cooperatively breeding families (Brown 1987, Emlen 1995). Selection for associating in families has been studied extensively for philopatric offspring participating in brood rearing (alloparenting: Brown 1987, Stacey & Koenig 1990, Koenig & Dickinson 2004), and the current evidence indicates that alloparental care is a selective trait offering inclusive fitness gains (Brown *et al.* 1982, Mumme 1992, Griffin & West 2003). However, there are many species in which young delay dispersal and live in groups but do not provide alloparental care (Ekman 2006).

Family groups are found within a wide variety of different social systems, and only in a few of these are they associated with alloparental care in the conventional sense (Table 12.2). By focusing on species with delayed dispersal and group living rather than alloparental care, the circle widens to find a general explanation for the evolution of delayed dispersal.

There are likely to be two main evolutionary paths selecting for delayed dispersal and family living. On the one hand, alloparental care could be the immediate factor selecting for family cohesion, and such fitness effects may be especially relevant to the maintenance of family living as historic legacy. On the other hand, the benefits accruing from philopatry and delayed dispersal may come either from the direct fitness gained through enhanced survival in family groups (e.g. better predator defence or food access), and/or from enhanced future personal reproduction. Survival benefits from cooperation among group-living kin are likely to be a better candidate for a fitness component selecting for family cohesion than the inclusive fitness gains from alloparental care. In that case, parental tolerance of retained offspring coupled with territoriality is likely to be a cornerstone of family cohesion in territorial species by providing the offspring benefits (e.g. safe haven) until they disperse. It provides an answer to the critical question of why home is the best place to wait for a breeding vacancy. Such survival benefits, arising from the immediate utility of family living, could indeed be relevant to its maintenance. Given that behaviour is plastic, the offspring may otherwise respond and leave because of the short-term costs of delayed dispersal, regardless of any future benefits of alloparental care.

The potential for group-living effects to select for delayed dispersal is evident from the variety of family groups that exist in the absence of cooperative breeding, although studies of vertebrate families have focused so far on quantifying the brood-rearing effect of extra individuals (Brown 1987, Emlen 1995, Hatchwell 1999). Group effects of relevance for survival, and in particular during the non-breeding season, such as predator protection, have attracted less attention, but they may nonetheless have a direct bearing on family living. Turning our attention to the latter group-living effects among family groups, and examining both cooperatively and non-cooperatively breeding species, will help us to gain an understanding of the variation in the length of time that offspring stay, and of the observed variations in sociality among many vertebrate species. A comprehensive approach to family cohesion should be the focus of future research. This can be achieved by incorporating the short- and long-term fitness consequences of delayed dispersal of offspring for both the offspring and their parents, and it is important to include species where the offspring do not provide parental care. The results of such research should reveal how natal philopatry may have evolved, and how it is maintained, in the absence of cooperative breeding.

Acknowledgements

We thank Michael Magrath and four anonymous reviewers for providing valuable comments on this review. Funding was provided by the Netherlands Organisation for Scientific Research (NWO – VICI) to JK (Grant 865–03–003) and by the Swedish Research Council (VR) to JE (Grant 621–2005–4493).

Suggested readings

Cezilly, F. ed. (2007) Cooperative breeding. *Behavioural Processes*, **76**, 61–182.

Ekman, J. (2006) Family living among birds. *Journal of Avian Biology*, **37**, 289–298.

Koenig, W. D. & Dickinson, J. L., eds. (2004) *Ecology and Evolution of Cooperative Breeding in Birds*. Cambridge: Cambridge University Press.

MacDonald, D. W. & Moehlman, P. D. (1982) Cooperation, altruism, and restraint in the reproduction of carnivores. In: *Perspectives in Ethology*, ed. P. P. G. Bateson & P. Klopfer. New York, NY: Plenum, pp. 433–467.

West, S. A., Griffin A. S. & Gardner, A. (2007) Evolutionary explanations for cooperation. *Current Biology*, **17**, 661–672.

References

Alonso, J. C., Bautista, L. M. & Alonso, J. A. (2004) Family-based territoriality vs flocking in wintering common cranes *Grus grus*. *Journal of Avian Biology*, **35**, 434–444.

Ancel, A., Visser, H., Handrich, Y., Masman, D. & Le Maho, Y. (1997) Energy saving in huddling penguins. *Nature*, **385**, 304–305.

Andersson, M. & Ahlund, M. (2000) Host–parasite relatedness shown by protein fingerprinting in a brood parasitic bird. *Proceedings of the National Academy of Sciences of the USA*, **97**, 13188–13193.

Andersson, M. & Waldeck, P. (2007) Host–parasite kinship in a female-philopatric bird population: evidence from relatedness trend analysis. *Molecular Ecology*, **16**, 2797–2806.

Arnold, K. E. & Owens I. P. F. (1998) Cooperative breeding in birds: a comparative test of the life history hypothesis. *Proceedings of the Royal Society B*, **265**, 739–745.

Arnold, K. E. & Owens, I. P. F. (1999) Cooperative breeding in birds: the role of ecology. *Behavioral Ecology*, **10**, 465–471.

Baglione, V., Marcos, J. M., Canestrari, D. *et al.* (2005) Does year-round territoriality rather than habitat saturation explain delayed natal dispersal and cooperative breeding in the carrion crow? *Journal of Animal Ecology*, **74**, 842–851.

Baglione, V., Canestrari, D, Marcos, J. M. & Ekman, J. (2006) Experimentally increased food resources in the natal territory promote offspring philopatry and helping in cooperatively breeding carrion crows. *Proceedings of the Royal Society B*, **273**, 1529–1535.

Balcombe, J. P. (1989) Non-breeder asymmetry in Florida scrub jays. *Evolutionary Ecology*, **3**, 77–79.

Barkan, C. P. L., Craig, J. L., Strahl, S. D., Stewart, A. M. & Brown, J. L. (1986) Social-dominance in communal Mexican jays *Aphelocoma ultramarina*. *Animal Behaviour*, **34**, 175–187.

Birkhead, T. R. (1991) *The Magpie: the Ecology and Behaviour of Black-billed and Yellow-billed Magpies*. London: Poyser.

Black, J. M. & Owen, M. (1987) Determinants of social rank in goose flocks: acquisition of social rank in young geese. *Behaviour*, **102**, 129–146.

Black, J. M. & Owen, M. (1989) Parent offspring relationships in wintering barnacle geese. *Animal Behaviour*, **37**, 187–198.

Brown, J. L. (1963) Aggressiveness, dominance, and social organization in the Steller's jay. *Condor*, **65**, 460–484.

Brown, J. L. (1969) Territorial behaviour and population regulation in birds, a review and re-evaluation. *Wilson Bulletin*, **81**, 293–329.

Brown, J. L. (1978a) Avian heirs of territory. *Bioscience*, **28**, 750–752.

Brown, J. L. (1978b) Avian communal breeding systems. *Annual Review of Ecology and Systematics*, **9**, 123–155.

Brown, J. L. (1987) *Helping and Communal Breeding in Birds: Ecology and Evolution*. Princeton, NJ: Princeton University Press.

Brown, J. L. & Brown, E. R. (1984) Parental facilitation: parent–offspring relations in communally breeding birds. *Behavioral Ecology and Sociobiology*, **14**, 203–209.

Brown, J. L., Brown, E. R., Brown, S. D. & Dow, D. D. (1982) Helpers: effects of experimental removal on reproductive success. *Science*, **110**, 207–214.

Burt, D. B. & Peterson, A. T. (1993) Biology of cooperatively breeding scrub jays (*Aphelocoma coerulescens*) of Oaxaca, Mexico. *Auk*, **1010**, 207–214.

Carmen, W. J. (2004) Behavioural ecology of the California scrubjay (*Aphelocoma californica*): a non-cooperative breeder with close cooperative relatives. *Studies in Avian Biology*, 28.

Cezilly, F., ed. (2007) Cooperative breeding. *Behavioural Processes*, **76**, 61–182.

Chapple, D. G. (2003) Ecology, life-history, and behavior in the Australian Scincid genus *Egernia*, with comments on the evolution of complex sociality in lizards. *Herpetological Monographs*, **17**, 145–180.

Clutton-Brock, T. H. (1991) *The Evolution of Parental Care*. Princeton, NJ: Princeton University Press.

Clutton-Brock, T. H. (2002) Breeding together: kin selection and mutualism in cooperative vertebrates. *Science*, **296**, 69–72.

Clutton-Brock, T. H., O'Riain, M. J., Brotherton, P. N. M. *et al.* (1999) Selfish sentinels in cooperative mammals. *Science*, **284**, 1640–1644.

Cockburn, A. (1998) Evolution of helping behavior in cooperatively breeding birds. *Annual Review of Ecology and Systematics*, **29**, 141–177.

Cockburn, A. (2003) Cooperative breeding in oscine passerines: does sociality inhibit speciation? *Proceedings of the Royal Society B*, **270**, 2207–2214.

Cockburn, A. (2004) Mating systems and sexual conflict. In: *Ecology and Evolution of Cooperative Breeding in Birds*, ed. W. D. Koenig & J. L. Dickinson. Cambridge: Cambridge University Press, pp. 81–101.

Cockburn, A. (2006) Prevalence of different modes of parental care in birds. *Proceedings of the Royal Society B*, **273**, 1375–1383.

Cockburn, A., Scott, M. P. & Dickman, C. R (1985) Sex ratio and intrasexual kin competition in mammals. *Oecologia*, **66**, 427–429.

Cockburn, A., Osmond, H. L., Mulder, R. A., Green, D. J. & Double, M. C. (2003) Divorce, dispersal, density-dependence and incest avoidance in the cooperatively breeding superb fairy-wren *Malurus cyaneus*. *Journal of Animal Ecology*, **72**, 198–202.

Covas, R. & Griesser, M. (2007) Life history and the evolution of family living in birds. *Proceedings of the Royal Society B*, **274**, 1349–1357.

Dahle, B. & Swenson, J. E. (2003) Family breakup in brown bears: are young forced to leave? *Journal of Mammalogy*, **84**, 536–540.

Dahlgren, J. (1990) Females choose vigilant males: an experiment with the monogamous gray partridge, *Perdix perdix*. *Animal Behaviour*, **39**, 646–651.

Daniels, S. J. & Walters, J. R. (2000) Between-year breeding dispersal in red-cockaded woodpeckers: multiple causes and estimated cost. *Ecology*, **81**, 2473–2484.

Derix, R., Van Hooff, J., De Vries, H. & Wensing, J. (1993) Male and female mating competition in wolves: female suppression vs. male intervention. *Behaviour*, **127**, 141–174.

Dickinson, J. L. & McGowan, A. (2005) Winter resource wealth drives delayed dispersal and family-group living in western bluebirds. *Proceedings of the Royal Society B*, **272**, 2423–2428.

Dickinson, J. L., Koenig, W. D. & Pitelka, F. A. (1996) Fitness consequences of helping behaviour in the western bluebird. *Behavioral Ecology*, **7**, 168–177.

Dierkes, P., Taborsky, M. & Kohler, U. (1999) Reproductive parasitism of broodcare helpers in a cooperatively breeding fish. *Behavioral Ecology*, **10**, 510–515.

Doerr, E. D. & Doerr, V. A. J. (2006) Comparative demography of treecreepers: evaluating hypotheses for the evolution and maintenance of cooperative breeding. *Animal Behaviour*, **72**, 147–159.

Double, C. M. & Cockburn, A. (2003) Subordinate superb fairy-wrens (*Malurus cyaneus*) parasitize the reproductive success of attractive dominant males. *Proceedings of the Royal Society B*, **270**, 379–384

Dugatkin, L. A. (1997) *Cooperation Among Animals: a Modern Perspective*. Oxford: Oxford University Press.

Duplessis, M. A., Siegfried, W. R. & Armstrong, A. J. (1995) Ecological and life-history correlates of cooperative breeding in South-African birds. *Oecologia*, **102**, 180–188.

Eden, S. F. (1987) Natal philopatry of the magpie *Pica pica*. *Ibis*, **129**, 470–490.

Eggers, S., Griesser, M., Andersson, T. & Ekman, J. (2005a) Nest predation and habitat change interact to influence Siberian jay numbers. *Oikos*, **111**, 150–158.

Eggers, S., Griesser, M. & Ekman, J. (2005b) Predator-induced plasticity in nest visitation rates in the Siberian jay (*Perisoreus infaustus*). *Behavioral Ecology*, **16**, 309–315.

Eggers, S., Griesser, M., Nystrand, M. & Ekman, J. (2006) Predation risk induces changes in nest-site selection and clutch size in the Siberian jay. *Proceedings of the Royal Society B-Biological Sciences*, **273**, 701–706.

Eikenaar, C., Richardson, D. S., Brouwer, L. & Komdeur, J. (2007) Parent presence, delayed dispersal, and territory acquisition in the Seychelles warbler. *Behavioral Ecology*, **18**, 874–879.

Eikenaar, C., Komdeur, J. & Richardson, D. S. (2008) Natal dispersal patterns are not associated with inbreeding avoidance in the Seychelles warbler. *Journal of Evolutionary Biology*, **21**, 1106–1116.

Ekman, J. (2006) Family living among birds. *Journal of Avian Biology*, **37**, 289–298.

Ekman, J. & Ericson, P. G. P. (2006) Out of Gondwanaland: the evolutionary history of cooperative breeding and social behaviour among crows, magpies, jays and allies. *Proceedings of the Royal Society B*, **273**, 1117–1125.

Ekman, J. & Griesser, M. (2002) Why offspring delay dispersal: experimental evidence for a role of parental tolerance. *Proceedings of the Royal Society B*, **269**, 1709–1713.

Ekman, J. & Rosander, B. (1992) Survival enhancement through food sharing – a means for parental control of natal dispersal. *Theoretical Population Biology*, **42**, 117–129.

Ekman, J., Sklepkovych, B. & Tegelstrom, H. (1994) Offspring retention in the Siberian jay (*Perisoreus infaustus*): the prolonged brood care hypothesis. *Behavioral Ecology*, **5**, 245–253.

Ekman, J., Bylin, A. & Tegelstrom, H. (1999) Increased lifetime reproductive success for Siberian jay (*Perisoreus infaustus*) males with delayed dispersal. *Proceedings of the Royal Society B*, **266**, 911–915.

Ekman, J., Eggers, S., Griesser, M. & Tegelstrom, H. (2001a) Queuing for preferred territories: delayed dispersal of Siberian jays. *Journal of Animal Ecology*, **70**, 317–324.

Ekman, J., Baglione, V., Eggers, S. & Griesser, M. (2001b) Delayed dispersal: living under the reign of nepotistic parents. *Auk*, **118**, 1–10.

Ekman, J., Eggers, S. & Griesser, M. (2002) Fighting to stay: the role of sibling rivalry for delayed dispersal. *Animal Behaviour*, **64**, 453–459.

Ekman, J., Dickinson, J. L., Hatchwell, B. J. & Griesser, M. (2004) Roles of extended parental investment and territory quality in the evolution and maintenance of delayed dispersal. In *Ecology and Evolution of Cooperative Breeding in Birds*, ed. W. D. Koenig & J. L. Dickinson. Cambridge: Cambridge University Press, pp. 35–47.

Emlen, S. T. (1982) The evolution of helping. 1. an ecological constraints model. *American Naturalist*, **119**, 29–39.

Emlen, S. T. (1991) The evolution of cooperative breeding in birds and mammals. In: *Behavioural Ecology: an Evolutionary Approach*, 3rd edn, ed. J. R. Krebs & N. B. Davies. Oxford: Blackwell, pp. 301–337.

Emlen, S. T. (1995) An evolutionary theory of the family. *Proceedings of the National Academy of Sciences of the USA*, **92**, 8092–8099.

Emlen, S. T. (1997) Predicting family dynamics in social vertebrates. In *Behavioural Ecology: an Evolutionary Approach*, 4th edn, ed. J. R. Krebs and N. B. Davies. Oxford: Blackwell, pp. 228–253.

Emlen, S. T. & Wrege, P. H. (1988) The role of kinship in helping decisions among white-fronted bee-eaters. *Behavioral Ecology and Sociobiology*, **23**, 305–315

Ens, B. J., Kersten, M., Brenninkmeijer, A. & Hulscher, J. B. (1992) Territory quality, parental effort and reproductive success of oystercatchers (*Haematopus ostralegus*). *Journal of Animal Ecology*, **61**, 703–715.

Ericson, P. G. P., Christidis, L., Cooper, A. *et al.* (2002) A Gondwanan origin of passerine birds supported by DNA sequences of the endemic New Zealand wrens. *Proceedings of the Royal Society B*, **269**, 35–241.

Faaborg, J. (1986) Reproductive success and survivorship of the Galapagos hawk *Buteo-galapagoensis*: potential costs and benefits of cooperative polyandry. *Ibis*, **128**, 337–347.

Fitzpatrick, J. W. & Woolfenden, G. E. (1984) The helpful shall inherit the scrub. *Natural History*, **93**, 55–63.

Fitzpatrick, J. W., Woolfenden, G. E. & McGowan, K. J. (1989) Sources of variation in lifetime fitness of Florida scrub jays. In: *Proceedings of the 19th International Ornithological Congress*, ed. H. Ouellet. Ottawa: University of Ottawa Press, pp. 876–891.

Ford, H. A., Bell, H., Nias, R. & Noske, R. (1988) The relationship between ecology and the incidence of cooperative breeding in Australian birds. *Behavioral Ecology and Sociobiology*, **22**, 239–249.

Frith, C. B., Frith, D. W. & Jansen, A. (1997) The nesting biology of the chowchilla, *Orthonyx spaldingii* (Orthonychidae). *Emu*, **97**, 18–30.

Fuchs, J., Fjeldså, J., Bowie, R. C. K., Voelker, G. & Pasquet, E. (2006) The African warbler genus *Hyliota* as a lost lineage in the Oscine songbird tree: molecular support for an African origin of the Passerida. *Molecular Phylogenetics and Evolution*, **39**, 186–197.

Gardner, J. L., Magrath, R. & Kokko, H. (2003) Stepping stones of life: natal dispersal in the group-living but noncooperative speckled warbler. *Animal Behaviour*, **66**, 521–530.

Gayou, D. C. (1986) The social system of the Texas green jay. *Auk*, **103**, 540–547.

Goodman, D. (1974) Natural selection and a cost ceiling on reproductive effort. *American Naturalist*, **108**, 247–268.

Green, D. J. & Cockburn, A. (2001) Post-fledging care, philopatry and recruitment in brown thornbills. *Journal of Animal Ecology*, **70**, 505–514.

Griesser, M. (2003) Nepotistic vigilance behavior in Siberian jay parents. *Behavioral Ecology*, **14**, 246–250.

Griesser, M. & Ekman, J. (2004) Nepotistic alarm calling in the Siberian jay, *Perisoreus infaustus*. *Animal Behaviour*, **67**, 933–939.

Griesser, M. & Ekman, J. (2005) Nepotistic mobbing behaviour in the Siberian jay, *Perisoreus infaustus*. *Animal Behaviour*, **69**, 345–352.

Griesser, M., Nystrand, M. & Ekman, J. (2006) Reduced mortality selects for family cohesion in a social species. *Proceedings of the Royal Society B*, **273**, 1881–1886.

Griesser, M., Nystrand, M., Eggers, S. & Ekman, J. (2007) Impact of forestry practices on fitness correlates and population productivity in an open-nesting bird species. *Conservation Biology*, **21**, 767–774.

Griffin, A. S. & West, S. A. (2003) Kin discrimination and the benefit of helping in cooperatively breeding vertebrates. *Science*, **302**, 634–636.

Griffin, A. S., Pemberton, J. M., Brotherton, P. N. M. *et al.* (2003) A genetic analysis of breeding success in the cooperative meerkat (*Suricata suricatta*). *Behavioral Ecology*, **14**, 472–480.

Hamilton, W. D. (1964a) The genetical evolution of social behaviour. I. *Journal of Theoretical Biology*, **7**, 1–16.

Hamilton, W. D. (1964b) The genetical evolution of social behaviour. II. *Journal of Theoretical Biology*, **7**, 17–52.

Hannon, S. J., Mumme, R. L., Koenig, W. D. & Pitelka, F. A. (1985) Replacement of breeders and within-group conflict in the cooperatively breeding acorn woodpecker. *Behavioral Ecology and Sociobiology*, **17**, 303–312.

Hardling, R. & Kokko, H. (2003) Life-history traits as causes or consequences of social behaviour: why do cooperative breeders lay small clutches? *Evolutionary Ecology Research*, **5**, 691–700.

Harrap, S. & Quinn, D. (1995) *Tits, Nuthatches and Treecreepers*. Cape Town: Russel Friedman.

Hatchwell, B. J. (1999) Investment strategies of breeders in avian cooperative breeding systems. *American Naturalist*, **154**, 205–219.

Hatchwell, B. J. & Komdeur, J. (2000) Ecological constraints, life history traits and the evolution of cooperative breeding. *Animal Behaviour*, **59**, 1079–1086.

Hawn, A. T., Radford, A. N. & Du Plessis, M. A. (2007) Delayed breeding affects lifetime reproductive success differently in male and female green woodhoopoes. *Current Biology*, **17**, 844–849.

Hockey, P. A. R., Dean, W. R. J. & Tyan, P. G. (2005) *Roberts Birds of Southern Africa*. Cape Town: John Voelcker Bird Book Fund.

Hoglund, J., Alatalo, R. V., Lundberg, A., Rintamaki, P. T. & Lindell, J. (1999) Microsatellite markers reveal the potential for kin selection on black grouse leks. *Proceedings of the Royal Society B*, **266**, 813–816.

Holmes, R. T., Frauenknecht, B. D. & Du Plessis, M. A. (2002) Breeding system of the Cape rockjumper, a South African fynbos endemic. *Condor*, **104**, 188–192.

Horrocks, J. A. & Hunte, W. (1986) Sentinel behaviour in vervet monkeys: who sees whom first. *Animal Behaviour*, **34**, 1566–1567.

Houston, A. I., Székely, T. & McNamara, J. M. (2005) Conflict over parental care. *Trends in Ecology and Evolution*, **20**, 33–38.

Jack, K. M. & Fedigan, L. (2004a) Male dispersal patterns in white-faced capuchins, *Cebus capucinus*. Part 1: patterns and causes of natal emigration. *Animal Behaviour*, **67**, 761–769.

Jack, K. M. & Fedigan, L. (2004b) Male dispersal patterns in white-faced capuchins, *Cebus capucinus*. Part 2: patterns and causes of secondary dispersal. *Animal Behaviour*, **67**, 771–782

Jansen, A. (1999) Home ranges and group-territoriality in chowchillas *Orthonyx spaldingii*. *Emu*, **99**, 280–290.

Kappeler, P. M. B. (2008) Genetic and ecological determinants of primate social systems. In: *Ecology of Social Evolution*, ed. J. Korb & J. Heinze. Cambridge: Cambridge University Press, pp. 225–243.

Keller, L. F. & Waller, D. M. (2002) Inbreeding effects in wild populations. *Trends in Ecology and Evolution*, **17**, 230–241.

Khan, M. Z. & Walters, J. R. (1997) Is helping a beneficial learning experience for red-cockaded woodpecker (*Picoides borealis*) helpers? *Behavioral Ecology and Sociobiology*, **41**, 69–73.

Kluyver, H. N. & Tinbergen, L. (1953) Territory and the regulation of density in titmice. *Archives Néerlandaises de Zoologie*, **10**, 265–287.

Koenig, W. D. & Dickinson, J. L., eds. (2004) *Ecology and Evolution of Cooperative Breeding in Birds*. Cambridge: Cambridge University Press.

Koenig, W. D. & Haydock, J. (2004) Incest and incest avoidance. In: *Ecology and Evolution of Cooperative Breeding in Birds*, ed. W. D. Koenig and J. L. Dickinson. Cambridge: Cambridge University Press, pp 142–156.

Koenig, W. D., Pitelka, F. A., Carmen, W. J., Mumme, R. L. & Stanback, M. T. (1992) The evolution of delayed dispersal in cooperative breeders. *Quarterly Review of Biology*, **67**, 111–150.

Koenig, W. D., Haydock, J. & Stanback, M. T. (1998) Reproductive roles in the cooperatively breeding acorn woodpecker: incest avoidance versus reproductive competition. *American Naturalist*, **151**, 243–255.

Koford, R. R., Bowen, B. S. & Vehrencamp, S. L. (1986) Habitat saturation in groove-billed anis (*Crotophaga sulcirostris*). *American Naturalist*, **127**, 317–337.

Kokko, H. (2007) Cooperative behaviour and cooperative breeding: what constitutes an explanation? *Behavioural Processes*, **76**, 81–85.

Kokko, H. & Ekman, J. (2002) Delayed dispersal as a route to breeding: territorial inheritance, safe havens, and ecological constraints. *American Naturalist*, **160**, 468–484.

Kokko, H. & Lundberg, P. (2001) Dispersal, migration, and offspring retention in saturated habitats. *American Naturalist*, **157**, 188–202.

Kokko, H., Johnstone, R. A. & Clutton-Brock, T. H. (2001) The evolution of cooperative breeding through group augmentation. *Proceedings of the Royal Society B*, **268**, 187–196.

Komdeur, J. (1992) Importance of habitat saturation and territory quality for evolution of cooperative breeding in the Seychelles warbler. *Nature*, **358**, 493–495.

Komdeur, J. (1996) Influence of helping and breeding experience on reproductive performance in the Seychelles warbler: a translocation experiment. *Behavioral Ecology*, **7**, 326–333.

Komdeur, J. & Edelaar, P. (2001) Male Seychelles warblers use territory budding to maximize lifetime fitness in a saturated environment. *Behavioral Ecology*, **12**, 706–715.

Komdeur, J. & Richardson, D. S. (2007) Molecular ecology reveals the hidden complexities of the Seychelles warbler. *Advances in the Study of Behavior*, **37**, 147–187.

Komdeur, J., Huffstadt, A., Prast, W. *et al.* (1995) Transfer experiments of Seychelles warblers to new islands: changes in dispersal and helping behaviour. *Animal Behaviour*, **49**, 695–708.

Leisler, B., Winkler, H. & Wink, M. (2002) Evolution of breeding systems in acrocephaline warblers. *Auk*, **119**, 379–390.

Ligon, J. D. & Burt, B. D. (2004) Evolutionary origins. In: *Ecology and Evolution of Cooperative Breeding in Birds*, ed. W. D. Koenig & J. L. Dickinson. Cambridge: Cambridge University Press, pp. 5–34.

Ligon, J. D., Ligon, S. H. & Ford, H. A. (1991) An experimental study of the basis of male philopatry in the cooperatively breeding superb fairy-wren *Malurus cyaneus*. *Ethology*, **87**, 134–148.

MacDonald, D. W. & Moehlman, P. D. (1982) Cooperation, altruism, and restraint in the reproduction of carnivores. In *Perspectives in Ethology*, ed. P. P. G. Bateson and P. Klopfer, pp. 433–467. New York: Plenum.

Macedo, R. H. & Bianchi, C. A. (1997) Communal breeding in tropical Guira cuckoos *Guira guira*: sociality in the absence of a saturated habitat. *Journal of Avian Biology*, **28**, 207–215.

Maynard Smith, J. (1964) Group selection and kin selection. *Nature*, **201**, 1145–1147.

Maynard Smith, J. (1977) Parental investment: a prospective analysis. *Animal Behaviour*, **25**, 1–9.

McGowan, K. J. & Woolfenden, G. E. (1989) A sentinel system in the Florida scrub jay. *Animal Behaviour*, **37**, 1000–1006.

Mulder, R. A. (1995) Natal and breeding dispersal in a co-operative, extra-group-mating bird. *Journal of Avian Biology*, **26**, 234–240.

Mumme, R. L. (1992) Do helpers increase reproductive success? An experimental analysis in the Florida scrub jay. *Behavioral Ecology and Sociobiology*, **31**, 319–328.

Newton, I. (1998) *Population Limitation in Birds*. London: Academic Press.

Newton, I., Davies, P. E. & Moss, D. (1994) Philopatry and population growth of red kites *Milvus milvus* in ales. *Proceedings of the Royal Society B*, **257**, 313–323.

Nilsson, J. A. & Smith, H. G. (1988) Effects of dispersal date on winter flock establishment and social-dominance in marsh tits *Parus palustris. Journal of Animal Ecology,* **57**, 917–928.

Nudds, T. D. (1978) Convergence of group size strategies by mammalian predators. *American Naturalist,* **112**, 957–960.

O'Riain, M. J., Jarvis, J. U. M., Alexander, R., Buffenstein, R. & Peeters, C. (2000) Morphological castes in a vertebrate. *Proceedings of the National Academy of Sciences of the USA,* **97**, 13194–13197.

Ostreiher, R. (2003) Is mobbing altruistic or selfish behaviour? *Animal Behaviour,* **66**, 145–149.

Pasinelli, G. & Walters, J. R. (2002) Social and environmental factors affect natal dispersal and philopatry of male red-cockaded woodpeckers. *Ecology,* **83**, 2229–2239.

Perrin, N. & Lehmann, L. (2001) Is sociality driven by the costs of dispersal or the benefits of philopatry? A role for kin-discrimination mechanisms. *American Naturalist,* **158**, 471–483.

Perrin, N. & Mazalov, V. (1999) Dispersal and inbreeding avoidance. *American Naturalist,* **154**, 282–292.

Pravosudova, E. V. & Grubb, T. C. (2000) An experimental test of the prolonged brood care model in the tufted titmouse (*Baeolophus bicolor*). *Behavioral Ecology,* **11**, 309–314.

Pruett-Jones, S. G. & Lewis, M. J. (1990) Sex-ratio and habitat limitation promote delayed dispersal in superb fairy-wrens. *Nature,* **348**, 541–542.

Pusey, A. E. & Packer, C. (1987) The evolution of sex-biased dispersal in lions. *Behaviour,* **101**, 275–310.

Rasa, O. A. E. (1979) Effects of crowding on the social relationships and behavior of the dwarf mongoose (*Helogale undulata rufala*). *Zeitschrift für Tierpsychologie-Journal of Comparative Ethology,* **49**, 317–329.

Rasa, O. A. E. (1986) Coordinated vigilance in dwarf mongoose family groups: the watchmans song hypothesis and the costs of guarding. *Ethology,* **71**, 340–344.

Rasa, O. A. E. (1989) The costs and effectiveness of vigilance behavior in the dwarf mongoose: implications for fitness and optimal group-size. *Ethology, Ecology and Evolution,* **1**, 265–282.

Reyer, H. U. (1984). Investment and relatedness: a cost/benefit analysis of breeding and helping in the pied kingfisher (*Ceryle rudis*). *Animal Behaviour,* **32**, 1163–1178.

Richardson, D. S., Burke, T. & Komdeur, J. (2002) Direct benefits explain the evolution of female biased cooperative breeding in the Seychelles warblers. *Evolution,* **56**, 2313–2321.

Richardson, D. S., Komdeur, J. & Burke, T. (2003) Altruism and infidelity among warblers. *Nature,* **422**, 580.

Robbins, A. M. & Robbins, M. M. (2005) Fitness consequences of dispersal decisions for male mountain gorillas (*Gorilla beringei beringei*). *Behavioral Ecology and Sociobiology,* **58**, 295–309.

Robinson, T. R. (2000) Factors affecting dispersal by song wrens (*Cyphorhinus phaeocephalus*): ecological constraints and demography. *The Quarterly Review of Biology,* **68**, 1–31.

Rood, J. P. (1990) Group size, survival, reproduction, and routes to breeding in dwarf mongooses. *Animal Behaviour,* **39**, 566–572.

Rowley, I. & Russell, E. (1989) Lifetime reproductive success in Malurus spendens, a co-operative breeder. In: *Proceedings of the 19th International Ornithological Congress,* ed. H. Ouellet. Ottawa: University of Ottawa Press, pp. 866–875.

Russell, A. F. & Hatchwell, B. J. (2001) Experimental evidence for kin-biased helping in a cooperatively breeding vertebrate. *Proceedings of the Royal Society B,* **268**, 2169–2174.

Russell, E. M. (1989) Cooperative breeding: a Gondwanan perspective. *Emu,* **89**, 61–62.

Safi K. & Kerth, G. (2007) Comparative analyses suggest that information transfer promoted sociality in male bats. *American Naturalist,* **170**, 465–472.

Schaffer, W. M. (1974) Selection for optimal life histories: effects of age structure. *Ecology,* **55**, 291–303.

Scott, D. K. (1980) Functional aspects of prolonged parental care in Bewick's swans. *Animal Behaviour,* **28**, 938–952.

Selander, R. K. (1964) Speciation in wrens of the genus *Campylorhynchos. University of California Publications in Zoology,* **74**, 1–305.

Sherman, P. W. (1985) Alarm calls of belding ground-squirrels to aerial predators – nepotism or self-preservation. *Behavioral Ecology and Sociobiology,* **17**, 313–323.

Shorey, L., Piertney, S., Stone, J. & J. Hoglund (2000) Fine-scale genetic structuring on *Manacus manacus* leks. *Nature,* **408**, 352–353.

Smiseth, P. T. & Moore, A. J. (2004) Behavioral dynamics between caring males and females in a beetle with facultative biparental care. *Behavioral Ecology,* **15**, 621–628.

Solomon, N. G. & French, J. A., eds. (1997) *Cooperative Breeding in Mammals.* Cambridge: Cambridge University Press.

Stacey, P. B. & Koenig, W. D., eds. (1990) *Cooperative Breeding in Birds: Long-term Studies of Ecology and Behaviour.* Cambridge: Cambridge University Press.

Stacey, P. B. & Ligon, J. D. (1987) Territory quality and dispersal options in the acorn woodpecker, and a challenge to the habitat-saturation model of cooperative breeding. *American Naturalist,* **130**, 654–676.

Stacey, P. B. & Ligon, J. D. (1991) The benefits-of-philopatry hypothesis for the evolution of cooperative breeding: variation in territory quality and group-size effects. *American Naturalist*, **137**, 831–846.

Støen, O.-G., Zedrosser, A., Wegge, P. & Swenson, J. E. (2006) Socially induced delayed primiparity in brown bears *Ursus arctos*. *Behavioral Ecology and Sociobiology*, **6**, 1–8.

Strickland, D. (1991) Juvenile dispersal in gray jays: dominant brood members expel siblings from natal territory. *Canadian Journal of Zoology*, **69**, 2935–2945.

Taborsky, M. (1994) Sneakers, satellites, and helpers: parasitic and cooperative behavior in fish reproduction. *Advances in the Study of Behavior*, **23**, 1–100.

Tchabovsky, A. & Bazykin, G. (2004) Females delay dispersal and breeding in a solitary gerbil, Meriones tamariscinus. *Journal of Mammalogy*, **85**, 105–112.

Vangen, K. M., Persson, J., Landa, A., Anderson, R. & Segerstrøm, P (2001) Characteristics of dispersal in wolverines. *Canadian Journal of Zoology*, **79**, 1641–1649.

Veltman, C. J. (1989) Flock, pair and group living lifestyles without cooperative breeding by Australian magpies. *Ibis*, **131**, 601–608.

Verbeek, N. A. M. & Butler, R. W. W. (1981) Cooperative breeding of the Nortwestern crow *Corvus caurinus* in British Columbia. *Ibis*, **123**, 183–189.

Walls, S. S. & Kenward, R. E. (1996) Movements of radio-tagged buzzards *Buteo buteo* in early life. *Ibis*, **140**, 561–568.

Walters, J. R., Copeyon, C. K. & Carter, J. H. (1992) Test of the ecological basis of cooperative breeding in red-cockaded woodpeckers. *Auk*, **109**, 90–97.

Weiss, B. M. & Kotrschal, K. (2004) Effects of passive social support in juvenile greylag geese (*Anser anser*): a study from fledging to adulthood. *Ethology*, **110**, 429–444.

West, S. A., Griffin, A. S. & Gardner, A. (2007) Evolutionary explanations for cooperation. *Current Biology*, **17**, 661–672.

Westneat, D. F. & Sherman, P. W. (1993) Parentage and the evolution of parental behavior. *Behavioral Ecology*, **4**, 66–77.

Wiley, R. H. & Rabenold, K. N. (1984) The evolution of cooperative breeding by delayed reciprocity and queuing for favorable social positions. *Evolution*, **38**, 609–621.

Wilson, E. O. (1975) *Sociobiology: the New Synthesis*. Cambridge, MA: Harvard University Press.

Woolfenden, G. E. & Fitzpatrick, J. W. (1984) *The Florida Scrub Jay: Demography of a Cooperative-Breeding Bird*. Princeton, NJ: Princeton University Press.

Woolfenden, G. E. & Fitzpatrick, J. W. (1986) Sexual asymmetries in the life history of the Florida scrub jay. In: *Ecological Aspects of Social Evolution*, ed. D. Rubenstein and R. W. Wrangham. Princeton, NJ: Princeton University Press, pp. 87–107.

Wright, J., Berg, E., De Kort, S. R., Khazin, V. & Maklakov, A. A. (2001a) Cooperative sentinel behaviour in the Arabian babbler. *Animal Behaviour*, **62**, 973–979.

Wright, J., Berg, E., De Kort, S. R., Khazin, V. & Maklakov, A. A. (2001b) Safe selfish sentinels in a cooperative bird. *Journal of Animal Ecology*, **70**, 1070–1079.

Zahavi, A. (1990) Arabian babbler: the quest for social status in a cooperative breeder. In: *Cooperative Breeding in Birds*, ed. P. B. Stacey and W. D. Koenig. Cambridge: Cambridge University Press, pp. 103–130.

Selections from a life in social selection

David C. Queller

Science is about theories and tests of theories, but it is not nearly as dry or as mechanical as that may seem to imply, especially in behavioural ecology. A life in science is also about career choices made, luck, interesting experiences and even fun. Here is a selection from my own career in studying social selection.

Wisest educational choice. Grad school at the University of Michigan. They had a policy of admitting the best students they could, and giving them time to find their advisors and research programme. I found Richard Alexander, though my first real interaction with him was when he thought I might have cribbed ideas for an essay I wrote for his class. Fortunately, as a good scientist, he could change his mind.

Luckiest educational choice. Grad school at the University of Michigan. Though I knew Alexander would be there, I did not know what an inspiring teacher he was. Nor did I know that he would be arranging semester-long visits, in my first three fall semesters at Michigan, by John Maynard Smith, Bill Hamilton and George Williams.

Favourite paper in grad school. Trivers' 1974 paper on parent–offspring conflict turned kin selection on its head by showing that it could describe conflict among relatives. Dick Alexander didn't think it could be true, but he changed his mind there too. This idea, when applied to social insects (first in Trivers & Hare 1976), made them much more interesting.

Favourite book in grad school. Richard Dawkins' *The Selfish Gene* (1976) showed how you could explain much of the social universe with a metaphor that imagines genes as calculating agents. You didn't even need to know which genes were involved!

Best pun. One of my first papers (Queller 1983) was about how the showiness of hermaphroditic milkweed *Asclepias exaltata* flowers was more about nasty male–male competition than about the cooperative good of getting male and female gametes together. I called this the *fleur-du-mâle* theory, evoking both the essential maleness of the floral display and Charles Baudelaire's *Fleurs du Mal* (*Flowers of Evil*). I figured a clever pun might just help get the manuscript into *Nature*. Too clever by half, as the Brits say, or maybe just too silly by half – they took the paper but made me drop the pun from the title. Just as well – the name never caught on, though the idea did.

Best collaboration. That's an easy one: most of my work has been carried out with my wife Joan Strassmann, who also got me switched from plant sociobiology to wasps. Fortunately we met after we had both established independent research reputations; otherwise tenure decisions might have hinged on separating out contributions that are inseparable. I also got three great kids out the deal.

Social Behaviour: Genes, Ecology and Evolution, ed. Tamás Székely, Allen J. Moore and Jan Komdeur. Published by Cambridge University Press. © Cambridge University Press 2010.

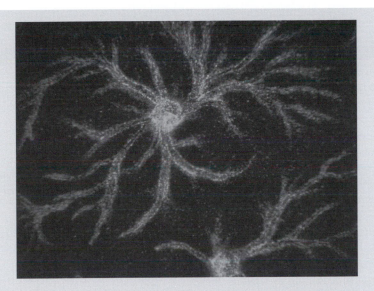

Labelled cells of the social amoeba *Dictyostelium discoideum* stream into an aggregation where 20% of them will sacrifice their lives in order to aid the dispersal of the others. Photo: Kevin Foster.

Best field site. Tuscany! I figured a career in biology might take me to interesting places, but I never expected Italy to be among them. But when our grad student Francesca Zacchi showed that cofoundresses of the paper wasp *Polistes dominulus* were often unrelated, we had the opportunity (nay, the duty!) to work on them. Actually the main field site was an old strip mine, but you still can't beat the whole package.

Best sign of seriousness of purpose (and serious mental derangement). Switching from wasps in Tuscany to slime moulds in Petri plates. A grad student who had no background in field biology made us think about lab projects, and we returned to an old idea of looking at the social amoeba *Dictyostelium discoideum* (Dicty for short; see also Chapter 13 and Amotz Zahavi's profile), made famous by John Bonner. After our early work showed interesting cooperation and cheating (Strassmann *et al.* 2000), we figured we could use this model organism to study real selfish genes. For example, we have recently found over 100 cheater mutations – actual selfish genes (Santorelli *et al.* 2008).

Most cited paper. One way to get cited is to name something, but having failed with the *fleurs du mâle* I succeeded with the next best – a method. Broadening previous work by Crozier and Pamilo, I was able to show how to estimate relatedness from genetic markers (Queller & Goodnight 1989). Estimating relatedness went from being the hard part of Hamilton's kin selection rule to estimate, to being the easy part.

Funniest paper. 'The spaniels of St Marx and the Panglossian paradox: a critique of a rhetorical programme' (Queller 1995). This was a response to Gould and Lewontin's famous 'Spandrels of San Marco' paper (1979) that attacked adaptationist thinking. George Williams was kind enough to risk slander charges by publishing it in the *Quarterly Review of Biology*, but Gould didn't sue; he simply called it 'jejune'. Read it, and you might disagree with my best-pun choice above.

Research I least imagined. The *D. discoideum* genome was already sequenced – that was part of the attraction – but now we are sequencing three or four related species. We already have sequenced two other strains of *D. discoideum* and, as sequencing costs plummet, we hope to sequence enough more to do population genetics across the genome. Why bother? We want to know if conflict leads to molecular arms races, and we want to find genes under balancing selection that contribute to either kin recognition or to frequency-dependent cooperation/cheating games.

Wildest scientific predictions. A good scientific theory makes risky predictions, and I have found a large set of very risky predictions of kin selection theory (Queller 2003). Following up on Trivers' ideas on parent–offspring conflict, David Haig constructed his genomic theory of imprinting (Haig 2000). Not only do offspring genes conflict with the mother; there can also be conflict between the offspring's genes according to whether they come from the mother or the father – I call them matrigenes and patrigenes. Patrigenes should be more aggressive in offspring conflicts with their mother, because patrigenes are less related to the mother. The haplodiploid social insects have numerous contexts for such intragenomic conflict. For example, one can predict that aggression between queens will be dominated by matrigenes in maternal half-sister honey bees, by patrigenes in full-sister *Polistes* wasps and by neither in unrelated ant cofoundresses. Similar sets of predictions can be made for worker egg laying, worker policing, sex ratios, queen replacement and many other contexts.

Biggest regret. Too many grant proposals written, but no books.

Bottom line. Select problems that fascinate you and will also be interesting to others. Don't be afraid to move in new directions or to change your mind. Collaborate: it really can pay to cooperate.

References

Dawkins, R. (1976) *The Selfish Gene*. Oxford: Oxford University Press.

Gould, S. J. & Lewontin, R. C. (1979) The spandrels of San Marco and the Panglossian paradigm: a critique of the adaptationist programme. *Proceedings of the Royal Society B*, **205**, 581–598.

Haig, D. (2000) The kinship theory of genomic imprinting. *Annual Review of Ecology and Systematics*, **31**, 9–32.

Queller, D. C. (1983) Sexual selection in a hermaphroditic plant. *Nature*, **305**, 706–707.

Queller, D. C. (1995) The spaniels of St Marx and the Panglossian paradox: a critique of a rhetorical programme. *Quarterly Review of Biology*, **70**, 485–489.

Queller, D. C. (2003) Theory of genomic imprinting conflict in social insects. *BMC Evolutionary Biology*, **3**, 15.

Queller, D. C. & Goodnight, K. F. (1989) Estimating relatedness using genetic markers. *Evolution*, **43**, 258–275.

Santorelli, L., Thompson, C., Villegas, E. *et al.* (2008) Facultative cheater mutants reveal the genetic complexity of cooperation in social amoebae. *Nature*, **451**, 1107–1110.

Strassmann, J. E., Zhu, Y. & Queller, D. C. (2000) Altruism and social cheating in the social amoeba, *Dictyostelium discoideum*. *Nature*, **408**, 965–967.

Trivers, R. L. (1974) Parent–offspring conflict. *American Zoologist*, **14**, 249–264.

Trivers, R. L. & Hare, H. (1976) Haplodiploidy and the evolution of the social insects. *Science*, **191**, 249–263.

13

Social behaviour in microorganisms

Kevin R. Foster

OVERVIEW

Sociobiology has come a long way. We now have a solid base of evolutionary theory supported by a myriad of empirical tests. It is perhaps less appreciated, however, that first discussions of social behaviour and evolution in Darwin's day drew upon single-celled organisms. Since then, microbes have received short shrift, and their full spectrum of sociality has only recently come to light. Almost everything that a microorganism does has social consequences; simply dividing can consume another's resources. Microbes also secrete a wide range of products that affect others, including digestive enzymes, toxins, molecules for communication and DNA that allows genes to mix both within and among species.

Many species do all of this in surface-attached communities, known as biofilms, in which the diversity of species and interactions reaches bewildering heights. Grouping can even involve differentiation and development, as in the spectacular multicellular escape responses of slime moulds and myxobacteria. Like any society, however, microbes face conflict, and most groups will involve instances of both cooperation and competition among their members. And, as in any society, microbial conflicts are mediated by three key processes: constraints on rebellion, coercion that enforces compliance, and kinship whereby cells direct altruistic aid towards clonemates.

13.1 Introduction

We must be prepared to learn some day, from the students of microscopical pond-life, facts of unconscious mutual support, even from the life of micro-organisms.

Kropotkin (1902).

The idea of sociality in the mere microbe can be met with a raised eyebrow and a smirk. Nevertheless, for as long as there has been evolutionary biology, and indeed sociology, microbes have featured in descriptions of social life. Prominent among these are the writings of Herbert Spencer, the social philosopher who coined the term *survival of the fittest* in the wake of Darwin's *Origin*. Spencer was widely responsible for popularising the notion of altruism in Victorian Britain (Auguste Comte probably first coined the term), and importantly used both humans and single-celled life to define altruism's nature (Dixon 2008).

Social Behaviour: Genes, Ecology and Evolution, ed. Tamás Székely, Allen J. Moore and Jan Komdeur. Published by Cambridge University Press. © Cambridge University Press 2010.

And it was not long before a near-modern perspective emerged at the hands of the eccentric Russian explorer and anarchist Peter Kropotkin. In what was arguably the first sociobiology text, Kropotkin ran the gamut of examples of biological cooperation. Many were inspired by his wanderings through frozen Siberia, but his imagination wandered further to include speculations on microbial life.

The concepts of altruism and cooperation in biology, therefore, were developed with the appreciation that they might be applied to even the smallest of organisms. From there, more familiar organisms took centre stage in the developing field of ethology (Chapter 1; Tinbergen 1963), which later became sociobiology (Hamilton 1964, Wilson 1975). In the last century the spectacularly social insects, cooperatively breeding vertebrates and, of course, we humans have been widely studied and drawn upon to test the core theories of social behaviour. The colourful chapters that comprise the majority of this book are a testament to this. But there was little word on the microbes. Until, that is, microbiologists started a revolution from within and challenged the oft prevailing view that the microorganism is a self-absorbed creature, swimming alone in the plankton. Researchers were finding that many species attach to surfaces, secrete structural polymers, and grow into large and sometimes diverse communities (Fig. 13.1; biofilms: Kolter

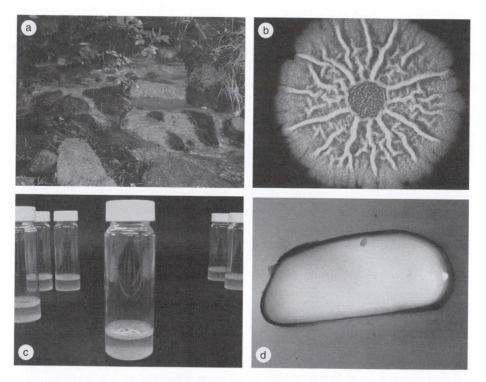

Figure 13.1 Microbial groups. (a) Large microbial biofilm in a Massachusetts river, USA. (b) Colony of the spore-forming bacteria *Bacillus subtilis* growing on agar. The cells secrete structural polymers that contribute to the wrinkly appearance. (c) Biofilm at the air–water interface in the bacterium *Pseudomonas fluorescens*, again formed with the help of extracellular polymer secretion. (d) Flocculation behaviour in the budding yeast *Saccharomyces cerevisiae*. A slice through a yeast 'floc' is shown, which forms after the yeast cells have aggregated (Smukalla *et al.* 2008). The floc has been treated with a toxin (ethanol). The dark area shows dead cells on the outside, but these protect the cells on the inside. Photos: (a) by the author, (b) by Hera Vlamakis, (c) by Andrew Spiers, (d) by Kevin Verstrepen.

& Greenberg 2006, Nadell *et al.* 2009). This led to a dramatic shift in perspective. Indeed the pendulum may have swung too far at first, with some descriptions bordering on the utopian: 'biofilms resemble the tissues formed by eukaryotic cells, in their physiological cooperativity and in the extent to which they are protected from variations in bulk phase conditions by a primitive homeostasis provided by the biofilm matrix' (Costerton *et al.* 1995). But with the close of the last century, the study of social behaviour in microorganisms bloomed, and most recently it has come to include sociobiologists, such as myself, who cut their teeth on studies of more classic social organisms (for me, it was the social wasps: Foster & Ratnieks 2001). And the microbes bring a valuable new perspective because, for the first time, we can hope to find the genes that underlie social behaviours and watch the emergent dynamics of social evolution (Foster *et al.* 2007).

But what exactly is a social behaviour in a microorganism? First things first; the use of *microorganism* here will mean a focus on species with individuals that we cannot see unaided and, in particular, the well-studied bacteria (Box 13.1). *Social behaviour* simply means a behaviour that affects another cell's evolutionary fitness (Table 13.1; Hamilton 1964, Wilson 1975), and the most interesting social behaviours are the ones that evolved *because* they affect others (West *et al.* 2007). Only if a behaviour evolved because of its social effects, or at least partly due to them, can it strictly be viewed as a social strategy. Consider a cell that secretes a waste product which harms another cell. One can probably safely assume that the act of secretion is the product of natural selection on the secreting cell, but the harm caused to the other cell may not be; it may simply be a by-product of natural selection to remove waste (Diggle *et al.* 2007a).

Box 13.1 Some key players in microbial social evolution

Dictyostelium discoideum – This slime mould or social amoeba is actually a member of a little-known kingdom, the Mycetozoa, which is the sister group of animals and fungi. *D. discoideum* is a bacterial predator that displays impressive multicellularity, aggregating upon starvation to form a multicellular slug and then a fruiting body, in which some cells die to hold the others aloft as spores (Fig. 13.6).

   Bacillus subtilis – A spore-forming soil bacterium that forms tough biofilms on agar and on the surface of growth medium (Fig. 13.1b). These biofilms show considerable differentiation, including isolated areas of spores and other areas containing cells that secrete the polymers that bind the group together. Under other lab conditions, *B. subtilis* cells will also diversify into competent and non-competent cells, and into chaining and single cells (see main text).

   Escherichia coli – The classical laboratory species, *E. coli* is found in the soil and, of course, in the digestive tracts of many healthy animals. *E. coli* displays evidence of cooperative entry into a dormant state upon starvation, and can carry a plasmid that poisons cells that do not possess it.

   Myxococcus xanthus – A striking example of convergent evolution with *D. discoideum*, this spore-forming soil bacterium will aggregate upon starvation to form a fruiting body. *M. xanthus* cells also secrete toxins that kill other cells within the fruiting body, other strains, and also species upon which it feeds. The latter process is sometimes associated with social motility, an example of group predation (Fig. 13.5a).

   Pseudomonas – *P. aeruginosa* is a pathogenic bacterium that is sometimes found in soil and often in the clinic (Fig. 13.2b). While best known for its ability to cause complications in the lungs of cystic fibrosis patients, it can cause problems in any

> **Box 13.1** Continued
>
> immunosuppressed patient. *P. aeruginosa* also forms robust biofilms (Fig. 13.4), displays quorum sensing, undergoes swarming motility, and secretes many shared products including siderophores that help with the uptake of iron. *P. fluorescens* is a generally non-pathogenic soil bacterium that also forms biofilms, most famously in the form of a mat on the surface of standing cultures in the laboratory (Fig. 13.1c).
>
> *Saccharomyces cerevisiae* – The workhorse of eukaryotic cell biology, the budding, brewer's or baker's yeast has been cultivated by humans for millennia. While laboratory strains are often grown in a manner that limits social behaviours, this species secretes several enzymes, will aggregate with other cells by flocculation (Fig. 13.1d), and can undergo pseudo-hyphal growth whereby growing cells do not separate after division and form long chains.
>
> *Vibrio* – *V. cholera* is the bacterium that causes cholera through the colonisation of the human intestine and the subsequent secretion of cholera toxin. Growth in the intestine and in the environment is often associated with biofilm formation and quorum sensing. The related species *V. fisheri* lives mutualistically in the light organ of the bobtail squid and produces light under quorum-sensing regulation.

The heart of this chapter is a review of the social behaviours of microorganisms, and the possible evolutionary benefits they carry to the cells that express them (section 13.2, *Form and function*). They range from the simple effects of growth rate through to complex multicellular development, with secretion, communication and genetic exchange in between. Some behaviours are downright selfish, but others have the appearance of cooperation, whereby the actions of one cell increase the reproductive fitness of another (Table 13.1; West *et al.* 2006). Identifying when behaviours are cooperative versus selfish – or the associated question of when they are a true social strategy versus a by-product of non-social traits – can be difficult for microbes. This is due in no small part to our limited understanding of microbial behaviours in nature. For example, when is it good, evolutionarily speaking, to be in a biofilm? Moreover, what really is a microbial group? A cell may sit in a massive biofilm but only ever affect its very nearest neighbours. So please take all interpretation herein with such caveats and questions in mind.

That said, many behaviours do seem to slow or even prevent a cell's division, which means a reduction in personal fitness. Keeping focus then not on the strain but on the individual cell, these behaviours have the hallmark of microbial altruism (Hamilton 1964, West

et al. 2007, Foster 2008), and even spite (Foster *et al.* 2001, Gardner *et al.* 2004) (see Table 13.1 for definitions). Finding microbial altruism, we are faced with the classic problem of sociobiology (Hamilton 1964, Wilson 1975): how can apparently selfless traits remain stable in the face of natural selection for conflict and cheating (Chapter 6)? Section 13.3, *Conflict resolution*, is dedicated to this question.

13.2 Form and function

13.2.1 Growth rate

A simple way to affect your neighbours is to steal their food. This is particularly easy when you share resources like carbon and oxygen as a microbe, and when these become growth-limiting the potential for conflict is clear (Ratnieks *et al.* 2006). Natural selection can favour cells that hungrily consume resources in order to obtain the lion's share, even though this may be inefficient and give poor future prospects (Kerr *et al.* 2006). At least mathematically, this is analogous to the ongoing clashes over fisheries, and air quality between laissez-faire capitalists on the one hand and environment-oriented interventionists on the other (the tragedy of the commons: Chapter 6, Rankin *et al.*

Table 13.1. Definitions of social behaviour based upon the effects on personal lifetime reproduction (direct fitness)

		Effect on *recipient*	
		Positive	Negative
Effect on *actor*	Positive	Mutual benefit	Selfishness
	Negative	Altruism	Spite
		Cooperation	***Competition/conflict***

2007). Many microbes have the ability to switch from aerobic respiration to fermentation, which produces energy more rapidly when oxygen is limited. However, fermentation is also inefficient and yields much less energy overall (Pfeiffer *et al.* 2001, Pfeiffer & Schuster 2005, Novak *et al.* 2006). Competing cells therefore are expected to more often make use of fermentation (MacLean & Gudelj 2006), while cooperative systems, including multicellular organisms, are more likely to be altruistically aerobic, whereby each cell slows its growth to allow other cells to have food in the future (Kreft 2004, Kreft & Bonhoeffer 2005).

High growth rate has many potential knock-on effects. One much discussed is the evolution of virulence, where rapid pathogen proliferation can mean trouble for a patient (Frank 1992). However, dividing rapidly will also tend to take resources away from cooperative traits like product secretion (Griffin *et al.* 2004), communication (Sandoz *et al.* 2007) and development (Velicer *et al.* 1998, Vulic & Kolter 2001); these are discussed below. When these systems are required for microbes to successfully attack the host, rapid growth can again lower ultimate yield, and lead to reduced, rather than increased, virulence (Brown *et al.* 2002, Foster 2005, Harrison *et al.* 2006).

13.2.2 Secreted products

Microbes secrete all manner of substances that physically and chemically alter their surroundings and their evolutionary fitness (Fig. 13.2). There are several ways out of a cell, including passive diffusion (Pearson *et al.* 1999), active pumps (Kostakioti *et al.* 2005), packaged in mini-membranes (vesicles: Mashburn-Warren & Whiteley 2006) and of course

when a cell bursts (Cascales *et al.* 2007). By secreting products, cells can create an environment that promotes growth – a simple form of niche construction (Lehmann 2006). For example, when cells of the budding yeast *Saccharomyces cerevisiae* get low on glucose, they secrete an enzyme called invertase that hydrolyses sucrose to liberate glucose and fructose (Greig & Travisano 2004).

Other secreted products bind and scavenge nutrients. The pathogen *Pseudomonas aeruginosa* is a fascinating but unpleasant bacterium that infects the lungs of patients with cystic fibrosis; a genetic disorder causing, amongst other symptoms, thickened airway mucus. *P. aeruginosa* relies on many secreted products for infection including siderophores (literally 'iron carriers' in Greek; Fig. 13.2). These dissolve insoluble iron and allow the bacterium to combat a common vertebrate response known as localised anaemia that reduces the iron in tissue (Jurado 1997). But the conflict lies not only with the patient. There is also the potential for infighting: mutants that neglect secretion are able to cheat those that do (Griffin *et al.* 2004), and the emergence of cheating can lead to reduced virulence in animal models (Harrison *et al.* 2006). It is interesting that the genetics underlying both yeast invertase and the siderophores display high variability (Greig & Travisano 2004, Smith *et al.* 2005). This may indicate shifting ecological demands (Brockhurst *et al.* 2007, Foster & Xavier 2007), or even an evolutionary arms race in which cooperators attempt to evolve products that cannot be used by cheaters (Tuemmler & Cornelis 2005).

But it is not all darkness and disease. Many microbes provide metabolic assistance by producing extracellular compounds or resources that their host

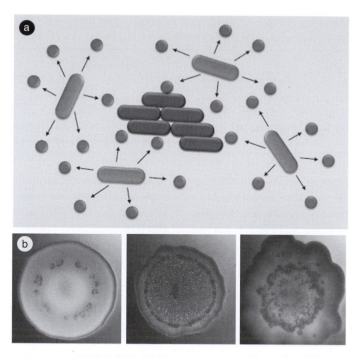

Figure 13.2 Secreted products in microbes. (a) Cooperative secreted products and cheating: the paler cells secrete a product that benefits all cells, but the darker cells do not, and save energy in the process. The darker cells cheat and outgrow the paler cells. (b) Different strains of the bacterium *Pseudomonas aeruginosa* growing on agar displaying different pigmentations that result, at least in part, from differences in pyoverdin (green, left) and pyocyanin (blue, middle) secretion, which both function in iron scavenging. The far-right strain also shows the characteristic spotting of viral-driven cell-lysis. Photos by the author.

organisms cannot make. This includes our own gut fauna, and also antifungal bacteria that protect leaf-cutter ant fungal gardens (Currie *et al.* 1999), light-producing *Vibrio fisheri* in fish and squid (Visick *et al.* 2000), and nitrogen-fixing bacteria or mycorrhizal fungi (Helgason & Fitter 2005) that provide nutrients for plants (Denison 2000). Cross-feeding among the microbes themselves also appears common, whereby the waste product of one species feeds another (Dejonghe *et al.* 2003), which, in turn, keeps the waste product at low levels and may improve their combined metabolism (Pfeiffer & Bonhoeffer 2004). With many species interacting, there is the potential for cross-feeding networks to reach dizzying complexity. One nice example occurs inside an insect, itself an exemplar of animal sociality: a termite. Termite society rests upon the ability to eat wood, and they are helped along by protozoa that break down cellulose

(Fig. 13.3; Noda *et al.* 2003). These protozoa in turn rely on bacteria, often spirochetes, that provide both metabolic assistance (Dolan 2001) and even motility (Tamm 1982, Wenzel *et al.* 2003, König *et al.* 2007). Meanwhile, some spirochetes rely on cross-feeding from yet other bacteria in the termite gut (Graber and Breznak 2005).

Shared products can also be structural. While not strictly secreted, the RNA virus φ6 produces proteins using the cellular machinery of its bacterial host. These proteins package the viral RNA in a protective coat and can be used by all viral RNAs such that cheater virus RNAs, which do not encode the proteins, can still be successfully packaged (Turner & Chao 1999, Brown 2001). While viruses coat themselves in rigid protein coats, bacteria instead use slime. More formally known as extracellular polymeric substances (EPS), the slimes found in bacterial biofilms

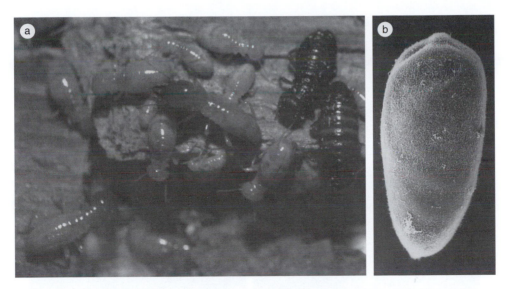

Figure 13.3 The symbioses inside termites, which feed on wood. (a) The host: the termite *Mastotermes darwiniensis*. (b) A symbiont, *Mixotricha paradoxa*, that helps to break down cellulose. The fur on the surface is actually the flagella of symbiotic spirochete bacteria that help it to swim around (König *et al.* 2007). Photos: (a) by Judith Korb, (b) by Helmut König.

are complex mixtures that probably protect the cells from various stresses (Crespi 2001, Velicer 2003, Hall-Stoodley *et al.* 2004, Foster 2005, Keller & Surette 2006, West *et al.* 2006). Slime may even allow one strain to smother and suffocate others in the quest for oxygen and nutrients, in the manner that a tree trunk allows one plant to grow tall and shade another (Fig. 13.4; Foster & Xavier 2007, Xavier & Foster 2007).

Although sinister, a bit of smothering is nothing compared to the favoured weapon in the microbial arsenal: secreted toxins. The toxin–antitoxin systems carried by many bacteria are probably the closest thing that microbes have to aggression (Chapter 7). In their simplest form, these systems comprise two neighbouring genes, one encoding a toxin (bacteriocin) that kills other strains, and the other an antitoxin, or immunity protein, that protects the toxin-producing strain. The cystic fibrosis pathogen *P. aeruginosa* carries multiple such toxin secretion systems, which evolve rapidly and may again be indicative of arms races (Smith *et al.* 2005). If *P. aeruginosa* is indeed involved in an arms race with other species, it appears to do well in the rankings: we find it near impossible to get accidental contamination of *P. aeruginosa*

cultures in our laboratory. Another interesting toxin–antitoxin system is found on a plasmid (a small, circular, extrachromosomal piece of DNA) carried by the well-known bacterium *Escherichia coli*. The toxin appears only to be released when some plasmid carriers burst, taking non-carrier cells down with them in dramatic fashion (Cascales *et al.* 2007), an example of evolutionary spite (Gardner *et al.* 2004). But it does not always end there, because the success of toxin-producing cells paves the way for a second strain that produces only the antitoxin and saves on the cost of the toxin. Then this second strain can be replaced by the original susceptible cell type that produces neither toxin nor antitoxin (Kerr *et al.* 2002), which means that toxin producers can reinvade, and so on. This non-transitive (rock–paper–scissors) relation can lead to cyclical dynamics that maintain all three types, and which may represent a general principle for the maintenance of biodiversity (Durrett & Levin 1997, Kerr *et al.* 2002, Reichenbach *et al.* 2007).

It is tempting to think that toxin–antitoxin systems always go hand in hand with conflict. Perhaps not; several examples have been instead interpreted in terms of cooperation, like that seen between the

338   **Kevin R. Foster**

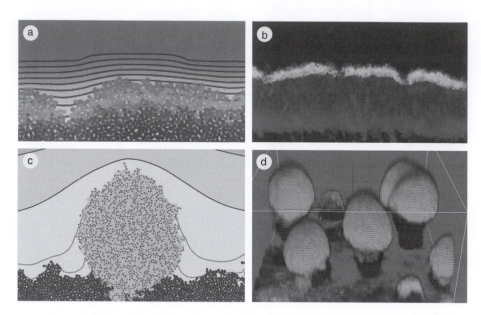

Figure 13.4 Nutrient competition and motility in bacterial biofilms. (a) An individual-based model of a microbial biofilm. The cells respire and in doing so create oxygen gradients (parallel lines) that slow the growth of cells deep in the biofilm (the paler cells are growing quickly and the darker ones slowly). (b) A biofilm of *P. aeruginosa* in which metabolically active cells have been stained yellow (the palest part of the image). (c) The effect of polymer secretion on success within a biofilm. The simulation shows cells that secrete a polymer and altruistically push their descendants up into the oxygen, which suffocates the cells beneath (shown dark) that do not secrete (Xavier & Foster 2007). (d) The effect of motility on success within a biofilm. Confocal image of a *P. aeruginosa* biofilm with a motile strain (pale) that moves towards the top of the biofilm and a non-motile strain (dark) that does not (Klausen *et al.* 2003). Images (a) and (c) from Joao Xavier, (b) from Phil Stewart, (d) from Tim Tolker-Nielsen.

germ and soma cells of your body. The *E. coli* chromosome contains the *mazEF* system (Metzger *et al.* 1988), where *E* encodes the antitoxin and *F* the toxin. This system has a clever feature: the two genes turn on and off together (they are an operon) but the toxin degrades more slowly than the antitoxin. This means that when the *mazEF* operon is deactivated, the levels of toxin and antitoxin in the cell will steadily decrease but, importantly, the antitoxin disappears first, leaving behind the toxin, and this kills the cell. What makes this clever is that various environmental stresses turn off the operon, including heat, DNA damage and virus attack, so that damaged cells will undergo lysis (Hazan *et al.* 2003). The process looks a lot like an altruistic behaviour – the weakened committing suicide to protect the strong – and there is evidence that *mazEF*-induced lysis of diseased cells

can inhibit the spread of viruses to healthy cells (Hazan and Engelberg-Kulka 2004). However, the benefits under other stresses are less clear (Tsilibaris *et al.* 2007), and more work is needed to dissect out the exact evolutionary pressures that drive the *mazEF* system and other toxin systems (Magnuson 2007). Critically, if lysis releases the toxin and kills non-carriers, like the colicins, then *mazEF* may also function in competition with other strains and species. Similar questions await the spore-forming bacterium *Bacillus subtilis* (Fig. 13.1b), which actively secretes a toxin that kills non-expressing cells in the surroundings (Gonzalez-Pastor *et al.* 2003, Dubnau & Losick 2006), and viral-induced cell death in *P. aeruginosa* biofilms (Fig. 13.2b; Allesen-Holm *et al.* 2006), which have both been interpreted as purely cooperative behaviours.

13.2.3 Communication

Microbes also use secretions to communicate with each other. Indeed, killing another cell with a toxin is a very simple, albeit rude, form of discourse. However, this would not, strictly speaking, be communication (or signalling) by some evolutionary definitions (Chapter 8), which demand that both producer and receiver benefit from their respective actions (Keller & Surette 2006, Diggle *et al*. 2007a). Such cooperative communication does seem likely in some systems, including the coordinated development of slime moulds discussed below, and perhaps the curious tendency of *S. cerevisiae* yeast cells to synchronise their intracellular physiologies, even though cell division is not synchronised (Tsuchiya *et al*. 2007). Microbes also display an impressive ability to detect the density of their own and other species through quorum sensing (literally, sensing who is around: Fuqua *et al*. 1994). Quorum sensing is found both in bacteria (Miller & Bassler 2001, Keller & Surette 2006, Diggle *et al*. 2007a) and in fungi (Hogan 2006), and involves a wide variety of secreted compounds known as autoinducers, including some packaged in vesicles (Mashburn & Whiteley 2005). All exploit the same simple principle: if cells secrete a chemical, then as cell density goes up, so will the local concentration of the chemical. By responding to the chemical, therefore, the cells can respond to their own density.

Quorum sensing was first characterised in *V. fisheri*, the glow-in-the-dark bacterium that lives in the sea, where it exists in a free-living form but also on and in squid and fish, whom it helps with behaviours like mate or prey attraction (Nealson *et al*. 1970, Fuqua *et al*. 1994). *V. fisheri* regulates luminescence with an autoinducer, an *N*-acylhomoserine lactone, such that the cells only turn on at high density in the host, and not when swimming in the sea. Moreover, this molecule works through a positive-feedback loop whereby it induces an increase in its own production. Since then, the name has spread to quorum-sensing molecules that do not autoinduce, and quorum sensing has been found to control a multitude of behaviours, including bacterial spore formation (Hagen *et al*. 1978, Gonzalez-Pastor *et al*. 2003, Dubnau & Losick 2006), biofilm formation (Davies *et al*. 1998), the

transition from a single-celled to a hyphal lifestyle in fungi (Hornby *et al*. 2001), DNA uptake and exchange (Piper *et al*. 1993, Magnuson *et al*. 1994, Havarstein *et al*. 1995) and many secreted products such as slime (EPS) (Hammer and Bassler 2003), iron-scavenging molecules (Stintzi *et al*. 1998) and toxins (van der Ploeg 2005).

Does quorum sensing always represent active communication from one cell to another? This is not yet clear. Some autoinducers may simply be waste products that did not evolve to allow secreting cells to communicate (Diggle *et al*. 2007a). In some cases, however, autoinducers have been shown to cost energy, which suggests that they do represent active and evolved communication. The cost also means that mute cells, which do not produce the signal, can cheat by listening in without paying the cost of communication, just as cells can cheat on a shared enzyme (Fig. 13.2a, Brown & Johnstone 2001, Diggle *et al*. 2007b). Other times it can pay to play deaf. Some *P. aeruginosa* strains from cystic fibrosis (CF) patients lack a functional copy of the autoinducer sensor protein LasR, which is required to respond to the autoinducer. Lacking the sensor protein stops cells producing cooperative products that may not be needed in the CF lung and, even if the products are needed, the *lasR* mutants can exploit the products of others (D'Argenio *et al*. 2007, Sandoz *et al*. 2007). Finally, strains unable to quorum sense in *V. cholerae* overproduce slime (EPS), which is thought to inhibit dispersal from biofilms but can provide a competitive advantage when it is better to stay put (Hammer & Bassler 2003, Nadell *et al*. 2008).

There is also the potential for communication among species. One quorum-sensing molecule, autoinducer-2 (AI-2), is produced by an amazingly diverse set of species, which opens the possibility of widespread interspecies communication (Federle & Bassler 2003). How often this represents active signalling on the part of secreting cells is not known (Keller & Surette 2006, Diggle *et al*. 2007a), but some species, including *P. aeruginosa*, respond to AI-2 even though they do not make it, which is at least consistent with the evolution of eavesdropping (Duan *et al*. 2003) (Chapter 8). When multiple species meet, there is also the possibility for devious manipulations (Keller

& Surette 2006): *E. coli* actively takes up AI-2, and thereby prevents *Vibrio cholerae* from secreting proteases that it uses during cholera gut infection (Xavier & Bassler 2005). Meanwhile, the dental bacterium *Veillonella atypica* secretes a compound that induces *Streptococcus gordonii* to release lactic acid, which *V. atypica* then feeds on (Egland *et al.* 2004).

13.2.4 Genetic exchange

The social behaviours of microorganisms include sex (Chapter 10). Indeed, eukaryotes like yeast are sexual creatures that undergo meiosis and mating to make recombinant progeny (Goddard *et al.* 2005). Although primarily asexual, bacterial cells also perform more limited DNA exchanges (Thomas & Nielsen 2005, Narra & Ochman 2006) via the environment, viruses and plasmids. A cell able to incorporate DNA from the environment into its genome is termed naturally competent (artificial competence means they will do it when forced by a persuasive lab scientist armed with electrodes or chemicals). Sometimes the act of DNA uptake itself may not be all that social; the cell performing the action may not affect the fitness of others. However, natural competence is often tightly associated with social traits.

V. cholerae becomes naturally competent when growing in a biofilm on arthropod exoskeletons (Meibom *et al.* 2005) and competence in *B. subtilis* involves both quorum-sensing (Magnuson *et al.* 1994) and differentiation (below). Perhaps the most interesting case, however, comes from *Streptococcus* species, which upon entering a competent state also activate multiple toxin–antitoxin systems (above) that selectively lyse surrounding cells that are not competent (Claverys *et al.* 2007). The evolution of DNA uptake is therefore intertwined with potential conflict among strains: the killing factors may both remove competing cells from the environment and also provide DNA for recombination. This adaptive story makes a lot of sense, but at the same time it has a curiously paradoxical aspect to it. Why kill another cell only to incorporate its DNA into your own and partially become it? The answer may lie in recognising that there can be differing evolutionary interests at different loci, and

some may favour killing-associated competence, while those that get replaced do not. A human analogy would be the occasions where a conquering nation incorporates some aspects of a subordinate's culture into its own, such as the Romans adopting Greek gods.

Transport of DNA between cells is even more directed when driven by plasmids (conjugation) and viruses (transduction). Plasmids are the relatively small circular pieces of DNA carried by bacteria. Despite their small size, plasmids exert a powerful influence on cell biology and are often able to engineer their own propagation, by inducing their cell to attach to another cell and make a channel through which a plasmid copy can pass (Thomas & Nielsen 2005). Many plasmids are benevolent and produce beneficial proteins, including antibiotic resistance genes, but others act like viruses, and spread within and among cells at a cost to their hosts (Eberhard 1990, Smith 2001, Paulsson 2002). And while plasmids show some specificity, they are often able to transfer their DNA to other species. One example is the tumour-inducing (TI) plasmid that makes the bacterium *Agrobacterium tumefaciens* into a plant pathogen. This plasmid has amazing abilities. It integrates fragments of its DNA into the plant's genome and induces the formation of a gall, which protects and feeds the bacteria. The plasmid also encodes its own quorum-sensing system, and at high quorum it will induce conjugation and transfer itself to other *A. tumefaciens* cells (Chilton *et al.* 1980, Piper *et al.* 1993). Transfers of viral and plasmid DNA between species, however, are not perfect and sometimes take host DNA along for the ride. This can have unintended but important consequences, such as mixing the DNA of prokaryotes and eukaryotes, which are otherwise separated by over a billion years of evolution (Gogarten & Townsend 2005, Thomas & Nielsen 2005).

13.2.5 Group formation

Social interactions are most intense when individuals live side by side in a group (Chapter 9), which for many microbes will mean a biofilm. Biofilms form when cells grow on a surface or attach to each other to form a living mat (Fig. 13.1) in which cells secrete all manner of products, including the slimy polymers that form a structural matrix around the cells (Fig. 13.4; Branda *et al.* 2005, Parsek & Greenberg 2005, Nadell *et al.* 2009). Interestingly, some strains turn on the slime at high density while others turn it off. Turning on at high density makes sense: slime will only be made in the biofilm and not when swimming around at low density, where slime presumably does not pay. But why do some species then turn it off again at even higher density? The answer may lie in dispersal. Negative regulation has been found in *V. cholerae*, which induces a short-lived acute infection that climaxes with dispersal en masse from the gut of the unfortunate patient. This need to disperse may favour strains that turn off the slime just before they leave, when they will no longer need it (Hammer & Bassler 2003, Nadell *et al.* 2008). Biofilms often also contain many species. *V. cholerae* must compete in the gut with many other species including *E. coli*, which can interfere with its quorum sensing, as we have seen (Xavier & Bassler 2005). The best studied multi-species biofilms, however, must be those growing upon your teeth as you read this. Dental plaque contains an amazing diversity of species (Kolenbrander 2000), including some that depend upon each other for attachment and growth (Palmer *et al.* 2001).

Living in a dense biofilm presents challenges, including intense nutrient competition that threatens to slow growth (Fig. 13.4a, b; Stewart 2003, Xavier & Foster 2007). So why make one? The answer is likely to vary between species (Hall-Stoodley & Stoodley 2005), but one common benefit is probably settling in a good place to live. A biofilm at an air–water interface has good access to oxygen and light (Fig. 13.1c; Rainey & Rainey 2003, Brockhurst *et al.* 2007), and attachment to solid surfaces can yield similar advantages, particularly given that cells will often attach reversibly and swim off if they end up in a bad spot (Sauer *et al.* 2002). Biofilm life also allows cells to condition the local environment to suit growth and communication (Parsek & Greenberg 2005, Keller & Surette 2006), and they are tough: biofilms are the scourge of industry and medicine, where they clog, contaminate and cake machines and people alike (Fux *et al.* 2005). This

suggests that the biofilm state provides considerable protection to its inhabitants, which can include resistance to antibiotics (Mah *et al.* 2003). Analogously, it has recently been shown in the yeast *S. cerevisiae* that flocculation, whereby cells aggregate together at high densities, provides protection against stresses and antifungal agents (Fig. 13.1d; Smukalla *et al.* 2008).

Bacterial biofilms can also be dynamic environments as strains struggle to get the best nutrients, both by altruistically pushing descendant cells with slime (above, Fig. 13.4c; Xavier & Foster 2007) and by active cell movement (Fig. 13.4d; Klausen *et al.* 2003). At its height, bacterial movement borders on mass exodus when dividing cells engage in a group migration away from high-density areas, in a process known as swarming. In nature, swarming may often be associated with dispersal from biofilms, and, like biofilm formation, swarming is often controlled by quorum sensing (Daniels *et al.* 2004): an exodus is best when it is really crowded. Furthermore, the cells appear to cooperate with one another to secrete products that ensure things go swimmingly, including digestive enzymes (Bindel Connelly *et al.* 2004) and chemicals that ease movement by reducing surface tension (biosurfactants: Kohler *et al.* 2000). In swarming *sensu stricto*, cells propel themselves with beating flagella (Harshey 2003), but they achieve similar ends by pulling themselves along with pili (the molecular equivalent of grappling hooks), and perhaps even by jetting slime out the back, jet-ski-like (Kaiser 2007). A single species can mix and match its methods: a strain of *Myxococcus xanthus* that had been mutated to stop pili-based swarming was able to re-evolve motility using a different mechanism (Fig. 13.5a; Velicer & Yu 2003). But not all microbes migrate outwards in this way. Some actively seek each other out and move together, and it is here that we find the pinnacle of microbial sociality, multicellular development.

13.2.6 Differentiation, diversification and development

Not all cells are equal. Many microbes can differentiate into distinct physiological states and morphologies. In the lab, differentiation events can be relatively

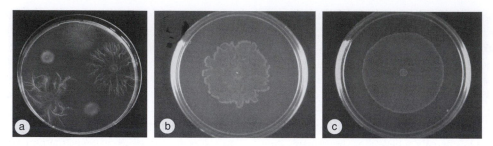

Figure 13.5 Swarming behaviours in bacteria. (a) Different swarming genotypes in the spore-forming bacterium *Myxococcus xanthus* (Velicer & Yu 2003). (b) Swarming cells in *Salmonella enterica*, which become elongated and carry many flagella for efficient propulsion (Kim *et al.* 2003). (c) A second strain of *Salmonella enterica* swarming. Photos: (a) by Greg Velicer, (b) and (c) by Wook Kim.

uniform, such as differentiation into swarming cells in *Salmonella enterica*, which become elongated and carry many flagella for efficient propulsion (Fig. 13.5b, c; Kim *et al.* 2003). But this can change in more complex environments. Cells bathed in oxygen at the surface of a biofilm may divide furiously while those below do little more than provide anchoring (Fig. 13.4a, b; Xu *et al.* 1998). Moreover, diversification into multiple cell types can occur without environmental gradients. One champion is *B. subtilis*, which can form both individual cells and chains of cells during growth, divide into competent and non-competent cells, and then form some spore cells that kill the others (above; Dubnau & Losick 2006). Another important example is the small subpopulations of dormant cells in many bacteria groups that are immune to many antibiotics (persister cells: Balaban *et al.* 2004, Keren *et al.* 2004, Gardner *et al.* 2007). Yeast diversify too: recent studies have shown bimodal expression of genes involved in phosphate uptake (Wykoff *et al.* 2007), and high variability in the tendency to become spores (Nachman *et al.* 2007). Finally, we also find microbial differentiation and diversification in symbioses. Some nitrogen-fixing bacteria in plant roots differentiate into swollen and terminal bacteriods that lose the ability to divide (Mergaert *et al.* 2006), while other cells in the surroundings remain viable and may even be altruistically fed by the differentiated cells (Denison 2000).

How do microbial cells diversify without external cues? The secret of course is *internal* variability. Nutritional state is one way to go. Recently divided cells in aggregates of the slime mould *Dictyostelium discoideum* are low on food, and as a consequence end up dead in a stalk rather than becoming reproductive spores (Fig. 13.6; David Queller's profile; Gomer & Firtel 1987). True randomness is another way to go. Entry into competence in *B. subtilis* is driven by a positive-feedback loop; once a cell starts down that road, there is no pulling out. However, entry is not guaranteed and appears to be driven by chance fluctuations in expression of the regulatory genes – the molecular equivalent of rolling dice (Suel *et al.* 2006). Another possibility in eukaryotes such as yeast is random acts of gene silencing by modification of DNA, or the nucleosomes that associate with DNA, which can suppress transcription (Rando & Verstrepen 2007). Or, more drastically, cells can undergo genetic changes to diversify their phenotypes. This appears to occur in *P. aeruginosa* biofilms, where multiple growth phenotypes appear from a single-type, and do so dependent upon *recA*, the gene central to DNA modification and repair (Boles *et al.* 2004). Finally, the tendency of the *S. cerevisiae* cells to stick to each other by flocculation is controlled by a gene with a large repeat sequence that makes flocculation evolve rapidly and reversibly (Fig. 13.1d; Verstrepen *et al.* 2005, Smukalla *et al.* 2008).

Why would a single strain diversify into multiple phenotypes? There is no doubt that some of the variability among cells is a simple by-product of unavoidable noise in cellular processes, and this must be kept in mind. But for cases that represent real evolutionary adaptations, there are two major explanations for

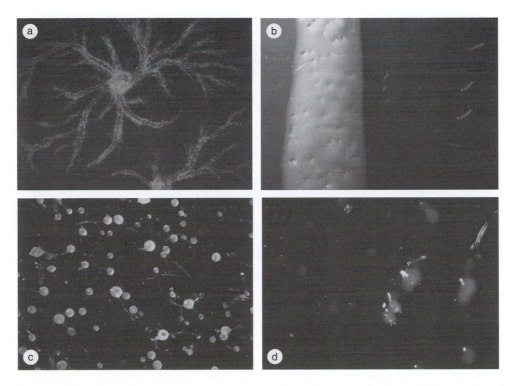

Figure 13.6 Social life, and strife, in the slime mould, or social amoeba, *Dictyostelium discoideum*. (a) Cells labelled with fluorescent beads that are streaming together to form an aggregate, which will then differentiate into a migrating slug. (b) Migrating slugs passing left to right through a strip of bacteria. In some hours, cells that were shed by the slugs will consume the bacteria and make new slugs (Kuzdzal-Fick *et al.* 2007), by which time the original slugs will have changed into fruiting bodies containing a stalk of dead cells that holds the rest up as reproductive spores. (c) Birds-eye view of a lawn of *D. discoideum* fruiting bodies. (d) Development in a *D. discoideum* cheater mutant. Alone, the mutant is unable to sporulate, but when mixed with the wild-type cells the mutant is competitively superior and produces more spores (Ennis *et al.* 2000, Gilbert *et al.* 2007). Photos by the author.

functional diversification. One idea is that cells are hedging their bets on the future (Kussell & Leibler 2005). That is, if there may or may not be an environmental catastrophe on the way, it can pay a strain to have some cells growing and others in a protected survival state as persisters (Balaban *et al.* 2004, Keren *et al.* 2004, Gardner *et al.* 2007). The other major overlapping explanation is a division of labour (Michod 2006). Microbes can divide their labour to perform a task, which might be bet-hedging or indeed something else, such as a division between polymer secretion and spore formation (Vlamakis *et al.* 2008). We, of course, are also living breathing testament to the

benefits of a division of labour – both in terms of the cells in your body and in our society.

The division of labour in microbial groups is most clear in development, whereby cells undergo a predictable series of changes over time. Simple development can occur without a division of labour. When short of food, for example, *E. coli* cells simultaneously slow their growth and transition into a dormant spore-like state (Vulic & Kolter 2001). The most convincing examples of development, however, include diversification and a division among cells between reproduction and other functions. This includes *B. subtilis* spore formation, but also some species that have evolved a dramatic way of getting out of a tight spot. When short of its bacterial prey, cells of the soil-dwelling slime mould *D. discoideum* (Kessin 2001, Shaulsky & Kessin 2007) secrete a signalling molecule (cyclic AMP) that induces the cells to stream together and differentiate into a multicellular slug that migrates towards heat and light (Fig. 13.6a). The slug sheds cells as it goes that colonise nearby patches (Fig. 13.6b; Kuzdzal-Fick *et al.* 2007) and near the soil surface transforms into a fruiting body, in which around a quarter of the cells die in a stalk that holds the other cells aloft as dispersing spores (Fig. 13.6c). Analogously, cells of the bacterium *Myxococcus xanthus*, also a bacterial predator, will aggregate upon food shortage to form a fruiting body containing spores (Julien *et al.* 2000). Again, many cells die in the process (Wireman & Dworkin 1977).

As with all social behaviours in microorganisms, with diversification and development comes potential evolutionary conflict. Indeed, whenever two neighbouring cells have a different phenotype, the chances are that one is doing better reproductively than the other. Natural selection, therefore, can favour cells that become the best type all the time, even though this may mess things up for everyone. Examples are seen in the slime moulds and myxobacteria, where single mutations can produce cheaters that over-produce spores in mixtures with other strains (Fig. 13.6d; Ennis *et al.* 2000, Velicer *et al.* 2000, Santorelli *et al.* 2008). But it also applies to the more simple cases, like the evolution of persister cells, which are dormant cells that suffer poor reproductive prospects, at least in the short term (Gardner *et al.* 2007). However, the fact that slime moulds still fruit and persisters persist tells us that disruptive mutants do not always win out. Why not? That comes next.

13.3 Conflict resolution

The social behaviours of microorganisms carry a variety of benefits, from regulating growth to maximise yield, through niche construction and communication, to the formation of dense protective groupings. Although the ability to cash in on these benefits will ultimately depend upon ecological conditions

(Brockhurst *et al.* 2007, Foster & Xavier 2007), broadly speaking these are the benefits that favour social life. But, as we have seen, group-level benefits alone may not be enough, and the potential for conflict looms large in the microbial world. But it is not all-out war, and mechanisms that limit conflicts must and do exist. The next sections review these mechanisms, dividing them up into *direct effects* – effects on the reproduction of the cell that performs the social action – and *indirect effects* – effects on cells that share genes with the focal cell (the structure is based upon Ratnieks *et al.* 2006, Gardner & Foster 2008 and references therein).

13.3.1 Direct effects: constraints and coercion

Non-enforced

As for herding wildebeest, if it is good to be in a group, then joining with other cells can simultaneously benefit the joiner and the joinees, which may mean limited conflict (Chapter 9). Increasing the size of a microbial group may often in this way confer benefits on all inhabitants: a large biofilm can provide better protection from the environment, and larger slime-mould slugs migrate further (Foster *et al.* 2002). Once in a group, though, there is the potential for things to turn nasty – a slime-mould cell may well benefit from other cells joining the slug (Fig. 13.6b), but not if they then force it to make a stalk (Santorelli *et al.* 2008). Mechanisms such as enforcement or genetic relatedness may then be needed to keep the peace (below). However, there are also reasons to believe that microbial groups, and indeed all social species, will tend to have intrinsic properties that moderate conflicts (Travisano & Velicer 2004).

If cooperative systems that avoid cheating persist longer than those that do not, over time there will be enrichment for systems with pre-existing constraints on the origin of cheaters (Foster *et al.* 2007, Rankin *et al.* 2007a). There are several mechanisms that might cause these constraints, including reduced mutation rate (below; Harrison & Buckling 2005, 2007) and genetic redundancy, whereby a cooperative trait is expressed by multiple genes (Foster *et al.* 2007). Another way is through the ubiquitous phenomenon of pleiotropy (each gene affecting multiple traits: Foster *et al.* 2004). For example, the group-wide entry into a dormant spore-like state in starving *E. coli* cultures (above) is sometime hijacked by the GASP mutant (growth at stationary phase: Vulic & Kolter 2001). Like a cancer, the mutant cells keep on growing under low nutrient conditions and replace the normal cells. However, this comes at a pleiotropic cost: long term the cheaters are compromised and probably doomed owing to poor acid tolerance, which prevents the cooperative trait being lost.

The gradual enrichment of constraints on cheater mutations, through pleiotropy or otherwise, may also be driven by shorter-term processes than trait or species persistence. As we will see below, some bacterial strains always have some cells that mutate into cheaters. When this harms the strain's prospects for founding new biofilms, selection will favour the evolution of genetic protection against cheater mutations, in the same way that multicellular organisms gain constraints on cancer mutations (Nunney 1999, Michod & Roze 2001). In this vein, natural selection for cooperation has been shown to lead to reduced global mutation rate in *P. aeruginosa* (below; Harrison & Buckling 2007). Constraints on cheating can also arise through an arms-race-like process in which a cheater strain paves the way for a new strain that can resist the cheater and others like it (Foster 2006). An experiment that mixed cheater strains with natural strains in the spore-forming bacterium *M. xanthus* caused some lab populations to go extinct (Fiegna *et al.* 2006). The cheater strains would rise to dominance, but this drove their own demise because they are impotent without the natural strains. However, in one case, a new mutant arose that could both outcompete the cheaters and form spores on its own: the system had evolved to constrain the cheaters.

Another process that can align evolutionary interests within a social group is niche separation. When strains or species compete, natural selection can favour individuals that specialise on a different resource than the competing species. This can have two knock-on effects. First, diversification may create a saturated environment where all niches are filled, which makes it more difficult for cheaters to arise, as has been seen in bacterial biofilms (Brockhurst *et al.* 2006). In addition, if two species no longer compete, the way is open for evolution of between-species cooperation. This occurs when species can exchange resources that are cheap for the donor but expensive for the recipient (Schwartz & Hoeksema 1998), e.g. a photosynthesiser exchanging organic carbon for inorganic carbon with a heterotroph (Kuhl *et al.* 1996). And a recent simulation suggested that natural selection operating on communities of microbes can promote such positive interactions (Williams & Lenton 2008). It requires that associations are fairly stable, however, so that the benefits from investing in the other species feed back on the investing cell or its descendants (partner-fidelity feedback: Sachs *et al.* 2004, Foster & Wenseleers 2006).

Enforced

In many societies, including our own, conflict is reduced by coercion that forces individuals to comply (Wenseleers & Ratnieks 2006). We understand relatively little of mechanisms of coercion in microbes, but there are some interesting candidates. One example is conjugation. If a cooperative secretion is encoded on a plasmid, then plasmid transfer will force other cells to secrete (Smith 2001). There is also toxin secretion in the bacteria *B. subtilis* (Gonzalez-Pastor *et al.* 2003) and *M. xanthus* (Wireman & Dworkin 1977) that kills some cells and provides nutrients for spore formation. One must be careful here, however, as toxin secretion can obviously also signify raw conflict, and not its resolution. We need more data before we can tell if, in nature, the secretion of these toxins really promotes the total reproduction of the bacterial group (conflict resolution: Ratnieks *et al.* 2006) or simply allows one strain to monopolise the resources of another (plain old conflict).

The role of enforcement is perhaps clearest in social behaviours that occur between species. There are many examples from symbioses, where a microbe lives in or on a host species and the host is able to select the microbial cells that help it the most (partner choice: Sachs *et al.* 2004, Foster & Wenseleers 2006). This includes fungus-growing ants that remove parasitic and foreign fungi (Currie & Stuart 2001, Mueller *et al.* 2004, Poulsen & Boomsma 2005) with the help of a streptomycete bacterium that secretes antifungals (Currie *et al.* 1999), and leguminous plants that direct resources to the roots with the most industrious nitrogen-fixing bacteria (Kiers *et al.* 2003, Simms *et al.* 2006). Even your intestine possesses mechanisms, some more subtle than others, which presumably tend to favour more cooperative bacteria and get rid of the less favourable ones. The subtle mechanisms include the still poorly understood effects of the immune system upon the microbial flora (Backhed *et al.* 2005, Ryu *et al.* 2008), and the less subtle mechanisms have been experienced by anyone who has travelled to a foreign country with a very different diet.

Successful coercion, however, requires that the recipient cannot easily escape its effects. Just as pleiotropy can internally constrain against cheating, it can also prevent escape from coercion. High-nutrient slime-mould cells (Fig. 13.6) induce low-nutrient cells to become stalk cells by secreting a chemical DIF-1, and avoiding DIF-1 is not an option: mutant cells that do not respond to DIF-1 also fail to enter the spore head to become spores (Foster *et al.* 2004). There are host–symbiont examples as well: the bobtail squid that hosts *V. fisheri* bacteria in its light organ creates an environment that enables fluorescent strains to outcompete non-fluorescent ones (Visick *et al.* 2000).

13.3.2 Indirect effects: kinship

Strain mixing

Personal benefits are an easy way to promote cooperation and make microbes behave as a unified group. However, just as important are benefits to related cells, or kin. Relatedness here means not genealogical relatedness, as in the statement 'rats and bats are related, they are both mammals', but rather relatedness among individuals within a species, as in 'I am related to my sister Gillian'. Simply put, if a group of microbes are recently derived from a single progenitor, their evolutionary interests are perfectly aligned,

like the cells in your body. This means that selection can lead to dramatically altruistic traits, like cell death, when this allows a cell to pass on the genes that they carry in common with other individuals (indirect genetic benefits: Chapter 6). It does not matter, evolutionarily speaking, which cells in a clonal group get to reproduce, so long as the group performs well overall.

The key theoretical corollary is that anything that breaks the genetic correlation among group members will promote competition and conflict (Hamilton 1964). This holds, whether the group is the bounded aggregation of a slime mould or a more nebulous biofilm, so long as grouping is defined by the scale of social interactions (Grafen 2007). The importance of genetic relatedness among cells is supported by several studies that have mixed up microbes. These have shown that mixing strains promotes rapid wasteful growth in bacterial viruses (Kerr *et al.* 2006) and the success of cheater mutants, which has been seen in many contexts including yeast enzyme secretion (Greig & Travisano 2004), *P. aeruginosa* iron scavenging (Griffin *et al.* 2004), *P. aeruginosa* quorum sensing (Diggle *et al.* 2007b), and the development of *M. xanthus* (Velicer *et al.* 2000) and *D. discoideum*, where a myriad cheater mutants have now been found (Ennis *et al.* 2000, Santorelli *et al.* 2008). But why does a cheater do better at low relatedness? Consider the fate of a rare cheater mutant that has just arisen in a natural population of slime moulds (Fig. 13.6; Gilbert *et al.* 2007). If many strains of *D. discoideum* mix together (low relatedness), the cheater cells will mostly meet cooperator cells and do well. But when aggregates form from a single strain, as they often do, the cheaters will have no one to exploit and will do badly: cheating does not pay when you are surrounded by relatives. Similar principles apply to multi-species cooperation, only now one needs not only low mixing *within* species, but also *between* species, because this allows enough time for investments in a partner species to provide feedback benefits (Foster & Wenseleers 2006).

One does not have to wait for evolutionary time scales to see strain mixing affecting microbial groups. This is particularly true when cells can pinpoint non-relatives, such as spitefully secreting a toxin to kill them (Gardner & West 2004, Gardner *et al.* 2004). With toxins, mixing immediately leads to problems: spore production is often decreased when *M. xanthus* strains are mixed (Fiegna & Velicer 2005) and mixing two bacteriocin-producing bacteria limits their ability to infect a host (Massey *et al.* 2004). The harmful effects of mixing can also be more subtle: slugs containing multiple strains of *D. discoideum* migrate poorly (Foster *et al.* 2002, Castillo *et al.* 2005).

If mixing is costly, then why do it? For some, the benefits of a large group will outweigh the costs, but others limit their mixing. A sister species of *D. discoideum*, *D. purpureum*, preferentially aggregates with cells of the same strain (Mehdiabadi *et al.* 2006), and strains of the bacterium *Proteus mirabilis* create an inhibition zone with other strains when swarming (Gibbs *et al.* 2008). In addition, so-called green-beard genes (Dawkins 1976), which code for cell-to-cell adhesion proteins, allow microbial cells that express the adhesion gene to preferentially associate with other expressing cells, while excluding non-expressers from aggregations. Such genes are likely to have promoted kinship in the early evolution of *D. discoideum* aggregation (Queller *et al.* 2003), and remain important today in *S. cerevisiae*, where only some strains express its key adhesion gene in natural populations (Smukalla *et al.* 2008). Quorum sensing can achieve similar effects. As we have seen, many beneficial secretions are only secreted when cells have grown to reach high density, which in biofilms may make a good proxy for being surrounded by relatives (Xavier & Foster 2007). And *B. subtilis* has taken this one step further by developing strain-specific quorum sensing (Tortosa *et al.* 2001, Ansaldi *et al.* 2002).

Mutation

One fundamental difference between microbes and more familiar social organisms such as insects, birds and mammals is probably the relative importance of mutation within groups (West *et al.* 2006). This is exemplified by the evolution of the bacterium *P. aeruginosa* in the cystic fibrosis lung (Smith *et al.* 2006). Over the years, strains arise that lose function in many genes important for normal social life, including

motility, attachment and, as we have seen, quorum sensing (D'Argenio *et al.* 2007, Sandoz *et al.* 2007). But mutation-driven evolution in microbes does not need years. Bacteria sitting in a flask on a bench will evolve cooperation and lose it again to cheating in a matter of days. One of the more friendly pseudomonads, *Pseudomonas fluorescens*, has a solitary smooth strain that swims around in the broth but will rapidly mutate to generate a second wrinkly strain, so-called because it secretes sticky stuff that makes its colonies look, well, wrinkly (Fig. 13.1b shows a similar case from another species). The wrinklies cooperate with each other and form a mat that suffocates the smooth cells below them (Fig. 13.1c), only to have new mutant smooth cells appear in their midst that sink the whole lot (Paul B. Rainey's profile; Rainey & Rainey 2003, Brockhurst *et al.* 2007) in a turbid tragedy of the commons (Rankin *et al.* 2007b).

Global mutation rate is also important. If mutation towards cheating occurs more often than towards cooperation, high mutation rate will tend to promote conflict: *Pseudomonas aeruginosa* strains that mutate rapidly (Oliver *et al.* 2000) produce more cheaters (Harrison & Buckling 2005). A high mutation rate then can reduce genetic relatedness in a group and lead to the emergence of cheaters and conflict. Moreover, the starting levels of genetic relatedness in a microbial group can interact with this process and affect the evolution of mutation rates. Growing strains of *P. aeruginosa* in isolation (high relatedness) favours a low mutation rate, because strains are less likely to produce cheater mutants that harm the group (Harrison & Buckling 2007). By contrast, growing mixtures of strains (low relatedness) can, at least temporarily, favour a higher mutation rate, as now the rise of cheater mutants harms not only the source strain but also its competitor. A bacterial group with a low relatedness among cells is prone to processes that drive relatedness even lower.

Mutation in key genes then can simultaneously reduce relatedness and produce cheaters that exploit others, even though cells may be genetically identical at every other locus. This brings us to an important point: when using relatedness to make evolutionary predictions about cooperation, one must focus on the locus or loci that cause the social action (Chapter 6). This is less of an issue in animal societies because sexual recombination means that, on average, relatedness is identical across the whole genome: any locus is a proxy for the loci that really matter. But in a mutating asexual microbe, the relatedness among cells can differ sharply at different loci, which suggests that the loci may also differ systematically in their evolutionary interests, creating within-genome conflicts (Burt & Trivers 2006, Helantera & Bargum 2007).

A candidate worthy of a little speculation in this regard is the reliable production of multiple growth phenotypes by *P. aeruginosa* within biofilms (Fig. 13.4; Boles *et al.* 2004). This appears to be genetically determined, and diversification makes biofilms tougher, suggesting that the majority of the loci in the genome, which do not alter, will benefit. However, if there are loci that must mutate to cause diversification, there is the potential for conflict among the resulting alleles, and also between these alleles and the rest of the genome. Examples such as this suggest that microbes may simultaneously indulge in the benefits of high relatedness at some loci (cooperation), while at the same time benefiting from variability at others (social heterosis: Nonacs & Kapheim 2007).

13.4 Conclusions and future directions

Recent years have seen the development of a host of so-called 'culture-independent' technologies for assessing microbial diversity. These detect a species directly from its RNA or DNA and remove the requirement that – in order to be detected – a species must grow in the laboratory setting. The new technologies have led to the realisation that many species were missed by traditional techniques and that natural microbial communities frequently contain hundreds of species living in close proximity. In many ways, therefore, the study of microbial behaviour and social interaction are only now beginning.

The newly recognised species diversity in microbial communities hints at an equally broad range of behavioural diversity that remains to be uncovered. There is therefore considerable scope for

taking both known and unknown species and simply documenting their social behaviours. Here I highlight three key questions that can be asked of a new microbial group, with the important caveat that any detailed study will always require that one can first get cells to grow in the laboratory setting. These questions are borrowed from a recent review on biofilms (Nadell *et al.* 2009).

Function: what are the constituent genes and phenotypes that drive microbial social traits? Identifying the genes that underlie social traits allows one to dissect complex group traits – like biofilms – into their constituent behaviours. This enables the systematic study of the costs and benefits of a given behaviour (below) and an assessment of the evolutionary forces acting upon traits by comparing DNA sequence variation within and between species (Smith *et al.* 2005).

Cooperation: what are the costs and benefits of microbial social behaviours? In order to understand the evolution of microbial behaviours, we need to identify which cells are affected by each behaviour. In particular, following the logic of Chapter 6, the two key questions are (1) what are the costs and benefits of a behaviour to the cell that expresses it, and (2) what are the costs and benefits of a behaviour to cells other than the individual that expresses it? A key experiment in this regard is to mix mutants that do not express a social trait with cells that do, in order to evaluate the potential for cheating (e.g. Gilbert *et al.* 2007). Only by asking such questions of a whole range of microbial behaviours will we get an idea of how many involve true altruism, whereby one cell helps another at a fitness cost to itself (Table 13.1).

Ecology: which strains and species are in natural microbial groups, and how are they arranged? We need a much better knowledge of microbial ecology in order to understand how costs and benefits measured in the laboratory translate into real fitness effects in the wild. An important start, which is well under way, is to identify the species and strains within natural communities. But to answer questions of social evolution one must go further still and assess the microscopic distribution of the different genotypes. While challenging, such fine-scale assessments in natural groups will provide estimates of genetic relatedness and, importantly, the spatial scale at which one can expect cells to act as a unified group of common interest (Fig. 13.2).

As you next stroll through a sun-dappled woodland, consider the humble microorganism. For they thrive all around us, be it on the surface of a water droplet, in the depths of the soil, or nestled inside the tiny pores of a leaf. Wherever they live, they are often packed together with many other species and strains. Here social interaction is rife: cells jostle for position, grab, secrete, poison and even shape-shift as the need arises. Only now is the true extent of the microbe's social sophistication becoming clear, and with it comes a rich opportunity to unravel the evolutionary paths that brought them there. But she who studies their societies faces a bewildering complexity, not only in terms of the diversity of those that interact, but also in the potential for rapid evolutionary responses when they do. There is some solace, however, in the knowledge that familiar principles of sociobiology are emerging from these microbial melees. Kinship, coercion and constraints are all important, and all-important. And in the end we know that each cell has its own interests at heart, and will act to safeguard the reproductive interest of itself and its clone-mates. There can be no doubt that microbial communities are shaped by the individual struggles that face all organisms, but there is room for some romanticism too. For with any struggle comes the benefit of alliances, familial or otherwise, that invest in a shared common good. Some microbes will even die for the cause, and rupturing to secrete a toxin can be simultaneously altruistic to those that are immune and spiteful to those that are not. In applying terms like altruism to microbes, however, we are met with something of a paradox. As Spencer realised long ago, the individual microorganism seems destined to be both selfish *and* altruistic because, in its eagerness to divide, it faces the ultimate metaphysical sacrifice: a loss of self.

The simplest beings habitually multiply by spontaneous fission. Physical altruism of the lowest kind, differentiating from physical egoism, may in this case be considered as not yet independent of it. For since the two halves which before fission constituted the individual, do not on dividing disappear, we must say that though the individuality of the parent infusorium or other protozoon is lost in ceasing to be single, yet the old individual continues to exist in each of the new individuals.

Herbert Spencer, *The Data of Ethics* (1879)

Acknowledgements

Many thanks to Anne Foster, John Koschwanez, Katharina Ribbeck, Thomas Dixon, Carey Nadell, Joao Xavier, Allan Drummond, Wook Kim, Beverly Neugeboren, Freya Harrison and two anonymous referees for comments and discussions. Thank you also to Helmut König, Greg Velicer, Kevin Versterpen, Judith Korb, Hera Vlamakis, Phil Stewart, Tim Tolker-Nielsen, Mike Brockhurst and Andrew Spiers for images. KRF is supported by National Institute of General Medical Sciences Center of Excellence Grant 5P50 GM 068763–01.

Suggested readings

Crespi, B. J. (2001) The evolution of social behavior in microorganisms. *Trends in Ecology and Evolution*, **16**, 178–183.

Keller, L. & Surette, M. G. (2006) Communication in bacteria: an ecological and evolutionary perspective. *Nature Reviews Microbiology*, **4**, 249–258.

Nadell, C. D., Xavier, J. & Foster, K. R. (2009) The sociobiology of biofilms. *FEMS Microbiology Reviews*, **33**, 206–224.

West, S. A., Griffin, A. S., Gardner, A. & Diggle, S. P. (2006) Social evolution theory for microorganisms. *Nature Reviews Microbiology*, **4**, 597–607.

References

Allesen-Holm, M., Barken, K. B., Yang, L. *et al.* (2006) A characterization of DNA release in *Pseudomonas aeruginosa* cultures and biofilms. *Molecular Microbiology*, **59**, 1114–1128.

Ansaldi, M., Marolt, D., Stebe, T., Mandic-Mulec, I. & Dubnau, D. (2002) Specific activation of the *Bacillus* quorum-sensing systems by isoprenylated pheromone variants. *Molecular Microbiology*, **44**, 1561–1573.

Backhed, F., Ley, R. E., Sonnenburg, J. L., Peterson, D. A. & Gordon, J. I. (2005) Host–bacterial mutualism in the human intestine. *Science*, **307**, 1915–1920.

Balaban, N. Q., Merrin, J., Chait, R., Kowalik, L. & Leibler, S. (2004) Bacterial persistence as a phenotypic switch. *Science*, **305**, 1622–1625.

Bindel Connelly, M., Young, G. M. & Sloma, A. (2004) Extracellular proteolytic activity plays a central role in swarming motility in *Bacillus subtilis*. *Journal of Bacteriology*, **186**, 4159–4167.

Boles, B. R., Thoendel, M. & Singh, P. K. (2004) Self-generated diversity produces 'insurance effects' in biofilm communities. *Proceedings of the National Academy of Sciences of the USA*, **101**, 16630–16635.

Branda, S. S., Vik, A., Friedman, L. & Kolter, R. (2005) Biofilms: the matrix revisited. *Trends in Microbiology*, **13**, 20–26.

Brockhurst, M. A., Hochberg, M. E., Bell, T. & Buckling, A. (2006) Character displacement promotes cooperation in bacterial biofilms. *Current Biology*, **16**, 2030–2034.

Brockhurst, M. A., Buckling, A. & Gardner, A. (2007) Cooperation peaks at intermediate disturbance. *Current Biology*, **17**, 761–765.

Brown, S. P. (2001) Collective action in an RNA virus. *Journal of Evolutionary Biology*, **14**, 821–828.

Brown, S. P. & Johnstone, R. A. (2001) Cooperation in the dark: signalling and collective action in quorum-sensing bacteria. *Proceedings of the Royal Society B*, **268**, 961–965.

Brown, S. P., Hochberg, M. E. & Grenfell, B. T. (2002) Does multiple infection select for raised virulence? *Trends in Microbiology*, **10**, 401–405.

Burt, A. & Trivers, R. L. (2006) *Genes in Conflict: the Biology of Selfish Genetic Elements*. Cambridge, MA: Harvard University Press.

Cascales, E., Buchanan, S. K., Duche, D. *et al.* (2007) Colicin biology. *Microbiology and Molecular Biology Reviews*, **71**, 158–229.

Castillo, D. I., Switz, G. T., Foster, K. R., Queller, D. C. & Strassmann, J. E. (2005) A cost to chimerism in *Dictyostelium discoideum* on natural substrates. *Evolutionary Ecology Research*, **7**, 263–271.

Chilton, M. D., Saiki, R. K., Yadav, N., Gordon, M. P. & Quetier, F. (1980) T-DNA from Agrobacterium Ti plasmid is in the nuclear DNA fraction of crown gall tumor cells. *Proceedings of the National Academy of Sciences of the USA*, **77**, 4060–4064.

Claverys, J. P., Martin, B. & Havarstein, L. S. (2007) Competence-induced fratricide in streptococci. *Molecular Microbiology*, **64**, 1423–1433.

Costerton, J. W., Lewandowski, Z., Caldwell, D. E., Korber, D. R. & Lappin-Scott, H. M. (1995) Microbial biofilms. *Annual Review of Microbiology*, **49**, 711–745.

Crespi, B. J. (2001) The evolution of social behavior in micro-organisms. *Trends in Ecology and Evolution*, **16**, 178–183.

Currie, C. R. & Stuart, A. E. (2001) Weeding and grooming of pathogens in agriculture by ants. *Proceedings of the Royal Society B*, **268**, 1033–1039.

Currie, C. R., Scott, J. A., Summerbell, R. C. & Malloch, D. (1999) Fungus-growing ants use antibiotic-producing bacteria to control garden parasites. *Nature*, **398**, 701–704.

Daniels, R., Vanderleyden, J. & Michiels, J. (2004) Quorum sensing and swarming migration in bacteria. *FEMS Microbiology Reviews*, **28**, 261–289.

D'Argenio, D. A., Wu, M., Hoffman, L. R. *et al.* (2007) Growth phenotypes of *Pseudomonas aeruginosa* lasR mutants adapted to the airways of cystic fibrosis patients. *Molecular Microbiology*, **64**, 512–533.

Davies, D. G., Parsek, M. R., Pearson, J. P. *et al.* (1998) The involvement of cell-to-cell signals in the development of a bacterial biofilm. *Science*, **280**, 295.

Dawkins, R. (1976) *The Selfish Gene*. Oxford: Oxford University Press.

Dejonghe, W., Berteloot, E., Goris, J. *et al.* (2003) Synergistic degradation of linuron by a bacterial consortium and isolation of a single linuron-degrading variovorax strain. *Applied and Environmental Microbiology*, **69**, 1532–1541.

Denison, R. F. (2000) Legume sanctions and the evolution of symbiotic cooperation by rhizobia. *American Naturalist*, **156**, 567–576.

Diggle, S. P., Gardner, A., West, S. A. & Griffin, A. S. (2007a) Evolutionary theory of bacterial quorum sensing: when is a signal not a signal? *Philosophical Transactions of the Royal Society B*, **362**, 1241–1249.

Diggle, S. P., Griffin, A. S., Campbell, G. S. & West, S. A. (2007b) Cooperation and conflict in quorum-sensing bacterial populations. *Nature*, **450**, 411–414.

Dixon, T. (2008) *The Invention of Altruism: Making Moral Meanings in Victorian Britain*. Oxford: Oxford University Press for the British Academy.

Dolan, M. F. (2001) Speciation of termite gut protists: the role of bacterial symbionts. *International Microbiology*, **4**, 203–208.

Duan, K., Dammel, C., Stein, J., Rabin, H. & Surette, M. G. (2003) Modulation of *Pseudomonas aeruginosa* gene expression by host microflora through interspecies communication. *Molecular Microbiology*, **50**, 1477–1491.

Dubnau, D. & Losick, R. (2006) Bistability in bacteria. *Molecular Microbiology*, **61**, 564–572.

Durrett, R. & Levin, S. (1997) Allelopathy in spatially distributed populations. *Journal of Theoretical Biology*, **185**, 165–171.

Eberhard, W. G. (1990) Evolution in bacterial plasmids and levels of selection. *Quarterly Review of Biology*, **65**, 3–22.

Egland, P. G., Palmer, R. J. & Kolenbrander, P. E. (2004) Interspecies communication in *Streptococcus gordonii-Veillonella atypica* biofilms: signaling in flow conditions requires juxtaposition. *Proceedings of the National Academy of Sciences of the USA*, **101**, 16917–16922.

Ennis, H. L., Dao, D. N., Pukatzki, S. U. & Kessin, R. H. (2000) *Dictyostelium* amoebae lacking an F-box protein form spores rather than stalk in chimeras with wild type. *Proceedings of the National Academy of Sciences of the USA*, **97**, 3292–3297.

Federle, M. J. & Bassler, B. L. (2003) Interspecies communication in bacteria. *Journal of Clinical Investigation*, **112**, 1291–1299.

Fiegna, F. & Velicer, G. J. (2005) Exploitative and hierarchical antagonism in a cooperative bacterium. *PLoS Biology*, **3** (11), e370.

Fiegna, F., Yu, Y. T., Kadam, S. V. & Velicer, G. J. (2006) Evolution of an obligate social cheater to a superior cooperator. *Nature*, **441**, 310–314.

Foster, K. R. (2005) Hamiltonian medicine: why the social lives of pathogens matter. *Science*, **308**, 1269–1270.

Foster, K. R. (2006) Sociobiology: the Phoenix effect. *Nature*, **441**, 291–292.

Foster, K. R. (2008) Behavioral ecology: altruism. In: *Encyclopedia of Ecology*. Oxford: Elsevier, pp. 154–159.

Foster, K. R. & Ratnieks, F. L. W. (2001) Paternity, reproduction and conflict in vespine wasps: a model system for testing kin selection predictions. *Behavioral Ecology and Sociobiology*, **50**, 1–8.

Foster, K. R. & Wenseleers, T. (2006) A general model for the evolution of mutualisms. *Journal of Evolutionary Biology*, **19**, 1283–1293.

Foster, K. R. & Xavier, J. B. (2007) Cooperation: bridging ecology and sociobiology. *Current Biology*, **17**, R319–321.

Foster, K. R., Wenseleers, T. & Ratnieks, F. L. W. (2001) Spite: Hamilton's unproven theory. *Annales Zoologici Fennici*, **38**, 229–238.

Foster, K. R., Fortunato, A., Strassmann, J. E. & Queller, D. C. (2002) The costs and benefits of being a chimera. *Proceedings of the Royal Society B*, **269**, 2357–2362.

Foster, K. R., Shaulsky, G., Strassmann, J. E., Queller, D. C. & Thompson, C. R. L. (2004) Pleiotropy as a mechanism to stabilize cooperation. *Nature*, **431**, 693–696.

Foster, K. R., Parkinson, K. & Thompson, C. R. (2007) What can microbial genetics teach sociobiology? *Trends in Genetics*, **23**, 74–80.

Frank, S. A. (1992) A kin selection model for the evolution of virulence. *Proceedings of the Royal Society B*, **250**, 195–197.

Fuqua, W. C., Winans, S. C. & Greenber, E. P. (1994) Quorum sensing in bacteria: the luxI family of cell density-responsive transcriptional regulators. *Journal of Bacteriology*, **176**, 269–275.

Fux, C. A., Costerton, J. W., Stewart, P. S. & Stoodley, P. (2005) Survival strategies of infectious biofilms. *Trends in Microbiology*, **13**, 34–40.

Gardner, A. & Foster, K. R. (2008) The evolution and ecology of cooperation: history and concepts. In: *Ecology of Social Evolution*, ed. J. Korb & J. Heinze. Berlin, Heidelberg: Springer Verlag, pp. 1–35.

Gardner, A. & West, S. A. (2004) Spite and the scale of competition. *Journal of Evolutionary Biology*, **17**, 1195–1203.

Gardner, A., West, S. A. & Buckling, A. (2004) Bacteriocins, spite and virulence. *Proceedings of the Royal Society B*, **271**, 1529–1535.

Gardner, A., West, S. A. & Griffin, A. S. (2007) Is bacterial persistence a social trait? *PLoS ONE*, **2** (1), e752.

Gibbs, K. A., Urbanowski, M. L. & Greenberg, E. P. (2008) Genetic determinants of self identity and social recognition in bacteria. *Science*, **321**, 256–259.

Gilbert, O. M., Foster, K. R., Mehdiabadi, N. J., Strassmann, J. E. & Queller, D. C. (2007) High relatedness maintains multicellular cooperation in a social amoeba by controlling cheater mutants. *Proceedings of the National Academy of Sciences of the USA*, **104**, 8913–8917.

Goddard, M. R., Godfray, H. C. & Burt, A. (2005) Sex increases the efficacy of natural selection in experimental yeast populations. *Nature*, **434**, 636–640.

Gogarten, J. P. & Townsend, J. P. (2005) Horizontal gene transfer, genome innovation and evolution. *Nature Reviews Microbiology*, **3**, 679–687.

Gomer, R. H. & Firtel, R. A. (1987) Cell-autonomous determination of cell-type choice in Dictyostelium development by cell-cycle phase. *Science*, **237**, 758.

Gonzalez-Pastor, J. E., Hobbs, E. C. & Losick, R. (2003) Cannibalism by sporulating bacteria. *Science*, **301**, 510–513.

Graber, J. R. & Breznak, J. A. (2005) Folate cross-feeding supports symbiotic homoacetogenic spirochetes. *Applied and Environmental Microbiology* **71**, 1883–1889.

Grafen, A. (2007) Detecting kin selection at work using inclusive fitness. *Proceedings of the Royal Society B*, **274**, 713–719.

Greig, D. & Travisano, M. (2004) The Prisoner's Dilemma and polymorphism in yeast SUC genes. *Proceedings of the Royal Society B*, **271**, S25–26.

Griffin, A. S., West, S. A. & Buckling, A. (2004) Cooperation and competition in pathogenic bacteria. *Nature*, **430**, 1024–1027.

Hagen, D. C., Bretscher, A. P. & Kaiser, D. (1978) Synergism between morphogenetic mutants of *Myxococcus xanthus*. *Developmental Biology*, **64**, 284–296.

Hall-Stoodley, L. & Stoodley, P. (2005) Biofilm formation and dispersal and the transmission of human pathogens. *Trends in Microbiology*, **13**, 7–10.

Hall-Stoodley, L., Costerton, J. W. & Stoodley, P. (2004) Bacterial biofilms: from the natural environment to infectious diseases. *Nature Reviews Microbiology*, **2**, 95–108.

Hamilton, W. D. (1964) The genetical evolution of social behaviour, I & II. *Journal of Theoretical Biology*, **7**, 1–52.

Hammer, B. K. & Bassler, B. L. (2003) Quorum sensing controls biofilm formation in *Vibrio cholerae*. *Molecular Microbiology*, **50**, 101–104.

Harrison, F. & Buckling, A. (2005) Hypermutability impedes cooperation in pathogenic bacteria. *Current Biology*, **15**, 1968–1971.

Harrison, F. & Buckling, A. (2007) High relatedness selects against hypermutability in bacterial metapopulations. *Proceedings of the Royal Society B: Biological Sciences*, **274**, 1341–1347.

Harrison, F., Browning, L., Vos, M. & Buckling, A. (2006) Cooperation and virulence in acute *Pseudomonas aeruginosa* infections. *BMC Biology*, **4**, 21.

Harshey, R. M. (2003) Bacterial motility on a surface: many ways to a common goal. *Annual Review of Microbiology*, **57**, 249–273.

Havarstein, L. S., Coomaraswamy, G. & Morrison, D. A. (1995) An unmodified heptadecapeptide pheromone induces competence for genetic transformation in *Streptococcus pneumoniae*. *Proceedings of the National Academy of Sciences of the USA*, **92**, 11140–11144.

Hazan, R. & Engelberg-Kulka, H. (2004) *Escherichia coli* mazEF-mediated cell death as a defense mechanism that inhibits the spread of phage P1. *Molecular Genetics and Genomics*, **272**, 227–234.

Hazan, R., Sat, B. & Engelberg-Kulka, H. (2003) *Escherichia coli* mazEF-mediated cell death is triggered by various stressful conditions. *Journal of Bacteriology*, **186**, 3663–3669.

Helantera, H. & Bargum, K. (2007) Pedigree relatedness, not greenbeard genes, explains eusociality. *Oikos*, **116**, 217–220.

Helgason, T. & Fitter, A. (2005) The ecology and evolution of the arbuscular mycorrhizal fungi. *Mycologist*, **19**, 96–101.

Hogan, D. A. (2006) Talking to themselves: autoregulation and quorum sensing in fungi. *Eukaryotic Cell*, **5**, 613–619.

Hornby, J. M., Jensen, E. C., Lisec, A. D. *et al.* (2001) Quorum sensing in the dimorphic fungus *Candida albicans* is mediated by farnesol. *Applied and Environmental Microbiology*, **67**, 2982–2992.

Julien, B., Kaiser, A. D. & Garza, A. (2000) Spatial control of cell differentiation in *Myxococcus xanthus*. *Proceedings of the National Academy of Sciences of the USA*, **97**, 9098–9103.

Jurado, R. L. (1997) Iron, infections, and anemia of inflammation. *Clinical Infectious Diseases*, **25**, 888–895.

Kaiser, D. (2007) Bacterial swarming: a re-examination of cell-movement patterns. *Current Biology*, **17**, R561–R570.

Keller, L. & Surette, M. G. (2006) Communication in bacteria: an ecological and evolutionary perspective. *Nature Reviews Microbiology*, **4**, 249–258.

Keren, I., Kaldalu, N., Spoering, A., Wang, Y. & Lewis, K. (2004) Persister cells and tolerance to antimicrobials. *FEMS Microbiology Letters*, **230**, 13–18.

Kerr, B., Riley, M. A., Feldman, M. W. & Bohannan, B. J. (2002) Local dispersal promotes biodiversity in a real-life game of rock–paper–scissors. *Nature*, **418**, 171–174.

Kerr, B., Neuhauser, C., Bohannan, B. J. M. & Dean, A. M. (2006) Local migration promotes competitive restraint in a host–pathogen 'tragedy of the commons'. *Nature*, **442**, 75–78.

Kessin, R. H. (2001) *Dictyostelium: Evolution, Cell Biology, and the Development of Multicellularity*. Cambridge: Cambridge University Press.

Kiers, E. T., Rousseau, R. A., West, S. A. & Denison, R. F. (2003) Host sanctions and the legume-rhizobia mutualism. *Nature*, **425**, 78–81.

Kim, W., Killam, T., Sood, V. & Surette, M. G. (2003) Swarm-cell differentiation in *Salmonella enterica* serovar typhimurium results in elevated resistance to multiple antibiotics. *Journal of Bacteriology*, **185**, 3111–3117.

Klausen, M., Aaes-Jorgensen, A., Molin, S. & Tolker-Nielsen, T. (2003) Involvement of bacterial migration in the development of complex multicellular structures in *Pseudomonas aeruginosa* biofilms. *Molecular Microbiology*, **50**, 61–68.

Kohler, T., Curty, L. K., Barja, F., van Delden, C. & Pechere, J.-C. (2000) Swarming of *Pseudomonas aeruginosa* is dependent on cell-to-cell signaling and requires flagella and pili. *Journal of Bacteriology*, **182**, 5990–5996.

Kolenbrander, P. E. (2000) Oral microbial communities: biofilms, interactions, and genetic systems. *Annual Review of Microbiology*, **54**, 413–437.

Kolter, R. & Greenberg, E. P. (2006) Microbial sciences: the superficial life of microbes. *Nature*, **441**, 300–302.

König, H., Frohlich, J., Li, L. *et al.* (2007) The flagellates of the Australian termite *Mastotermes darwiniensis*: identification of their symbiotic bacteria and cellulases. *Symbiosis*, **44**, 1–65.

Kostakioti, M., Newman, C. L., Thanassi, D. G. & Stathopoulos, C. (2005) Mechanisms of protein export across the bacterial outer membrane. *Journal of Bacteriology*, **187**, 4306–4314.

Kreft, J. U. (2004) Biofilms promote altruism. *Microbiology*, **150**, 2751–2760.

Kreft, J. U. & Bonhoeffer, S. (2005) The evolution of groups of cooperating bacteria and the growth rate versus yield trade-off. *Microbiology*, **151**, 637–641.

Kropotkin, P. A. (1902) *Mutual Aid: a Factor of Evolution*. New York, NY: McClure Philips.

Kuhl, M., Glud, R. N., Ploug, H. & Ramsing, N. B. (1996) Microenvironmental control of photosynthesis and photosynthesis-coupled respiration in an epilithic cyanobacterial biofilm. *Journal of Phycology*, **32**, 799–812.

Kussell, E. & Leibler, S. (2005) Phenotypic diversity, population growth, and information in fluctuating environments. *Science*, **309**, 2075–2078.

Kuzdzal-Fick, J. J., Foster, K. R., Queller, D. C. & Strassmann, J. E. (2007) Exploiting new terrain: an advantage to sociality in the slime mold *Dictyostelium discoideum*. *Behavioral Ecology*, **18**, 433.

Lehmann, L. (2006) The evolution of trans-generational altruism: kin selection meets niche construction. *Journal of Evolutionary Biology*, **20**, 181–189.

MacLean, R. C. & Gudelj, I. (2006) Resource competition and social conflict in experimental populations of yeast. *Nature*, **441**, 498–501.

Magnuson, R., Solomon, J. & Grossman, A. D. (1994) Biochemical and genetic characterization of a competence pheromone from *B. subtilis*. *Cell*, **77**, 207–216.

Magnuson, R. D. (2007) Hypothetical functions of toxin-antitoxin systems. *Journal of Bacteriology*, **189**, 6089–6092.

Mah, T. F., Pitts, B., Pellock, B. *et al.* (2003) A genetic basis for *Pseudomonas aeruginosa* biofilm antibiotic resistance. *Nature*, **426**, 306–310.

Mashburn, L. M. & Whiteley, M. (2005) Membrane vesicles traffic signals and facilitate group activities in a prokaryote. *Nature*, **437**, 422–425.

Mashburn-Warren, L. M. & Whiteley, M. (2006) Special delivery: vesicle trafficking in prokaryotes. *Molecular Microbiology*, **61**, 839–846.

Massey, R. C., Buckling, A. & ffrench-Constant, R. (2004) Interference competition and parasite virulence. *Proceedings of the Royal Society B*, **271**, 785–788.

Mehdiabadi, N. J., Jack, C. N., Farnham, T. T. *et al.* (2006) Social evolution: kin preference in a social microbe. *Nature*, **442**, 881–882.

Meibom, K. L., Blokesch, M., Dolganov, N. A., Wu, C.-Y. & Schoolnik, G. K. (2005) Chitin induces natural competence in *Vibrio cholerae*. *Science*, **310**, 1824–1827.

Mergaert, P., Uchiumi, T., Alunni, B. *et al.* (2006) Eukaryotic control on bacterial cell cycle and differentiation in the Rhizobium–legume symbiosis. *Proceedings of the National Academy of Sciences of the USA*, **103**, 5230–5235.

Metzger, S., Dror, I. B., Aizenman, E. *et al.* (1988) The nucleotide sequence and characterization of the relA gene of *Escherichia coli*. *Journal of Biological Chemistry*, **263**, 15699–15704.

Michod, R. E. (2006) The group covariance effect and fitness trade-offs during evolutionary transitions in individuality. *Proceedings of the National Academy of Sciences of the USA*, **103**, 9113–9117.

Michod, R. E. & Roze, D. (2001) Cooperation and conflict in the evolution of multicellularity. *Heredity*, **86**, 1–7.

Miller, M. B. & Bassler, B. L. (2001) Quorum sensing in bacteria. *Annual Review of Microbiology*, **55**, 165–199.

Mueller, U. G., Poulin, J. & Adams, R. M. M. (2004) Symbiont choice in a fungus-growing ant (Attini, Formicidae). *Behavioral Ecology*, **15**, 357–364.

Nachman, I., Regev, A. & Ramanathan, S. (2007) Dissecting timing variability in yeast meiosis. *Cell*, **131**, 544–556.

Nadell, C. D., Xavier, J. B., Levin, S. A. & Foster, K. R. (2008) The evolution of quorum sensing in bacterial biofilms. *PLoS Biology*, **6** (1), e14.

Nadell, C. D., Xavier, J. & Foster, K. R. (2009) The sociobiology of biofilms. *FEMS Microbiology Reviews*, **33**, 206–224.

Narra, H. P. & Ochman, H. (2006) Of what use is sex to bacteria? *Current Biology*, **16**, R705–R710.

Nealson, K. H., Platt, T. & Hastings, J. W. (1970) Cellular control of the synthesis and activity of the bacterial luminescent system. *Journal of Bacteriology*, **104**, 313–322.

Noda, S., Ohkuma, M., Yamada, A., Hongoh, Y. & Kudo, T. (2003) Phylogenetic position and in situ identification of ectosymbiotic spirochetes on protists in the termite gut. *Applied and Environmental Microbiology*, **69**, 625–633.

Nonacs, P. & Kapheim, K. M. (2007) Social heterosis and the maintenance of genetic diversity. *Journal of Evolutionary Biology*, **20**, 2253–2265.

Novak, M., Pfeiffer, T., Lenski, R. E., Sauer, U. & Bonhoeffer, S. (2006) Experimental tests for an evolutionary trade-off between growth rate and yield in *E. coli*. *American Naturalist*, **168**, 242–251.

Nunney, L. (1999) Lineage selection and the evolution of multistage carcinogenesis. *Proceedings of the Royal Society B*, **266**, 493–498.

Oliver, A., Canton, R., Campo, P., Baquero, F. & Blazquez, J. (2000) High frequency of hypermutable *Pseudomonas aeruginosa* in cystic fibrosis lung infection. *Science*, **288**, 1251–1254.

Palmer, R. J., Kazmerzak, K., Hansen, M. C. & Kolenbrander, P. E. (2001) Mutualism versus independence: strategies of mixed-species oral biofilms in vitro using saliva as the sole nutrient source. *Infection and Immunity*, **69**, 5794–5804.

Parsek, M. R. & Greenberg, E. P. (2005) Sociomicrobiology: the connections between quorum sensing and biofilms. *Trends in Microbiology*, **13**, 27–33.

Paulsson, J. (2002) Multileveled selection on plasmid replication. *Genetics*, **161**, 1373–1384.

Pearson, J. P., Van Delden, C. & Iglewski, B. H. (1999) Active efflux and diffusion are involved in transport of *Pseudomonas aeruginosa* cell-to-cell signals. *Journal of Bacteriology*, **181**, 1203–1210.

Pfeiffer, T. & Bonhoeffer, S. (2004) Evolution of cross-feeding in microbial populations. *American Naturalist*, **163**, E126–135.

Pfeiffer, T. & Schuster, S. (2005) Game-theoretical approaches to studying the evolution of biochemical systems. *Trends in Biochemical Sciences*, **30**, 20–25.

Pfeiffer, T., Schuster, S. & Bonhoeffer, S. (2001) Cooperation and competition in the evolution of ATP-producing pathways. *Science*, **292**, 504–507.

Piper, K. R., von Bodman, S. B. & Farrand, S. K. (1993) Conjugation factor of *Agrobacterium tumefaciens* regulates Ti plasmid transfer by autoinduction. *Nature*, **362**, 448–450.

Poulsen, M. & Boomsma, J. J. (2005) Mutualistic fungi control crop diversity in fungus-growing ants. *Science*, **307**, 741–744.

Queller, D. C., Ponte, E., Bozzaro, S. & Strassmann, J. E. (2003) Single-gene greenbeard effects in the social amoeba *Dictyostelium discoideum*. *Science*, **299**, 105–106.

Rainey, P. B. & Rainey, K. (2003) Evolution of cooperation and conflict in experimental bacterial populations. *Nature*, **425**, 72–74.

Rando, O. J. & Verstrepen, K. J. (2007) Timescales of genetic and epigenetic inheritance. *Cell*, **128**, 655–668.

Rankin, D. J., López-Sepulcre, A., Foster, K. R. & Kokko, H. (2007a) Species-level selection reduces selfishness through competitive exclusion. *Journal of Evolutionary Biology*, **20**, 1459–1468.

Rankin, D. J., Bargum, K. & Kokko, H. (2007b) The tragedy of the commons in evolutionary biology. *Trends in Ecology and Evolution*, **22**, 643–651.

Ratnieks, F. L. W., Foster, K. R. & Wenseleers, T. (2006) Conflict resolution in insect societies. *Annual Review of Entomology*, **51**, 581–608.

Reichenbach, T., Mobilia, M. & Frey, E. (2007) Mobility promotes and jeopardizes biodiversity in rock–paper–scissors games. *Nature*, **448**, 1046–1049.

Ryu, J.-H., Kim, S.-H., Lee, H.-Y. *et al.* (2008) Innate immune homeostasis by the homeobox gene caudal and commensal-gut mutualism in *Drosophila*. *Science*, **319**, 777–782.

Sachs, J. L., Mueller, U. G., Wilcox, T. P. & Bull, J. J. (2004) The evolution of cooperation. *Quarterly Review of Biology*, **79**, 135–160.

Sandoz, K. M., Mitzimberg, S. M. & Schuster, M. (2007) Social cheating in *Pseudomonas aeruginosa* quorum sensing. *Proceedings of the National Academy of Sciences of the USA*, **104**, 15876–15881.

Santorelli, L. A., Thompson, C. R. L., Villegas, E. *et al.* (2008) Facultative cheater mutants reveal the genetic complexity of cooperation in social amoebae. *Nature* **451**, 1107.

Sauer, K., Camper, A. K., Ehrlich, G. D., Costerton, J. W. & Davies, D. G. (2002) *Pseudomonas aeruginosa* displays multiple phenotypes during development as a biofilm. *Journal of Bacteriology*, **184**, 1140–1154.

Schwartz, M. W. & Hoeksema, J. D. (1998) Specialization and resource trade: biological markets as a model of mutualisms. *Ecology*, **79**, 1029–1038.

Shaulsky, G. & Kessin, R. H. (2007) The cold war of the social amoebae. *Current Biology*, **17**, R684–692.

Simms, E. L., Taylor, D. L., Povich, J. *et al.* (2006) An empirical test of partner choice mechanisms in a wild legume-rhizobium interaction. *Proceedings of the Royal Society B*, **273**, 77–81.

Smith, E. E., Sims, E. H., Spencer, D. H., Kaul, R. & Olson, M. V. (2005) Evidence for diversifying selection at the pyoverdine locus of *Pseudomonas aeruginosa*. *Journal of Bacteriology*, **187**, 2138–2147.

Smith, E. E., Buckley, D. G., Wu, Z. *et al.* (2006) Genetic adaptation by *Pseudomonas aeruginosa* to the airways of cystic fibrosis patients. *Proceedings of the National Academy of Sciences of the USA*, **103**, 8487–8492.

Smith, J. (2001) The social evolution of bacterial pathogenesis. *Proceedings of the Royal Society B*, **268**, 61–69.

Smukalla, S., Caldara, M., Pochet, N. *et al.* (2008) FLO1 is a variable green beard gene that drives biofilm-like cooperation in budding yeast. *Cell*, **135**, 727–737.

Spencer, H. (1879) *The Data of Ethics*. London: Williams & Norgate.

Stewart, P. S. (2003) Diffusion in biofilms. *Journal of Bacteriology*, **185**, 1485–1491.

Stintzi, A., Evans, K., Meyer, J. M. & Poole, K. (1998) Quorum-sensing and siderophore biosynthesis in *Pseudomonas aeruginosa*: lasR/lasI mutants exhibit reduced pyoverdine biosynthesis. *FEMS Microbiology Letters*, **166**, 341–345.

Suel, G. M., Garcia-Ojalvo, J., Liberman, L. M. & Elowitz, M. B. (2006) An excitable gene regulatory circuit induces transient cellular differentiation. *Nature*, **440**, 545–550.

Tamm, S. L. (1982) Flagellated ectosymbiotic bacteria propel a eucaryotic cell. *Journal of Cell Biology*, **94**, 697–709.

Thomas, C. M. & Nielsen, K. M. (2005) Mechanisms of, and barriers to, horizontal gene transfer between bacteria. *Nature Reviews Microbiology*, **3**, 711–721.

Tinbergen, N. (1963) On aims and methods of ethology. *Zeitschrift für Tierpsychologie*, **20**, 410–433.

Tortosa, P., Logsdon, L., Kraigher, B., Itoh, Y., Mandic-Mulec, I. & Dubnau, D. (2001) Specificity and genetic polymorphism of the *Bacillus* competence quorum-sensing system. *Journal of Bacteriology*, **183**, 451–460.

Travisano, M. & Velicer, G. J. (2004) Strategies of microbial cheater control. *Trends in Microbiology*, **12**, 72–78.

Tsilibaris, V., Maenhaut-Michel, G., Mine, N. & Van Melderen, L. (2007) What is the benefit to *Escherichia coli* of having multiple toxin-antitoxin systems in its genome? *Journal of Bacteriology*, **189**, 6101–6108.

Tsuchiya, M., Wong, S. T., Yeo, Z. X. *et al.* (2007) Gene expression waves. Cell cycle independent collective dynamics in cultured cells. *FEBS Journal*, **274**, 2878–2886.

Tuemmler, B. & Cornelis, P. (2005) Pyoverdine receptor: a case of positive darwinian selection in *Pseudomonas aeruginosa*. *Journal of Bacteriology*, **187**, 3289–3292.

Turner, P. E. & Chao, L. (1999) Prisoner's dilemma in an RNA virus. *Nature*, **398**, 441–443.

van der Ploeg, J. R. (2005) Regulation of bacteriocin production in *Streptococcus mutans* by the quorum-sensing system required for development of genetic competence. *Journal of Bacteriology*, **187**, 3980–3989.

Velicer, G. J. (2003) Social strife in the microbial world. *Trends in Microbiology*, **11**, 330–337.

Velicer, G. J. & Yu, Y. T. N. (2003) Evolution of novel cooperative swarming in the bacterium *Myxococcus xanthus*. *Nature*, **425**, 75–78.

Velicer, G. J., Kroos, L. & Lenski, R. E. (1998) Loss of social behaviors by *Myxococcus xanthus* during evolution in an unstructured habitat. *Proceedings of the National Academy of Sciences of the USA*, **95**, 12376–12380.

Velicer, G. J., Kroos, L. & Lenski, R. E. (2000) Developmental cheating in the social bacterium *Myxococcus xanthus*. *Nature*, **404**, 598–601.

Verstrepen, K. J., Jansen, A., Lewitter, F. & Fink, G. R. (2005) Intragenic tandem repeats generate functional variability. *Nature Genetics*, **37**, 986–990.

Visick, K. L., Foster, J., Doino, J., McFall-Ngai, M. & Ruby, E. G. (2000) *Vibrio fischeri* lux genes play an important role in colonization and development of the host light organ. *Journal of Bacteriology*, **182**, 4578–4586.

Vlamakis, H., Aguilar, C., Losick, R. & Kolter, R. (2008) Control of cell fate by the formation of an architecturally complex bacterial community. *Genes and Development*, **22**, 945.

Vulic, M. & Kolter, R. (2001) Evolutionary cheating in *Escherichia coli* stationary phase cultures. *Genetics*, **158**, 519–526.

Wenseleers, T. & Ratnieks, F. L. (2006) Enforced altruism in insect societies. *Nature*, **444**, 50.

Wenzel, M., Radek, R., Brugerolle, G. & König, H. (2003) Identification of the ectosymbiotic bacteria of *Mixotricha paradoxa* involved in movement symbiosis. *European Journal of Protistology*, **39**, 11–23.

West, S. A., Griffin, A. S., Gardner, A. & Diggle, S. P. (2006) Social evolution theory for microorganisms. *Nature Reviews Microbiology*, **4**, 597–607.

West, S. A., Griffin, A. S. & Gardner, A. (2007) Social semantics: altruism, cooperation, mutualism, strong reciprocity and group selection. *Journal of Evolutionary Biology*, **20**, 415–432.

Williams, H. T. P. & Lenton, T. M. (2008) Environmental regulation in a network of simulated microbial ecosystems. *Proceedings of the National Academy of Sciences of the USA*, **105**, 10432–10437.

Wilson, E. O. (1975) *Sociobiology: the New Synthesis.* Cambridge, MA: Harvard University Press.

Wireman, J. W. & Dworkin, M. (1977) Developmentally induced autolysis during fruiting body formation by *Myxococcus xanthus. Journal of Bacteriology,* **129**, 798–802.

Wykoff, D. D., Rizvi, A. H., Raser, J. M., Margolin, B. & O'Shea, E. K. (2007) Positive feedback regulates switching of phosphate transporters in *S. cerevisiae. Molecular Cell,* **27**, 1005–1013.

Xavier, J. B. & Foster, K. R. (2007) Cooperation and conflict in microbial biofilms. *Proceedings of the National Academy of Sciences of the USA,* **104**, 876–881.

Xavier, K. B. & Bassler, B. L. (2005) Interference with AI-2-mediated bacterial cell-cell communication. *Nature,* **437**, 750–753.

Xu, K. D., Stewart, P. S., Xia, F., Huang, C.-T. & McFeters, G. A. (1998) Spatial physiological heterogeneity in *Pseudomonas aeruginosa* biofilm is determined by oxygen availability. *Applied and Environmental Microbiology,* **64**, 4035–4039.

The de novo evolution of cooperation: an unlikely event

Paul B. Rainey

My interest in the evolution of diversity in microbial populations began more than 20 years ago. For the first 10 of those years I was oblivious to the fact that one of the most dramatic forms to emerge during the course of selection experiments, the so-named wrinkly spreader (WS) type, owed its success to cooperation among individual cells. Rather ashamedly, despite having recognised the novelty of what I had witnessed, it took me another 10 years to get round to publishing this work. Perhaps, however, an attempt to publish in the early 1990s, in the absence of studies that gave credibility to the microcosm experiments (see Chapter 13), would have met with limited success.

There was no eureka moment of realisation, although with hindsight there ought to have been. I was aware that WS genotypes formed cellular mats that grew at the air–liquid interface of broth-filled microcosms (Rainey & Travisano 1998). I was also aware that the ability to occupy the air–liquid interface was the secret of their evolutionary success (the broth phase rapidly become anaerobic due to microbial growth). Most tellingly, I was aware that the mats sank into the broth when they became old and heavy. It should therefore have been obvious that cells growing at the air–liquid interface had to be connected to neighbouring cells and, via connections to the neighbours of neighbours, ultimately to be cemented firmly to the edge of the glass

vial. However, it was not until genetic analysis of the defining features of WS revealed the central importance of a cellulosic polymer (Spiers *et al.* 2002) that I realised that this polymer was 'glue', and that the glue was the substance that made the connections. More profound, though, was recognition (backed by several lines of experimental evidence) that the mutations that caused over-production of the glue reduced the fitness of individual WS cells (Knight *et al.* 2006). And yet the WS mutants increased in frequency. The cause of their success had to lie in some benefit that accrued above the level of the individual cell. The mat of course was the answer: the mat is the cumulative product of the cooperative interactions of millions of cells. By working together, the cells in the mat are able to colonise a niche unavailable to the ancestral type. In colonising this new niche, the cells of the mat are rewarded with an abundance of oxygen (Rainey & Rainey 2003).

As the significance of what had been observed became clear, I began to wonder about the extent to which WS evolution conformed to theoretical predictions. My initial focus was on explanations for the evolution of cooperation. In the case of WS evolution, interactions among kin (promoted by spatial structure) were of central importance and I saw no need, or evidence, to invoke selection among groups (not that the latter cannot happen). Subsequent investigations turned to the downside

Social Behaviour: Genes, Ecology and Evolution, ed. Tamás Székely, Allen J. Moore and Jan Komdeur. Published by Cambridge University Press. © Cambridge University Press 2010.

357

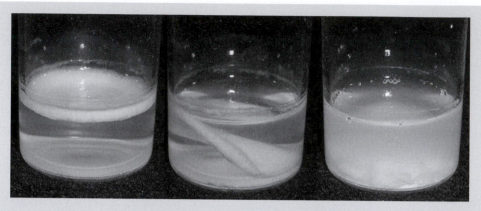

The rise, the fall and the outright destruction of a simple undifferentiated group. Left: the wrinkly spreader mat is the cumulative product of the cooperative interactions of millions of cells. By working together, the cells in the mat colonise the air–liquid interface – a niche that is unavailable to the ancestral (broth-colonising) type. In colonising this new niche the cells of the mat are rewarded with an abundance of oxygen. Middle: when the mat becomes too heavy it collapses into the broth (it is not buoyant); the collapse is hastened by the presence of cheating genotypes that grow like a cancer within the mat, adding no structural strength but reaping the benefits (access to oxygen). Right: a mat is far more than the sum of the individual parts. This photo was taken immediately after disturbing (with a brief shake) a microcosm with an intact mat. The mat breaks into many pieces (just visible on the bottom) and does not spontaneously reform. While a mat will eventually re-emerge, it will do so by a process of growth and development from just a single cell.

of cooperation: the inevitable conflict between the interests of individuals and groups. If cooperation (as I claimed) was costly, then theory predicted the emergence of cheats that would hasten the demise of newly emergent cooperating groups. A search for cheating types revealed mutants that grew as a cancer within the mat. Analysis of these cheaters showed that they no longer over-produced the polymer, and as a consequence they grew faster than the cooperating types. They enjoyed the benefits of group membership (access to oxygen), but they did not contribute to mat strength, which meant the collapse of WS groups. A classic tragedy of the commons (see Chapter 6).

The profound nature of WS evolution and the demise of these groups perhaps explain why the obvious was overlooked for so long. One does not expect to observe, directly and in real time, the de novo evolution of cooperation – that is, the evolution of cooperation from an ancestral type that behaves selfishly and has no capacity for social behaviour. This is the evolution of cooperation in a deeply profound and primordial sense. As such, WS evolution provides an opportunity to study the emergence of cooperation in a way that is not possible through the study of an organism, or group, in which cooperation or sociality evolved some time in the past, in response to unknown selective conditions and with unknowable genetic causes.

Of course direct observation of cooperation opens the door to many interesting possibilities. For a start it becomes possible to assign causality in terms of the selective conditions (Rainey & Rainey 2003), the genetic events (Bantinaki *et al.* 2007), their phenotypic consequences (Spiers *et al.* 2002, Goymer *et al.* 2006), and so forth. It also shifts the level of inquiry to embrace new kinds of questions. One question that continues to intrigue me is the point at which the costs of cooperation to individual cells are traded against the benefit gained at the group level. Does this occur after the first cell division (when two cells are joined), or after a single layer of cells has spread across the surface and attached to the vial edge, or at some intermediate point? What is the dynamic? And what about development and emergence? As is evident in the accompanying photo, the mat is far more than the product of the sum of the individual cooperating cells: the success of the group is intimately linked to the development of the mat. What theory incorporates development into our understanding of cooperation?

As a final point I mention an emerging fascination: the further evolution of groups (see also Chapter 6). At first glance, group selection experiments are straightforward: the experimenter imposes selection for some group-level property, for example mat strength. This involves the experimenter deciding before the experiment on the particular property of the group that s/he will select for; it also involves the experimenter acting as the means of group reproduction. We have performed such group selection experiments with dramatic group-level responses, including the evolutionary emergence of differentiation and a division of labour (M. McDonald & P. B. Rainey, unpublished), but in reality I feel these experiments fall short of the mark. The dissatisfaction stems from the fact that the experimenter must define the group-level trait upon which to select, and must also be the means of group reproduction. This precludes the evolution of groups in ways that would see a genuine improvement in the Darwinian fitness of groups. As I have explained elsewhere, simple groups, such as WS mats, lack a crucial element of individuality: the ability to reproduce as a collective (P. B. Rainey & B. Kerr, unpublished; Rainey 2007). This curtails the ability of groups to participate in the process of evolution by natural selection. And yet groups must have participated in this process.

My pondering of this problem through the eyes of an experimentalist has led to the realisation of a simple way forward which involves nothing other than recognising that the WS group and the cheaters that arise from it comprise a rudimentary life cycle – the mat being synonymous with soma and the cheat a kind of germ line. The success of the two stages is intimately linked. Rightly or wrongly, given an appropriate set of ecological conditions, it does become possible for selection to act very powerfully on the higher-level collective, with the cells of the lower level being integral to this process. Our experiments continue ...

Principles that have guided my research:
(1) curiosity
(2) the predictive power of Darwin's theory of evolution by natural selection
(3) the desire to provide a mechanistic explanation for the evolution of individuality

References

Bantinaki, E., Kassen, R., Knight, C. *et al.* (2007) Adaptive divergence in experimental populations of *Pseudomonas fluorescens*. III. Mutational origins of wrinkly spreader diversity. *Genetics*, **176**, 441–453.

Goymer, P., Kahn, S. G., Malone, J. G. *et al.* (2006) Adaptive divergence in experimental populations of *Pseudomonas fluorescens*. II. Role of the GGDEF regulator, WspR, in evolution and development of the wrinkly spreader phenotype. *Genetics*, **173**, 515–526.

Knight, C. G., Zitzmann, N., Prabhakar, S. *et al.* (2006) Unravelling adaptive evolution: how a single point mutation affects the protein co-regulation network. *Nature Genetics* **38**, 1015–1022.

Rainey, P. B. (2007) Unity from conflict. *Nature*, **446**, 616.

Rainey, P. B. & Rainey, K. (2003) Evolution of cooperation and conflict in experimental bacterial populations. *Nature*, **425**, 72–74.

Rainey, P. B. & Travisano, M. (1998) Adaptive radiation in a heterogeneous environment. *Nature*, **394**, 69–72.

Spiers, A. J., Kahn, S. G., Bohannon, J., Travisano, M. & Rainey, P. B. (2002) Adaptive divergence in experimental populations of *Pseudomonas fluorescens*. I. Genetic and phenotypic bases of wrinkly spreader fitness. *Genetics*, **161**, 33–46.

14

Social environments, social tactics and their fitness consequences in complex mammalian societies

Marion L. East and Heribert Hofer

Overview

In this chapter we outline proximate processes that favour group formation and lead to the emergence of social structure in mammalian societies, particularly complex societies. We operationally define a mammalian society as complex if its social structure includes social coalitions, social alliances or social queues – well known from primates, elephants and cetaceans but also present in, for instance, some carnivores, bats, rodents and ungulates. We consider how social structure can lead to a disparity in the benefits and costs acquired by group members, and how this leads to conflicts of interest between them. We detail the social and reproductive tactics that individuals use when conflicts arise, and consider the fitness consequences associated with these tactics. We illustrate most key points using observational studies of free-ranging mammals, because experimental studies are rare, and we draw examples from a broad range of social systems and mammalian orders.

14.1 Introduction

How do complex societies emerge from a life in groups? Living in groups inevitably results in conflicts of interest between group members. The specific forms of these conflicts are likely to affect the strategies to cope with them. Not only will the details of these strategies shape the social relationships we can observe, they may be the consequences of evolutionary processes, and are likely to have resulted in the social complexity described for many mammalian societies. We seek to tackle these issues by discussing both theoretical and observational studies, considering the contribution of important physiological mechanisms and focusing on the fitness consequences of traits relevant to group living, particularly social and reproductive tactics. The fitness consequences of social and reproductive tactics are important because there is growing evidence that social factors can be a force of natural selection as potent as environmental or ecological factors such as predation, competition, food resources, shelter or pathogens.

We begin by considering the value of group formation, which provides the opportunity to gather social information. We then consider how group formation provides the opportunity to share social goods, under

Social Behaviour: Genes, Ecology and Evolution, ed. Tamás Székely, Allen J. Moore and Jan Komdeur. Published by Cambridge University Press. © Cambridge University Press 2010.

which conditions cooperative behaviour improves an individual's efficiency of resource acquisition, and which mechanisms of individual recognition assist an individual's life in a group. This is followed by a discussion of how social structure emerges within groups, which mechanisms produce an individual's social status, how valuable social relationships and social networks are developed and maintained, and to what extent brain size is a cause or a consequence of social complexity. We then consider important physiological mechanisms and evolutionary consequences of reproductive tactics and review the consequences of sexual selection, particularly sexual conflict and female mate choice, within a social environment.

14.2 Social information

To exploit opportunities and avoid danger, individuals need to gather information and select between the options open to them. Gathering information requires time and energy and may involve risks. The gathering of personal information will be limited by constraints on time and resources and by the trial-and-error nature of such information gathering (Dall *et al.* 2005). By forming groups, animals can access public information (social information), a benefit thought to be a key driving force in social evolution (Danchin *et al.* 2004).

Public information may be inadvertently passed between animals (inadvertent social information). Several studies on fish and birds have demonstrated inadvertent information exchange and have called this a bystander effect (Dugatkin 2001, Chase *et al.* 2002) or social eavesdropping (Earley & Dugatkin 2002, Peake 2005). A mammalian example involves pregnant female mice *Mus musculus* housed next to conspecifics infected with a non-contagious pathogen (*Babesia microti*) that produced offspring

which mounted an accelerated immune response to *B. microti* infection as adults (Curno *et al.* 2009).

Public information also includes the intentional transmission of information with the use of specific signals evolved for this purpose (e.g. see section 14.4). Social signals need not always be reliable, and may even be deceitful and designed to manipulate social partners (see sections 14.3.2 and 14.10.4). For this reason, animals in groups require strategies to decide how best to allocate effort to gathering their own information (personal information) and when to rely on personal information or social information obtained from observing the behaviour of others (Dall *et al.* 2005).

Imitation of behavioural patterns learnt through the exchange of social information can result in the development of traditions passed across generations, leading to the formation of distinct cultures within particular animal groups or populations, such as the culture of foraging with a marine sponge in the bottlenose dolphin *Tursiops truncatus* (Krützen *et al.* 2005).

14.3 Social goods and cooperation

Social goods arise when individuals invest in cooperative activities that provide benefits to group members, or when members refrain from activities that generate conflict within the society (Frank 1995). The efficiency of many essential activities can be increased by cooperation, thereby providing fitness benefits that exceed those obtained in the absence of cooperation. Activities that have been shown to benefit from cooperation include foraging, resource defence, protection against predation and the collective rearing of young (Box 14.1). Thus, sociality provides many benefits but it also entails costs (Chapter 9; Alexander 1974, Bertram 1978, Walters & Seyfarth 1986), such as an increased chance of infection by pathogens (e.g. Pontier *et al.* 1998, East *et al.* 2001).

Box 14.1 Social environments and offspring survival

Cooperative care of offspring is one important benefit of social life. For example, female sperm whales *Physeter macrocephalus* hunt at depths that their young calves cannot reach. As a result, young calves are left at the surface, where they are

Box 14.1 Continued

vulnerable to attack by large sharks and killer whales *Orcinus orca*. When vulnerable calves are present in a foraging group, females stagger their deep dives to reduce the time calves are unattended by an adult at the surface (Whitehead 1996). As babysitting is considered to be a cultural trait in sperm whales, matrilines that take up babysitting have an advantage compared to those that do not, with potentially profound effects on the evolution and genetic structure of the population (Whitehead 1998, 1999). As some females within sperm whale groups are unrelated (Mesnick 2001) it would be interesting to know whether related and unrelated females are equally willing to cooperate in babysitting activities.

Female family group members of African savanna elephants *Loxodonta africana* also cooperate to guard young calves against predator attacks and to care for calves while their mothers rest or feed (Lee 1987). Babysitting probably explains improved calf survival with both increased family group size and the number of carers per family (Lee 1989). Similarly, in banded mongooses *Mungos mungo*, where pups are produced synchronously in a group, pup survival increases with the number of available babysitters (Cant 2003).

Even without communal or cooperative care, sociality itself may be sufficiently important to benefit offspring. Silk *et al.* (2003) studied the effect of strong social bonds among female savanna baboons *Papio cynocephalus* on the fitness of adult females. In these baboons, sociality of adult females was positively associated with infant survival to one year of age, and this effect was independent of social status, group membership or environmental conditions.

Although sociality itself or cooperative care of offspring may increase offspring survival, being reared in a social environment need not always be beneficial. For example, juvenile spotted hyenas *Crocuta crocuta* reared in communal dens are occasionally killed by female group members (Hofer & East 1995, White 2007). Infanticide of offspring of subordinate females by the dominant breeding female has also been observed in several cooperative-breeding mammals such as the African wild dog *Lycaon pictus* (Malcolm & Martin 1982), the dwarf mongoose *Helogale parvula* (Rood 1980) and the common marmoset *Callithrix jacchus* (Digby 1995). Fetuses of subordinate females in wolf *Canis lupus* packs have a lower chance of survival when packs suffer nutritional constraints (Hillis & Mallory 1996).

When the benefits and costs of group living are unequally distributed among group members, conflicts of interest between group members will arise (Chapter 9; Alexander 1974, Walters & Seyfarth 1986), and relationships between group members are likely to be asymmetric. In the coming sections we discuss under which conditions cooperation can evolve, how conflicts arise, how asymmetric relationships can lead to a stable social structure, which factors stabilise social structure and determine an individual's social position, and how animals respond to conflicts by trading biological goods, forming alliances, queuing, actively submitting, or avoiding conflicts altogether.

14.3.1 The evolution of cooperative behaviour

The evolution of cooperative behaviours among related animals has received much attention (Chapters 1, 4 and 6). Such behaviour includes altruism, a behaviour that is costly to the actor and beneficial to the recipient. It has been most successfully explained by the theory of kin selection (Hamilton 1964a, 1964b). There is considerable empirical evidence consistent with this theory (e.g. Griffin & West 2003, Chapais & Berman 2004).

Among unrelated animals with symmetrical relationships, altruism was first explained by Trivers' (1971) model of reciprocal altruism and later by the model of the prisoner's dilemma (Chapters 4 and 6; Michael Taborsky's profile; Axelrod & Hamilton 1981). Although the idea of reciprocal altruism is appealing, it has rarely been described in free-ranging social mammals, and each case appears open to alternative explanations. A study claiming to demonstrate reciprocal altruism among male baboons *Papio anubis* (Packer 1977) drew heavy criticism (Noë 1990), and is probably best viewed as an example of simple cooperation (Bercovitch 1988). A second, often cited, example are groups of female vampire bats *Desmodus rotundus* sharing a communal roost who also share blood meals by regurgitation to close kin and to individuals which may or may not be related but for which there is a high expectation of future encounters (Wilkinson 1984). Without measures of degrees of genetic relatedness amongst females that share blood meals (Wilkinson 1985) it is unclear whether this behaviour really is reciprocal altruism.

In the natural world, few relationships are symmetrical, and therefore an alternative approach has been developed to explain intraspecific cooperation in asymmetrical relationships – the *biological market models* (Ronald Noë's profile; Noë & Hammerstein 1994). These models can be applied to a range of situations, yet surprisingly their use has been limited. In these models, traders exchange commodities of mutual benefit, partner choice occurs through competition within trader classes (with preference for partners that offer the highest value for a particular commodity), and cheats cannot prosper. Although conflict is expected to arise between trading partners over the exchange value of a commodity, commodities are inalienable and cannot be obtained by force (Noë & Hammerstein 1995).

Henzi and Barrett (2002) applied a biological market approach to the study of social dynamics among female chacma baboons *Papio ursinus*. In accordance with expected market effects, they found that females seeking access to young (termed handlers) were prepared to groom mothers with young to gain access to infants, and as the availability of infants declined the duration of infant-related grooming by handlers increased, suggesting that animals were prepared to pay more for a scarce commodity. In contrast, dominant females used their high social status to immediately gain access to infants, thus obtaining the commodity by force and violating an assumption of biological market models. Other studies have suggested that dominance, coercion and punishment may act as market forces (Clutton-Brock & Parker 1995) and generate market effects (Barrett & Henzi 2001).

14.3.2 Cheating as a social tactic

Individuals that do not contribute to but still gain from social goods have been termed cheaters (Frank 1995). For example, in African lions *Panthera leo*, female pride members cooperate in the defence of their group territory against neighbouring prides, and skirmishes between prides may be costly in terms of physical injuries. Simulated territorial intrusions provided experimental evidence that some female pride members consistently cheated by never being among the first to approach simulated intruders (Heinsohn & Packer 1995).

Cheating is expected because individual selection is likely to be stronger than kin selection or selection through reciprocal altruism. When cheaters significantly reduce or destroy social goods, a conflict of interest will arise between cheaters and group members that do not cheat. Hardin's (1968) 'tragedy of the commons' analogy has been used to study such social dilemmas (Milinski *et al.* 2002, Rankin *et al.* 2007). Punishment of cheaters can be a mechanism that would prevent social goods from being destroyed (Clutton-Brock & Parker 1995, Frank 1995). However, when punishment is costly, individuals may gain little by punishing cheaters (Hauert *et al.* 2007), and for this reason acts of punishment should not be costly, or should provide increased benefits to those that exercise punishment (Gardner & West 2004). Diminishing returns obtained from social goods may also prevent selfish cheaters from destroying social goods (Rankin *et al.* 2007).

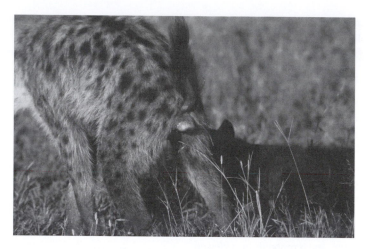

Figure 14.1 'Over-pasting' scent on grass stalks previously scent-marked by another group member helps spotted hyenas to concoct a group odour badge. Photo: M. L. East and H. Hofer.

14.4 Recognition of group members: a prerequisite for social life

The formation and functioning of a social group requires members of a group to recognise other group members and to distinguish these from non-group members. Group members may be known by the recognition of individual identity cues that are learnt through repeated encounters (Tibbetts & Dale 2007), or by the detection of a distinct group membership badge (Bradbury & Vehrencamp 1998).

Evidence for individual identity cues has been described in many social mammals in vocalisations (e.g. primates, Cheney & Seyfarth 1980, 1999; carnivores, East & Hofer 1991a, 1991b, Holekamp *et al.* 1999, Insley 2001; elephants, McComb *et al.* 2003; bats, Behr & von Helversen 2004; cetaceans, Sayigh *et al.* 2007) and olfactory signals (Bradbury & Vehrencamp 1998, Wyatt 2003, Burgener *et al.* 2009).

Group membership badges, in the form of group-specific calls, occur in species as diverse as the greater spear-nosed bat *Phyllostomus hastatus* (Boughman & Wilkinson 1998) and the killer whale *Orcinus orca* (Yurk *et al.* 2002, Riesch *et al.* 2006). Group-specific odours have been identified in naked mole-rat *Heterocephalus glaber* colonies (O'Riain & Jarvis 1997), maternal colonies of Bechstein's bat *Myotis*

bechsteinii (Kamran & Kerth 2003), beaver *Castor fiber* groups (Sun & Müller-Schwarze 1998) and spotted hyena *Crocuta crocuta* clans (Burgener *et al.* 2008).

How is a group identity badge formed, and how is it acquired by group members? In colonies of Bechstein's bat and the naked mole-rat, a group odour is concocted by the exchange of scent between individuals in close physical contact. In the spotted hyena, a group odour is concocted by remote exchange when group members collect scent deposited by other group members on vegetation. One group member pastes (Kruuk 1972) their fatty anal gland secretion on a grass stalk, and this is then acquired by another group member that over-pastes this scent mark with its own scent gland protruded (Burgener *et al.* 2008; Fig. 14.1).

14.5 The emergence of social structure

Stable social structure, in the form of a dominance hierarchy, is thought to emerge when individuals learn, through repeated contests, which group members they win contests against and which they will lose against. At least two important aspects characterise dominance hierarchies: their linearity and the level of dominance that individuals exert over other group members. Dominance hierarchies are termed *linear* (or transitive) if individual *A* is dominant over *B*, *B* is dominant over *C* and *A* is also dominant over *C*, and *non-linear* (or intransitive) if this does not hold (i.e. *A* is dominant over *B*, *B* is dominant over *C* and *C* is dominant over *A*). '*A* is dominant over *B*' is usually held to imply that in contests between *A* and *B*, *A* will always win. There are also dominance hierarchies in which *A* only wins more than 50% but less than 100% of encounters; then dominance ranks are known as *cardinal* dominance ranks (Boyd & Silk 1983).

Once social order has emerged, a reduction in contests between group members and increased social stability would be expected, to the benefit of both subordinate and dominant contestants (Bernstein 1981, Chase *et al.* 1994, Broom 2002). If individuals learn their relative social position through repeated contests, individual recognition of group members is a prerequisite for the emergence of a stable social structure (Barnard & Burk 1979). To what extent individual recognition really facilitates or hinders the emergence of stable linear dominance hierarchies is still a matter of theoretical debate (Hemelrijk 2000, Dugatkin & Earley 2004).

We now discuss the key processes that help form social structures – aggression, training to become a winner or loser, active submission and the avoidance of conflicts – before considering more complex processes that determine social status such as coalitions, alliances and social queues.

14.5.1 Social dominance and aggression

In both behavioural science and common usage, the term *aggression* is applied to a range of behaviours (Chapter 7). In a strict sense, aggression is any behaviour used with the intent to cause physical injury (Hinde 1974). In a broader sense, aggression is assertive behaviour that may not have the intent of causing direct physical harm but is detrimental to an opponent in other ways (Wingfield *et al.* 2006). Although sometimes used interchangeably, *social dominance* is not identical with aggression, nor is it defined by it (Fedigan 1982). This is because aggression without subsequent submission by an opponent does not indicate social dominance – a point that perhaps receives insufficient attention.

14.5.2 Training to become a winner (or loser)

There are several possible mechanisms individuals might use to assess the dominance of other group members. An important concept in this context is the idea that winning an encounter trains an individual to increase its chance to win the next encounter, and conversely, an individual that loses an encounter becomes more likely to lose the next – the trained winner or loser effect. The trained winner and loser effect is likely to play an important role in the emergence of stable dominance hierarchies in mammalian societies (Barnard & Burk 1979, Chase *et al.* 1994, Bonabeau *et al.* 1996, Dugatkin 1997). Trained winner and loser effects have not been experimentally studied in free-ranging social mammals, but an elegant experiment in nestling blue-footed boobies *Sula nebouxii* demonstrated a substantial trained winner and loser effect (Drummond & Canales 1998) and subsequently showed that training of winning and losing occurs along two, largely separate, axes of learning (Valderrábano-Ibarra *et al.* 2007). It is conceivable that the trained winner or loser effect is also part of the mechanism that ensures rank inheritance (i.e. social position of offspring with regard to that of the parent) in many social mammals (see section 14.6.4 and Box 14.2).

14.5.3 Active submission

Active submission (submission in the absence of assertive behaviour by an opponent) is a useful tactic for subordinates because it communicates a lack of intent to challenge the status quo, thereby reducing the need for dominants to assert their status. For example, in the cooperatively breeding meerkat *Suricata suricatta*, the oldest female helper in a group submits to the dominant breeding female at a higher frequency than that at which the helper receives assertive behaviour from her (Kutsukake & Clutton-Brock 2006). In the spotted hyena, a female-dominated species where females are often and incorrectly portrayed as hyper-aggressive (Goymann *et al.* 2001a, East & Hofer 2002), subordinates initiate ritualised greeting ceremonies to actively signal submission to dominants. During greetings, subordinates of

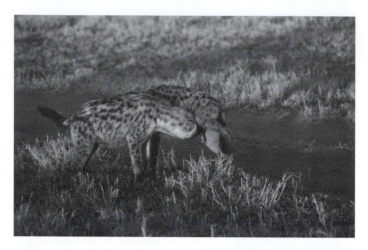

Figure 14.2 In greeting ceremonies, spotted hyenas actively signal their submission by a variety of gestures, including erecting the penis (males) or penile clitoris (females). Photo: M. L. East and H. Hofer.

both sexes use a quintessentially male gesture (Fig. 14.2) to signal submission (East *et al.* 1993).

14.5.4 Avoidance of conflict

Subordinates can avoid situations in which conflicts with dominants are likely (Aureli & de Waal 2000). This tactic is probably frequently used by subordinates in fission–fusion societies in which individuals and small subgroups are spatially separated for much of the time, as is the case in chimpanzee *Pan troglodytes* groups (Goodall 1986), elephants (Moss & Poole 1983), bottlenose dolphins (Wells 2003), African lions (Schaller 1972) and spotted hyenas (see below). Avoidance of conflict may also be a useful tactic in species that live in groups in which group members normally maintain relatively close proximity, such as meerkats (Kutsukake & Clutton-Brock 2008).

The fitness consequence of conflict avoidance has rarely been assessed. One example is provided by commuting spotted hyenas in the Serengeti National Park, Tanzania. Subordinates face increased competition for food with dominant group members when the main prey species migrate out of the group territory. Subordinates avoid conflict by travelling long distances (up to 70 km in one direction) to forage in areas with large concentrations of migratory

prey (Hofer & East 1993a, 1993b). This tactic carries the physiological consequence of increased corticosteroid levels for lactating females (Goymann *et al.* 2001b), decreased offspring growth and survival, intensified sibling rivalry and an increased chance of facultative siblicide in twin litters (Hofer & East 1997, 2008, Golla *et al.* 1999). Such conflict avoidance is consistent with models of the expected distribution of animals in relation to resource and competitor distribution (Fretwell & Lucas 1970, Sutherland & Parker 1985, Sutherland 1996).

14.6 Determinants of social status

Social status is the position of an individual in a society. This position may be the outcome of many processes and factors. Traditionally, scientists measured social status by recording an individual's submissive response to group members during pair-wise (dyadic) interactions, and scored status as a rank. In our discussion, we will refer to rank, because this is what most studies measure. However, it should be borne in mind that an individual's rank may emerge not only as the result of dyadic interactions but also by other processes such as support from coalition or alliance partners.

There is an intrinsic assumption in much of the theoretical and some of the empirical literature that body size determines the social status of an individual. Theoreticians often use size as a shorthand to introduce an asymmetry between contestants (Chapter 4; Maynard Smith & Parker 1976) but in empirical studies an effect of size on status should be demonstrated rather than assumed. A defining feature of complex mammalian societies is that dominance is the result of several, more subtle traits than relative body size. We therefore focus on processes and factors other than intrinsic factors that determine social status in mammals. Those that we discuss below include the social context of interactions, social queues, recruitment of support (coalitions and alliances), rank inheritance and the ability to recognise third-party relationships. We note that these processes still do not receive the full attention they deserve from field workers or theoreticians, possibly because their contributions are more difficult to detect and a challenge to investigate.

14.6.1 Social context

The rank of an individual may depend on the social context of an interaction. For instance, in the domestic cat *Felis catus*, males dominate females in most social contexts, yet females dominate males in dyadic interactions in feeding situations (Bonanni *et al.* 2007). Female dominance in feeding situations probably results from payoff asymmetries (Noë *et al.* 1991, Lewis 2002) in relation to the value of food and the cost of winning or losing. Males are likely to pay significant fitness costs by winning contests over food against females which invest heavily (in terms of gestation and lactation) in the male's offspring (Bonanni *et al.* 2007). A similar explanation has been proposed for female dominance in lemurs (Young *et al.* 1990).

14.6.2 Social queues

In some social mammals, social status, access to breeding territories or access to mates is determined by the order in which animals join a group or locate a receptive female. The first animal present has the highest rank, later arrivals obtain lower ranks, and the most recent animal to join holds the lowest rank. Animals advance in social status when higher-ranking animals drop out of the queue. Because a queue is not based on any individual trait, it is an arbitrary convention and therefore considered by theoreticians to be an inherently unstable arrangement, because it is open to cheating (Maynard Smith 1982). Yet the longest observed social queue, among 20 or more immigrant male spotted hyenas, is also the most stable queue known for animal societies (East & Hofer 2001). Evolutionary game theory (Chapter 4) suggests that the stability of queues is improved if (1) cheaters are punished, (2) fitness benefits are shared amongst queue members, thereby reducing the advantage of advancing within the queue, and (3) the total fitness benefits from reaching the top are lower than the costs associated with queue jumping (Maynard Smith 1982).

Queues are little appreciated yet widespread, as subordinates of both sexes queue for breeding positions in many societies with reproductive suppression (see below) and males often queue for territories on leks (Kokko *et al.* 1998, Kokko & Johnstone 1999). Other well studied social and reproductive queues include male thirteen-lined ground squirrels *Spermophilus tridecemlineatus* (Schwagmeyer & Parker 1990) and sac-winged bats *Saccopteryx bilineata* (Voigt & Streich 2003).

14.6.3 Recruitment of support

One reason why social status does not necessarily depend on body size is that social life provides the possibility for contestants to recruit support from other group members in short-term coalitions or long-term alliances. The ability of a contestant to recruit support is important, because it is likely that the winner of a contest will be the contestant that recruits the largest number of supporters (Bygott *et al.* 1979, Maynard Smith 1982, Hofer & East 1993b).

In many social mammals, groups have a matrilineal structure in which females stay within their natal group (philopatry) and form social bonds with female relatives, whereas males typically disperse from their natal groups (Greenwood 1980). This matrilineal structure favours the recruitment of support amongst females (e.g. Harcourt & de Waal 1992, Silk *et al*. 2003). There are also examples of alliances forged between related and unrelated males (Bygott *et al*. 1979, Connor *et al*. 1999, Möller & Beheregaray 2004, van Schaik *et al*. 2004). The importance of social support is demonstrated in several primate species, where coalitions of subordinate females may successfully challenge otherwise socially dominant males (Smuts 1986).

14.6.4 Rank inheritance

In many primates, some carnivores and some rodents, offspring acquire a social position very close to that of a parent, a phenomenon termed rank inheritance (Holekamp & Smale 1991). When social dominance provides fitness benefits, it may sometimes be passed onto offspring – the silver-spoon effect (Hofer & East 2003). If the correlation in social status between parents and offspring is sufficiently close, optimal life-history decisions differ significantly from standard predictions (Leimar 1996). For instance, if philopatric daughters in a polygynous matrilineal society inherit maternal social status but dispersing sons do not (as in many macaque species), high-ranking females ought to bias maternal investment in favour of daughters rather than sons (Leimar 1996), even if the usual prediction (Trivers & Willard 1973) suggests a bias in favour of sons.

The traditional mechanism to explain rank inheritance has been parental behavioural support of offspring during interactions with other group members. Parents successfully support offspring against group members that the parents themselves dominate, and thus offspring gain a rank close to that held by their parents (Hausfater *et al*. 1982, Horrocks & Hunte 1983). Box 14.2 contains a case study of the emergence of offspring rank under rank inheritance.

Box 14.2 Ontogenetic determinants of social status

Female mammals provide the environment in which their offspring develop from conception through gestation to weaning, and as a result mothers have a considerable effect on the expression of their offspring's phenotype (Chapter 2). Maternal effects on the expression of offspring phenotype are mediated through different interconnected pathways that include physiological, behavioural and genetic components (Bernardo 1996, Rossiter 1996, Mousseau & Fox 1998, Wolf *et al*. 1998).

In birds, cross-fostering experiments of eggs and chicks have disentangled maternal effects on the emergence of offspring phenotype (Griffith *et al*. 1999, Verboven *et al*. 2003). Recently, we used natural cases of adoption by surrogate mothers of 13 spotted hyena litters shortly after birth to test which of three possible pathways best explained the emergence of social dominance in adopted offspring (East *et al*. 2009). In all 13 litters, both the genetic and surrogate mothers were members of the clan in which the adopted cub was reared until weaning, came from a wide range of ranks, and in 12 cases both mothers were still alive when the adopted offspring obtained adulthood at two years of age. Thus the social environment in which adopted offspring were raised was similar to the one they would have experienced with their genetic mother, except that the maternal environmental effects of the genetic mother were replaced with the corresponding effects of the surrogate mother shortly after birth.

The spotted hyena is one of several social mammals that exhibit *rank inheritance* (Holekamp & Smale 1991, Engh *et al*. 2000). At adulthood, daughters obtain a social position in the linear dominance hierarchy similar to and below that of their mother, as do non-reproductive sons before they emigrate or become reproductively

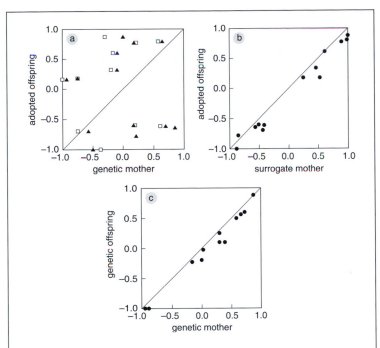

Figure 14.3 Using natural cases of adoption by surrogate mothers of spotted hyena litters shortly after birth to test which maternal pathway (genetic, endo-crine or behavioural support) best explains the emergence of social rank: the standardised rank of adopted spotted hyenas at adulthood in relation to (a) the standardised rank of their genetic mother when the adopted young reached adulthood (genetic pathway, □) or the standardised rank of their genetic mother on the date they were born (endocrine pathway, ▲); (b) the standardised rank of their surrogate mother at the time when the adopted young reached adulthood (behavioural support pathway); (c) the standardised rank of control cubs at adulthood (raised in the same cohort as the adopted cubs) in relation to the standardised rank of the genetic mother of the control cub when the control cub reached adulthood. Standardised ranks express ranks at positions of equal distance from the lowest rank of –1 via median rank at 0 to the highest rank at +1. The line indicates where the standardised rank of the adopted individual is identical with that of its (a, c) genetic or (b) surrogate mother.

active in their natal group (Smale *et al.* 1993, East & Hofer 2001). Because dominant females have priority of access to resources, their offspring benefit from the silver-spoon effect through faster growth and higher survival than offspring of subordin-ate females (Hofer & East 2003).

We examined three pathways by which mothers may influence the ability of their offspring to compete for social status at adulthood (East *et al.* 2009):

(1) The direct transfer of maternal genes that predispose offspring to be roughly as competitive as their mother within a similar social environment (Chapter 2; Moore 1993, Moore *et al.* 1997).

Box 14.2 Continued

(2) Maternal rank-related exposure of a fetus to maternal androgens during gestation, such that dominant mothers with higher concentrations of circulating androgens provide their developing fetuses with higher exposure to maternal androgens than more subordinate mothers. Elevated androgen exposure is supposed to result in aggressive offspring better able to compete for rank than offspring of lower-ranking females that experienced lower prenatal androgen exposure (Dloniak *et al.* 2006a).

(3) Maternal behavioural support during interactions with group members, which provides offspring with a competitive advantage during interactions with group members that are subordinate to their mother.

The genetic and endocrine pathways predict that offspring obtain a similar rank as their genetic mother. The maternal behavioural support pathway predicts that offspring will assume a rank at adulthood just below that held by their surrogate mother (Hausfater *et al.* 1982, Horrocks & Hunte 1983, Holekamp & Smale 1991). Adopted offspring did not gain a position in the dominance hierarchy when reaching adulthood similar to that held by their genetic mother on that date (genetic pathway). Adopted offspring also did not obtain a rank at adulthood close to that held by their genetic mother at the end of gestation (endocrine pathway). Adopted cubs did, however, obtain a rank at adulthood close to, and below that, of their surrogate mother (East *et al.* 2009; Fig. 14.3). Thus the evidence is consistent with the hypothesis that the emergence of offspring social status was influenced by maternal behavioural support rather than direct maternal genetic effects or maternal hormonal effects as the key factor determining rank inheritance in hyenas.

14.6.5 Knowledge of third-party relationships

Individuals in mammalian societies are likely to monitor social interactions between group members to gain information about their relative competitive ability. Such a bystander effect and social eavesdropping (see section 14.2 and Chapter 8) probably play an important role in the emergence of mammalian social hierarchies.

If an animal recognises the relationship between two other animals, it is considered to have the ability to recognise *third-party relationships*. Recognition of third-party relationships was initially suggested to occur in primates (Tomasello & Call 1997), and several studies on primates have been interpreted as providing evidence of this process. Range and Noë (2005) cautioned that behavioural patterns interpreted as recognition of third-party relationships might be equally well explained by animals applying simple rules of thumb. They argued that intervention in a

contest by an animal that outranks both participants does not necessarily show recognition of third-party relationships; it might simply be that the intervening animal knows that it outranks both contestants. Similarly, consistent support of the higher-ranking contestant need not indicate knowledge of the rank relationship between contestants – perhaps animals apply the simple rule 'always support the winner of the contest', which will be the dominant animal in most cases. Range and Noë (2005) noted that their results on triadic interactions in free-ranging sooty mangabeys *Cercocebus atys* could be interpreted as demonstrating either the existence of third-party recognition or the application of simple behavioural rules; and that the use of simple rules does not imply that more complex cognitive processes cannot or do not occur, only that they may not be necessary if simple rules suffice. They note that simple heuristics (e.g. Todd & Gigerenzer 2000) suggest that humans apply relatively simple rules during cooperative interactions, and that similar rules may determine cooperative interactions in many mammalian societies. Clearly, whether or not social mammals have the ability to recognise third-party relationships has important implications for how we interpret the formation of coalitions and its cognitive basis.

Clear evidence for the recognition of third-party relationships in primates comes from playback experiments in which female bystanders looked towards the mother whose infant's distress screams were experimentally broadcast (Cheney & Seyfarth 1980, 1999, Bergman *et al.* 2003). Engh *et al.* (2005) provided evidence that spotted hyenas may recognise third-party relationships, with individuals more likely to attack relatives of their opponents than low-ranking animals unrelated to their opponents.

14.7 Valuable social relationships and social networks

The fitness benefit (or loss) associated with interactions with one group member is unlikely to equal that associated with interactions with another group member. For this reason, animals in stable social groups are expected to learn to preferentially seek interactions with group members that provide benefits and avoid interactions with less beneficial group members (Hamilton 1964a, 1964b, Barnard & Burk 1979, Axelrod & Hamilton 1981).

Numerous studies provide evidence that mammalian group members interact more frequently with specific group members (Dunbar 1991, Cheney 1992, East *et al.* 1993, Barrett *et al.* 1999, Wells 2003; see discussion of biological markets in section 14.3.1). Few studies demonstrate fitness benefits obtained from social partner preferences, possibly because benefits are difficult to measure, or acquired in the long term. This may in future be improved by applying social network analysis (Chapter 9), recently used to describe the network of social interactions in several mammals (bottlenose dolphin, Lusseau 2003; killer whale, Williams & Lusseau 2006; Galapagos sea lion *Zalophus wollebaeki*, Wolf *et al.* 2007). For instance, in the long-tailed manakin *Chiroxiphia linearis*, a lek-

mating bird, a long-term study used social network analysis to identify the fitness consequences of individual social competence (McDonald 2007). It is likely that analyses of social networks will be much used in future to reveal complex social tactics and their fitness consequences (McDonald 2007, Croft *et al.* 2008, Wey *et al.* 2008).

14.8 Social complexity, sexual selection, brains and evolution

Both complexity of social life and the challenges provided by sexual conflict (see section 14.10.2) for successful reproductive strategies may have interacted with brain size in social mammals. The *social brain hypothesis* posits that individuals with a larger brain have a selective advantage in complex social groups. The *expensive sexual tissue hypothesis* suggests that a trade-off between expensive tissues may select for smaller brain size under strong sexual selection. Predictions of both hypotheses have yet to be tested on the same taxonomic group.

14.8.1 The social brain hypothesis

It has been proposed that an increase in the complexity of social life may have led to the evolution of large brains and the enlargement of the neocortex in social mammals, particularly in primates (Humphrey 1976, Barton & Dunbar 1997, Dunbar & Shultz 2007). Selection for large brains to allow for improved management and manipulation of social relationships in large social groups has become known as the social brain hypothesis (Dunbar 1998) and has been tested on a number of social mammals (Dunbar & Shultz 2007) using the comparative approach (Chapter 5; Harvey & Pagel 1991). There is evidence that managing female social relationships in primates is a greater cognitive challenge than managing male relationships, since the number of females per primate group is correlated with neocortex volume, whereas the number of males per group is not (Lindenfors *et al.* 2007).

Not all species fit the social brain hypothesis (Cheney & Seyfarth 2007). For instance, the prosimian

with the relatively largest brain is a solitary species, the aye-aye *Daubentonia madagascariensis*
(van Schaik & Deaner 2003). Van Schaik and Deaner
(2003) queried whether the social brain hypothesis
did identify the main selective pressure on cognitive
evolution, because large brains are costly to grow and
maintain even if they provide cognitive benefits, and
they argued that tests of the social brain hypothesis
ought to take a species' life history into account.

Because life-history features of mammals covary
with maximum lifespan, van Schaik and Deaner
(2003) investigated the relationship between relative
brain mass and maximum lifespan. Longevity positively correlated with brain mass in primates and
with encephalisation in eutherian mammals after
removing one outlier, the bats (Chiroptera) – a group
in which the energetic cost of flight may limit brain
size (see below). Theoretically, the usually vulnerable
juvenile phase of life is expected to be short (Charnov
1991), and a slow life history is expected in species with
a low mortality and an advantage to delayed reproduction in terms of producing better-quality young
(Stearns 1992). With this in mind, van Schaik and
Deaner (2003) summarised four non-exclusive ideas to
explain delayed reproduction in long-lived mammal
species and how these traits might relate to brain size.
(1) Large-brained mammals delay reproduction until
their brain and cognitive abilities are fully developed,
because immature nervous systems do not function at
an adult level. (2) A large brain provides the delayed
benefit of reduced mortality in adult life, thus allowing
a slowing down of life history. (3) Brain development
is impaired by shortages in nutrients and energy, and
hence selection for large brains would be expected in
species with a slow life history because rapid brain
development during periods of shortage would produce adults with poorly developed brains or cognitive
disabilities. (4) Fitness benefits gained after the brain
has developed, such as reduced mortality from predation, will be greater in species with a slow life history.

These ideas suggest that brains and life histories
evolved together, and that not all mammals with
slow life histories would have evolved large brains,
although large-brained mammals must have slow life
histories. It appears to us that this idea will benefit
further from a consideration of general physiological

arguments. For instance, there is evidence of a
physiological constraint on the rate of body tissue
production, and evidence that such rates vary with
respect to lifestyle and life history of a species (Sibly
& Brown 2007).

14.8.2 The expensive sexual tissue hypothesis

The possible role of sexual selection in brain-size
evolution has received little attention. As brain tissue is expensive to produce and maintain, and sexually selected traits may also be expensive, energetic
trade-offs might constrain brain size in species that
heavily invest in costly sexual organs, ornaments or
armaments (Pitnick *et al*. 2006). This expensive sexual tissue hypothesis was tested in bats, a group in
which testis mass ranges from 0.1% to 8.4% of body
mass, compared to a range of 0.02–0.75% of body
mass in primates. Pitnick *et al*. (2006) found a negative covariation between brain size and testis size
in echolocating bats, suggesting a trade-off between
these metabolically expensive organs. No evidence
of trade-off was found in fruit-eating bats, possibly
because they might be less energetically constrained
than echolocating species. Pitnick *et al*. (2006) noted
that extreme investment in testes in bats does not
reduce longevity (in bats about 3.5 times longer than
in non-flying placental mammals of similar size), and
thus does not require a reduction in somatic maintenance. In general, bat species with promiscuously
mating females have relatively small brains. Male
promiscuity has no influence on brain dimensions
compared to monogamous and polygynous species
and, contrary to the expectation of the social brain
hypothesis, there was a strong trend towards diminishing brain size as complexity in roosting group
composition increased (Pitnick *et al*. 2006).

14.9 Reproduction in a social environment

In the final sections of this chapter we consider how
group life influences reproduction in social mammals

in terms of reproductive skew, sexual selection and sexual conflict. We describe how male and female mating tactics evolved in response to these factors and the fitness benefits derived from them. Many aspects of reproduction are likely to be influenced by social life (Chapters 10, 11 and 12). The presence of several or many potential breeding partners in a social group increases the potential for individuals of both sexes to copulate with multiple mates, and this is likely to favour sexual selection for traits that provide fitness advantages during competitive interactions over access to mates, during mate choice and when sexual conflicts arise.

Gestation and lactation ensure that female mammals typically invest more in the production of offspring than males, and, as a result, males are less constrained than females in terms of their potential rate of reproduction. Consequently, in many social mammals the operational sex ratio (reproductively active males per receptive females) is biased towards males, and this bias is expected to favour sexual selection for traits preferred by females, and traits that provide an advantage during contests over access to mates (Clutton-Brock & Vincent 1991, Shuster & Wade 2003). Female preference need not focus on exaggerated male displays. Females may discriminate between male traits favoured by natural selection such as vigour or longevity, and may prefer male traits that decrease the chance of inbreeding (Lehmann & Perrin 2003, Höner *et al.* 2007). Although it is sometimes assumed that male traits which provide an advantage during direct male–male contests, such as size or fighting ability, are traits also favoured by female mate choice, this should be tested rather than assumed (East *et al.* 2003). Sexual selection is expected to operate not only before copulation (Darwin 1871) but also after copulation – in terms of sperm competition and cryptic female mate choice (Parker 1970, Smith 1984, Eberhard 1998, Birkhead & Møller 1998).

Indirect measures of the success of reproductive tactics such as copulations or mate guarding are often unreliable indicators of reproductive success and tend to underestimate the importance of female mate choice. Today, empirical studies can directly establish reproductive success by applying molecular genetic methods. One important caveat concerns the use of molecular genetic methods to investigate mate choice or the degree of within-litter multiple paternity in social mammals with reproductive skew among females. These methods will yield biased results if offspring are genetically sampled only after most juvenile mortality has occurred, because better survival of offspring of high-quality females will skew observed mate-choice patterns towards those of high-quality females – and in reality these may substantially differ from those of low-quality females (East *et al.* 2003).

14.10 Reproductive tactics

In most social mammals, reproductive benefits are rarely shared equally among group members (Lacey & Sherman 1997). Theoretical models of reproductive skew seek to explain social evolution by considering why some individuals (typically socially dominant animals) obtain higher reproductive benefits than others (social subordinates), and why subordinates remain members of a group even though their reproductive benefits are low. Such models consider the degree of reproductive skew in relation to ecological constraints which might influence an animal's propensity to leave a group as its reproductive benefits are reduced (Johnstone 2000, Magrath & Heinsohn 2000, Kokko 2002).

14.10.1 Social dominance, reproductive skew and 'power'

What determines the degree of reproductive skew in social groups? It may arise from random processes (Sutherland 1985) or result from social dynamics between group members (Keller & Reeve 1994). For example, social harassment of subordinates by dominants may induce physiological stress that inhibits ovulation or implantation, result in infant loss, or exclude subordinates from resources essential for reproduction (Clutton-Brock *et al.* 1986, Rhine *et al.* 1988, Holekamp *et al.* 1996).

Two basic types of models have been proposed to explain differences in reproductive skew (Keller & Reeve 1994, Clutton-Brock 1998, Reeve & Keller 2001). *Concession* models assume that dominants yield reproductive concessions to subordinates if the dominant breeder receives sufficient benefits from the subordinate, and subordinates remain group members if they gain greater benefits from staying than leaving. *Limited-control* models assume that dominants do not have (total) control over whether or not subordinates are able to breed.

When testing predictions from these models with empirical data (Magrath & Heinsohn 2000), one key assumption of the models should be tested first, the assumption concerning which group member(s) control reproductive skew (Johnstone 2000, Kokko 2002). For example, a lack of breeding by subordinates may be explained by incest avoidance rather than social control by dominants. In a naked mole-rat colony, death of a dominant female halts reproduction until a non-group female immigrates into the colony, because female colony members will not mate with closely related males in the colony (Clarke *et al.* 2001). Similarly, long-term demography of African wild dog *Lycaon pictus* packs in the Serengeti ecosystem suggests that inbreeding avoidance determines pack dynamics following the death of either the top (alpha) breeding male or female. When the alpha female dies, her breeding partner loses the alpha-male breeding position, all adult females disperse, and one of the youngest sexually mature natal males assumes the alpha position and awaits the arrival of an immigrant female to form a new pack. When the alpha male dies, a young natal male assumes the alpha-male position and again all female pack members disperse, leaving the males and any pups behind to await the immigration of a female to form a new breeding pack (Burrows 2004).

Beekman *et al.* (2003) suggested that because the reproduction optima of group members differ, the reproductive characteristics of a group may not be fully explained by reproductive-skew models. They proposed that consideration of *power*, defined as the ability to control reproduction when conflict exists, might clarify mechanisms that determine whose interests prevail, and mentioned examples of biological idiosyncrasies of different taxa that may influence power relations. Infanticide, musth in elephants, concealed ovulation, multiple mating by females or unusual reproductive anatomies could all be viewed as traits which shift the balance of power.

They acknowledged that whilst heuristically a useful tool, the concept of power cannot be easily integrated into testable hypotheses (Beekman *et al.* 2003).

Low female reproductive skew

Female reproductive success may be strongly influenced by access to resources required for the successful rearing of offspring. When access to essential resources cannot be monopolised by dominant females, low reproductive skew is expected. Reproductive skew among female members of bottlenose dolphin groups is small, perhaps because resources in their marine environment cannot be easily monopolised (Wells 2003). Even when dominant females can monopolise resources, as in some vervet monkey *Cercopithecus aethiops* groups, reproductive success may not be correlated with female rank if there is a high rate of predation on offspring across all ranks (Cheney *et al.* 1988). Dominant female savanna baboons can also monopolise access to preferred food resources, yet female social status and reproductive success are correlated in only some but not all baboon populations (Altmann *et al.* 1988).

High female reproductive skew

In some social mammals, one or at most two dominant females monopolise reproduction and all other female subordinates are reproductively suppressed (Lacey & Sherman 1997). Examples include the naked mole-rat (Faulkes & Abbott 1997), the Damaraland mole-rat *Cryptomys damarensis* (Bennett *et al.* 1997, Clarke *et al.* 2001), the meerkat (O'Riain *et al.* 2000, Clutton-Brock *et al.* 2001), the dwarf mongoose *Helogale parvula* (Creel *et al.* 1992), the banded mongoose *Mungos mungo* (Cant 2003), at least ten canid species (Moehlman & Hofer 1997) and several callitrichid primates (French 1997, Abbott *et al.* 1998). In these species, dispersal appears to be constrained, relatedness within breeding groups is high, alloparental care is provided by group members of both sexes, there are even morphologically different breeding casts in some mole-rats (Keller & Reeve 1994, Abbott *et al.* 1998) and subordinate females are reproductively suppressed by specific neuroendocrine or behavioural pathways rather than 'stressed' by dominants (Abbott *et al.* 1998), unlike species in which several females breed per group (Lacey & Sherman 1997, Hofer & East 1998).

All species with one dominant breeder exhibit a high degree of reproductive skew, even though subordinate females occasionally reproduce. In the dwarf mongoose, offspring of subordinate females will only survive if they are born at roughly the same time as the dominant female's litter and are successfully mixed with the dominant female's offspring. This confusion tactic results in 15% of juveniles being the genetic offspring of subordinate females. Subordinate males are more successful, siring 25% of juveniles in their group (Creel & Waser 1994, Keane *et al.* 1994). In African wild dog packs, the pups of beta females survive if they do not compete with pups of the alpha female for regurgitated food from helpers. Genetic studies of female reproductive success in this species are limited (Creel & Creel 2002). Observations suggest that most litters (75% of 57 litters) are produced by alpha females (Burrows 1995). The degree of reproductive skew among male pack members is unknown.

14.10.2 Sexual conflict

In many mammal societies, the evolutionary interests of females differ sufficiently from those of males to result in conflict between the sexes (Chapter 10; Parker 1979). Sexual conflict is expected to favour male tactics that manipulate female mate choice through direct and indirect male–male competition and by increasing the cost of female mate choice through coercion and harassment. In response, females are expected to evolve counter-tactics to reduce the detrimental effects of manipulative males (Parker 1979, Clutton-Brock & Parker 1995, Gowaty 1996).

Although the concept of sexual conflict was introduced decades ago, studies on sexual selection have been mostly limited to male–male competition (for reviews see Andersson 1994, Bradbury & Vehrencamp 1998). Box 14.3 reviews a key physiological component of male–male contests relevant to male reproductive tactics – the ability of males to respond to challenges from competing males – and demonstrates that group structure and other social factors influence testosterone concentrations and the ability of individuals to respond to social challenge.

Box 14.3 The physiology of male reproductive tactics

A key physiological aspect in male reproduction is spermatogenesis and the ability to rise to challenges from competitors. In both processes, androgens, in particular testosterone, play an essential role. The *challenge hypothesis* (Wingfield *et al.* 1990, 2006) has provided a useful framework to predict how androgen levels are likely to vary as a function of mating system, male–male aggression and parental care.

The challenge hypothesis states that in seasonal breeders testosterone levels rise at the start of the breeding season from a non-breeding baseline to a higher breeding baseline. In breeding systems with high paternal care, testosterone levels should only rise above breeding baseline levels if males are challenged by competitors. In mating systems with little paternal care and males seeking multiple copulations, testosterone levels should remain at a high elevation throughout the breeding season to facilitate behaviour appropriate for intense male–male competition over access to females. The challenge hypothesis assumes that androgen responsiveness (the ratio between breeding-season maximum and breeding baseline elevation) in both types of mating system is mainly a response to prevailing levels of social challenge. In its most recent development, the challenge hypothesis posits that androgen responses to seasonality and those associated with social challenges may be viewed as different types of responses (Goymann *et al.* 2007).

Box 14.3 Continued

The challenge hypothesis has been tested in many taxa, including social mammals. Empirical results were generally consistent with it (Hirschenhauser & Oliveira 2006, Wingfield *et al.* 2006). For instance, in multi-male, multi-female groups of ring-tailed lemurs *Lemur catta*, males seek multiple matings during the mating season, and male–male competition increased during the mating period, as did faecal testosterone levels. Outside the mating period, male testosterone levels were reduced to non-breeding baseline levels independent of a male's social position or age (Gould & Ziegler 2007). Similar results were obtained from other multi-male, multi-female seasonally breeding lemurs such as Verreaux's sifaka *Propithecus verreauxi* (Brockmann *et al.* 2001) and red-fronted lemur *Eulemur rufifrons* (Ostner *et al.* 2002).

In social species with multi-male, multi-female groups that breed throughout the year, males may need to balance the potential benefit of elevated testosterone levels associated with reproduction (particularly male–male competition for access to females) against the possible cost of maintaining such elevated levels throughout the year (Folstad & Karter 1992). Spotted hyenas breed throughout the year, and mid- to high-ranking males consort (shadow and defend) with females (East *et al.* 2003). As predicted, males that seek to monopolise access to females by defending them against approaches by competing males had elevated plasma testosterone (Goymann *et al.* 2003). Similarly, Dloniak *et al.* (2006b) found a positive association between reproductive aggression and elevated faecal androgen levels in immigrant males.

Of interest are also the exceptions. For instance, in cooperatively breeding species such as the dwarf mongoose *Helogale parvula* (Creel *et al.* 1993) and the African wild dog *Lycaon pictus* (Creel *et al.* 1997), androgen levels did not increase during the breeding season in either dominant or subordinate males as predicted, despite increased male–male aggression among dwarf mongooses. In African wild dogs, rates of aggression among male pack members declined during mating periods, even though some contests escalated and resulted in wounding (Creel & Creel 2002). Both species are characterised by reproductive suppression, a factor that played no role in the original formulation of the challenge hypothesis (Wingfield *et al.* 1990).

Few studies have adopted sexual conflict theory in a consequent manner. Sexual conflict is a useful framework for investigating sex-specific social and reproductive tactics in mammalian societies precisely because it predicts conflicts beyond precopulatory male–male competition. For this reason we will focus on reproductive tactics from the point of view of sexual conflict and female mate choice, and start with a case study on spotted hyenas. Spotted hyenas are interesting in this context because, unlike most social mammals, spotted hyena society is female-dominated, and most subordinates of both sexes reproduce. Social status, age and tenure influence reproductive opportunities, resulting in a complex

mating system. We will outline this complexity as revealed by long-term field studies in East Africa.

Mate choice and power asymmetries between the sexes

Most female spotted hyenas select their mating partner from within their group, and may have 10 or more potential mates to choose between. Reproductively active males are usually immigrants, but some males become long-term breeding males within their natal group (East & Hofer 2001). There is no breeding season; receptive females occur throughout the year. High female investment in singleton or twin litters and a lack of paternal care (Hofer & East 1993c, 2003) predict that females should exercise a high degree of mate choice (Parker 1983). The unusual anatomy of females (Glickman *et al.* 2005) allows them to exercise strong mate choice, because males require the full cooperation of females to achieve intromission (East *et al.* 1993, 2003).

Because the penile clitoris carries fitness costs in terms of likely stillbirths (Frank *et al.* 1995) we suspect that the persistence of this large organ provides females with a fitness benefit outweighing its cost (East *et al.* 1993, East & Hofer 1997). This benefit may be strong female mate choice, tipping the balance of power (*sensu* Beekman *et al.* 2003) in favour of females. We strongly doubt that this shift in power was achieved by females becoming androgenised and larger than males, as suggested by Frank *et al.* (1995) and Frank (1997), because (1) testosterone concentrations in female spotted hyenas are the same as in other female mammals (including *Homo sapiens*) and an order of magnitude lower than those of reproductively active males (Goymann *et al.* 2001a); (2) there are no significant differences and rather a large overlap in skeletal body measures between the sexes (East & Hofer 2002).

Male spotted hyena reproductive tactics

Male spotted hyenas compete for access to females but rarely use physical contests (Kruuk 1972, East & Hofer 2001). Immigrant males observe strict queuing conventions (Kokko *et al.* 1998), i.e. male status rises with tenure and males rarely fight. Males breeding in their natal groups do not queue but rapidly obtain high status in the male hierarchy, possibly as a result of the trained winner effect (East & Hofer 2001). Males above median rank strongly prefer to shadow (follow females for periods between hours and days) or defend (deterring other males from approaching females) high-ranking females (East & Hofer 2001). High-ranking females are high-quality mates, providing higher fitness benefits than lower-ranking females (Hofer & East 2003). Males invest considerable effort in shadowing and defending high-quality females, whether or not they are reproductively receptive, probably to foster long-term relationships with them and to prevent lower-status males

from doing so. Even though socially dominant males attempt to monopolise high-quality females, they fail to do so effectively, as shown by the lack of correlation between the ranks of sires and those of mothers. Thus, regardless of the tactics of socially dominant males to monopolise high-ranking females, these females are able to exercise strong mate choice (East *et al.* 2003).

Female mate-choice rules: a mechanism to avoid costly inbreeding

In spotted hyena groups, older females are more tolerant of long-tenured than short-tenured males, whereas young females are more tolerant of short-tenured males (East & Hofer 2001). This age-related asymmetry in female response to males reflects female mate-choice patterns, as offspring of young females are mostly sired by short-tenured males and those of older females by long-tenured males (East *et al.* 2003, Höner *et al.* 2007). Preference by young breeding females for short-tenured sires is probably a female mating tactic to avoid costly inbreeding with their long-lived fathers (East & Hofer 2001, Höner *et al.* 2007). The conventional idea (Van Horn *et al.* 2008) that females might prefer immigrant males apparently does not apply to spotted hyenas (Höner *et al.* 2008).

Individual males or male coalitions that coerce or severely harass females increase female mate-choice costs, thereby potentially decreasing female choosiness (East & Hofer 2001). As coercion and harassment are not necessarily confined to receptive periods of females, these tactics may signal the behaviour a female could expect if she is located when receptive. In the short term, coercion and harassment is an unsuccessful male tactic, as offspring of females are rarely sired by males which coerced or harassed them (East *et al.* 2003). In the long term, females may occasionally copulate with known coercive males, if the cost of rejecting such a male at that instant is too high.

In the commuting Serengeti population, both males and females face considerable costs of mate choice when clan members forage a long distance (up to 70 km) from the clan territory (Hofer & East 1993b). During these periods, the pool of mating partners inside a clan territory will be limited (East & Hofer

2001, Hofer & East 1993c). Because of strong male preference for high-quality females, the cost of mate choice (in terms of distance travelled, energy and time) for low-quality females is likely to be relatively high. This higher cost of mate choice for lower-quality females, coupled with a low reproductive rate and male coercion or harassment, might prompt such females to accept mates of poor quality rather than forgo a receptive cycle. Females that accept a mate of unknown or low quality would be expected to mate multiply, to dilute the detrimental effect of this decision on their offspring (Johnstone *et al.* 1996). This may explain why low-ranking Serengeti females produce more multiple-paternity litters than high-ranking females (East *et al.* 2003).

Female spotted hyenas prefer males that display friendly and unthreatening behaviours, and probably require considerable evidence of a male's friendly intent before considering him a desirable mate (East *et al.* 1993, East & Hofer 2001). Because a friendly relationship with a female is a non-transferable resource, males stand to gain little from physical contests with competing males (Maynard Smith 1982), and thus strong female mate choice may explain the low level of male–male aggression in this species. Because reproductive success is not monopolised by socially dominant males but shared across 'queuing' males, this may stabilise the male hierarchy (Maynard Smith 1982, Kokko & Johnstone 1999), despite the large number of queuing males (East & Hofer 2001).

Female mate choice and male-biased dispersal

In many social mammals, dispersal is male-biased (Greenwood 1980). This may be an adaptive response to female mate choice evolved to avoid costly inbreeding with close relatives, even though dispersal carries costs (Parker 1979, Perrin & Mazalov 1999, Lehmann & Perrin 2003). Empirical studies of social mammals indicate that dispersal decreases the chance of inbreeding (Pusey & Wolf 1996). Direct social learning may help females avoid mating with direct kin, as in the black-tailed prairie dog *Cynomys ludovicianus* (Hoogland 1982). In many long-lived social mammals, daughters reproduce in groups containing their fathers

but generally appear to avoid mating with them. Preference by young female spotted hyenas for males of short tenure provides a simple rule that avoids close inbreeding with a long-lived and unknown father (or elder brothers, if present). Such a preference suggests that when a male starts his reproductive career, he should select a social group with the largest number of young females, as this is the female age class most likely to accept him as a mate. Testing this idea using the entire population (eight clans) of spotted hyenas on the floor of the Ngorongoro Crater, Tanzania, Höner *et al.* (2007) showed that most males started their reproductive careers in the clans with the highest number of young females, and males that did so had a significantly and substantially higher long-term reproductive success than males that reproduced in other clans. Because the majority of males disperse to join clans with high numbers of young females, male dispersal was an adaptive response to female mate choice. The number of competing males in a group, measured in terms of either males per female or total number of males in the male social queue, did not influence dispersal decisions (Höner *et al.* 2007).

Similarly, in coastal groups of bottlenose dolphins, where long-term philopatry to natal areas has been observed in both males and females (Connor *et al.* 1999, Wells 2003), genetic evidence suggests that philopatry is far stronger in females than in males, and that some males disperse when their breeding prospects in new areas are better than in their home area (Möller & Beheregaray 2004).

14.10.3 Sexual selection and female mate choice in bats

In the greater horseshoe bat *Rhinolophus ferrumequinum*, female mate choice has led to close kinship and may have promoted female sociality (Rossiter *et al.* 2001). Male greater horseshoe bats occupy underground territories that are spatially segregated from female breeding colonies (Rossiter *et al.* 2006). The reproductive success of males thus depends on receptive females choosing to visit particular males. High female mate fidelity across years means that offspring from different litters are typically full siblings. As female relatives more often share breeding partners than expected by chance, relatedness amongst jointly roosting females is enhanced and exceeds 0.3 among first-order and second-order relatives (Rossiter *et al.* 2005). Strong female mate choice and high male longevity result in a high degree of male reproductive skew. Rossiter *et al.* (2006) reported that just three males sired a fifth of all colony offspring born in a decade, whereas 62% of males did not sire any pups.

In contrast to many social mammals, female sac-winged bats disperse from natal colonies, probably to avoid mating with their long-lived fathers. Males remain in their natal colony as non-territorial males, queuing for a territory within the colony to become vacant (Voigt & Streich 2003, Nagy *et al.* 2007). While hovering, territorial males fan odour from their wing sacs over females resting in their territory (Voigt & von Helversen 1999) and produce a courtship song (Behr & von Helversen 2004). Small territorial males have a higher reproductive success than larger territorial males, possibly due to the competitive advantage provided by a smaller size during aerial courtship (Voigt *et al.* 2005). Although territorial males sire more offspring than non-territorial males in day roosts, territorial males do not monopolise paternity of offspring born in their territory, siring only about 30% of these juveniles (Heckel & von Helversen 2003, Voigt *et al.* 2005).

14.10.4 Limiting male monopolies: mechanisms favouring cryptic female mate choice

Several traits are usually considered to increase male reproductive success by helping to monopolise mating opportunities. With the availability of new molecular techniques, evidence mounts that in complex societies female responses to these traits reduce or limit male monopolies and provide an opportunity for cryptic female choice, i.e. postcopulatory processes by which females may choose amongst received ejaculates which sperms should fertilise their eggs.

Oestrus synchrony

Synchrony of oestrus among female group members may be driven by ecological factors that favour reproduction within a narrowly defined breeding season. It may also be a female tactic to reduce the ability of males to monopolise females, thus effectively decreasing reproductive skew among males (Ims 1989, Owens & Thompson 1994, Say *et al.* 2001). In ring-tailed lemur *Lemur catta* groups, females socially dominate males and oestrus is synchronised within a two-week period. During this time there is intense male–male competition for access to oestrus females and the male dominance hierarchy is disrupted (Sauther 1991). Females mate promiscuously, sometimes with males of neighbouring groups. Oestrus synchrony and promiscuity of females probably facilitate cryptic female mate choice, and has driven selection for large testes. Male ring-tailed lemurs have the largest relative testis size of any strepsirhine primate (Kappeler 1997).

Promiscuous mating and cryptic female mate choice is likely to promote greater vigour in and survival of offspring than would be expected in the absence of promiscuity (Zeh & Zeh 1997, Tregenza & Wedell 2000). For example, in the grey mouse lemur *Microcebus murinus* there is evidence that promiscuous mating results in cryptic mate choice for sires which provide offspring with a higher number of supertypes of the major histocompatibility complex (MHC) that are different from those of the mother, a higher degree of microsatellite heterozygosity, and a higher amino acid distance to the MHC of the mother, than randomly assigned males (Schwensow *et al.* 2008).

When oestrus synchrony provides males with numerous mating opportunities, they should discriminate between available mates when the variance in female quality is large. Under these conditions, males should prefer high-quality over low-quality females, as in the thirteen-lined ground squirrel (Schwagmeyer & Parker 1990). Male choosiness for high-quality females and competition between females for high-quality males also occurs in other social mammals with oestrus synchrony, such as Soay sheep *Ovis aries* (Preston *et al.* 2005) and topi *Damaliscus lunatus* (Bro-Jørgensen 2007).

Copulatory plugs and sperm competition

After successful copulation, ring-tailed lemur males appear to attempt to delay females from copulating with other males by inserting a copulatory plug in the vagina (Sauther *et al.* 1999). Penile spines in this species may therefore facilitate the removal of the copulatory plug (Sauther 1991, Parga 2003). Copulatory plugs occur in other social mammals, including deer mice *Peromyscus maniculatus* (Dewsbury 1988) and the polygynous Mexican free-tailed bat *Tadarida brasiliensis* (McCracken & Wilkinson 2000). A comparative study of the size of testes and male accessory reproductive glands in rodents (Ramm *et al.* 2005) found a positive association between relative testes size and the prevalence of within-litter multiple paternity, and between the degree of sperm competition and the relative size of the seminal vesicles and anterior prostate gland, two accessory glands used to produce copulatory plugs. This suggests that promiscuity by females may drive selection for males to produce larger copulatory plugs.

Spatial separation of females

Spatial separation of receptive females may also be a factor that limits the ability of males to monopolise females. Musth in African savanna elephants *Loxodonta africana* (Poole 1987) is a phenomenon that probably evolved to assist male elephants to locate and compete for widely spaced receptive females (Poole 1989). Musth duration increases with age from a few days or weeks in young males to a median period of 81 days in males of 46–50 years of age (Poole 1989). Male reproductive success is influenced by musth and age, with the majority of calves (74%) sired by males in musth, and males between 45 and 50 years of age siring offspring at an average annual rate six times that of males of 30 years of age (Hollister-Smith *et al.* 2007). Male harassment of females may cause females to seek the protection of larger, older, dominant bulls, thereby increasing the desirability of these males (Poole 1989) and skewing male reproductive success in their favour (Hollister-Smith *et al.* 2007).

As in several other long-lived mammals, including spotted hyenas and sac-winged bats, female preference for relatively long-lived males may be a good choice, as these males demonstrate an ability to survive (Kokko & Lindström 1996).

Male infanticide and female mate choice

Infanticide by unrelated males has been observed in a wide range of social mammals (e.g. Hausfater & Hrdy 1984; see Sarah Hrdy's profile) and interpreted as a male mating tactic to make females become reproductively receptive, once their dependent juveniles have been killed (Hrdy 1977). This form of male–male competition results in strong sexual conflict between potentially infanticidal males and mothers of vulnerable offspring. Infanticide would be selected against if males mistakenly killed their own offspring. Females might reduce the opportunity for infanticide by confusing the paternity of their offspring by copulating with more than one male (Hrdy 1977, Gomendio *et al.* 1998).

In closely bonded social groups with oestrus synchrony, females easily confuse paternity by copulating with several males. When oestrus is asynchronous, females that signal their receptivity are likely to attract several mating partners, and thus the paternity of their offspring may also be confused. If females can conceal receptivity, they may be able to copulate with preferred males when receptive and confuse their offspring's paternity by copulating when they are not receptive. Therefore, in social mammals, promiscuous behaviour by females may decrease male aggression to offspring and simultaneously provide the benefit of precopulatory or cryptic mate choice (Gomendio *et al.* 1998, Hrdy 2000, Jennions & Petrie 2000).

14.11 Conclusions and future directions

In this chapter we have summarised aspects of the social life of mammals that influence individual fitness, introduced theoretical models that help explain the evolution of social life, considered some of the proximate mechanisms that facilitate social and reproductive tactics, and described behavioural mechanisms that may play a role in the genesis of social structure and complex mammalian societies. We have also outlined behavioural tactics employed by individuals in these societies to foster cooperation with group members and avoid conflict. All these topics are discussed in a massive body of literature, of which only a fraction has been cited here. Yet there is still much that we do not understand about why mammals live in groups, or which factors lead to their different social structures, dispersal patterns, mating systems and reproductive tactics.

We think that a better understanding of how societies are formed and operate will require a deeper understanding of the fitness consequences of various aspects of the social environment. Some recent studies point the way (e.g. Silk *et al.* 2003, Silk 2007, McDonald 2007). Measuring fitness consequences is challenging, because their effects might only be apparent after long-term monitoring of interrelated aspects of the social environment. Here, recent developments of accurate short-term measures of fitness may help (e.g. Coulson *et al.* 2006). More information is needed on the fitness consequences of multi-partner interactions in the context of both cooperation and conflict and how these are influenced by different demographic conditions, or reproductive and life-history stages.

In this chapter we have refrained from discussing the many studies that searched for aspects to distinguish human societies from those of primates, or primate societies from those of non-primates, to emphasise and identify the special qualities of primates (and within them, humans). In terms of social strategies, many of these attempts have been futile because the argument 'only primates have it' has sooner or later been disproved (Cheney & Seyfarth 2007). In terms of the cognitive (and implied physiological) underpinnings of social strategies, there has been a tendency to favour complex explanations rather than to search for simple rules of thumb (Todd & Gigerenzer 2000, Range & Noë 2005, Höner *et al.* 2007), consider non-adaptive explanations, or simply play devil's advocate (Bshary *et al.* 2002, 2007). The field will advance more rapidly if more researchers seriously consider such alternative explanations for behaviours in complex mammalian societies.

Acknowledgements

We thank Wolfgang Goymann, Oliver Höner, Ronald Noë, Simone Sommer and Wolfgang Wickler for helpful comments on earlier drafts, Cornelia Greulich, Beate Peters, Dagmar Thierer and Kerstin Wilhelm for their assistance, and the Leibniz Institute for Zoo and Wildlife Research, the Deutsche Forschungsgemeinschaft, the Fritz-Thyssen-Stiftung, the Stifterverband der Deutschen Wissenschaft, and the Max Planck Society for their support of our research.

Suggested readings

The following books and articles address essential issues for the understanding of complex societies by providing key results, important methods or a thoughtful, critical look at the conceptual development of the field, thereby stimulating many new research questions.

Conceptual foundations for and methods of social analysis in complex societies

Whitehead, H. (2008) *Analyzing Animal Societies: Quantitative Methods for Vertebrate Social Analysis.* Chicago, IL: University of Chicago Press.

Social and cognitive tactics

Cheney, D. L. & Seyfarth, R. M. (2007) *Baboon Metaphysics.* Chicago, IL: University of Chicago Press.

Accurate short-term measures of fitness

Coulson, T., Benton, T. G., Lundberg, P. *et al.* (2006) Estimating individual contributions to population growth: evolutionary fitness in ecological time. *Proceedings of the Royal Society B,* **273**, 547–555.

Sex allocation in complex societies

Leimar, O. (1996) Life-history analysis of the Trivers and Willard sex-ratio problem. *Behavioral Ecology,* **7**, 316–325.

Reproductive conflicts and power

Beekman, M., Komdeur, J. & Ratnieks, F. L. W. (2003) Reproductive conflicts in social animals: who has power? *Trends in Ecology and Evolution*, **18**, 277–282.

Sexual conflict

Gowaty, P. A. (1996) Battle of the sexes and origins of monogamy. In: *Partnerships in Birds*, ed. J. M. Black. Oxford: Oxford University Press, pp. 21–52.

References

Abbott, D. A., Saltzman, W., Schultz-Darken, N. J. & Tannenbaum, P. L. (1998) Adaptations to subordinate status in female marmoset monkeys. *Comparative Biochemistry and Physiology C*, **119**, 261–274.

Alexander, R. D. (1974) The evolution of social behaviour. *Annual Review of Ecology and Systematics*, **5**, 325–383.

Altmann, J., Altmann, S. & Hausfater, G. (1988) Determinants of reproductive success in savannah baboons (*Papio cynocephalus*). In: *Reproductive Success*, ed. T. H. Clutton-Brock. Chicago, IL: University of Chicago Press, pp. 403–418.

Andersson, M. (1994) *Sexual Selection*. Princeton, NJ: Princeton University Press.

Aureli, F. & de Waal, F. B. M. (2000) *Natural Conflict Resolution*. Berkeley, CA: University of California Press.

Axelrod, R. & Hamilton, W. D. (1981) The evolution of cooperation. *Science*, **211**, 1390–1396.

Barnard, C. & Burk, T. (1979) Dominance hierarchies and the evolution of individual recognition. *Journal of Theoretical Biology*, **81**, 65–73.

Barrett, L. & Henzi, S. P. (2001) The utility of grooming in baboon troops. In: *Economics in Nature. Social Dilemmas, Mate Choice and Biological Markets*, ed. R. Noë, J. A. R. A. M. van Hooff & P. Hammerstein. Cambridge: Cambridge University Press, pp. 119–145.

Barrett, L., Henzi, S. P., Weingrill, T., Lycett, J. E. & Hill, R. A. (1999) Market forces predict grooming reciprocity in female baboons. *Proceedings of the Royal Society B*, **266**, 665–670.

Barton, R. & Dunbar, R. I. M. (1997) Evolution of the social brain. In *Machiavellian Intelligence II*, ed. R. Byrne & A. Whiten. Cambridge: Cambridge University Press, pp. 240–263.

Beekman, M., Komdeur, J. & Ratnieks, F. L. W. (2003) Reproductive conflicts in social animals: who has power? *Trends in Ecology and Evolution*, **18**, 277–282.

Behr, O. & von Helversen, O. (2004) Bat serenades: complex courtship songs of the sac-winged bat (*Saccopteryx bilineata*). *Behavioral Ecology and Sociobiology*, **56**, 106–115.

Bennett, N. C., Faulkes, C. G. & Spinks, A. C. (1997) LH responses to single doses of exogenous GnRH by social Mashona mole-rats: a continuum of socially induced infertility in the family Bathyergidae. *Proceedings of the Royal Society B*, **264**, 1001–1006.

Bercovitch, F. B. (1988) Coalitions, cooperation and reproductive tactics among adult male baboons. *Animal Behaviour*, **36**, 1198–1209.

Bergman, T. J., Beehner, C. J., Cheney, D. L. & Seyfarth, R. M. (2003) Hierarchial classification by rank and kinship in baboons. *Science*, **302**, 1234–1236.

Bernardo, J. (1996) Maternal effects in animal ecology. *American Zoologist*, **36**, 83–105.

Bernstein, I. S. (1981) Dominance: the baby and the bathwater. *Behavioral and Brain Sciences*, **4**, 419–457.

Bertram, B. (1978) Living in groups: predators and prey. In: *Behavioural Ecology: an Evolutionary Approach*, ed. J. R. Krebs & N. B. Davies. Oxford: Blackwell, pp. 64–96.

Birkhead, T. R. & Møller A. P., eds. (1998) *Sperm Competition and Sexual Selection*. London: Academic Press.

Bonabeau, E., Theraulaz, G. & Deneubourg, J.-L. (1996) Mathematical model of self-organizing hierarchies in animal societies. *Bulletin of Mathematical Biology*, **58**, 661–717.

Bonanni, R., Cafazzo, S., Fantini, C., Pontier, D. & Natoli, E. (2007) Feeding-order in an urban feral domestic cat colony: relationship to dominance rank, sex and age. *Animal Behaviour*, **74**, 1369–1379.

Boughman, J. W. & Wilkinson, G. S. (1998) Greater spearnosed bats discriminate group mates by vocalizations. *Animal Behaviour*, **55**, 1717–1732.

Boyd, R. & Silk, J. B. (1983) A method for assigning cardinal dominance ranks. *Animal Behaviour*, **31**, 45–58.

Bradbury, J. W. & Vehrencamp, S. L. (1998) *Principles of Animal Communication*. Sunderland, MA: Sinauer Associates.

Brockmann, D. K., Whitten, P. L., Richard, A. F. & Benander, B. (2001) Birth season testosterone levels in male Verrauxi's sifaka, *Propithecus verreauxi*: insights into socio-demographic factors mediating seasonal testicular function. *Behavioral Ecology and Sociobiology*, **49**, 117–127.

Bro-Jørgensen, J. (2007) Reversed sexual conflict in a promiscuous antelope. *Current Biology*, **17**, 2157–2161.

Broom, A. (2002) A unified model of dominance hierarchy formation and maintenance. *Journal of Theoretical Biology*, **219**, 63–72.

Bshary, R., Wickler, W. & Fricke, H. W. (2002) Fish cognition: a primate's eye view. *Animal Cognition*, **5**, 1–13.

Bshary, R., Salwiczek, L. H. & Wickler, W. (2007) Social cognition in non-primates. In: *The Oxford Handbook of Evolutionary Psychology*, ed. R. I. M. Dunbar & L. Barrett. Oxford: Oxford University Press, pp. 83–101.

Burgener, N., East, M. L., Hofer, H. & Dehnhard, M. (2008) Do spotted hyena scent marks code for clan membership? In: *Chemical Communication in Vertebrates XI*, ed. J. Hurst, R. Beynon and D. Müller-Schwarze. Berlin, New York: Springer-Verlag, pp. 169–177.

Burgener, N., East, M. L., Hofer, H. & Dehnhard, M. (2009) Does anal scent signal identity in the spotted hyena? *Animal Behaviour*, **77**, 707–715.

Burrows, R. (1995) Demographic changes and social consequences in wild dogs, 1964–1992. In: *Serengeti II: Dynamics, Management and Conservation of an Ecosystem*, ed. A. R. E. Sinclair & P. Arcese. Chicago, IL: University of Chicago Press, pp. 400–420.

Burrows, R. (2004) Pack cohesion in the African wild dog, *Lycaon pictus*, and a 'young-male first' protocol in the acquisition of dominance. *Advances in Ethology*, **38**, 124.

Bygott, J. D., Bertram, B. C. R. & Handy, J. P. (1979) Male lions in large coalitions gain reproductive advantages. *Nature*, **282**, 839–841.

Cant, M. A. (2003) Patterns of helping effort in co-operatively breeding banded mongooses (*Mungos mungo*). *Journal of Zoology London*, **259**, 115–121.

Chapais, B. & Berman, C. M. (2004) *Kinship and Behavior in Primates*. New York, NY: Oxford University Press.

Charnov, E. L. (1991) Evolution of life history variation among female mammals. *Proceedings of the National Academy of Sciences of the USA*, **88**, 1134–1137.

Chase, I., Bartolomeo, C. & Dugatkin, L. A. (1994) Aggressive interactions and inter-contest interval: how long do winners keep winning? *Animal Behaviour*, **48**, 393–400.

Chase, I. D., Tovey, C., Spangler-Martin, D. & Manfredonia, M. (2002) Individual differences versus social dynamics in the formation of animal dominance hierarchies. *Proceedings of the National Academy of Sciences of the USA*, **99**, 5744–5749.

Cheney, D. L. (1992) Intragroup cohesion and intergroup hostility: the relation between grooming distribution and intergroup competition among female primates. *Behavioral Ecology*, **3**, 334–345.

Cheney, D. L. & Seyfarth, R. M. (1980) Vocal recognition in free-ranging vervet monkeys. *Animal Behaviour*, **28**, 362–367.

Cheney, D. L. & Seyfarth, R. M. (1999) Recognition of other individuals' social relationships by female baboons. *Animal Behaviour*, **58**, 67–75.

Cheney, D. L. & Seyfarth, R. M. (2007) *Baboon Metaphysics*. Chicago, IL: University of Chicago Press.

Cheney, D. L., Seyfarth, R. M., Andelman S. J. & Lee, P. C. (1988) Reproductive success in vervet moneys. In: *Reproductive Success*, ed. T. H. Clutton-Brock. Chicago, IL: University of Chicago Press, pp. 384–402.

Clarke, F. M., Miethe, G. H. & Bennett, N. C. (2001) Reproductive suppression in female Damaraland mole-rats *Cryptomys damarensis*: dominant control or self-restraint? *Proceedings of the Royal Society B*, **268**, 899–909.

Clutton-Brock, T. H. (1988) *Reproductive Success: Studies of Individual Variation in Contrasting Breeding Systems*. Chicago, IL: University of Chicago Press.

Clutton-Brock, T. H. (1998) Reproductive skew, concession and limited control. *Trends in Ecology and Evolution*, **13**, 288–292.

Clutton-Brock, T. H. & Parker, G.A. (1995) Sexual coercion in animal societies. *Animal Behaviour*, **49**, 1345–1365.

Clutton-Brock, T. H. & Vincent, A. C. J. (1991) Sexual selection and the potential reproductive rates of males and females. *Nature*, **351**, 58–60.

Clutton-Brock, T. H., Albon, S. D. & Guinness, F. E. (1986) Great expectations: dominance, breeding success and offspring sex ratios in red deer. *Animal Behaviour*, **34**, 460–471.

Clutton-Brock, T. H., Brotherton, P. N. M., Russell, A. F. *et al.* (2001) Cooperation, conflict and concession in meerkat groups. *Science*, **291**, 478–481.

Connor, R., Heithaus, M. & Barre, L. (1999) Superalliance of bottlenose dolphins. *Nature*, **397**, 571–572.

Coulson, T., Benton, T. G., Lundberg, P. *et al.* (2006) Estimating individual contributions to population growth: evolutionary fitness in ecological time. *Proceedings of the Royal Society B*, **273**, 547–555.

Creel, S. & Creel, N. M. (2002) *The African Wild Dog: Behavior, Ecology and Conservation*. Princeton, NJ: Princeton University Press.

Creel, S. & Waser, P. M. (1994) Inclusive fitness and reproductive strategies in dwarf mongooses. *Behavioral Ecology*, **5**, 339–348.

Creel, S., Creel, N. M., Wildt, D. E. & Montfort, S. L. (1992) Behavioural and endocrine mechanisms of reproductive suppression in Serengeti dwarf mongooses. *Animal Behaviour*, **43**, 231–245.

Creel, S., Wildt, D. E. & Monfort, S. L. (1993) Aggression, reproduction, and androgens in wild dwarf mongooses: a test of the challenge hypothesis. *American Naturalist*, **141**, 816–825.

Creel, S., Creel, N. M., Mills, M. G. L. & Monfort, S. L. (1997) Rank and reproduction in cooperatively breeding African wild dogs: behavioural and endocrine correlates. *Behavioral Ecology*, **8**, 298–306.

Croft, D. P., James, R. & Krause, J. (2008) *Exploring Animal Social Networks*. Princeton, NJ: Princeton University Press.

Curno, O., Behnke, J. M., McElligott, A. G., Reader, T. & Barnard, C. J. (2009) Mothers produce less aggressive sons with altered immunity when there is a threat of disease during pregnancy. *Proceedings of the Royal Society B*, **276**, 1047–1054.

Dall, S. R. X., Giraldeau, L.-A., Olsson, O., McNamara, J. M. & Stephens, D. W. (2005) Information and its use in evolutionary ecology. *Trends in Ecology and Evolution*, **20**, 187–193.

Danchin, É., Giraldeau, L.-A., Valone, T. J. & Wagner, R. H. (2004) Public information: from nosy neighbors to cultural evolution. *Science*, **305**, 487–491.

Darwin, C. (1871) *The Descent of Man, and Selection in Relation to Sex*. London: John Murray.

Dewsbury, D. A. (1988) A test of the role of copulatory plugs in sperm competition in deer mice (*Peromyscus maniculatus*). *Journal of Mammalogy*, **69**, 854–857.

Digby, L. J. (1995) Infant care, infanticide and female reproductive strategies in polygynous groups of common marmosets (*Calithrix jacchus*). *Behavioral Ecology and Sociobiology*, **37**, 51–61.

Dloniak, S. M., French, J. A. & Holekamp, K. E. (2006a) Rank related maternal effects of androgens on behaviour in wild spotted hyaenas. *Nature*, **440**, 1190–1193.

Dloniak, S. M., French, J. A. & Holekamp, K. E. (2006b) Faecal androgen concentrations in adult male spotted hyaenas, *Crocuta crocuta*, reflect interactions with socially dominant females. *Animal Behaviour*, **71**, 27–37.

Drummond, H. & Canales, C. (1998) Dominance between booby nestlings involves winner and loser effects. *Animal Behaviour*, **55**, 1669–1676.

Dugatkin, L. A. (1997) Winner effects, loser effects and the structure of dominance hierarchies. *Behavioral Ecology*, **8**, 583–587.

Dugatkin, L. A. (2001) Bystander effects and the structure of dominance hierarchies. *Behavioral Ecology*, **12**, 348–352.

Dugatkin, L. A. & Earley, R. L. (2004) Individual recognition, dominance hierarchies and winner and loser effects. *Proceedings of the Royal Society B*, **271**, 1537–1540.

Dunbar, R. I. M. (1991) Functional significance of social grooming in primates. *Folia Primatologica*, **57**, 121–131.

Dunbar, R. I. M. (1998) The social brain hypothesis. *Evolutionary Anthropology*, **6**, 178–190.

Dunbar, R. I. M. & Shultz, S. (2007) Evolution in the social brain. *Science*, **317**, 1344–1347.

Earley, R. L. & Dugatkin, L. A. (2002) Eavesdropping on visual cues in green swordtail (*Xiphophorus helleri*) fights: a case for networking. *Proceedings of the Royal Society B*, **269**, 943–952.

East, M. L. & Hofer, H. (1991a) Loud calling in a female-dominated mammalian society: I. Structure and composition of whooping bouts of spotted hyaenas, *Crocuta crocuta*. *Animal Behaviour*, **42**, 637–649.

East, M. L. & Hofer, H. (1991b) Loud calling in a female-dominated mammalian society: II. Behavioural contexts and functions of whooping of spotted hyaenas, *Crocuta crocuta*. *Animal Behaviour*, **42**, 651–669.

East, M. L. & Hofer, H. (1997) The peniform clitoris of female spotted hyaenas. *Trends in Ecology and Evolution*, **12**, 401–402.

East, M. L. & Hofer, H. (2001) Male spotted hyenas (*Crocuta crocuta*) queue for status in social groups dominated by females. *Behavioral Ecology*, **12**, 558–568.

East, M. L. & Hofer, H. (2002) Conflict and cooperation in a female dominated society: a reassessment of the 'hyper-aggressive' image of spotted hyenas. *Advances in the Study of Behavior*, **31**, 1–30.

East, M. L., Hofer, H. & Wickler, W. (1993) The erect 'penis' as a flag of submission in a female-dominated society: greetings in Serengeti spotted hyenas. *Behavioral Ecology and Sociobiology*, **33**, 355–370.

East, M. L., Hofer, H., Cox, J. H. *et al.* (2001) Regular exposure to rabies virus and lack of symptomatic disease in Serengeti spotted hyenas. *Proceedings of the National Academy of Sciences of the USA*, **98**, 15026–15031.

East, M. L., Burke, T., Wilhelm, K., Greig, C. & Hofer, H. (2003) Sexual conflict in spotted hyenas: male and female mating tactics and their reproductive outcome with respect to age, social status and tenure. *Proceedings of the Royal Society B*, **270**, 1247–1254.

East, M. L., Höner, O. P., Wachter, B. *et al.* (2009) Maternal effects on offspring social status in spotted hyenas. *Behavioral Ecology*, **20**, 478–483.

Eberhard, W. G. (1998) Female roles in sperm competition. In: *Sperm Competition and Sexual Selection*, ed. T. R. Birkhead & A. P. Møller. London: Academic Press, pp. 91–116.

Engh, A. L., Esch, K., Smale, L. & Holekamp, K. E. (2000) Mechanisms of maternal 'rank inheritance' in the spotted hyena, *Crocuta crocuta*. *Animal Behaviour*, **60**, 323–332.

Engh, A. L, Siebert, E. R., Greenberg, D. A. & Holekamp, K. E. (2005) Patterns of alliance formation and post-conflict aggression indicate spotted hyenas recognize third party relationships. *Animal Behaviour*, **69**, 209–217.

Faulkes, C. G. & Abbott, D. H. (1997) The physiology of a reproductive dictatorship: regulation of male and female reproduction by a single breeding female in colonies of naked mole-rats. In: *Cooperative Breeding in Mammals*, ed. N. G. Solomon & J. A. French. Cambridge: Cambridge University Press, pp. 267–301.

Fedigan, L. M. (1982) *Primate Paradigms: Sex Roles and Social Bonds*. Chicago, IL: University of Chicago Press.

Folstad, I. & Karter, A. J. (1992) Parasites, bright males, and the immunocompetence handicap. *American Naturalist*, **139**, 603–622.

Frank, L. G. (1997) Evolution of genital masculinization: why do female hyaenas have such a large 'penis'? *Trends in Ecology and Evolution*, **12**, 58–62.

Frank, L. G., Weldele, M. L. & Glickman, S. E. (1995) Masculinization costs in hyaenas. *Nature*, **377**, 584–585.

Frank, S. A. (1995) Mutual policing and repression of competition in the evolution of cooperative groups. *Nature*, **377**, 520–522.

French, J. A. (1997) Proximate regulation of singular breeding in callitrichid primates. In: *Cooperative Breeding in Mammals*, ed. N. Solomon & J. A. French. Cambridge: Cambridge University Press, pp. 34–75.

Fretwell, S. D. & Lucas, H. L. (1970) On territorial behaviour and other factors influencing habitat distribution in birds. *Acta Biotheoretica*, **19**, 16–36.

Gardner, A. & West, S. A. (2004) Cooperation and punishment, especially in humans. *American Naturalist*, **164**, 753–764.

Glickman, S. E., Short, R. V. & Renfree, M. B. (2005) Sexual differentiation in three unconventional mammals: spotted hyenas, elephants and tammar wallabies. *Hormones and Behavior*, **48**, 403–417.

Golla, W., Hofer, H. & East, M. L. (1999) Within-litter sibling aggression in spotted hyaenas: effect of maternal nursing, sex and age. *Animal Behaviour*, **58**, 715–726.

Gomendio, M., Harcourt, A. H. & Roldán, E. R. S. (1998) Sperm competition in mammals. In: *Sperm Competition and Sexual Selection*, ed. T. R. Birkhead and A. P. Møller, London: Academic Press, pp. 667–755.

Goodall, J. (1986) *The Chimpanzees of Gombe: Patterns of Behavior*. Cambridge, MA: Harvard University Press.

Gould, L. & Ziegler, T. E. (2007) Variation in fecal testosterone levels, inter-male aggression, dominance rank and age during mating and post-mating periods in wild adult male ring-tailed lemurs (*Lemur catta*). *American Journal of Primatology*, **69**, 1325–1339.

Gowaty, P. A. (1996) Battle of the sexes and origins of monogamy. In: *Partnerships in Birds*, ed. J. M. Black. Oxford: Oxford University Press, pp. 21–52.

Goymann, W., East, M. L. & Hofer, H. (2001a) Androgens and the role of female 'hyperaggressiveness' in spotted hyenas (*Crocuta crocuta*). *Hormones and Behavior*, **39**, 83–92.

Goymann, W., East, M. L., Wachter, B. *et al.* (2001b) Social, state-dependent and environmental modulation of faecal corticosteroid levels in free-ranging female spotted hyaenas. *Proceedings of the Royal Society B*, **268**, 2453–2459.

Goymann, W., East, M. L. & Hofer, H. (2003) Defense of females, but not social status, predicts plasma androgen levels in male spotted hyenas. *Physiological and Biochemical Zoology*, **76**, 586–593.

Goymann, W., Landys, M. M. & Wingfield, J. C. (2007) Distinguishing seasonal androgen responses from male-male androgen responsiveness – revisiting the Challenge Hypothesis. *Hormones and Behavior*, **51**, 463–476.

Greenwood, P. J. (1980) Mating systems, philopatry and dispersal in birds and mammals. *Animal Behaviour*, **28**, 1140–1162.

Griffin, A. S. & West, S. A. (2003) Kin discrimination and the benefits of helping in cooperatively breeding vertebrates. *Science*, **302**, 634–636.

Griffith, S. G., Owens, I. P. F. & Burke, T. (1999) Environmental determination of a sexually selected trait. *Nature*, **400**, 358–360.

Hamilton, W. D. (1964a) The genetical evolution of social behaviour I. *Journal of Theoretical Biology*, **7**, 1–16.

Hamilton, W. D. (1964b) The genetical evolution of social behaviour II. *Journal of Theoretical Biology*, **7**, 17–52.

Harcourt, A. H. & de Waal, F. B. M. (1992) Cooperation and conflict: from ants to anthropoids. In: *Coalitions and Alliances in Humans and Other Animals*, ed. A. H. Harcourt & F. B. M. de Waal. Oxford: Oxford University Press, pp. 493–511.

Hardin, G. (1968) The tragedy of the commons. *Science*, **162**, 1243–1248.

Harvey, P. H. & Pagel, M. D. (1991) *The Comparative Method in Evolutionary Biology*. Oxford: Oxford University Press.

Hauert, C., Traulsen, A., Brandt, H., Nowak, M. A. & Sigmund, K. (2007) Via freedom to coercion: the emergence of costly punishment. *Science*, **316**, 1905–1907.

Hausfater, G. & Hrdy, S. B. (1984) *Infanticide: Comparative and Evolutionary Perspectives*. New York, NY: Aldine.

Hausfater, G., Altmann, J. & Altmann, S. (1982) Long-term consistency of dominance relations among female baboons (*Papio cynocephalus*). *Science*, **217**, 752–755.

Heckel, G. & von Helversen, O. (2003) Genetic mating system, relatedness and the significance of harem associations in the bat *Saccopteryx bilineata*. *Molecular Ecology*, **12**, 219–227.

Heinsohn, R. & Packer, C. (1995) Complex cooperative strategies in group-territorial African lions. *Science*, **269**, 1260–1262.

Hemelrijk, C. K. (2000) Towards the integration of social dominance and spatial structure. *Animal Behaviour*, **59**, 1035–1048.

Henzi, S. P. & Barrett, L. (2002) Infants as a commodity in a baboon market. *Animal Behaviour*, **63**, 915–921.

Hillis, T. L. & Mallory, F. F. (1996) Fetal development in wolves (*Canis lupus*) of the Keewatin District, Northwest Territories, Canada. *Canadian Journal of Zoology*, **74**, 2211–2218.

Hinde R.A. (1974) *Biological Bases of Human Social Behaviour.* New York, NY: McGraw-Hill.

Hirschenhauser, K. & Oliveira, R. F. (2006) Social modulation of androgens in male vertebrates: meta-analyses of challenge hypothesis. *Animal Behaviour*, **71**, 265–277.

Hofer, H. & East, M. L. (1993a) The commuting system of Serengeti spotted hyaenas: how a predator copes with migratory prey. I. Social organization. *Animal Behaviour*, **46**, 547–557.

Hofer, H. & East, M. L. (1993b) The commuting system of Serengeti spotted hyaenas: how a predator copes with migratory prey. II. Intrusion pressure and commuters' space use. *Animal Behaviour*, **46**, 559–574.

Hofer, H. & East, M. L. (1993c) The commuting system of Serengeti spotted hyaenas: how a predator copes with migratory prey. III. Attendance and maternal care. *Animal Behaviour*, **46**, 575–589.

Hofer, H. & East, M. L. (1995) Population size, population dynamics and commuting system of Serengeti spotted hyenas. In: *Serengeti II: Dynamics, Management and Conservation of an Ecosystem*, ed. A. R. E. Sinclair & P. Arcese. Chicago, IL: University of Chicago Press, pp. 332–363.

Hofer, H. & East, M. L. (1997) Skewed offspring sex ratios and sex composition of twin litters in Serengeti spotted hyaenas (*Crocuta crocuta*) are a consequence of siblicide. *Applied Animal Behavior Science*, **51**, 307–316.

Hofer, H. & East, M. L. (1998) Biological conservation and stress. *Advances in the Study of Behavior*, **27**, 405–525.

Hofer, H. & East, M. L. (2003) Behavioral processes and costs of co-existence in female spotted hyenas: a life history perspective. *Evolutionary Ecology*, **17**, 315–331.

Hofer, H. & East, M. L. (2008) Siblicide in Serengeti spotted hyenas: a long-term study of maternal input and cub survival. *Behavioral Ecology and Sociobiology*, **62**, 341–351.

Holekamp, K. E. & Smale, L. (1991) Dominance acquisition during mammalian social development: the 'inheritance' of maternal rank. *American Zoologist*, **31**, 306–317.

Holekamp, K. E., Smale, L. & Szykman, M. (1996) Rank and reproduction in female spotted hyenas. *Journal of Reproduction and Fertility*, **108**, 229–237.

Holekamp, K. E., Boydston, E. E., Szykman, M. *et al.* (1999) Vocal recognition in the spotted hyaena and its possible implications regarding the evolution of intelligence. *Animal Behaviour*, **58**, 383–395.

Hollister-Smith, J. A., Poole, J. H., Archie, E. A. *et al.* (2007) Age, musth and paternity success in wild male African elephants, *Loxodonta africana*. *Animal Behaviour*, **74**, 287–296.

Hoogland, J. L. (1982) Prairie dogs avoid extreme inbreeding. *Science*, **215**, 1639–1641.

Höner, O. P., Wachter, B., East, M. L. *et al.* (2007) Female mate choice drives the evolution of male-biased dispersal in a social mammal. *Nature*, **448**, 798–801.

Höner, O. P., Wachter, B., East, M. L. *et al.* (2008) Do female hyenas choose mates based on tenure? Reply to Van Horn *et al. Nature*, **454**, E2.

Horrocks, J. & Hunte, W. (1983) Maternal rank and offspring rank in vervet monkeys: an appraisal of the mechanisms of rank acquisition. *Animal Behaviour*, **31**, 772–782.

Hrdy, S. B. (1977) Infanticide as a primate reproductive strategy. *American Scientist*, **65**, 40–49.

Hrdy, S. B. (2000) The optimal number of fathers: evolution, demography, and history in the shaping of female mate preferences. *Annals of the New York Academy of Sciences*, **907**, 75–96.

Humphrey, N. K. (1976) The social function of intellect. In: *Growing Points in Ethology*, ed. P. P. G. Bateson & R. A. Hinde. Cambridge: Cambridge Univeristy Press, pp. 303–317.

Ims, R. A. (1989) The potential for sexual selection in males: effect of sex ratio and spatial temporal distribution of receptive females. *Evolutionary Ecology*, **3**, 338–352.

Insley, S. J. (2001) Mother–offspring vocal recognition in northern fur seals is mutual but asymmetrical. *Animal Behaviour*, **61**, 129–137.

Jennions, M. D. & Petrie, M. (2000) Why do females mate multiply? A review of the genetic benefits. *Biological Reviews*, **75**, 21–64.

Johnstone, R. A. (2000) Models of reproductive skew: a review and synthesis. *Ethology*, **106**, 5–26.

Johnstone, R. A., Reynolds, J. D. & Deutsch, J. C. (1996) Mutual mate choice and sex differences in choosiness. *Evolution*, **50**, 1382–1391.

Kamran, S. & Kerth, G. (2003) Secretions of the interaural gland contain information about individuality and colony membership in the Bechstein's bat. *Animal Behaviour*, **65**, 363–369.

Kappeler, P. K. (1997) Intrasexual selection and testis size in strepsirhine primates. *Behavioral Ecology*, **8**, 10–19.

Keane, B., Waser, P., Creel, S., Creel, N. M., Elliott, L. F. & Minchella, D. J. (1994) Subordinate reproduction in dwarf mongooses. *Animal Behaviour*, **47**, 65–75.

Keller, L. & Reeve, H. K. (1994) Partitioning of reproduction in animal societies. *Trends in Ecology and Evolution*, **9**, 98–103.

Kokko, H. (2002) Are reproductive skew models evolutionary stable? *Proceedings of the Royal Society B*, **270**, 265–270.

Kokko, H. & Johnstone, R. A. (1999) Social queuing in animal societies: a dynamic model of reproductive skew. *Proceedings of the Royal Society B*, **266**, 571–578.

Kokko, H. & Lindström, J. (1996) Evolution of female preference for old males. *Proceedings of the Royal Society B*, **263**, 1533–1538.

Kokko, H., Lindström, J., Alatalo, R. V. & Rintamäki P. T. (1998) Queuing for territory position in the lekking black grouse (*Tetrao tetrix*). *Behavioral Ecology*, **9**, 376–383.

Krützen, M., Mann, J., Heithaus, M. R. *et al.* (2005) Cultural transmission of tool use in bottlenose dolphins. *Proceedings of the National Academy of Sciences of the USA*, **102**, 8939–8943.

Kruuk, H. (1972) *The Spotted Hyena*. Chicago, IL: University of Chicago Press.

Kutsukake, N. & Clutton-Brock, T. H. (2006) Aggression and submission reflect reproductive conflict between females in cooperatively breeding meerkats *Suricata suricatta*. *Behavioral Ecology and Sociobiology*, **59**, 541–548.

Kutsukake, N. & Clutton-Brock, T. H. (2008) Do meerkats engage in conflict management following aggression? Reconciliation, submission and avoidance. *Animal Behaviour*, **75**, 1441–1453.

Lacey, E. A. & Sherman, P. W. (1997) Cooperative breeding in naked mole-rats: implications for vertebrate and invertebrate sociality. In: *Cooperative Breeding in Mammals*, ed. N. G. Solomon & J. A. French. Cambridge: Cambridge University Press, pp. 267–301.

Lee, P. C. (1987) Allomothering among African elephants. *Animal Behaviour*, **35**, 278–291.

Lee, P. C. (1989) Family structure, communal care, and female reproductive effort. In: *Comparative Socioecology*,

ed. V. Standen & R. A. Foley. Oxford: Blackwell Scientific Publications, pp. 323–340.

Lehmann, L. & Perrin, N. (2003) Inbreeding avoidance through kin recognition: choosy females boost male dispersal. *American Naturalist*, **162**, 638–652.

Leimar, O. (1996) Life-history analysis of the Trivers and Willard sex-ratio problem. *Behavioral Ecology*, **7**, 316–325.

Lewis, R. J. (2002) Beyond dominance: the importance of leverage. *Quarterly Review of Biology*, **77**, 149–164.

Lindenfors, P., Nunn, C. L. & Barton, R. A. (2007) Primate brain architecture and selection in relation to sex. *BMC Biology*, **5**, 20.

Lusseau, D. (2003) The emergent properties of a dolphin social network. *Proceedings of the Royal Society B*, **270**, S186–188.

Magrath, R. D. & Heinsohn, R. G. (2000) Reproductive skew in birds: model, problems and prospects. *Journal of Avian Biology*, **31**, 247–258.

Malcolm, J. R. & Marten, K. (1982) Natural selection and the communal rearing of pups in African wild dogs. *Behavioral Ecology and Sociobiology*, **10**, 1–13.

Maynard Smith, J. (1982) *Evolution and the Theory of Games*. Cambridge: Cambridge University Press.

Maynard Smith, J. & Parker, G. A. (1976) The logic of asymmetric contests. *Animal Behaviour*, **24**, 159–175.

McComb, K., Reby, D., Baker, L., Moss, C. & Sayialel, S. (2003) Long-distance communication of acoustic cues to social identity in African elephants. *Animal Behaviour*, **65**, 317–329.

McCracken, G. F. & Wilkinson, G. S. (2000) Bat mating systems. In: *Reproductive Biology of Bats*, ed. E. G. Crichton & P. H. Krutzch. London: Academic Press, pp. 321–362.

McDonald, D. B. (2007) Predicting fate from early connectivity in a social network. *Proceedings of the National Academy of Sciences of the USA*, **104**, 10910–10914.

Mesnick, S. L. (2001) Genetic relatedness in sperm whales: evidence and cultural implications. *Behavioral and Brain Sciences*, **24**, 346–347.

Milinski, M., Semmann, D. & Krambeck, H.-J. (2002) Reputation helps solve the 'tragedy of the commons'. *Nature*, **415**, 424–426.

Moehlman, P. D. & Hofer, H. (1997) Cooperative breeding, reproductive suppression, and body mass in canids. In: *Cooperative Breeding in Mammals*, ed. N. Solomon and J. A. French. Cambridge: Cambridge University Press, pp. 76–128.

Möller, L. M. & Beheregaray, L.B. (2004) Genetic evidence for sex-biased dispersal in resident bottle-nosed dolphins (*Tursiops aduncus*). *Molecular Ecology*, **13**, 1607–1612.

Moore, A. J. (1993) Towards an evolutionary view of social dominance. *Animal Behaviour*, **46**, 594–596.

Moore, A. J., Brodie, E. D. & Wolf, J. B. (1997) Interacting phenotypes and the evolutionary process: I. Direct and indirect genetic effects of social interactions. *Evolution*, **51**, 1352–1362.

Moss, C. J. & Poole, J. (1983) Relationships and social structure of African elephants. In: *Primate Social Relationships: an Integrated Approach*, ed. R. Hinde. Oxford: Blackwell Scientific Press, pp. 315–325.

Mousseau, T. A. & Fox, C. W. (1998) The adaptive significance of maternal effects. *Trends in Ecology and Evolution*, **13**, 403–407.

Nagy, M., Heckel, G., Voigt, C. C. & Mayer, F. (2007) Patrilineal social system drives female dispersal in a polygynous bat. *Proceedings of the Royal Society B*, **274**, 3019–3025.

Noë, R. (1990) A veto game played by baboons: a challenge to the use of the Prisoner's Dilemma as a paradigm for reciprocity and cooperation. *Animal Behaviour*, **39**, 78–90.

Noë, R. & Hammerstein, P. (1994) Biological markets: supply and demand determines the effect of partner choice in cooperation, mutualism and mating. *Behavioral Ecology and Sociobiology*, **35**, 1–11.

Noë, R & Hammerstein, P. (1995) Biological markets. *Trends in Ecology and Evolution*, **10**, 336–339.

Noë, R., van Schaik, C. P. & van Hooff, J. A. R. A. M. (1991) The market effect: an explanation for pay-off asymmetries among collaborating animals. *Ethology*, **87**, 97–118.

O'Riain, M. J. & Jarvis, J. U. M. (1997) Colony member recognition and xenophobia in the naked mole-rat. *Animal Behaviour*, **53**, 487–498.

O'Riain, M. J, Bennett, N. C., Brotherton, P. N. M., McIlrath, G. M. & Clutton-Brock, T. H. (2000) Reproductive suppression and inbreeding avoidance in wild populations of cooperatively breeding meerkats (*Suricata suricatta*). *Behavioral Ecology and Sociobiology*, **48**, 471–477.

Ostner, J., Kappeler, P. M. & Heistermann, M. (2002) Seasonal variation and social correlates of androgen excretion in male red-fronted lemurs (*Eulemur fulvus rufus*). *Behavioral Ecology and Sociobiology*, **52**, 485–495.

Owens, I. P. F. & Thompson D. B. A. (1994) Sex differences, sex ratios and sex roles. *Proceedings of the Royal Society B*, **258**, 93–99.

Packer, C. (1977) Reciprocal altruism in *Papio anubis*. *Nature*, **265**, 441–443.

Parga, J. A. (2003) Copulatory plug displacement evidences sperm competition in *Lemur catta*. *International Journal of Primatology*, **24**, 889–899.

Parker, G. A. (1970) Sperm competition and its evolutionary consequences in insects. *Biological Reviews*, **45**, 525–567.

Parker, G. A. (1979) Sexual selection and sexual conflict. In: *Sexual Selection and Reproductive Competition in Insects*, ed. M. S. Blum & N. A. Blum. New York, NY: Academic Press, pp. 123–166.

Parker, G. A. (1983) Mate quality and mating decisions. In: *Mate Choice*, ed. P. P. G. Bateson. Cambridge: Cambridge University Press, pp. 141–166.

Peake, T. M. (2005) Eavesdropping in communication networks. In: *Animal Communication Networks*, ed. P. K. McGregor. Cambridge: Cambridge University Press, pp. 13–37.

Perrin, N. & Mazalov, V. (1999) Dispersal and inbreeding avoidance. *American Naturalist*, **154**, 282–292.

Pitnick, S., Jones, K. E. & Wilkinson, G. S. (2006) Mating system and brain size in bats. *Proceedings of the Royal Society B*, **273**, 719–724.

Pontier, D., Fromont, E., Courchamp, F., Artois, M. & Yoccoz, N. G. (1998) Retroviruses and sexual size dimorphism in domestic cats (*Felis catus* L.). *Proceedings of the Royal Society B*, **265**, 167–173.

Poole, J. H. (1987) Rutting behaviour in African elephants: the phenomenon of musth. *Behaviour*, **102**, 283–316.

Poole, J. H. (1989) Announcing intent: the aggressive state of musth in African elephants. *Animal Behaviour*, **37**, 140–152.

Preston, B. T., Stevenson, I. R., Pemberton, J. M., Coltman, D. W. & Wilson, K. (2005) Male mate choice influences female promiscuity in Soay sheep. *Proceedings of the Royal Society B*, **272**, 365–373.

Pusey, A. & Wolf, M. (1996) Inbreeding avoidance in animals. *Trends in Ecology and Evolution*, **11**, 201–206.

Ramm, S. A., Parker, G. A. & Stockley, P. (2005) Sperm competition and the evolution of male reproductive anatomy in rodents. *Proceedings of the Royal Society B*, **272**, 949–955.

Range, F. & Noë, R. (2005) Can simple rules account for the pattern of triadic interactions in juvenile and adult female sooty mangabeys? *Animal Behaviour*, **69**, 445–452.

Rankin, D. J., Bargum, K. & Kokko, H. (2007) The tragedy of the commons in evolutionary biology. *Trends in Ecology and Evolution*, **22**, 643–651.

Reeve, H. K. & Keller, L. (2001) Tests of reproductive-skew models in social insects. *Annual Review of Entomology*, **46**, 347–385.

Rhine, R. J., Wasser, S. K. & Norton, G. W. (1988) Eight-year study of social and ecological correlates of mortality among immature baboons of Mikumi National Park, Tanzania. *American Journal of Primatology*, **16**, 199–212.

Riesch, R., Ford, J. K. & Thomsen, F. (2006) Stability and group specificity of stereotyped whistles in resident killer whales, *Orcinus orca*, off British Columbia. *Animal Behaviour*, **71**, 79–91.

Rood, J. P. (1980) Mating relationships and breeding suppression in the dwarf mongoose. *Animal Behaviour*, **28**, 143–150.

Rossiter, M. C. (1996) Incidence and consequences of inherited environmental effects. *Annual Review of Ecology and Systematics*, **27**, 451–476.

Rossiter, S. J., Jones, G., Ransome, R. D. & Barratt, E. M. (2001) Outbreeding increases offspring survival in wild greater horseshoe bats (*Rhinolophus ferrumequinum*). *Proceedings of the Royal Society B*, **268**, 1055–1061.

Rossiter, S. J., Ransome, R. D., Faulkes, C. G., Le Comber, S. C. & Jones G. (2005) Mate fidelity and intra-lineage polygyny in greater horseshoe bats. *Nature*, **437**, 408–411.

Rossiter, S. J., Ransome, R. D., Faulkes, C. G., Dawson, D. A. & Jones, G. (2006) Long-term paternity skew and the opportunity for selection in a mammal with reversed sexual size dimorphism. *Molecular Ecology*, **15**, 3035–3043.

Sauther, M. L. (1991) Reproductive behavior of free-ranging *Lemur catta* at Beza Mahafaly Special Reserve, Madagascar. *American Journal of Physical Anthropology*, **84**, 463–477.

Sauther, M. L., Sussman, R. W. & Gould, L. (1999) The socioecology of the ring-tailed lemur: thirty-five years of research. *Evolutionary Anthropology*, **8**, 120–132.

Say, L., Pontier, D. & Natoli, E. (2001) Influence of oestrus synchronization on male reproductive success in the domestic cat (*Felis catus* L.). *Proceedings of the Royal Society B*, **268**, 1049–1053.

Sayigh, L. S., Carter Esch, H., Wells, R. S. & Janik, V. M. (2007) Facts about signature whistles of bottlenose dolphins, *Tursiops truncatus*. *Animal Behaviour*, **74**, 1631–1642.

Schaller, G. B. (1972) *The Serengeti Lion: a Study of Predator-Prey Relations*. Chicago, IL: University of Chicago Press.

Schwagmeyer, P. L. & Parker, G. A. (1990) Male mate choice as predicted by sperm competition in thirteen-lined ground squirrels. *Nature*, **348**, 62–64.

Schwensow, N., Eberle, M. & Sommer, S. (2008) Compatibility counts: MHC-associated mate choice in a wild promiscuous primate. *Proceedings of the Royal Society B*, **275**, 555–564.

Shuster, S. M. & Wade, M. J. (2003) *Mating Systems and Strategies*. Princeton, NJ: Princeton University Press.

Sibly, R. M. & Brown, J. H. (2007) Effects of body size and life-style on evolution of mammal life histories. *Proceedings of the National Academy of Sciences of the USA*, **104**, 17707–17712.

Silk, J. B. (2007) Social components of fitness in primate groups. *Science*, **317**, 1347–1351.

Silk, J. B., Alberts, S. C. & Altmann, J. (2003) Social bonds of female baboons enhance infant survival. *Science*, **302**, 1231–1234.

Smale, L., Frank, L. G. & Holekamp, K. E. (1993) Ontogeny of dominance in free-living spotted hyaenas: juvenile rank relations with adult females and immigrant males. *Animal Behaviour*, **46**, 467–477.

Smith, R. L. (1984) *Sperm Competition and the Evolution of Animal Mating Systems*. New York, NY: Academic Press.

Smuts, B. B. (1986) Gender, aggression, and influence. In: *Primate Societies*, ed. B. B. Smuts, D. L. Cheney, R. M. Seyfarth, R. W. Wrangham & T. T. Struhsaker. Chicago, IL: University of Chicago Press, pp. 400–412.

Stearns, S. C. (1992) *The Evolution of Life Histories*. Oxford: Oxford University Press.

Sun, L. & Müller-Schwarze, D. (1998) Anal gland secretion codes for family membership in beavers. *Behavioral Ecology and Sociobiology*, **44**, 199–208.

Sutherland, W. J. (1985) Chance can produce a sex difference in variance in mating success and explain Bateman's data. *Animal Behaviour*, **33**, 1349–1352.

Sutherland, W. J. (1996) *From Individual Behaviour to Population Ecology*. Oxford: Oxford University Press.

Sutherland, W. J. & Parker, G. (1985) Distribution of unequal competitors. In: *Behavioural Ecology*, ed. R. M. Sibly and R. H. Smith. Oxford: Blackwell, pp. 255–273.

Tibbetts, E. A. & Dale, J. (2007) Individual recognition: is it good to be different. *Trends in Ecology and Evolution*, **22**, 529–537.

Todd, P. M. & Gigerenzer, G. (2000) Précis of simple heuristics that make us smart. *Behavioral and Brain Science*, **23**, 727–741.

Tomasello, M. & Call, J. (1997) *Primate Cognition*. Oxford: Oxford University Press.

Tregenza, T. & Wedell, N. (2000) Genetic compatibility, mate choice and patterns of parentage: invited review. *Molecular Ecology*, **9**, 1013–1027.

Trivers, R. L. (1971) The evolution of reciprocal altruism. *Quarterly Review of Biology*, **46**, 35–57.

Trivers, R. L. & Willard, D. E. (1973) Natural selection of parental ability to vary the sex ratio of offspring. *Science*, **179**, 90–92.

Valderrábano-Ibarra, C., Brumon, I. & Drummond, H. (2007) Development of a linear dominance hierarchy in nestling birds. *Animal Behaviour*, **74**, 1705–1714.

Van Horn, R. C., Watts, H. E. & Holekamp, K. E. (2008) Do female hyaenas choose mates based on tenure? *Nature*, **454**, E1.

van Schaik, C. P. & Deaner, R. O. (2003) Life history and cognitive evolution in primates. In: *Animal Social Complexity*, ed. F. B. M. de Waal & P. L. Tyack, Cambridge, MA: Harvard University Press, pp. 5–25.

van Schaik, C., Pandit, S. A. & Vogel, E. R. (2004) A model for within-group coalitionary aggression among males. *Behavioral Ecology and Sociobiology*, **57**, 101–109.

Verboven, N. M., Monaghan, P., Evans, D. M. *et al.* (2003) Maternal condition, yolk androgens and offspring performance: a supplementary feeding experiment in the lesser black-backed gull (*Larus fuscus*). *Proceedings of the Royal Society B*, **270**, 2223–2232.

Voigt, C. C. & Streich, W. J. (2003) Queuing for harem access in colonies of the sac-winged bat. *Animal Behaviour*, **65**, 149–156.

Voigt, C. C. & von Helversen, O. (1999) Storage and display of odor by male *Saccopteryx bilineata* (Chiroptera; Emballonuridae). *Behavioral Ecology and Sociobiology*, **47**, 29–40.

Voigt, C. C., Heckel, G. & Mayer, F. (2005) Sexual selection favours small and symmetric males in the polygynous greater sac-winged bat *Saccopteryx bilineata* (Emballonuridae, Chiroptera). *Behavioral Ecology and Sociobiology*, **57**, 457–464.

Walters, J. R. & Seyfarth, R. M. (1986) Conflict and cooperation. In: *Primate Societies*, ed. B. B. Smuts, D. L. Cheney, R. M. Seyfarth, R. W. Wrangham & T. T. Struhsaker. Chicago, IL: University of Chicago Press, pp. 306–317.

Wells, R. S. (2003) Dolphin social complexity: lessons from long-term study and life history. In: *Animal Social Complexity*, ed. F. B. M. de Waal & P. L. Tyack, Cambridge, MA: Harvard University Press, pp. 32–56.

Wey, T., Blumstein, D. T., Shen, W. & Jordan, F. (2008) Social network analysis of animal behaviour: a promising tool for the study of sociality. *Animal Behaviour*, **75**, 333–344.

White, P. A. (2007) Costs and strategies of communal den use vary by rank for spotted hyaenas, *Crocuta crocuta*. *Animal Behaviour*, **73**, 149–156.

Whitehead, H. (1996) Babysitting, dive synchrony, and indications of alloparental care in sperm whales. *Behavioral Ecology and Sociobiology*, **38**, 237–244.

Whitehead, H. (1998) Cultural selection and genetic diversity in matrilineal whales. *Science*, **282**, 1708–1711.

Whitehead, H. (1999) Cultural and genetic evolution in whales. *Science*, **284**, 2055.

Wilkinson, G. S. (1984) Reciprocal food sharing in vampire bats. *Nature*, **308**, 181–184.

Wilkinson, G. S. (1985) The social organization of the common vampire bat. II. Mating system, genetic structure, and relatedness. *Behavioral Ecology and Sociobiology*, **17**, 123–134.

Williams, R. & Lusseau D. (2006) A killer whale social network is vulnerable to targeted removals. *Biology Letters*, **2**, 497–500.

Wingfield, J. C., Hegner, R. E., Dufty, A. M. & Ball, G. F. (1990) The 'challenge hypothesis': theoretical implications for the patterns of testosterone secretion, mating systems and breeding strategies. *American Naturalist*, **136**, 829–846.

Wingfield, J. C., Moore, I. T., Goymann, W., Wacker, D. & Sperry, T. (2006) Contexts and ethology of vertebrate aggression: Implications for the evolution of hormone-behavior interactions. In: *Biology of Aggression*, ed. R. Nelson. Oxford: Oxford University Press, pp. 179–210.

Wolf, J. B., Brodie, E. D., Cheverud, J. M., Moore, A. J. & Wade, M. J. (1998) Evolutionary consequences of indirect genetic effects. *Trends in Ecology and Evolution*, **13**, 64–69.

Wolf, J. B. W., Mawdsley, D., Trillmich, F. & James, R. (2007) Social structure in a colonial mammal: unravelling hidden structural layers and their foundations by network analysis. *Animal Behaviour*, **74**, 1293–1302.

Wyatt, T. D. (2003) *Pheromones and Animal Behaviour*. Cambridge: Cambridge University Press.

Young, A. L., Richard, A. F. & Aiello, L. C. (1990) Female dominance and maternal investment in strepsirhine primates. *American Naturalist*, **135**, 473–488.

Yurk, H., Barrett-Lennard, L., Ford, J. K. B. & Matkin, C.O. (2002) Cultural transmission within maternal lineages: vocal clans in resident killer whales in southern Alaska. *Animal Behaviour*, **62**, 1103–1119.

Zeh, J. A. & Zeh, D. W. (1997) The evolution of polyandry. II. Post-copulatory defences against genetic incompatibility. *Proceedings of the Royal Society B*, **264**, 69–75.

Evolutionary genetics and social behaviour: changed perspectives on sexual coevolution

Michael G. Ritchie

Studies of the evolutionary genetics of sexual behaviour have undergone major changes in the last few decades (see Chapters 2 and 10). There have been many great successes in identifying and analysing the influence of single genes, but also an increasing realisation that sexual coevolution and social interactions can influence the evolution of sexual communication systems in unpredictable ways.

When I was a zoology student at the University of Edinburgh in the early 1980s, studying the evolutionary genetics of behaviour seemed an interesting and reasonably tractable project. Lectures in genetics, particularly by Trudy Mackay and Doug Falconer, had impressed upon us that traits like morphology or milk yield in cows were influenced by too many genes to ever identify, so a statistical approach to partitioning genetic and environmental effects (heritability) was necessary. Lectures on the evolution of behaviour, particularly from Linda Partridge and Aubrey Manning, had shown how the genetic control of behaviour had itself evolved, and that the amount of genetic variation for traits was a key to understanding behavioural evolution. So, for example, females exert sexual selection on males by choosing mates based upon traits which evolve in a manner equivalent to milk yield in cows. These traits are correlated with fitness (for indirect genetic benefits, or 'good genes'). However, mutual coevolution between male and female traits was particularly important. Fisher's runaway process of sexual selection elegantly demonstrated that coevolution between male sexual behaviours and female preferences could lead to rapid evolution of both, and indirectly cause speciation by sexual selection (see also Chapter 19). This intersection between genetics, behaviour and the origin of species sparked my curiosity and defined the arena of research which I wished to work in.

These main interests have not changed much despite the intervening decades – perhaps I lack imagination. But how have our notions about the evolutionary genetics of sexual interactions changed? 'Good genes' theories of sexual selection have come and perhaps gone. If I was to choose one topic which has undergone a rethink to the extent that we might need to change our 'way of seeing things', I would highlight how the mutual coevolution thought to underlie sexual behavioural interactions has been replaced by the realisation that coevolution is often sexually antagonistic: males and females have different evolutionary interests, and the lack of resolution between these alters the evolutionary dynamics of such social interactions (Arnqvist & Rowe 2005). Does this provide a 'new paradigm' for understanding inter-sexual interactions (Tregenza et al. 2006)? That conflict rather than cooperation underlies sexual

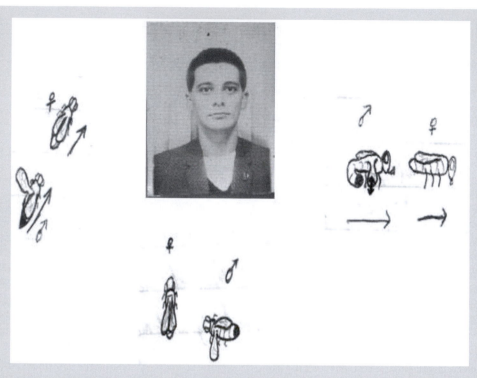

Edinburgh Zoology undergraduate M. G. Ritchie produced some woeful illustrations of fly courtship behaviour when he first saw it in 1982. But he did notice that *Drosophila melanogaster* and *D. simulans* showed interesting subtle differences, which sparked an interest in behaviour and speciation.

interactions is not a radically new idea – perhaps the first landmark paper was Parker's (1979), though others recognised the issue before this.

The study that I would highlight as having had most impact on me was Bill Rice's (1996) study 'Sexually antagonistic male adaptation triggered by experimental arrest of female evolution'. An arresting title, and the opening two sentences made any reader interested in the evolution of sexual interactions sit up and take note: 'Each sex is part of the environment of the other sex. This may lead to perpetual coevolution between the sexes, when adaptation by one sex reduces the fitness of the other.' Any cosy notion of coevolution is immediately challenged, but another important change is that our idea of the environment, and

environmental variation, is also subtly shifted here. In this experiment Rice took advantage of rearranged fly chromosomes to 'freeze' a female genotype and allow a pool of male genotypes to evolve against this environment, which they mated with and passed genes through. Rice cycled out non-recombined male genotypes, and parcelled out some male chromosomes to allow genetic recombination. After 30 generations of evolution male genotypes were fitter than controls with these females, better able to induce females to re-mate and more capable at sperm competition against control males – but this came at the expense of the female genotype, which showed increased mortality as a result of mating with the experimental males. In this very clever experiment females were a static genetic environment that males evolved to adapt to, and exploit.

This is all a logical consequence of the 1970s rejection of group selectionist arguments in favour of selfish genes, but ethologists had seemed slow to drop the notion that sexual reproduction was cooperative or that sexual communication served some beneficial mutual stimulation (indeed, some biologists still seem reluctant to discard such ideas). The implications of viewing sexual interactions as antagonistic rather than neutral or beneficial coevolution are still being explored. Rice and colleagues have likened the new view of sexual coevolution to a dance in which both male and female genotypes are moving, taking step by step exploitation and counter-exploitation moves, in a 'chase-away' rather than runaway scenario. Many features of courtship have needed recent re-interpretation. For example, nuptial gifts that males give to females during courtship or copulation may be much less benign than previously imagined, and females may evolve discrimination against these inducements or any unwanted side effects they bring. Components of semen may be toxic to females, through undesirable effects on female physiology, either as a side-product of sperm competition or because they manipulate female fecundity. Traumatic insemination, where intromission directly damages the female, is being found to be more common than previously imagined, even in very familiar species of *Drosophila*. Sexually antagonistic coevolution may influence major steps in evolution such as the nature of sex chromosomes or features of speciation (though sexual conflict can either accelerate or inhibit speciation, depending on how it acts). It may also have a major impact upon genomic architecture. Unlike in Bill Rice's flies, the alleles involved in adaptation of one gender are constantly being cycled and recombined through both sexes. Genomic studies are revealing that sex-biased expression of loci, which will counter expression of alleles beneficial to only one sex or to the other, is extremely widespread. About 30% of loci in the fruit fly show sex-biased expression; these loci are amongst the fastest-diverging between species, and probably include the best candidates for so-called 'speciation genes'.

Viewing interacting social partners as part of the environment also has profound implications for quantitative genetics or heritability. The 'good genes' models of sexual selection dominated studies of behavioural ecology and sexual selection for decades. Sexually antagonistic selection is a means of maintaining abundant genetic variation, but its value in increasing mean offspring fitness may be nil. Detailed studies of genetic variation within natural populations have suggested that the genetic covariance between male and female fitness may be indistinguishable from -1 (Foerster *et al.* 2007), so much of the genetic variation beneficial to females is detrimental to males, and vice versa. The idea that social interactions form part of the environment that behaviour evolves within has been formalised within quantitative genetics in the concept of 'indirect genetic effects' (see Chapters 1 and 2). Social interactions (in the form of inter- or intrasexual selection, aggression, competition, communication, dominance, etc.) are ubiquitous in sociobiology. The environment therefore includes the genetic variation of the interacting individuals and itself evolves in response to the evolution of the focal animal. Partitioning sources of variance has never been a simple exercise, but non-additive effects such as indirect genetic effects can have unexpected effects on the effective heritability of social behaviours. The dynamics of these effects, their magnitude and ubiquity are only beginning to be explored (Moore & Pizarri 2005). While we are making fantastic progress in identifying single genes with large effects on behaviour, the real sea changes in evolutionary studies of behaviour genetics are perhaps going to involve studies in the darker recesses of quantitative genetics – non-additive interaction effects between loci and between gene effects and the social environment.

I suggest the following principles for evolutionary studies of behavioural genetics:

- Be integrative. Modern research programmes are usually laboratory-bound mechanistic reductionist studies or evolutionary, but the two are synergistic.
- Genes evolve within populations and vary in space and time. Population genetics is essential to understanding why genes vary, or why one is now fixed.
- Welcome variation. Look at how individuals and species vary and try to understand why.
- Single-gene approaches are fantastic for understanding the function and mechanism of gene action, but genes never act on their own. Genes evolve because of their genotype-by-environment interactions and epistasis: these are not an analytical inconvenience.
- Never, ever, study only one species.

References

Arnqvist, G. & Rowe, L. (2005) *Sexual Conflict*. Princeton, NJ: Princeton University Press

Foerster, K., Coulson, T., Sheldon, B. C. *et al.* (2007) Sexually antagonistic genetic variation for fitness in red deer. *Nature*, **447**, 1107–1109.

Moore, A. J. & Pizzari, T. (2005) Quantitative genetic models of sexual conflict based on interacting phenotypes. *American Naturalist*, **165**, S88–97.

Parker, G. A. (1979) Sexual selection and sexual conflict. In: *Sexual Selection and Reproductive Competition in Insects,* ed. M. S. Blum & N. A. Blum . New York, NY: Academic Press, pp. 123–166.

Rice, W. R. (1996) Sexually antagonistic male adaptation triggered by experimental arrest of female evolution. *Nature*, **381**, 232–234.

Tregenza, T., Wedell, N. & Chapman, T. (2006) Sexual conflict: a new paradigm? *Philosophical Transactions of the Royal Society B*, **361**, 229–234. [Plus other articles in this special issue.]

15

Social behaviour in humans

Ruth Mace

Overview

The behavioural ecological approach, and in some cases a cultural evolutionary approach, has enabled us to address a number of key questions in the evolution of human social behaviour. What were our ancestral families like, did we breed cooperatively, and how has that contributed to our life-history evolution? Why is there diversity in human cultural norms between societies, especially in marriage and kinship systems? What evolutionary mechanisms underpin the unique abilities of humans to coordinate actions between large numbers of only distantly related individuals – individual natural selection or group-level cultural selection? This is far from an exhaustive list of topics in a huge field, but these have been selected because they all illustrate examples of human behaviours that have at least some uniquely human characteristics.

Human social systems are unique, no doubt due to our cognitive capacity. Our life history suggests a long period of learning and slow growth (childhood), which is associated with the cognitive development of our large brains, followed by a period of intense levels of parental investment in numerous offspring who are fed through technologically advanced methods which children generally cannot entirely master until they are at least teenagers. Husbands, grandmothers and other members of the social group can all help defray the costs of rearing multiple costly offspring; although there is still some disagreement about which individuals are most important; it probably depends on ecology. There seems little doubt now that our life history is one adapted to transferring massive resources down the generations, to enable this technological lifestyle, although there is still no consensus on whether menopause is an adaptation to child and grandchild care.

There is also debate about how humans form much larger groups, including ethno-linguistic groups of many hundreds or thousands of unrelated individuals. Whilst there is no doubt that we do this, whether this is an emergent property of strategic decision rules selected for at the level of the individual, or the result of some form of multi-level selective forces, remains a matter of debate. There is no doubt, however, that we are social. We need to live not just with our families but in a wider grouping. Warfare was exceptionally common in our history and prehistory, so numbers of associates were always needed, be it to defend women from being raided, or to protect territory and later property. Whether social emotions such as a sense of fairness evolved in these conditions and govern economic behaviour today is a moot point.

Social Behaviour: Genes, Ecology and Evolution, ed. Tamás Székely, Allen J. Moore and Jan Komdeur. Published by Cambridge University Press. © Cambridge University Press 2010.

15.1 Introduction to human behavioural ecology

Human behavioural ecology is the study of fitness costs and benefits of human actions, and how they vary with ecological conditions. Human behaviour is highly plastic, and differs between groups and between individuals according to the environment in which they find themselves at any particular time. This is true of all animal behaviour, but in humans the picture is further complicated by the fact that our cognitive abilities enable us to be cultural beings, whose environment is cultural as well as ecological. Social norms vary from culture to culture and seem to constrain the ability of individuals to make independent decisions about how to behave. The fact that cultural traits can be inherited in non-Mendelian ways can, at least in theory, lead to some behaviours evolving that we would not expect to see in non-cultural animals, especially group-level actions (Boyd & Richerson 1985). Here I will show how the behavioural ecological approach, and in some cases a cultural evolutionary approach, has addressed key questions in the evolution of human social behaviour.

When anthropology departments talk about biological anthropology, they are generally referring to a group of people studying the evolutionary ecology, behaviour and genetics of extant apes, hominin fossils and small-scale human societies. The rationale for this grouping of diverse topics is phylogenetic. But in the realm of social behaviour, humans are worlds apart from their great ape cousins. We don't think like them, we don't live like them and we don't behave like them. Apes can learn from each other, but the capacity in non-human primates for cumulative cultural evolution is very limited. Apes perform better than most other animal species at a range of cognitive tasks, including making and manipulating simple tools, but have lost any right to claim exclusivity in this task given findings about corvids such as the Caledonian crow *Corvus moneduloides* (Hunt & Gray 2003, Weir & Kacelnik 2006). Chimpanzees *Pan troglodytes* can hunt, but they rarely share their kills, and almost never share with unrelated males. Primates live in a diverse range of social groupings, often with large

numbers of female kin living together, but few show strong bonds outside the mother–offspring dyad, and most of them have a social system with little in common with human social groups.

The essential unit of human social structure is the monogamous pair. This is social monogamy rather than strict monogamy, in that monogamy may be more or less serial and mating strategies may be more or less polygynous, but human females can generally be described as associated with (married to) a particular male at any one time in their adult life. Several dependent and costly offspring, which usually reside in a central location, need to be provisioned (to a greater or lesser extent) by both parents, or by one parent with help from the extended family. In this respect, the behavioural ecology of human families has as much in common with that of the birds (Chapter 11) as it does with most other primates.

In hunter–gatherer societies, families are embedded in bands of several families (Kelly 1995), and such grouping may enhance defence, food security, mating opportunities and other social functions. Hunting is often a communal activity, and large prey items are almost always shared amongst the whole band. Gathered products are not necessarily shared. Bands often periodically come together in larger groupings of several hundred individuals, often for ceremonies, such as club-fights in the Ache of Paraguay (Hill & Hurtado 1996), which provide opportunities for display and mate choice beyond the band. In most societies, women tend to leave their natal group to live with patrilocal relatives after marriage (which varies from a formal to an informal arrangement), although women can often stay with the matrilocal family until after the first child has been born (Marlowe 2004). These wider groupings are embedded within an ethnic group usually defined by a unique language, that can range in size from a few hundred to many thousands of individuals.

15.2 Are humans cooperative breeders?

Human life histories show strong differences from that of other great apes – much longer childhoods (i.e. late onset of puberty and reproduction), then short inter-birth intervals, low adult mortality, and a long period of post-reproductive life, especially for females. This combination of life-history traits poses a central problem for women: that of raising several dependent children simultaneously. The human birth interval of about three years in natural-fertility populations is out of line with that of other great apes of similar body size. The orang-utan *Pongo* spp., for example, has an inter-birth interval of about eight years, and the chimpanzee four to five years (Galdikas & Wood 1990). Only gibbons *Hylobates lar* (less than 25% the body mass of humans) have a three-year inter-birth interval. Most anthropologists now agree that human females are capable of such rapid reproduction because of the support they receive from other family members. Work on the transfer of resources between family members has helped to establish the view that children are especially costly in humans, requiring much more sustained parental investment than, for example, do chimpanzees (Kaplan & Lancaster 2003). The 'traditional view' of the family has been that help for the mother comes from the father – hence the human pair bond is based on mutual interdependence of husband and wife to raise their children. In hunter–gatherer societies, the division of labour is nearly always such that men bring back meat to the band, while women gather mainly plant resources. However, the observation that the number of calories brought back from gathered foods often exceeds that from hunting, combined with the fact that meat is often shared widely throughout the band rather than strictly within the nuclear family (Kaplan & Hill 1985, Hawkes *et al.* 1997, 2001), has led to the suggestion that women are not necessarily dependent on men to raise their family (Hawkes *et al.* 1997).

If the human life history poses a problem for women, then it may also provide the solution. Human females spend a relatively high proportion of their lives in a non-reproductive state, so both pre- and post-reproductive individuals may be available to help mothers in raising offspring at relatively little cost to their own reproduction. Grandmothers, in particular, may provide an alternative to, or complement, paternal care, as has now been shown in about 20 different studies (Sear & Mace 2008). If grandmothers are helping to support their children's children, then two unusual features of human female life history – menopause and high birth rates – can potentially be explained at once. It is striking that mothers typically reach menopause as daughters reach reproductive age, and mothers die as their daughters reach menopause. Menopause may be an adaptation to enable grandmaternal support, which in turn enables a high human birth rate (Hawkes *et al.* 1998, Shanley & Kirkwood 2001). Mothers may also use the labour of their older children, particularly daughters, to spread the costs of raising offspring. The extended juvenile period of human young may enable the economic contributions of older children to ameliorate the costs of large family size, although this effect has only been shown in agricultural societies (Lee & Kramer 2002).

Given that we clearly evolved as hunter–gatherers, information on who supports the family in foraging societies is of especial interest. However, empirical studies on hunter–gatherer communities are data-limited, due to both the small number of such societies that survive and the small number of individuals living in something approaching a hunter–gatherer lifestyle within those societies. This may have contributed to the fact that a consensus view on the relative importance of fathers as compared to grandmothers has not emerged.

Much of the evidence in the debate over whether fathers or grandmothers are key helpers to mothers came from nutritional studies. Hawkes *et al.* (1997) point out that in the Hadza of Tanzania, children with older female relatives in their band are better nourished, and their data suggest that the hunting season is not actually a particularly good time of year for children. Some studies on foraging strategies in the Ache of Paraguay and in the Hadza highlight the fact that total calories and energy return rates from gathering often equal or even exceed those from hunting (Hill *et al.* 1987, Blurton Jones *et al.* 2000, Marlowe 2003). But Hill, Kaplan and others (Hill & Kaplan 1993, Gurven & Kaplan 2006) have argued that the nature of the food brought back by males is superior and very important, leading them to conclude that the contribution of males to family nutrition is significant, perhaps around 80% of the calories (though note that an important contribution by males to the diet does not necessarily imply that fathers are directly provisioning their families, as meat is shared). As an extreme example, Arctic hunters such as the Inuit are almost entirely dependent on hunted food brought in by men. In the coldest areas, babies and young children could barely survive outside in winter, and thus females are dependent on their spouses for almost everything. Marlowe (2003) shows that male provisioning occurs at critical times in the Hadza, such as when a woman's foraging is handicapped because she recently gave birth.

The variability in the findings suggests that the ecology of the system influences the relative importance of fathers, grandmothers, and potentially other kin such as siblings or older offspring, in the rearing of human children. This should come as no surprise to evolutionary ecologists. Unfortunately, few hunter–gatherer studies can generate large enough sample sizes to estimate important determinants of rare events like mortality, or low-variance measures like fertility. Most populations for which such data are available are farmers, not hunter–gatherers, but historical populations or farmers in less developed countries do share with hunter–gatherers characteristics such as high workloads, high disease burdens and high reproductive rates. Whilst most populations for which such data are available are/were growing rather than stable, the same can be said of contemporary hunter–gatherer populations too, so demographic datasets from such farming populations remain useful databases with which to test hypotheses about human life history.

Our study of rural Gambia was one of few in which both detailed longitudinal data on matrilineal and patrilineal kin and data on child nutrition were available for a non-contracepting population. We were able to show that mothers, maternal grandmothers (Fig. 15.1) and older sisters were significant contributors to both child survival and nutrition, whereas patrilineal relatives, including fathers, were not (Sear *et al.* 2000, 2002). However, patrilineal kin did enhance female fertility (Sear *et al.* 2003, Allal *et al.* 2004). This illustrates a trade-off we might predict due to the asymmetric cost of reproduction for each lineage. In

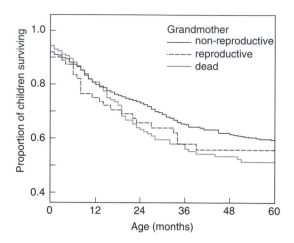

Figure 15.1 In rural Gambia, having a living, non-reproductive maternal grandmother enhanced the survival prospects of children between the ages of 1 and 4, compared to when the maternal grandmother was dead. The beneficial effect was much reduced in the few cases where the grandmother was still reproducing herself. From Sear *et al.* (2000, 2002).

natural-fertility populations, where costs of reproduction are high, women have traded off reproductive rate against mortality risk – and the optimal balance in that trade-off will be at a higher reproductive rate for the patriline (including the father) than it is for the matriline (Mace & Sear 2005).

For the patriline, the death of a spouse is obviously disadvantageous to the family, but she can nonetheless be replaced through remarriage. For the matriline, the death of a woman is the end of her line.

Looking over the full range of similar studies, the pattern of matrilineal kin help observed in rural Gambia is common. Across all societies from which data are available, mothers were universally important, and maternal grandmothers usually improved child survival; the few studies of elder sisters show that they are also helpful. However, the importance of fathers and paternal grandparents for child survival was more variable – although their contribution may be in wealth inheritance, or other benefits that occur later and are not necessarily reflected in childhood mortality rates (Sear & Mace 2008).

There is little evidence that one particular family structure has been of paramount importance throughout human history. For example, foragers in the Old World tend to rely relatively more on gathering and have lower male contributions to the diet than New World foragers (Marlowe 2005). It seems reasonable to assume that human family systems have always been somewhat flexible and responsive to ecological conditions, as are those of many other species (Chapter 12).

15.3 Evolution of human life history

I introduced the previous section by describing the unusual features of human female life history – late puberty, short birth spacing and menopause. It is as if the female fertile period of life has been compressed into the middle of life, with a late start and an early end. Do kin effects tell us anything important about the evolution of these human female life-history characteristics? That grandmothers appear to be almost universally beneficial across societies in improving the fitness of their relatives does provide some support for the grandmother hypothesis for menopause, but we still cannot be entirely certain that menopause evolved because of its fitness benefits. It may be that grandmothers invest in their grandchildren because they are unable to continue having children of their own, and investing in grandchildren is better than investing in nothing at all; it may even be a means by which to reduce competition with younger kin for the resources required to breed (Cant & Johnstone 2008).

Mathematical modelling is useful to examine whether a particular trait is likely to have evolved given a set of life-history parameters; we do not have real women without menopause whose fitness we can examine empirically. Several attempts to build quantitative models in which women can compensate for lost fertility in later life through enhancing the fitness of children and grandchildren have failed to find fitness benefits sufficiently large to favour menopause at the age of 50 years (Hill & Hurtado 1991), which has contributed to a belief that grandparental and parental care are significant selective forces on human

longevity, but not necessarily on the timing of menopause (Hawkes *et al*. 1998). However, this argument also relies on the notion that the fertile span is somehow constrained, for which there is no evidence. Shanley and Kirkwood (2001) argue that menopause at a slightly older age could be favoured if a range of selective forces are combined, including an increase in maternal mortality with age, as well as grandmaternal effects both on grandchild survival and on their daughters' fertility (and these latter effects need to be large). When using Shanley and Kirkwood's model with data from a natural mortality and fertility population in the Gambia (Shanley *et al*. 2007), we found that grandmaternal effects on child survival are particularly important. The reasons for this lie in the fact that selection is derived from the size of the effect of a loss of kin, combined with how likely that loss is to occur. Whilst maternal deaths posed more serious risks to the child, they were rare (due to low mortality in reproductive-age adults), whereas grandmaternal deaths were common; hence the total number of child deaths caused by grandmaternal deaths per year exceeded those caused by maternal deaths. The model, which is one of the few to incorporate the full life history (necessary because changing one aspect of life history necessarily alters selective forces on other areas of the life course), shows that the grandmother effect is therefore a far more potent selective force on menopause than maternal or other effects (Shanley *et al*. 2007).

A shift towards modelling the mortality schedules and ageing patterns of our species, rather than a specific component of human life history such as menopause, has suggested that many peculiarities of human life history, including a long juvenile period, long lifespan and post-reproductive life, may hinge on intergenerational transfers and conflicts not just with grandmothers, but all transfers and competitive interactions between older and younger individuals (Kaplan & Robson 2002, Lee 2003, Johnstone & Cant 2008). The mathematical framework needed to address these problems continues to develop. Such models would also benefit from more information on the parameters needed to inform these models: effect sizes for kin help and kin competition across a number of different populations would illustrate the relative importance of mothers, fathers and grandmothers.

15.4 Families as systems of wealth inheritance

Since the adoption of agriculture, human social systems have been largely shaped by the existence of exceedingly important resources (such as fields or livestock) that can be owned (by individuals or by groups), and passed down to future generations. Access to such resources greatly influences the future reproductive success of descendants. Systems of wealth inheritance are fundamentally linked with systems of marriage and the associated transfers of wealth at marriage, and thus marriage and descent systems are products of the socioeconomic system on which societies are based. As is well known to behavioural ecologists, if males are able to monopolise access to a bit of land that has the resources required for breeding, then that resource can be used to attract females, who will mate polygynously if need be to acquire that resource. Resource-defence polygyny, not dissimilar to that described in birds (where males compete to defend the resources females need to reproduce, and females distribute themselves over the resources, such that males who are defending more productive resources acquire more mates), is also common in humans. As in other species, such polygynous systems can only really emerge where there are sufficient resources for females to raise their children without a great deal of individual help from fathers. Resources such as livestock are particularly associated with polygynous marriage and male-biased wealth inheritance (Hartung 1982). If the number of grandchildren can be enhanced more by leaving livestock to sons (enabling them to marry earlier and more often) than to daughters, which is the case under resource-based polygyny, then patrilineal wealth-inheritance norms doing just that will emerge (Mace 1996).

This is usually the case in livestock-keeping groups. In such systems, men find themselves competing for the heritable resources (a competition that is often resolved by parents between brothers through systems such as primogeniture – where the eldest sons are the only ones to inherit the estate – or between unrelated individuals by warfare and livestock raiding). Those males that are successful in the competition will find themselves able to attract numerous wives; wives reside with the patriline, often far from their parents (patrilocal residence). Parents will benefit from the competition for females by demanding a brideprice (a payment from the groom's family to that of the bride) before releasing their daughters for marriage (hopefully also thereby ensuring that she marries a wealthy man). Such systems tend to leave women rather politically powerless, as wealth is held in the hands of males, and marriage becomes binding as parents are unwilling (or unable) to relinquish the resources they have acquired in brideprice should the marriage be unsuccessful, making divorce almost impossible.

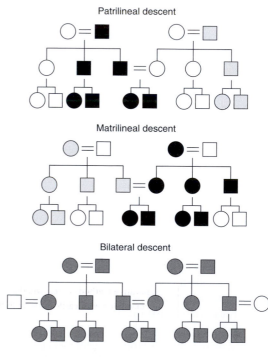

Figure 15.2 Diagram of lineal descent and kinship systems common in human societies. Shaded shapes indicate members of the lineage. □, male; ○, female.

Within lineal family systems (Fig. 15.2), patriliny is by far the most common, but a significant minority (about 17%) of systems described in the *Ethnographic Atlas* of world cultures (Murdock 1967), are matrilineal. Here marriage bonds are often weak, with women frequently marrying several husbands over the course of their lives, and resources are passed down the female line. The extent to which power resides with the males in the matriline or within the nuclear family varies, but residency is normally matrilocal (with mothers and sisters), with farms or gardens passed down from mothers to daughters (marriage generally not entitling males to land ownership, and sometimes not to control over children). There is some evidence that children may benefit from resources being more in the control of their mothers than of their fathers (Leonetti *et al.* 2005).

The ecology that is predictive of matriliny is those systems where resources cannot be monpolised by males to attract females. In Africa it is strongly associated with the absence of livestock (Holden & Mace 2003; Box 15.1). African farms are often not land-limited but labour-limited, so whereas livestock offer females the promise of resources relatively easily accumulated, land that is only of value after months of back-breaking labour in the fields does not generally provide men with the opportunity to monopolise large areas to attract polygynous mates. Women will only remain married to men as long as they help them work the land. In other parts of the world matriliny has been associated with high male mortality rates (either in warfare, as in some matrilineal native American groups, or with ocean fishing, as in the Pacific). Whatever the underlying ecology, women in matrilineal systems rely on mothers, daughters and sisters to support their family, as help from males is often transitory. Paternity uncertainty tends to be high in matrilineal systems, although the extent to which this is a cause or consequence of matrilineal descent systems is a matter of debate.

Box 15.1 Using phylogenetic comparative methods to study human cultural evolution: the coevolution of cattle keeping and matriliny

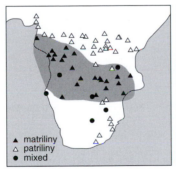 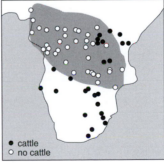

(1) Matrilineal groups in Africa are roughly coincident with an area where cattle are not kept, in the tsetse belt. Holden and Mace (2003) used phylogenetic comparative methods to test whether the social system of patrilineal descent was coevolving with cattle keeping in the Bantu-speaking populations. This work illustrates how language data can be used to make phylogenetic trees of population history, at least in some language groups, and that these can be used to test functional hypotheses about coevolution in the same way that biologists have used phylogenetic comparative methods to test adaptive hypotheses using cross species comparisons (Chapter 5).

Box 15.1 Continued

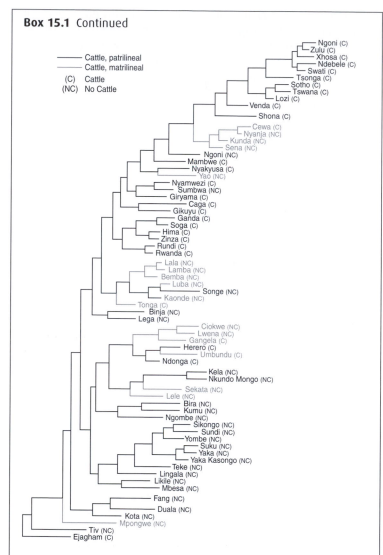

Cattle, patrilineal
Cattle, matrilineal
(C)   Cattle
(NC)   No Cattle

(2) This tree was built using language similarity in a maximum-parsimony tree-building algorithm to ascertain the historical relationships between groups (Holden & Mace 2003). The phylogenetic groupings match well those that linguists and archaeologists have identified.

(3) Using the phylogenetic comparative method DISCRETE (Pagel 1994), rates of transition between states are estimated, to show that there is coevolution between descent systems and cattle keeping. The model compares a model of dependent coevolution of descent system and cattle keeping (L_D) with a model of cattle and descent system evolving independently of each (L_I), and finds that the model of correlated evolution shown in this flow diagram is a significantly

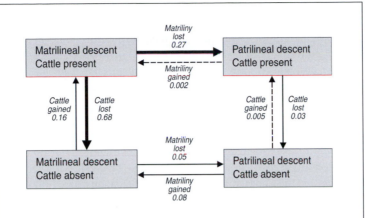

$L_I = -62.52$ $L_D = -56.80$ LR = 5.72, $p = 0.02$

better fit. The thickness of the arrows indicates the rate of change (big arrows and higher rates mean that change happens fast).

These results show that matrilineal-descent groups who keep cattle are unstable, and either they rapidly lose the cattle or the group changes descent system to patriliny. Patrilineal groups with cattle are stable. Thus there is evidence that matrilineal descent systems are associated with lack of cattle. Furthermore, these methods can do more than estimate correlated evolution, as the rates of transition between states shows that it is much more likely that matrilineal groups without cattle first gained cattle and then became patrilineal, rather than first becoming patrilineal and then gaining cattle (the latter is extremely unlikely to occur). Therefore the likely direction of causation is that a change in the subsistence system changes the social system rather than vice versa.

Monogamous marriage, associated with strong, usually lifelong marriage partnerships, is most common in Europe and parts of Asia. It was the most probable ancestral marriage system of the IndoEuropeans, thus long pre-dating the world religions that went on to enforce it (Fortunato *et al.* 2006). Monogamy generates competition between females for mates. This is because, for the wife, in polygynous societies a rich husband with many other wives may be little better than a poor husband with one wife, but in monogamous societies the benefits of a wealthy man's resources are monopolised by one woman and her children. Dowry payments (wealth transfers from the bride's family to that of the groom) then emerge (Gaulin & Boster 1990). The evolutionary ecological bases of human monogamy are not fully understood, but I shall assume that it is based on the need for biparental care and lifelong investment in offspring. The inheritance of land for farming is probably an important consideration in monogamy, as appreciated by Goody (1976). Over the last century, human fertility rates (that is number of offspring born) have plummeted in Western countries, followed by South America and Asia, and now Africa is also experiencing rapid fertility decline. This process remains something of an evolutionary puzzle, but it may well be an extension of the need for high levels of parental investment that at first gave rise to the monogamous marriage system (Mace 2007); monogamy is also now becoming the norm even in countries that were previously polygynous, as the world becomes a more crowded and competitive place.

There are few cases of human polyandrous societies, where one woman marries several men, who are usually brothers. The best-known case is that of the Tibetans, where farmland is limited to small areas on the valley floors and the arid mountains of the Himalayas leave nowhere for farms to expand into (Crook & Crook 1988). Parents could not afford to provide all their sons with a farm without dividing the farm into unsustainably small plots, so all sons unite to marry a single wife, and raise one family only (this has some parallels to primogeniture, such as was common in historical Europe). Younger brothers do badly out of this arrangement, and tend to leave and remarry monogamously if other job opportunities (such as working for government) emerge. Polyandry can be seen as the extreme end of a spectrum of marriage systems in lowest-productivity areas where men need to help the most, with monogamy in intermediate-productivity areas and polygyny in higher-productivity areas where men need to help the least (Marlowe 2000).

Human social systems are incredibly diverse. However, this is not a reason to abandon the toolkit of evolutionary ecology. Quite the opposite: the evolutionary ecological approach can tell us as much about the ecological systems that generate different social systems in humans as they can in other species. Methods such as phylogenetic comparative methods can also be applied to test these hypotheses about cultural or bio-cultural evolution (Chapter 5; Mace & Pagel 1994). Cultural traits are heritable, and traits such as language can be used to build trees of population history (Mace *et al.* 2005). Optimality models can help us determine optimal subsistence strategies, just as has been done in other species.

However, there are also clear theoretical differences to be taken into account when studying human behaviour, particularly important being the insight that because culture is heritable it can provide an additional path of inheritance. Dual inheritance (gene and culture coevolutionary) models were pioneered by Boyd and Richerson (1985) and others. Because cultural traits are not inherited in a Mendelian manner,

cultural evolution may lead to the evolution of some kinds of behaviour that cannot be explained without including cultural traits in an evolutionary model. In particular, biased transmission of traits (i.e. preferential transmission from successful persons, or preferential transmission of the most common form) could underlie the emergence of group-level differences that are relatively persistent, and some have argued that this enables forms of cultural group selection that may underpin our uniquely human capacity to organise behaviour at levels well beyond the family unit (Richerson & Boyd 1999).

15.5 Cooperation beyond the family

Human society, whilst built on families, is also characterised by all families being part of a wider ethnic (or clan-based) group. Even in small-scale tribal societies, ethnic groups of at least 600 individuals were normal, and groups were often much larger. In evolutionary terms, it is puzzling why individuals feel a strong identity associated with this wider grouping, which in the past was associated with high levels of coordinated actions such as warfare. Warfare in chimpanzees, or spotted hyenas *Crocuta crocuta*, is on a much smaller scale and involves related individuals, and thus is not really comparable to human wars. We may also cooperate in other tasks, such as common property management, the enforcement of laws or the raising of orphaned children, and share a range of beliefs and rituals across society. As has already been mentioned, hunter–gatherers share food well beyond the nuclear family within hunter–gatherer bands. Reciprocal systems of bride exchange and trade can extend across wide groupings.

Are we hypersocial animals? Recent work suggested we have emotions based on fair sharing of resources. Economic games have shown that even in single-interaction and anonymous games, individuals appear to be willing to share and expect to be shared with in a 'fair' way (Henrich *et al.* 2001). Individuals playing 'ultimatum games' (a game from experimental economics where a pot of money is given to one player who can share it with another at a particular split, but

only if the other person accepts the offer) will sometimes reject offers even it means no material gain for
themselves and a loss for the other player. Such spiteful behaviour is thought to underlie the tendency of
individuals in the game to make offers typically of up
to half the original allocation of money.

A number of theoretical models have been
advanced to explain this apparently irrational
behaviour. Assuming kin selection and simple reciprocal altruism do not apply to such single encounters with unidentified persons, two main types of
explanation have been proposed. One set is based on
indirect reciprocity (Nowak & Sigmund 2005), which
relies on establishing a reputation for fair play; but
this cannot be important in economic games if players truly believe that their decisions are anonymous,
which is how the game is generally played, so this
could only be an explanation if one does not really
believe the premise of the game. The other explanation relies on various forms of group-level selection
on cultural traits (Boyd & Richerson 1985, Boyd *et al.*
2003, Guzman *et al.* 2007); indeed, the appearance of
economic game data that have been interpreted as
showing a possibly innate sense of fairness has led
to more support emerging for cultural group selection, although it remains a controversial concept.
However, although there is now evidence of cross-
cultural variation in the way people play games, both
in small-scale (Henrich *et al.* 2005) and large-scale
societies (Herrmann *et al.* 2008), behavioural ecology of cross-societal variation has still hardly been
addressed, with the exception of studies by Gurven
(2004) and Marlowe and Berbesque (2008).

Humans are unique in being able to have social
systems based on reputation, due to our cognitive
ability. Whilst individual red deer *Cervus elaphus* or
chimpanzees may strike fear into their opponents,
who may remember not to challenge them again
as a result of defeats, in human society we not only
remember who is powerful but also talk about it to
others. The ability to gossip enables the reputation of
a large number of individuals to be learnt even when
we have not directly witnessed their behaviours, be
it altruistic or aggressive. If having a reputation for
altruism increases the likelihood of receiving favours

in future, the altruistic behaviour can spread. This
system of indirect reciprocity means that the person
who provides a benefit in return is not necessarily the
same person whom you helped in establishing your
reputation. It is not clear exactly how many people's
reputations we can remember – surely no more than
about 100 – yet many human social systems extend
beyond this size.

The concept of family honour is common, so we
may take a short cut by tarring all members of one
family with the same brush to save ourselves the cognitive costs of remembering which individuals can be
trusted and which cannot. (Extremely violent measures can be taken in some cultures against individuals who are thought to threaten the honour of their
family, and so-called honour killings of young women
who are deemed not to have married suitable partners remains a risk even today in some ethnic groups,
with the killing typically conducted by a close family member). It still seems unlikely, however, that a
system based on remembering individual or family
reputations could underlie coordinated action in tribal groups of many hundreds or thousands of individuals without the aid of modern technology. eBay,
Napster and other such computerised systems can of
course record an almost unlimited number of reputations, allowing indirect reciprocal systems to emerge
in very large groups.

The second set of models relies on some kind of
group-level cultural selection. Group selection is
not thought to be important in genetic selection –
even very low levels of inter-group migration destroy
the integrity of groups, such that 'altruistic' groups
would quickly be invaded by less altruistic individuals (Chapter 6). However, if altruistic behaviour
is cultural, then pressures such as conformity, and
especially punishment of non-conformists, can stabilise the differences between groups and allow
selection to occur at the level of the group (Boyd &
Richerson 1985). Such models have not yet been subject to much empirical testing (Bowles 2006), and do
rely on low levels of migration between groups, which
may be unrealistic. Models including punishment,
often altruistic punishment (i.e. some individuals are
willing to pay a cost to punish those who transgress

cultural norms), can generate high levels of cooperative behaviour and conformism in quite large groups (Guzman *et al.* 2007).

All human cultures have some form of religious beliefs, even if some have recently lost those beliefs. Some anthropologists associated our cognitive capacity to be sensitive to punishment, and to avoid it through conforming to local norms, with multilevel selection and with religion (Wilson & Sober 1994). Fear of divine punishment could help enforce group cohesion through cultural group selection, albeit usually backed up by more earthly forms of punishment (ranging from social exclusion to execution for non-conformists). Whereas in small-scale societies norms are enforced by neighbours or local clan leaders, nation states have developed much higher levels of rule enforcement (police and justice systems based on secular or religious laws) that can serve to maintain culture norms of coordinated and often cooperative relations between very large numbers of unrelated people living in cities of millions of persons. Of course the emergence of such control systems does allow powerful individuals to invent laws that benefit themselves, if they maintain control over the enforcement system, and such systems do not require any special explanation beyond an unequal distribution of power.

15.6 Proximate mechanisms

The hormonal, neurological and genetic bases of social behaviour are reviewed elsewhere in this volume (Chapters 1, 2, 3, 11 and 17). We experience the physiological processes though a range of emotions. Emotions such as shame and guilt may not be found in other species. It seems our brains have evolved to enable us to be highly social animals that live in a group with a set of norms with which we have to comply (Fessler & Haley 2003). However, whilst we assist our own infants and other kin irrespective of who is watching, social behaviour towards unrelated individuals may not be so selfless. Charities and law-enforcement agencies have long appreciated the role of visibility in helping to encourage altruism

and deter rule breaking. Generous behaviour in economic games, or donations into honesty boxes, can be influenced by as little as an image of a pair of eyes (Haley & Fessler 2005, Bateson *et al.* 2006). This does not so much suggest an innately moral system, but more that fear of punishment or loss of reputation is a strong reason to be fair, or to conform to social norms of no obvious benefit to ourselves or our immediate family. Such findings, unfortunately, do not enable us to distinguish between models for the evolution of cooperative social norms via indirect reciprocity (which relies on individual-level selection), or cultural group-selection models that include punishment. Indeed, both could be important. However, it is always going to be difficult to prove some kind of group-level effect if an individual-level effect is also important.

If humans have social emotions that are species-typical, we can assume that they have a genetic basis. Social and cognitive disorders such as autism do appear to be highly heritable. The extent to which quantitative genetics can help us understand variation between individuals within the normal range of behaviour is difficult in any species (see Chapter 2), and perhaps especially so in humans, where culture is clearly so influential in helping to determine behaviour. The definition of a complex behavioural trait is in itself a problem (Chapter 16) – consider, for example, the controversies that have raged over trying to measure and work out the heritability of IQ. Clearly, humans cannot be subjected to the kinds of experiments or breeding programmes available to those working on other species. Twin studies have been useful, but even these throw up difficulties of correctly estimating the effects of shared environment. Devlin and others showed how correctly accounting for the shared environment of the womb, even for twins separated at birth, led to a substantial reduction in the estimated heritability of IQ (Devlin *et al.* 1997). The extent to which humans are reliably social or antisocial in economic games has yet to be determined: whilst it is certainly likely that there is real variation in personality, exactly which personality traits are measured in economic games is not always without ambiguity. Whether such variation can be reliably defined and then correlated with genetic markers has yet to be shown.

15.7 Conclusions and future directions

Applying a behavioural ecological approach, and in some cases a cultural evolutionary approach, to the study of human social behaviour has answered many questions. It is now clear that highly developed cognitive abilities and human culture, along with extended parental care, have influenced our social systems. It is less clear, however, which individuals are most important to the structure of the group. The question of how humans form much larger groups also remains unresolved, and prompts a debate concerning individual versus group-level cultural selection.

Finally, the theoretical approach best applied to understanding the origins and maintenance of human social evolution has itself been a matter for debate (Laland & Brown 2002). Most social scientists rejected evolutionary approaches to human social behaviour throughout the twentieth century, and many still do, but thankfully now evolutionary anthropologists, biologists, economists, demographers and psychologists are emerging, and to some extent are combining forces, to help answer the many questions that are still outstanding.

Acknowledgements

Thank-you to Clare Holden, Fiona Jordan and Rebecca Sear for help with the figures, and for general discussions over the years on the topics covered.

Suggested readings

Boyd, R. & Richerson, P. J. (2005) *The Origin and Evolution of Cultures*. Oxford: Oxford University Press.

Cronk, L., Chagnon, N. & Irons, W., eds. (2000) *Adaptation and Human Behavior: an Anthropological Perspective*. New York, NY: Aldine de Gruyter.

Dunbar, R. I. M. & Barrett, L., eds. (2006) *The Oxford Handbook of Evolutionary Psychology*. Oxford: Oxford University Press.

Hill, K. & Hurtado, A. M. (1996) *Ache Life History: the Ecology and Demography of a Foraging People*. New York, NY: Aldine de Gruyter.

Laland, K. & Brown, G. (2002) *Sense and Nonsense*. Oxford: Oxford University Press.

Mace, R., Holden, C. J. & Shennan, S., eds. (2005) *The Evolution of Cultural Diversity: a Phylogenetic Approach*. Walnut Creek, CA: Left Coast Press.

References

Allal, N., Sear, R., Prentice, A. M. & Mace, R. (2004) An evolutionary model of stature, age at first birth and reproductive success in Gambian women. *Proceedings of the Royal Society B*, **271**, 465–470.

Bateson, M., Nettle, D. & Roberts, G. (2006) Cues of being watched enhance cooperation in a real-world setting. *Biology Letters*, **2**, 412–414.

Blurton Jones, N. G., Marlowe, F., Hawkes, K. & O'Connell, J. F. (2000) Paternal investment and hunter–gatherer divorce rates. In: *Adaptation and Human Behaviour: an Anthropological Perspective*, ed. L. Cronk, N. Chagnon & W. Irons. New York, NY: Aldine de Gruyter, pp. 69–89.

Bowles, S. (2006) Group competition, reproductive leveling, and the evolution of human altruism. *Science*, **314**, 1569–1572.

Boyd, R. & Richerson, P. J. (1985) *Culture and the Evolutionary Process*. Chicago, IL: University of Chicago Press.

Boyd, R., Gintis, H., Bowles, S. & Richerson, P. J. (2003) The evolution of altruistic punishment. *Proceedings of the National Academy of Sciences of the USA*, **100**, 3531–3535.

Cant, M. A. & Johnstone, R. A. (2008) Reproductive conflict and the separation of reproductive generations in humans. *Proceedings of the National Academy of Sciences of the USA*, **105**, 5332–5336.

Crook, J. H. & Crook, S. J. (1988) Tibetan polyandry: problems of adaptation and fitness. In: *Human Reproductive Behaviour: a Darwinian Perspective*, ed. L. Betzig, M. Borgerhoff Mulder & P. Turke. Cambridge: Cambridge University Press, pp. 97–114.

Devlin, B., Daniels, M. & Roeder, K. (1997) The heritability of IQ. *Nature*, **388**, 468–471.

Fessler, D. M. T. & Haley, K. J. (2003) The strategy of affect: emotions in human co-operation. In: *Genetic and Cultural Evolution of Co-operation*, ed. P. Hammerstein. Cambridge, MA: MIT Press, pp. 7–36.

Fortunato, L., Holden, C. & Mace, R. (2006) From bridewealth to dowry? A Bayesian estimation of ancestral states of marriage transfers in Indo-European groups. *Human Nature*, **17**, 355–376.

Galdikas, B. M. F. & Wood, J. W. (1990) Birth spacing patterns in humans and apes. *American Journal of Physical Anthropology*, **83**, 185–191.

Gaulin, S. J. C. & Boster, J. S. (1990) Dowry as female competition. *American Anthropologist*, **92**, 994–1005.

Goody, J. (1976) *Production and Reproduction*. Cambridge: Cambridge University Press.

Gurven, M. (2004) Economic games among the Amazonian Tsimane: exploring the roles of market access, costs of giving, and cooperation on pro-social game behavior. *Experimental Economics*, **7**, 5–24.

Gurven, M. & Kaplan, H. (2006) Determinants of time allocation across the lifespan: a theoretical model and an application to the Machiguenga and Piro of Peru. *Human Nature*, **17**, 1–49.

Guzman, R. A., Rodriguez-Sickert, C. & Rowthorn, R. (2007) When in Rome, do as the Romans do: the coevolution of altruistic punishment, conformist learning, and cooperation. *Evolution and Human Behavior*, **28**, 112–117.

Haley, K. J. & Fessler, D. M. T. (2005) Nobody's watching? Subtle cues affect generosity in an anonymous economic game. *Evolution and Human Behavior*, **26**, 245–256.

Hartung, J. (1982) Polygyny and the inheritance of wealth. *Current Anthropology*, **23**, 1–12.

Hawkes, K., O'Connell, J. F. & Jones, N. G. B. (1997) Hadza women's time allocation, offspring provisioning and the evolution of long postmenopausal life spans. *Current Anthropology*, **38**, 551–578.

Hawkes, K., O'Connell, J. F., Jones, N. G. B., Alvarez, H. & Charnov, E. L. (1998) Grandmothering, menopause and the evolution of human life histories. *Proceedings of the National Academy of Sciences of the USA*, **95**, 1336–1339.

Hawkes, K., O'Connell, J. F., & Blurton-Jones, N. G. (2001) Hadza meat sharing. *Evolution and Human Behavior*, **22**, 113–142.

Henrich, J., Boyd, R., Bowles, S. *et al.* (2001) In search of *Homo economicus*: behavioral experiments in 15 small-scale societies. *American Economic Review*, **91**, 73–78.

Henrich, J., Boyd, R., Bowles, S. *et al.* (2005) 'Economic man' in cross-cultural perspective: behavioral experiments in 15 small-scale societies. *Behavioral and Brain Sciences*, **28**, 795–855.

Herrmann, B., Thoni, C. & Gächter, S. (2008) Antisocial punishment across societies. *Science*, **319**, 1362–1367.

Hill, K. & Hurtado, A. M. (1991) The evolution of premature reproductive senescence and menopause in human females: an evaluation of the 'grandmother hypothesis'. *Human Nature*, **2**, 313–350.

Hill, K. & Hurtado, A. M. (1996) *Ache Life History: the Ecology and Demography of a Foraging People*. New York, NY: Aldine de Gruyter.

Hill, K. & Kaplan, H. (1993) On why male foragers hunt and share food. *Current Anthropology*, **34**, 701–706.

Hill, K., Kaplan, H., Hawkes, K. & Hurtado, A. M. (1987) Foraging decisions among Ache hunter-gatherers: new data and implications for optimal foraging models. *Ethology and Sociobiology*, **8**, 1–36.

Holden, C. J. & Mace, R. (2003) Spread of cattle led to the loss of matrilineal descent in Africa: a coevolutionary analysis. *Proceedings of the Royal Society B*, **270**, 2425–2433.

Hunt, G. R. & Gray, R. D. (2003) Diversification and cumulative evolution in New Caledonian crow tool manufacture. *Proceedings of the Royal Society B*, **270**, 867–874.

Johnstone, R. A. & Cant, M. A. (2008) Sex differences in dispersal and the evolution of helping and harming. *American Naturalist*, **172**, 318–330.

Kaplan, H. & Hill, K. (1985) Food sharing among Ache foragers: tests of explanatory hypotheses. *Current Anthropology*, **26**, 223–246.

Kaplan, H. & Lancaster, J. (2003) An evolutionary and ecological analysis of human fertility, mating patterns and parental investment. In: *Offspring: Human Fertility Behavior in Biodemographic Perspective*, ed. K. W. Wachter & R. A. Bulatao. Washington, DC: National Academies Press, pp. 170–223.

Kaplan, H. S. & Robson, A. J. (2002) The emergence of humans: the coevolution of intelligence and longevity with intergenerational transfers. *Proceedings of the National Academy of Sciences of the USA*, **99**, 10221–10226.

Kelly, R. L. (1995) *The Foraging Spectrum: Diversity in Hunter–Gatherer Lifeways*. Washington, DC: Smithsonian Institution Press.

Laland, K. & Brown, G. (2002) *Sense and Nonsense*. Oxford: Oxford University Press.

Lee, R. D. (2003) Rethinking the evolutionary theory of aging: transfers, not births, shape social species. *Proceedings of the National Academy of Sciences of the USA*, **100**, 9637–9642.

Lee, R. D. & Kramer, K. L. (2002) Children's economic roles in the Maya family life cycle: Cain, Caldwell, and Chayanov revisited. *Population and Development Review*, **28**, 475–499.

Leonetti, D. L., Nath, D. C., Hemam, N. S. & Neill, D. B. (2005) Kinship organisation and the impact of grandmothers on reproductive success among matrilineal Khasi and patrilineal Bengali of northeast India. In: *Grandmotherhood: the Evolutionary Significance of the Second Half of Female Life*, ed. E. Voland, A. Chasiotis & W. Schiefenhovel. New Brunswick, Rutgers University Press, pp. 194–214.

Mace, R. (1996) Biased parental investment and reproductive success in Gabbra pastoralists. *Behavioral Ecology and Sociobiology*, **38**, 75–81.

Mace, R. (2007) The evolutionary ecology of human family size. In: *The Oxford Handbook of Evolutionary Psychology*, ed. R. I. M. Dunbar and L. Barrett. Oxford: Oxford University Press, pp. 383–396.

Mace, R. & Pagel, M. (1994) The comparative method in anthropology. *Current Anthropology*, **35**, 549–564.

Mace, R. & Sear, R. (2005) Are humans co-operative breeders? In: *Grandmotherhood: the Evolutionary Significance of the Second Half of Female Life*, ed. E. Voland, A. Chasiotis & W. Schiefenhovel. New Brunswick, NJ: Rutgers University Press, pp. 143–159.

Mace, R., Holden, C. J. & Shennan, S., eds. (2005) *The Evolution of Cultural Diversity: a Phylogenetic Approach*. Walnut Creek, CA: Left Coast Press.

Marlowe, F. (2000) Paternal investment and the human mating system. *Behavioural Processes*, **51**, 45–61.

Marlowe, F. W. (2003) A critical period for provisioning by Hadza men – implications for pair bonding. *Evolution and Human Behavior*, **24**, 217–229.

Marlowe, F. W. (2004) Marital residence among foragers. *Current Anthropology*, **45**, 277–284.

Marlowe, F. W. (2005) Hunter–gatherers and human evolution. *Evolutionary Anthropology*, **14**, 54–67.

Marlowe, F. W. & Berbesque, J. C. (2008) More 'altruistic' punishment in larger societies. *Proceedings of the Royal Society B*, **275**, 587–590.

Murdock, G. P. (1967) *Ethnographic Atlas*. Pittsburgh, PA: University of Pittsburgh Press.

Nowak, M. A. & Sigmund, K. (2005) Evolution of indirect reciprocity. *Nature*, **437**, 1291–1298.

Pagel, M. 1994. Detecting correlated evolution on phylogenies: a general method for the comparative analysis of discrete characters. *Proceedings of the Royal Society B*, **255**, 37–45.

Richerson, P. J. & Boyd, R. (1999) Complex societies: the evolutionary origins of a crude superorganism. *Human Nature*, **10**, 253–289.

Sear, R. & Mace, R. (2008) Who keeps children alive? A review of the effects of kin on child survival. *Evolution and Human Behavior*, **29**, 1–18.

Sear, R., Mace, R. & McGregor, I. A. (2000) Maternal grandmothers improve the nutritional status and survival of children in rural Gambia. *Proceedings of the Royal Society B*, **267**, 1641–1647.

Sear, R., Steele, F., McGregor, I. A. & Mace, R. (2002) The effects of kin on child mortality in rural Gambia. *Demography*, **39**, 43–63.

Sear, R., Mace, R. & McGregor, I. A. (2003) A life-history approach to fertility rates in rural Gambia: evidence for trade-offs or phenotypic correlations? In: *The Biodemography of Human Reproduction and Fertility*, ed. J. L. Rodgers & H. P. Kohler. Boston, MA: Kluwer, pp. 135–160.

Shanley, D. P. & Kirkwood, T. B. L. (2001) Evolution of the human menopause. *BioEssays*, **23**, 282–287.

Shanley, D. P., Sear, R., Mace, R. & Kirkwood, T. B. L. (2007) Testing evolutionary theories of menopause. *Proceedings of the Royal Society B*, **274**, 2943–2949.

Weir, A. A. S. & Kacelnik, A. (2006) A New Caledonian crow (*Corvus moneduloides*) creatively re-designs tools by bending or unbending aluminium strips. *Animal Cognition*, **9**, 317–334.

Wilson, D. S. & Sober, E. (1994) Reintroducing group selection to the human behavioral sciences. *Behavioral and Brain Sciences*, **17**, 585–608.

Genes and social behaviour: from gene to genome to 1000 genomes

Gene E. Robinson

Which comes first – passion for the scientific question or passion for the organism? For most biologists I think it's the former, but for me it was the latter. I became smitten with honey bees at the age of 18 and have never looked back.

Once immersed in study, the question did come: how can a honey bee, with a brain the size of a grass seed, create a collective organisation in which all tasks are divided efficiently but flexibly among as many as 50 000 individuals? Honey bee division of labour is a spectacular example of social behaviour; trying to understand its mechanisms and evolution has motivated most of the research in my laboratory over the years and also has led periodically to rewarding expeditions into new scientific terrains.

After starting with behavioural and endocrine analyses as a graduate student at Cornell University with Roger Morse, my postdoctoral studies with Robert Page at Ohio State University demonstrated for the first time heritable influences on division of labour (Robinson & Page 1988). Then mechanistic studies in my own lab at the University of Illinois revealed striking differences in brain chemistry and brain structure between bees performing different jobs, raising the possibility that these changes were orchestrated by changes in brain gene expression (Withers *et al.* 1993). To enhance our ability to discover insights into the mechanisms and evolution of this form of social behaviour, I decided in the mid 1990s to initiate a molecular component to our research programme.

An early project involved *foraging* (*for*), first identified by Marla Sokolowski's laboratory as a gene that causes behavioural differences in *Drosophila melanogaster* (see Chapter 1). We also found a connection between *for* and behaviour, but in honey bees there is an intriguing twist. In *Drosophila* it is allelic variation that matters, whereas in honey bees it is the real-time regulation of *for* expression. The expression of this gene in the brain increases as the bee shifts from working in the hive to foraging outside, and treatments that activate *for* expression cause precocious foraging behaviour (Robinson *et al.* 2005).

for was the first gene found to affect division of labour, but the laboratory work proved slow and arduous, requiring the gene to be cloned from scratch. On top of that, studying social behaviour naturalistically is hard. One must obtain large sample sizes and multiple replications to deal with the variation inherent in field biology, which includes lack of controlled climate conditions and the use of wild-type, non-inbred, strains. And all this work for just one gene! It is obvious that something as complex as division of labour must involve many genes, working together in a variety of networks. I started

Social Behaviour: Genes, Ecology and Evolution, ed. Tamás Székely, Allen J. Moore and Jan Komdeur. Published by Cambridge University Press. © Cambridge University Press 2010.

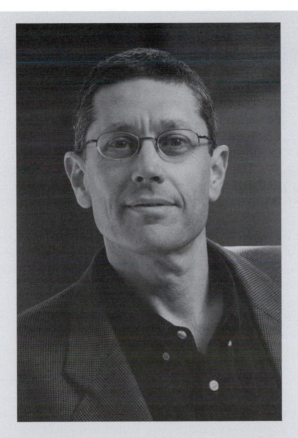

Gene E. Robinson. Photo: L. Brian Stauffer.

to worry that molecular biology and social behaviour would not make a good match.

Fortunately, a sabbatical at Hebrew University in the laboratory of molecular neurobiologist Hermona Soreq in 1996 afforded me the time to read and reflect on this problem. I came across a paper from Patrick Brown's laboratory (Schena *et al*. 1995) and started learning about the emerging field of genomics. I was impressed with the vast increase in efficiency and scope of genomics relative to traditional molecular biology. Aha! This is the marriage that needs to be made – genomics and social behaviour! My lab created a set of over 5000 bee brain expressed sequence tags (gene fragments) and used them to build a microarray to measure the expression of thousands of genes at the same time (Whitfield *et al*. 2003). Sequencing the whole genome by the National Institutes of Health's Human Genome Research Institute soon followed, further empowering the honey bee as a model for sociogenomics.

Important discoveries have been made with the bee genome sequence, demonstrating the value of genomic information to the study of social life. For example, we found that honey bees possess all the genes necessary for epigenetic regulation of gene expression (Wang *et al*. 2006), the first such case for an insect. This led to elegant work by Ryszard

Maleszka and colleagues showing that caste determination relies upon epigenetics to regulate the distinct programmes of gene expression that underlie development of either a worker or queen from a totipotent larva (Kucharski *et al.* 2008).

So far the study of social behaviour has had to rely on just a few genome sequences – far too few to resolve some key issues. For example, we discovered that some *cis*-regulatory elements are more prevalent in the promoter regions of socially regulated genes in the honey bee than in their *Drosophila* orthologues (Sinha *et al.* 2006). Is this a hint of a *cis*-regulatory code for social behaviour, or a feature of hymenopteran or dipteran biology? To answer this question requires multiple hymenopteran genomes, from both social and non-social species. One tried and true method of biological inquiry is the comparative method – we infer evolutionary changes by studying diverse extant species. To do this with genomic information requires having sequenced genomes from many different species.

We are now on the threshold of a new era, in which it will be possible to obtain whole genome sequences for any and all species of interest. This is because of the strong drive to develop faster and cheaper sequencing methods for diagnostic medicine, but all of biology stands to benefit handsomely.

Inexpensive genome sequences are around the corner. When the '$1000 human genome' is achieved, I hope the scientific community has in place a compelling vision to ensure maximum benefit from this milestone for all of biology. What a boon to all types of research if we sequenced the genomes of hundreds of selected species to cover all of animal phylogeny! And the prospect of this mountain of sequence should spur bioinformaticians to create radically new bioinformatics tools to better mine all those genomes for knowledge. The following is a taste of some of the possibilities for social behaviour in the '1000 animal genome' era.

One insight into the connection between genes and social behaviour is that genes involved in solitary behaviour are also used in evolution for social behaviour (Robinson *et al.* 2005). *for* is a good example; this gene has been implicated in the regulation of foraging behaviour in ants, bees, flies, worms, and mammals, so far. It is important to identify such evolutionarily labile molecular pathways, to pinpoint how and why various components of these pathways – both genes and regulatory regions – are more labile than others, and to understand how they figure in social evolution. Social insects will likely feature prominently in this endeavour because they and their close relatives span the full range of sociality, from solitary to eusocial, and they have evolved eusociality multiple times independently. Having the genome sequences for 25–50 of them, which I predict will occur within 5–10 years, will provide a strong foundation for the 'solitary to social' paradigm.

A second insight into the connection between genes and social behaviour is that the genome is highly sensitive to social influence, measured in terms of effects on brain gene expression (Robinson *et al.* 2008). Social regulation of brain gene expression has a powerful influence on behaviour. We must understand how social influences are perceived, processed and ultimately transformed into signals in the nucleus of brain neurons to orchestrate transcriptional activity and neural plasticity. We also need to discover the basis for individual and species variation in this process, and how it relates to the evolution and diversity of social behaviour. As I asked above, is there a *cis*-regulatory code for social behaviour? A histone code? We can answer this when we obtain multiple sets of genome sequences for key model social-behaviour species – songbirds, cichlid fish, social insects, voles and other rodents – together with the genome sequences of their related social, less social, and non-social taxa. Vertebrate genomes tend to be larger than most insect genomes, but soon sequencing costs will be low enough to blur these differences. Genomics, proteomics and bioinformatics can then be used to provide the information necessary to elucidate social regulation of gene expression.

E. O. Wilson (1975) wrote that 'social behavior is the phenotype that is furthest away from DNA.' But in the rapidly approaching 1000-animal-genome era, elucidating the intricate and varied connections between the two will lead to a profound transformation in our understanding of the mechanisms and evolution of social life.

These are some of the highlights of my research and vision for the future:

- Understanding the mechanisms and evolution of division of labour in honey bee colonies has been the primary pursuit in my laboratory.
- Genetic, endocrine, neurochemical and neuroanatomical analyses led to the initiation of molecular studies of division of labour in the mid 1990s.
- Molecular studies have so far revealed two important general insights into the connection between genes and social behaviour: (1) genes involved in solitary behaviour are also used in evolution for social behaviour; and (2) the genome (specifically brain gene activity) is highly sensitive to social influence.
- Studies of candidate genes gave way to building resources for genomic analysis, including sequencing of the honey bee genome.
- The Honey Bee Genome Project has led to many important discoveries by several laboratories that bear on the understanding of social life, including our findings of a fully functioning epigenetic (CpG methylation) system and hints of a cis-regulatory code for social behaviour.
- Soon it will be possible to obtain whole genome sequences for any and all species of interest, which will provide new powerful tools to further elucidate the mechanisms and evolution of division of labour in bees and other social insects, and many other forms of social behaviour as well.

I thank S. E. Fahrbach, M. B. Sokolowski, A. L. Toth and A. J. Moore for comments that improved this essay. Research from my laboratory mentioned here has been funded by grants from the National Science Foundation, National Institutes of Health and the University of Illinois Sociogenomics Initiative.

References

Kucharski, R., Maleszka, J., Foret, S. & Maleszka, R. (2008) Nutritional control of reproductive status in honeybees via DNA methylation. *Science*, **319**, 1827–1830.

Robinson, G. E. & Page, R. E. (1988) Genetic determination of guarding and undertaking in honey-bee colonies. *Nature*, **333**, 356–358.

Robinson, G. E., Grozinger, C. M. & Whitfield, C. W. (2005) Sociogenomics: social life in molecular terms. *Nature Reviews Genetics*, **6**, 257–270.

Robinson, G. E., Fernald, R. D. & Clayton, D. F. (2008) Genes and social behavior. *Science*, **322**, 896–900.

Schena, M., Shalon, D., Davis, R. W. & Brown P. O. (1995) Quantitative monitoring of gene expression patterns with a complementary DNA microarray. *Science*, **270**, 467–70.

Sinha, S., Ling, X., Whitfield, C. W., Zhai, C. & Robinson, G. E. (2006) Genome scan for cis-regulatory DNA motifs associated with social behavior in honey bees. *Proceedings of the National Academy of Sciences of the USA*, **103**, 16352–16357.

Wang, Y., Jorda, M., Jones, P. L. *et al.* (2006) Functional CpG methylation system in a social insect. *Science*, **314**, 645–647.

Whitfield, C. W., Cziko, A.-M. & Robinson, G. E. (2003) Gene expression patterns in the brain predict behavior in individual honey bees. *Science*, **302**, 296–299

Wilson, E. O. (1975) *Sociobiology: the New Synthesis*. Cambridge, MA: Harvard University Press.

Withers, G. S., Fahrbach, S. E. & Robinson, G. E. (1993) Selective neuroanatomical plasticity and division of labour in the honey bee (*Apis mellifera*). *Nature*, **364**, 238–240.

PART III

Implications

16

Personality and individual social specialisation

Denis Réale and Niels J. Dingemanse

Overview

Animals differ in their behaviour, as humans differ in personality. Animal personality represents consistent behavioural individual differences over time and across contexts, and/or correlations between different types of behaviour. In many animal species, individuals differ in activity, aggressiveness, risk-taking and exploratory behaviour, and these behaviours are often positively correlated with each other. We therefore expect that personality affects social behaviour, and that social behaviour also influences personality. New discoveries about the evolutionary ecology of personality suggest exciting research opportunities on the effects of personality on the fate of individuals in social contexts, and on the influences of social interactions on development and evolution of personality.

Studying personality in a social context can provide new insights in the study of social behaviour because it allows us to consider one important question: are social groups composed of individuals with varying degrees of specialisation? Here we consider that the degree of specialisation of an individual for a given trait corresponds to the range of phenotypic expression of that trait for that individual relative to its population. A specialist for a trait is limited in its range of expression of that trait relative to its population, whereas a generalist expresses the whole range of phenotypic variation observed for that trait in the population.

In this chapter we suggest that studies on personality should include not only individual variation in the average value of a trait, but also a measure of the degree of specialisation of each individual. We review current knowledge on both proximal and ultimate causes of individual variation and degree of specialisation. We then highlight new research directions on the links between personality, degree of specialisation and social behaviour. We discuss specific examples in the context of personality research including begging, parental style and offspring development, dispersal, dominance, mating strategies and group living.

16.1 Introduction

Anyone who observes animals long enough will notice that individuals behave predictably over time and across situations. Individuals within a population – whether it be a population of ants, sunfish, octopuses, tits, hyenas or humans – show consistent differences in their level of activity, sensation seeking, attraction

Social Behaviour: Genes, Ecology and Evolution, ed. Tamás Székely, Allen J. Moore and Jan Komdeur. Published by Cambridge University Press. © Cambridge University Press 2010.

to novelty, or their willingness to fight against or to avoid conspecifics, among other types of behaviours (Gosling 2001). Psychologists have been studying this variation for a long time and have named it personality (Gosling 2001). Discoveries on animal personality are raising new questions about the implication of personality on the ecology of animal populations, particularly their social systems.

Behavioural ecologists have been very successful at answering the question why animals behave the way they do by assuming that animal behaviours are adaptations. These behaviours result from long-term selection pressures that have adjusted the responses of animals to specific situations (e.g. high predation versus low predation risk). Animals in a population should show the 'optimal phenotype' of a trait: the value of the trait that maximises the ratio of benefits over costs in terms of fitness (Krebs & Davis 1997, Danchin *et al.* 2008). Personality ecologists are interested in answering the question why individual animals differ consistently in their behavioural response to the same stimulus.

Behavioural expressions of personality can be measured and are called temperament or personality traits (Réale *et al.* 2007). In humans, most personality traits can be associated with social interactions (Pervin *et al.* 2005), which is not surprising considering the social species we are. Instead of discussing the literature on human personality and social behaviours, we focus on the ill-studied link between personality and social behaviours in other animals. Despite recent progress on the evolutionary ecology of personality traits (Clark & Ehlinger 1987, Wilson *et al.* 1994, Sih *et al.* 2004, Dingemanse & Réale 2005, Réale *et al.* 2007), our knowledge of the evolutionary ecology of personality in a social context is still limited. Animal personality in a social context is thus like a new continent to discover.

In this chapter we first discuss the concept of personality, and the physiological (i.e. proximate) and evolutionary (i.e. ultimate) reasons that lead to personality differences within populations. We then suggest that in order to study personality differences in a population, we should consider not only differences in the average value of a behaviour among individuals

(generally called *behavioural profile*), but also how individuals differ in their variation around their average behaviour, which we call *degree of specialisation*. We thus explain here how in a social context looking at individual differences (in means and degree of specialisation) may provide insights on a neglected aspect of social behaviour: whether groups are composed of *specialists* or *generalists*. We review empirical studies on social behaviour over the lifetime of individual animals and outline how personality might affect (1) offspring solicitation, maternal care and the offspring behavioural ontogeny, (2) dispersal, (3) the acquisition of dominance ranks, (4) mating strategies and (5) social roles, including conflicts and cooperation among individuals in a group. Our aim is to present exemplary studies that illustrate each topic, and to discuss potential areas for future research on personality and degree of specialisation in the context of animal groups.

16.2 The concept of personality

Personality traits can be characterised by two main features: individual behavioural consistency over time and environmental conditions, and potentially the correlations with other behavioural traits (Réale *et al.* 2007; Box 16.1). Individual behavioural consistency means that an individual maintains its rank for a behavioural phenotype relative to the phenotypes of other individuals in the population, not that this individual always shows the same phenotypic value (Fig. 16.1). The maintenance of individual ranks in a behavioural trait across environments is also called a *behavioural carryover* (Sih *et al.* 2004). For example, in sunfish salamanders *Ambystoma barbouri* a behavioural carryover exists because individuals that are the most active in an environment without predators also show the highest level of activity in an environment with predators (Sih *et al.* 2003). Note that if we assume that two different ages can be analogous to two different environments, the consistency of a personality trait over time can be considered a developmental behavioural carryover. Personality traits may (or may not) be correlated with each other (Wilson *et al.* 1994, Sih *et al.* 2004, Réale *et al.* 2007).

Box 16.1 What is personality?

There are numerous definitions of personality or temperament (Réale *et al.* 2007). For example, personality has been defined as *'an individual's set of behavioural tendencies'* (Penke *et al.* 2007). For Réale *et al.* (2007) personality and temperament could be considered as 'the phenomenon that individual behavioural differences are consistent over time and/or across situations'. In humans, for example, the five-factor model of personality proposed by psychologists decomposes personality into five main dimensions: (1) openness to new experiences, (2) conscientiousness, (3) extraversion, (4) agreeableness and (5) emotional stability or neuroticism (Gosling 2001). Each dimension is built up from a multivariate factor analysis based on questionnaires that ask people to describe their reactions or emotions in specific contexts. This means that the five main personality dimensions are composed of a set of correlated behavioural reactions or emotions in specific contexts.

Personality dimensions are observed in various animal species with different degrees of complexity. Primates may show similar personality dimensions as humans, while simpler personality dimensions are assumed to be found in insects and other invertebrates (Gosling 2001). Réale *et al.* (2007) recently proposed to classify animal personality (or temperament) dimensions into five categories: (1) activity, (2) exploration, (3) boldness, (4) aggressiveness, (5) sociability. Although the last two dimensions are clearly operational in a social context, other personality dimensions may also play a role in how an individual interacts with conspecifics and affect the dynamics of social interactions.

Is behavioural variation always personality? There could be many reasons for animals to show individual behavioural variation consistently, and these differences do not necessarily correspond to personality differences per se. For example, individuals change their behaviour throughout ontogeny (e.g. social status in social mammals or age polyphenism in social insects), and male mammals are generally more aggressive than females of the same species. Although all these examples correspond to consistent behavioural differences within a population, we do not consider them personality. Similarly, our definition of personality does not include within-individual behavioural variation based on reproductive status (e.g. aggressiveness increases during the period of offspring care in species that defend their progeny) or body condition, because over a sufficiently long period of time these differences may not be persistent. However, in a statistical analysis, the step that takes reproductive status into account must be done with caution if individuals with different personalities have different reproductive outputs.

As evolutionary biologists, we are primarily interested in personality traits because individual behavioural differences can be caused by heritable differences of genetic or maternal origin. The heritability of a trait represents the portion of the variance measured for that trait in a population (i.e. phenotypic variance) that is caused by additive genetic variance. That variance reflects the total effect of a number of genes with additive effects, while the individual effects of each of these genes are negligible (Falconer & Mackay 1996). The concept of heritability is important if we want to understand the evolution of personality traits, as genetic information is transmitted from generation to generation and results in evolutionary change in a population. Maternal effects, and effects caused by environmental conditions shared by a limited set of individuals (e.g. families), could be other sources

Box 16.1 Continued

of individual variation in personality in a population (Réale *et al.* 2007). Maternal effects have been shown to play a strong role in the evolution of quantitative traits (see Chapter 2).

The occurrence of personality differences in a population is generally estimated by using the repeatability for a trait measured two or more times per individual. Repeatability (the proportion of total phenotypic variation attributable to differences between individuals: Falconer & Mackay 1996) indicates how predictable the behaviour is. Predictability of an individual's personality from observation of its behaviour early in life can be illustrated by a positive correlation between a behaviour at a given life stage and the same behaviour at a later stage (there are other ways of estimating repeatability with more than two replicates per individual: see Lessells & Boag 1987, Martin & Réale 2008). When repeatability equals one, it is possible to predict exactly the behavioural value of each individual at the second life stage from the value at its first life stage. With a repeatability of zero, it is impossible to make any prediction.

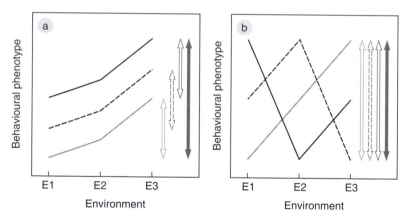

Figure 16.1 (a) Behaviour measured for three individuals in three different environments (E_1, E_2 and E_3). Individual behavioural consistency is represented by the fact that the variation among individuals (solid double arrow) is larger than the variation within any individual (the three hollow double arrows). Note the presence of phenotypic plasticity: the three individuals express different behavioural phenotypes according to the environment. (b) The three individuals vary their behavioural phenotype according to the environment, but there is no way to predict what each of them will do in one environment based on the information from another environment. Furthermore, within-individual variation is as large as among-individual variation (repeatability = 0).

Consistency of behavioural phenotypes across contexts and the correlation between behavioural traits are called *behavioural syndromes* as well (Clark & Ehlinger 1987, Sih *et al.* 2004). Behavioural syndromes are indicated by a positive phenotypic correlation between two behavioural traits (Sih *et al.* 2004). For example, it has been shown that the most aggressive three-spined sticklebacks *Gasterosteus aculeatus* were also the boldest ones in front of a predator (Huntingford 1976), and that the most aggressive North American red squirrels *Tamiasciurus hudsonicus* were also the most active and the most explorative (Boon *et al.* 2007).

16.3 The proximate and evolutionary causes of personality

The existence of individual personality differences in wild animal populations has led people to question what evolutionary causes were responsible for the maintenance of that behavioural variation (Dingemanse & Réale 2005). Two major hypotheses have been proposed, the *constraint* hypothesis and the *adaptive* hypothesis (Wilson *et al.* 1994, Sih *et al.* 2004, Bell 2005, Dingemanse & Réale 2005, Réale *et al.* 2007). The first corresponds to a proximate approach, whereas the second corresponds to an ultimate approach.

The first hypothesis considers that the correlation between two personality traits results from a common gene–physiology–behaviour pathway, and this correlation acts as a constraint on the independent evolution of personality traits (Sih *et al.* 2004). Neuroendocrinological individual differences have been shown to influence the differential expression of a suite of behavioural traits among individuals in many animals (Chapter 3; Koolhaas *et al.* 1999, Adkins-Regan 2005, Groothuis & Carere 2005). At the genetic level, pleiotropy (i.e. one gene is involved in the expression of two different traits) or linkage disequilibrium (i.e. a gene involved in the expression of one trait is located on the chromosome near a gene involved in the expression of another trait) are generally the two mechanisms considered to be responsible for the resulting genetic correlation (Roff 1997, Lynch & Walsh 1998). The constraint hypothesis poses that two traits are associated at both the phenotypic and genetic level so that the phenotypic value of the first trait, associated with high fitness, corresponds to a phenotypic value for the second trait that is related to low fitness, thus generating an evolutionary trade-off (Roff & Fairbairn 2007). The trade-off leads to the evolution of either a single optimal combination of the two traits, or a fitness ridge with multiple combinations of the two traits characterised by the same fitness.

Recent models have considered that the evolution of personality traits and behavioural syndromes could have evolved as an adaptive response of behavioural traits within the constraint of a trade-off between life-history traits (Biro & Stamps 2008). For example, Mangel and Stamps (2001) showed that the trade-off between growth and survival can maintain individual variation in growth rate in species with indeterminate growth, based on which Stamps (2007) reasoned that any behaviour contributing to this trade-off should differ between individuals differing in growth rate. For instance, if aggressiveness and boldness both facilitate increased growth at the cost of increased mortality, we would expect that the trade-off selects for individual differences in and correlations between these two personality traits (the aggressiveness–boldness syndrome). Wolf *et al.* (2007) have proposed a formal model based on the same type of relationship between personality and life-history strategies. In their example, bold and aggressive individuals should be characterised by a rapid development and an early age at first reproduction, and should die rapidly, whereas shy and non-aggressive individuals should show a slower development, start reproducing later, spread their reproductive effort over a longer period of life, and die at an older age. Some empirical studies support the hypothesised link between personality and life history (Armitage 1986, Réale *et al.* 2000, Biro *et al.* 2004, Boon *et al.* 2007; but see Dingemanse *et al.* 2004). If so, this would mean that we can predict, to a certain extent, the fate of individuals with different personalities. Moreover, given the link between life history, personality and social role, general ecological conditions may affect the proportion of individuals of different personality types, which may in turn affect the structure and the dynamics of social groups and create new selection pressures.

According to the second hypothesis, natural selection favours specific combinations of personality traits, which is at the origin of the genetic–phenotypic correlation between these traits (Bell & Sih 2007, Dingemanse *et al.* 2007). For example, the correlation between boldness and aggressiveness in the three-spined stickleback is strong in populations living sympatrically with fish predators compared to populations where predators are absent (Dingemanse *et al.* 2007), and experiments have confirmed that predation can generate this correlation (Bell & Sih 2007).

The maintenance of personality differences can also be caused by spatial or temporal heterogeneity in environmental conditions. Such environmental heterogeneity creates different selection pressures that favour different personality types at different times, or in different areas (Dingemanse *et al.* 2004, Both *et al.* 2005, Boon *et al.* 2007). Game theory has provided an evolutionary explanation for the phenotypic variation in behaviour especially in a social context (Chapter 4; Maynard Smith 1982). Game-theoretic models define an evolutionarily stable strategy (ESS) at which no mutant using a different behavioural strategy can invade the population. In such a game, the fitness payoff of a particular strategy may decrease with the proportion of individuals playing this strategy in the population. Game-theoretic models, therefore, can explain the coexistence of alternative strategies within a population (Brockmann 2001, Giraldeau & Dubois 2008, Oliveira *et al.* 2008). Game-theoretic models can be applied to the evolution of social behaviour in a context of frequency-dependent selection, where the optimal strategy depends on the frequency of individuals in the population showing a particular strategy (e.g. hawk versus dove, Maynard Smith 1982; scrounging versus producing while foraging, Giraldeau & Dubois 2008).

Personality differences in a population can also be explained by individual experiences of a particular condition during development and learning that lead to the fixation of specific behaviour or tasks over ontogeny (West-Eberhard 2003, Hemelrijk & Wiantia 2005). For example, learning is at the origin of the diet diversity among individuals of a given species (Giraldeau 1984, Bolnick *et al.* 2003). Learning and the conditions that an individual experiences during its development could also have an effect on the development of other behavioural tendencies.

16.4 Personality, degree of specialisation, and the importance of individual social roles

As we have seen above, personality generally implies that an individual shows some consistency in its behaviours, or that an individual does not express the whole range of phenotypic variation of a trait observed in its population for the environmental conditions measured (Fig. 16.1). Testing for individual behavioural consistency in a population should thus be a first step in every study on personality (Réale *et al.* 2007). Personality traits are generally characterised by repeatability values around 0.30–0.50 (Réale *et al.* 2007). Repeatability provides a good index of individual consistency at the level of the population. However, it does not provide any information on the degree of specialisation of a particular individual within this population. Highly consistent individuals will increase the estimate of repeatability, and less consistent individuals will decrease this estimate. Up until now, people have characterised the personality of an individual using the average value of a behavioural trait. The variance around this average value has rarely been considered (but see Carere *et al.* 2005a, Sinn *et al.* 2008, Wolf *et al.* 2008, Dingemanse *et al.* 2009).

We suggest that looking at both average values and within-individual variance in a behaviour can provide new insights in the study of social behaviour, because it allows us to consider one important question: are social groups composed of individuals differing in degree of specialisation? We consider that the degree of specialisation of an individual for a given trait corresponds to the range of phenotypic expression of that trait for that individual relative to its population. Individuals with a high degree of specialisation – or highly consistent individuals – will show negligible individual phenotypic variation relative to that of the population, whereas individuals with a low degree of specialisation will express the whole phenotypic variation observed in the population for that trait (Box 16.2). Therefore, individual variation in the degree of specialisation equates to individual variation in plasticity (or individual-by-environment interaction; see below).

The idea of specialisation is not new. However, we believe it provides a clear link between personality ecology and other fields of research such as the study of phenotypic plasticity (De Witt 1998, Schlichting & Pigliucci 1998, West-Eberhard 2003,

Box 16.2 How to measure the degree of specialisation?

One way of obtaining information on individual specialisation is to calculate what we call the *coefficient of relative plasticity* (*CRP*) of a trait for each individual. The *CRP* represents the ratio of an individual's variance (V_i) for the trait over the overall phenotypic variance (V_p) of the population ($CRP = V_i/V_p$). In other words, *CRP* provides a standardised index of individual variation for a given trait relative to its population. This index is appropriate when the trait is repeatable (i.e., when the trait is not repeatable, measuring relative plasticity of individuals is not appropriate), and when there is no sampling bias according to environmental conditions, because environmental conditions that an individual experiences are partly responsible for the variation around the mean of the trait. This requirement could be difficult to fulfil in the wild, where one can rarely control for environmental conditions. Thus if some individuals experience more variable environmental conditions than others,

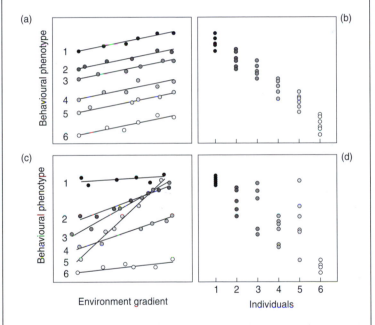

Hypothetical examples of individual variation in slope and intercept of a behavioural trait as a function of an environmental gradient (a and c), and the projection of these data in the absence of information on environmental conditions (b and d). In a and b the population is composed of individuals that vary in their mean values for the behaviour, but show similar and high consistencies (i.e. none of them expresses the whole phenotypic variation observed in the population for that behaviour). In c and d, by contrast, the population is composed of individuals that vary in their mean for the behaviour and in their degree of specialisation (slope in c or coefficient of consistency in d). Repeatability is expected to be higher in b than in d.

Box 16.2 Continued

the difference in *CRP* between individuals could reflect this bias rather than an actual difference in consistency. Random bias relative to an individual's mean will increase errors in the relationship between consistency and other characteristics.

When it is known which environmental factor affects the behaviour of interest, one can use a random regression approach to test for individual differences in slopes of the behaviour as a function of the environment (Nussey *et al.* 2007, Dingemanse *et al.* 2007, Martin & Réale 2008). Non-significant variation caused by random slopes would indicate that individuals have similar degrees of specialisation in the population (figure a). In contrast, a significant random slope effect would indicate that individuals differ in their reaction to change in the environment and show different degrees of specialisation (figure c). Individual slopes estimated from the random regression thus provide individual estimates of the degree of specialisation: the degree of specialisation decreases with the steepness of the slope. Figure a is intentionally simplified. Actual data rarely show such a clear pattern of parallel individual lines. Statistical testing is necessary to infer behavioural consistency in a population. However, it should be clear that a significant repeatability does not imply that all the individuals are consistent.

Another way of testing for the presence of specialists in a population is to estimate the genetic correlation of a trait across environments. A trait measured on individuals experiencing two different environmental conditions could be considered as two different traits from a quantitative genetic point of view (Falconer & Mackay 1996). Quantitative geneticists use the genetic correlation of the trait across the two environments to validate this hypothesis. If the genetic correlation is equal to 1, then in principle all the genes affecting the trait in one environment are affecting the trait in the same way in the other environment. It also indicates that the population is composed of specialist genotypes. However, a correlation lower than 1 indicates a genotype-by-environment interaction, and therefore variation in the degree of specialisation in the population. Therefore a decrease in genetic correlation would indicate a decrease in the proportion of specialists in the population.

Nussey *et al.* 2007), or of the coexistence of specialists and generalists (Giraldeau 1984, van Tienderen 1991, Wilson & Yoshimura 1994, Bolnick *et al.* 2003, Leimar 2005). Few studies have documented both individual and genetic variation in plasticity of personality traits, implying that personality is linked to specialisation (Dingemanse *et al.* 2009, Bouwman *et al.* unpublished).

According to the definition of personality, individuals exhibit limited phenotypic plasticity (Wilson *et al.* 1994, Sih *et al.* 2004). By phenotypic plasticity

of a trait we mean the ability of a genotype (e.g. an individual) to express a range of phenotypes according to the environment (Schlichting & Pigliucci 1998). In terms of phenotypic plasticity, the coexistence of individuals with different degrees of specialisation implies that these individuals differ in their plastic response to environmental changes, also called individual-by-environment interaction (Nussey *et al.* 2007). It is important to note that being a specialist does not mean showing no phenotypic plasticity; a specialist can change its behaviour according to the environment, but it expresses only a limited portion of the whole phenotypic variation of its population (Box 16.2). Consideration of individual degrees of specialisation may stimulate empirical research on the costs and limitations of phenotypic plasticity (De Witt 1998, De Witt et al. 1998). In the case of behavioural traits, this should help us understand the evolution of personality (Dall et al. 2004, McElreath & Strimling 2006, Wolf et al. 2008).

Other links can be made between degree of specialisation and tactics in game-theoretic models (Dall et al. 2004). First, game-theoretic models do not systematically address whether individuals can switch in a reversible way from one strategy to another depending on environmental conditions (i.e. conditional strategy), or whether each individual expresses only one strategy during its lifetime (i.e. fixed strategy: Bergstrom & Godfrey-Smith 1998, Dall et al. 2004). It is possible, however, to consider the coexistence of conditional or fixed strategies with game theory and therefore to question the existence of personality differences within a population (Dall et al. 2004, Plaistow et al. 2004, Wolf et al. 2007, 2008). There is an important difference between the conditional and fixed strategies, and this difference lies in the degree of reversibility of phenotypic plasticity of an individual (Brockmann 2001). In the case of a conditional strategy, and when individuals can express the full range of tactics (i.e. in a mixed ESS), individuals can show reversible phenotypic plasticity during their life; they do not show personality differences, and show a low degree of specialisation. In the case of a fixed strategy, the frequency of individuals using each strategy varies across generations; individuals thus show extreme personalities and could be considered specialists. Reality probably lies somewhere in between these two extremes, and by studying personality differences we have a good opportunity to study the conditions that favour the evolution of specialisation. Second, some of the best-known game-theoretical models deal with discrete strategies (play Hawk or Dove, care for the brood or desert) and seek to establish how these strategies may coexist in a population. Other game-theoretic models, however, are continuous

(Chapter 4). Personality traits generally show continuous variation. It is conceptually possible to generalise the insights of the game-theoretic approach to traits with continuous distribution. However, thus far few game-theory models have explained the maintenance of a continuum of behavioural traits (but see Wolf et al. 2007, 2008).

Ecologists and evolutionary biologists have studied ecological factors at the origin of the evolution and coexistence of trophic specialist and generalist species, or genotypes within a species (Giraldeau 1984, van Tienderen 1991, Wilson & Yoshimura 1994, Bolnick et al. 2003, Leimar 2005, Wolf et al. 2008). These studies are linked with our idea of degree of specialisation. We believe, however, that in the context of personality differences we can extend the concept of specialisation to individuals within a species and to situations more diverse than trophic specialisations only. The concept of degrees of specialisation need not restrict us to thinking in terms of a small number of discrete morphs (phenotypic polymorphism), but allows for the possibility that populations can be composed of a continuum in individual degrees of specialisation (Dingemanse et al. 2009, Bouwman et al. unpublished).

Begging, dispersal, dominance, cooperation, mate choice and parental behaviours have all been subject to much attention from behavioural ecologists (Danchin et al. 2008; Chapters 6, 7, 10, 11, 12 and 18). However, considering personality and the degree of specialisation in a social context helps us to consider a social group as an aggregation of individuals with different abilities, limitations and interests. In other words, individuals may not be randomly interchangeable but have specific social roles according to their personality. Furthermore, in order to study social behaviour it is essential to remember that in a given social situation individuals with different personalities will not have the same fitness payoff. Consequently, the dynamics of a group will depend on the types of individuals that compose the group. These differences among individuals in a social context may be important in explaining group cohesion, group movements, the dynamics of group structure, and the fate of individuals within the group.

16.5 Personality and the fate of individuals within their social group

In this section we will review empirical evidence for the role of personality in the social roles an individual can play, and for the coexistence of individuals with variable degrees of specialisation in a population. We focus on the evidence for links between social behaviours and personality traits, and address the three following questions: (1) Is there evidence for consistent individual differences in social behaviour? (2) Are these differences linked with classic personality traits measured in other contexts (e.g. boldness, aggressiveness, activity, exploration and sociability)? (3) Is there evidence for the coexistence of individuals with varying degrees of specialisation for the social behaviour studied?

16.5.1 Personality, level of solicitation as an offspring and parental style

The study of parental care and offspring development through independence has been an important and fruitful topic in behavioural ecology over the last 30 years (Chapter 11; Clutton-Brock 1991). This large array of research has benefited from the influential work of Trivers (1972, 1974) on parental investment and parent–offspring conflict. Both parents and offspring play an active role in the dynamics of parent–offspring interactions (Agrawal *et al.* 2001, Lock *et al.* 2004, Kölliker 2005).

Differences among offspring in how much they beg for parental care depend on whether they are from the same family or different families. For example, genetic influences on offspring solicitations are well established for diverse species (for reviews see Kölliker & Richner 2001, Kölliker 2005). Although there is a lot of evidence that offspring behaviour affects parental care (Clutton-Brock 1991), the role of offspring personality on the outcome of parental care, investment, and parent–offspring conflict should receive more attention. It is likely that variation in aggressiveness, activity or boldness among sibs within or between litters or broods could affect the level of parental investment provided to each of these offspring. If a behavioural

syndrome exists, relatively aggressive/active offspring may obtain more food from their parents than less aggressive/active offspring. When resources are limited we may thus expect strong selection favouring aggressiveness within the nest.

The effects of offspring personality on the outcome of parent–offspring conflict may be complicated by the fact that patterns of maternal care are also affected by the personality of the mother (see below). Positive or negative genetic correlations have been found between maternal care and offspring solicitation, which has been explained as the result of coevolution between these two traits (Chapter 2; Kölliker 2005). It may thus be very important to consider the role of personality in the relationship between parents and their offspring in future research. Furthermore, given that personality is heritable (Réale *et al.* 2007), we should expect that half-sibs may show more dissimilar personalities than full sibs. This may have serious consequences in the level of competition within a litter or brood. In the same way, it would be interesting to ask whether individual offspring differ in how they adjust their level of solicitation with variation in food provisioning.

We have more evidence for individual consistency in parental styles in animals, especially in primates (see Fairbanks 1996 for a review), but also in guinea pigs *Cavia aperea* (Albers *et al.* 1999), house mice *Mus musculus* (Benus & Rondig 1996) and domestic sheep *Ovis aries* (Dwyer & Lawrence 1998; see review by Grandison 2005). Furthermore, there are numerous studies showing genetic effects on maternal care and performance (Grandison 2005, Kölliker & Richner 2001), and several quantitative trait loci associated with maternal behaviour have been isolated (Peripato & Cheverud 2002). Female primates generally show two independent maternal dimensions called protectiveness and rejection. In rhesus monkeys *Macaca mulatta* females differ consistently in the way they spend time in contact with their infant, initiate those contacts, and reject the infant (Berman 1990). Similarly, in vervet monkeys *Cercopithecus aethiops* Fairbanks (1996) reported across-year repeatability of 0.69 and 0.59 for protectiveness and rejection scores, respectively. Both maternal protectiveness and rejection can vary in degree as a response to eco- logical factors, such as a risky social context, body condition and female experience. For example, cap- tive females generally increase their protectiveness in the presence of new males (Fig. 16.2). However, most phenotypic variation observed is caused by consistent differences among females (Fairbanks 1996). Interestingly, Fairbanks' results suggest that females differ in their degrees of specialisation for protectiveness.

Maternal style has been proposed as a personality trait (Réale *et al.* 2007), and a question is therefore whether maternal style is linked with other personal- ity traits (Fairbanks & McGuire 1993, Réale *et al.* 2007). Few studies have provided evidence for such links. One good example is the study by Benus and Rondig (1996), who compared maternal behaviour between two lines of mice artificially selected for their aggres- siveness (SAL, for short attack latency, versus LAL, for long attack latency), thereby documenting individual variation in maternal behaviour. If two traits are gen- etically correlated with each other, artificial selection on one trait should induce phenotypic (and genetic) changes in the other trait (Falconer & Mackay 1996). A difference in another trait assessed in bidirectionally selected lines, therefore, reveals the genetic associ- ation between that trait and the trait under selection. SAL mice spent more time nursing their pups than LAL mice. They also licked their pups more than LAL mothers, a behaviour known to play an important role in pups' development (Meaney 2001). LAL moth- ers spent more time resting alone than SAL ones. Thus nursing, licking, and resting alone are genetically correlated with attack latency.

Links between personality and mothering style and maternal ability have also been found in domestic breeds (Boissy *et al.* 2005, Grandison 2005). In general, high docility and low fearfulness are positively related to good maternal performance. Another example comes from a recent study by Boon *et al.* (2007), who found that aggressiveness and activity in female North American red squirrels were repeatable and positively correlated. In years of poor food abundance, aggressive females experienced higher offspring mortality within the nest than under years of high food abundance. Less aggressive females showed less variation in offspring mortality with food availability. Juvenile growth rate decreased with female activity during years with low food abundance but increased with activity during years of high food abundance. These results suggest

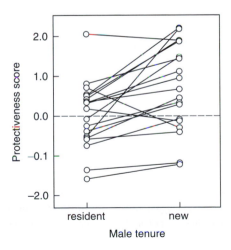

Figure 16.2 Increase in maternal protectiveness in vervet monkeys *Cercopithecus aethiops* in a stable group and in the presence of new males. Although most females increase their protectiveness in the presence of new males, they vary in their adjustment, which suggests the occurrence of different degrees of specialisation for this 'maternal protectiveness' trait. After Fairbanks (1996).

that relatively aggressive/active females are specialists of rich environments, whereas maternal performance of less aggressive/active females was less sensitive to variation in food abundance (Boon *et al.* 2007). Similarly, among great tits *Parus major* breeding for the first time in their lives, female exploratory tendencies (Dingemanse *et al.* 2002) predict the probability of nest failure (Both *et al.* 2005). As in the squirrels, the relatively explorative/aggressive animals appeared to be bad mothers and experienced more nest failures. These two studies show that female personality can affect the recruitment in the population in interaction with an environmental condition such as food abundance.

16.5.2 Maternal style and the development of offspring personality

Does maternal style play an important role in the development of offspring personality? There is experimental and observational evidence that maternal care affects the behaviour of offspring adults (Cameron *et al.* 2005). Numerous studies on primates indicate some correlates between mothering style and offspring personality (Fairbanks 1996). For example, in Japanese macaques *Macaca fuscata* infants of less protective mothers were more explorative and more sociable than those of highly protective mothers (Bardi & Huffman 2002). Similarly, Schino *et al.* (2001) found that maternal rejection was related to less fearful and anxious offspring as a grown-up adult.

Correlational studies cannot, however, be used to evaluate whether genetic or maternal effects (i.e. differences in mothering styles) are most important in explaining the link between maternal style and offspring personality. One may argue that because genes affecting maternal style might also affect personality traits such as sociability and anxiety, one should find a positive correlation between maternal style and offspring personality without implying any direct causal influence. Three approaches have been used to investigate this issue.

The first and most commonly used approach is to experimentally change the degree of maternal care. For example, as indicated above, mothers differ in the

level of maternal care, and it has been shown that a reduction in food provisioning and increased sibling competition increase aggressiveness in birds from lines selected for fast exploration but not in birds from lines selected for slow exploration (Carere *et al.* 2005b). In a recent study of blue tits *Cyanistes caeruleus* Arnold *et al.* (2007) fed one sibling in each brood with taurine, an amino acid present in large quantities in spiders, and compared its behaviour with that of a control chick of the same brood when both had become adults. Taurine-fed chicks were bolder than control ones. These experiments indicate that parents can influence the personality of their offspring by changing the level of care provided to them. However, such experiments are not feasible in all species; they can be performed more easily, for example, on birds than on mammals. Furthermore, they may create changes that are more important than natural variation in maternal style or care, and therefore they do not provide information on the relative importance of parental effects.

The second approach to unravel maternal from genetic effects is to cross-foster offspring between families, and to estimate the offspring's resemblance to both the biological and the foster mother (Table 16.1). For example, Maestripieri (2003) used this approach in a group of rhesus monkeys to tease apart genetic from maternal effects on personality of their daughters. Female sociability and aggression during the first three years of life was similar to that of their biological mother and unrelated to the behaviour of the foster mother, suggesting that genetic influences but not rearing effects by the foster parent play a role in these personality traits. In contrast, Francis *et al.* (1999) showed that in the rat *Rattus norvegicus* maternal effects could affect the pups' reaction to stress later in life. Female rats differ in maternal behaviour (e.g. licking and grooming pups, and nursing time spent in an arched-back position). Francis and colleagues formed two groups of females called low and high LG-ABN (for licking/grooming and arched-back nursing) respectively. Fearfulness and maternal behaviour of female rats were more similar to that of their foster mothers than to that of their biological mothers.

Table 16.1. Evidence for genetic or maternal effects on personality traits

Species	Traits	Method [a]	Maternal effects	Genetic effects	Reference
Japanese macaque *Macaca fuscata*	Fearfulness/ anxiety	PC	Yes	?	Schino *et al.* 2001
Japanese macaque *Macaca fuscata*	Exploration/ sociability	PC	Yes	?	Bardi & Huffman 2002
Rhesus macaque *Macaca mulata*	Sociability/ aggression	CF	No	Yes	Maestripieri 2003
Rat *Rattus norvegicus*	Anxiety	CF	No	Yes	Wigger *et al.* 2001
Rat *Rattus norvegicus*	Novelty seeking/ anxiety	CF	No	Yes	Stead *et al.* 2006
Rat *Rattus norvegicus*		CF	Yes	No	Francis *et al.* 1999
White-footed mouse *Peromyscus leucopus* and California mouse *P. californicus*	Aggressiveness (attack latency)	CF	Yes	?	Bester-Meredith & Marler 2001
German shepherd dog *Canis familiaris*	Playfulness/ aggressiveness/ curiosity/chase-proneness	PA	No	Yes	Strandberg *et al.* 2005
Cattle *Bos taurus*	Docility	PA	No	Yes	Beckman *et al.* 2007
Domestic sheep *Ovis aries*	Emotional reactivity	PA	No	Yes	Boissy *et al.* 2005
Bighorn sheep *Ovis canadensis*	Docility/boldness	PA	No	Yes	Réale *et al.* 2009
Zebra finch *Taeniopygia guttata*	Aggressiveness	PA [b]	Yes	Yes	Forstmeier *et al.* 2004
Three-spined stickleback *Gasterosteus aculeatus*	Exploration/ activity	PA	No	Yes	Dingemanse *et al.* 2009

[a] PC, phenotypic correlation; CF, cross-fostering; PA, pedigree analysis using the animal model.
[b] Pedigree analysis included cross-fostered individuals.

Finally, the genetic and maternal influences on offspring behaviour may also be tested using breeding experiments or with information from the pedigree of a population. Recent quantitative genetic experiments have found substantial heritability but negligible maternal effects on the variance of personality traits in animals (Table 16.1). Standard full-sib/half-sib experiments revealed heritable variation in stickleback personality, but no parental effects (Dingemanse *et al.* 2009). Forstmeier *et al.* (2004), however, found strong maternal effects on male aggressiveness in zebra finches *Taeniopygia guttata*. In another quantitative genetic experiment, van Oers *et al.* (2004) crossed individuals from two lines of great tits artificially selected for early exploration and backcrossed F$_1$ individuals with individuals from parental lines. They found that maternal effects were negligible compared to additive genetic effects for boldness, exploration and early exploratory behaviour, suggesting once again that despite potential maternal effects, the personality of an individual was strongly influenced by genes.

The preceding studies were, notably, conducted in laboratory-bred birds that did not experience the full range of potential environmental influences that might result in maternal effects. In the wild, for instance, female great tits that have fast-exploring social mates do deposit higher levels of yolk androgens in their eggs compared to females mated with slow-exploring social mates (Dingemanse *et al.* unpublished). Because experimental manipulation of yolk androgens affects personality (Groothuis *et al.* 2005), and females with different personalities deposit different levels of yolk androgens in their eggs (Groothuis *et al.* 2008), the work on the great tits implies that maternal effects influence personality in the wild. Overall, there is a need for experiments that could control both genetic and maternal influences on the development of offspring personality.

16.5.3 Personality and dispersal

Natal dispersal – the movement between the place of birth and the place of first breeding – is a major determinant of the dynamics and genetic structure of populations (Hamilton & May 1977, Johnson & Gaines 1990, Whitlock 2001). There are various reasons why some individuals disperse and others do not (Chapter 12). For instance, dispersal may allow an individual to avoid breeding with related individuals (inbreeding-depression avoidance), or to avoid competition for resources, such as breeding habitat, food and mates (Clobert *et al.* 2001). In many animals, dispersal decisions appear to be shaped in part by social interactions between individuals. Dispersal is thus often considered to be condition-dependent, implying the existence of a dispersal generalist phenotype. Zero heritability of dispersal tendency in some birds (Wheelwright & Mauck 1998, Pasinelli & Walters 2002) and mammals (Waser & Jones 1989) suggests that it is largely environmentally determined. However, accumulating evidence shows that multiple dispersal specialists do coexist in other species, as shown by substantial heritable variation in insects, birds and rodents (Kent & Rankin 2001, Hansson *et al.* 2003, Krackow 2003, Pasinelli *et al.* 2004, Duckworth & Badyaev 2007, Saastamoinen 2008).

Recent studies show that dispersal ability covaries predictably with certain personality traits (Fraser *et al.* 2001, Dingemanse *et al.* 2003, Cote & Clobert 2007, Duckworth & Badyaev 2007). Dispersal appears particularly linked with exploratory or aggressive behaviour, two traits that are often part of the same behavioural syndrome (Réale *et al.* 2007). Exploration might facilitate efficient information gathering in novel environments, and aggressiveness might facilitate successful recruitment into the breeding population following dispersal. In great tits, offspring from fast-exploring parents disperse and breed further from their place of birth than offspring from slow-exploring parents (Dingemanse *et al.* 2003). In these birds, slow-exploring, non-dispersing individuals seem to cope better with social stress and are generally dominant over fast explorers prior to territory settlement (Dingemanse & de Goede 2004). In other species, such as western bluebirds *Sialia mexicana*, male aggressiveness is heritable and genetically linked with dispersal ability (Duckworth & Badyaev 2007). The latter species has expanded its range over the last decades, and natural selection favours aggressiveness only in the invasion front. On the other hand, low aggressiveness is favoured in established populations, as a result of the trade-off between aggressiveness and territory defence and paternal care (Duckworth 2006). In wild house mice, dispersal tendency is linked to explorative behaviour but neither to anxiety nor to individual variation in kin preference (Krackow 2003). Similarly, highly sociable animals are expected to be less dispersive, as shown for lizards and marmots (Armitage 1986, Cote & Clobert 2007).

The study of the coexistence of specialised and generalist dispersers within the same population is relatively difficult, because most animals show natal dispersal only once in their lifetime. Therefore repeatability of dispersal or individual variation in the variance of dispersal decisions along a given environmental gradient (i.e. local density) cannot be studied (Nussey *et al.* 2007). It is therefore only possible to study the specific dispersal decisions of different genotypes in response to change in the environment (i.e. genotype-by-environment interaction: Chapters 1 and 2, Nussey *et al.* 2007).

Some quantitative genetic methods using pedigree information can allow one to estimate the variance in the probability of dispersal as a function of the environment (Falconer & Mackay 1996). That is, we can treat dispersal in one environment (e.g. low competition) as a different trait from dispersal in another environment (e.g. high competition), and calculate via the pedigree the heritabilities of both traits as well as the cross-environment genetic correlation (r_A) between those traits. The latter parameter can be used to evaluate the existence of generalist and specialist genotypes (see Box 16.2). In summary, individuals could only be considered as specialists (i.e. they disperse or not), whereas at the genotypic level it may be possible to show the coexistence of specialists and generalists.

16.5.4 Personality and dominance

Dominance and personality are intertwined. The aggression shown by an individual depends both on intrinsic (i.e. genetic or epigenetic) effects and on the behaviour expressed by the opponent (i.e. indirect genetic effects: Chapter 2, Wilson *et al.* 2009). Dominance results from repeated interactions between individuals (Chapters 7 and 14), and is best defined as 'an attribute of the pattern of repeated agonistic interactions between two individuals, characterized by a consistent outcome in favour of the same dyad member and default yielding response of its opponent rather than escalation' (Drews 1993). An individual's dominance rank therefore depends both on the characteristics of that individual and on those of the other individuals with whom it is competing. Dominance hierarchies are shaped by aggressiveness, winner effects (the change in probability of winning future fights following winning), and loser effects (the change in probability of losing fights following a severe loss) of all individual players (Chapter 14; Chase *et al.* 1994, Dugatkin 1997). Therefore both behavioural (e.g. aggressiveness) and physiological traits (e.g. level of corticosterone produced in response to losing) may affect an individual's dominance rank.

Although we might expect that, according to personality, individuals may show different dispositions that affect their dominance position, the link between personality and dominance may not be as simple as expected. For example, in the great tit, fast explorers occupy either top or bottom dominance positions, whereas slow explorers acquire predominantly middle positions (Verbeek *et al.* 1999). Fast-exploring individuals are more aggressive and generally acquire high dominance ranks in newly formed aviary groups (Drent & Marchetti 1999, Verbeek *et al.* 1999). However, following a defeat, fast explorers show less elevated corticosterone levels (Fig. 16.3; Carere *et al.* 2001, 2003), and suffer more from loser effects than slow explorers (Verbeek 1998). On the other hand, slow explorers increase their rank by preferentially attacking higher ranked birds that have suffered from repeated loss (Verbeek 1998).

The latter results were supported in the field, where fast-exploring birds have lowest dominance rank among non-territorial birds, but highest dominance rank among territorial birds (Dingemanse & de Goede 2004). Evidence that individuals with different personalities show differential stress responses (Koolhaas *et al.* 1999) raises the question of how we should interpret the consequences of social conflicts. In the absence of data on personality, information on the production of a stress hormone such as cortisol in an organism following a social conflict may lead to spurious conclusions.

As most fast explorers are able to acquire a top dominant position only when they are rare, the great tit example illustrates potential negative frequency-dependent selection acting on personality, though modelling still needs to test this idea in an explicit mathematical framework. Work on pigs *Sus scrofa* further illustrates the notion of frequency-dependent success of different personalities (D'Eath & Burn 2002). In this domestic species, interactions between two aggressive individuals were more likely to result in injuries compared to interactions of other combinations of personalities (two non-aggressive pigs, one aggressive versus one non-aggressive pig), implying that social interactions play a key role in understanding the maintenance of variation in personality.

As with dispersal behaviour, it might prove relatively difficult to study the occurrence of specialists

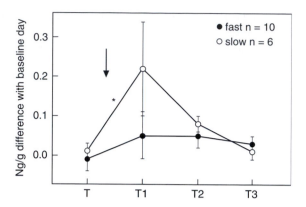

Figure 16.3 Changes in corticosterone level in faecal samples after a social challenge (i.e. confrontation with an aggressive resident male) in two lines of great tits *Parus major* artificially selected for different personalities. Slow birds had a significant increase in their level of stress hormones after the challenge, whereas fast birds did not. After Carere *et al.* (2003).

and generalists with regard to dominance in field conditions. Individuals acquire a specific rank after a series of repeated agonistic interactions with conspecifics. However, in artificially selected lines of great tits (see above) slow explorers show limited plasticity and can be regarded as individuals that specialise in middle positions. In contrast, fast explorers acquire either high or low dominance positions depending on their individual history, and can therefore be regarded as generalists. Therefore, an important avenue for future research will be to address which conditions favour a mix of specialists and generalists, and which conditions favour their environmental versus genetic determination.

16.5.5 Personality and mating strategies

Given that animal personality affects an individual's reactions to challenging, stressful situations, it seems reasonable to hypothesise that personality should play a role in an individual's ability to compete for access to mates, mate choice and mating behaviour. In humans, for example, male extroverts have more extra-pair matings, female extroverts change partners more often than introvert individuals, and both have a higher risk of hospitalisation for accidents (Nettle 2005). The ways in which personality affects mating behaviour in animals have been studied in a few cases.

A good example of a link between personality and mating strategies is provided by the side-blotched lizard *Uta stansburiana*. In this species, males of three throat-colour morphs corresponding to six different genotypes show alternative strategies (Sinervo & Lively 1996). Large and aggressive orange males usurp territories, medium-size blue males perform mate guarding, whereas small-size yellow males mimic females and use a sneaker strategy (Sinervo & Lively 1996). Orange males disperse further than other male types, and cooperation among unrelated blue males permits them to reduce the chance of orange males to usurp their territories (Sinervo & Clobert 2003).

The three alternative strategies are maintained over generations as a result of frequency-dependent selection, in a rock–paper–scissors evolutionarily strategy, whereby each morph outperforms another, and is in turn beaten by the third morph (Sinervo & Lively 1996). This lizard population is composed of specialists, and no male is able to switch from one strategy to another during his lifetime. In bighorn sheep *Ovis canadensis*, paternity analyses and quantitative genetic studies demonstrated a link between reproductive success and male personality (Réale *et al.* 2009). Bighorn sheep show a promiscuous mating system, and males overtly compete for access to and fertilisation of receptive females. Age and horn length have a strong impact on the ability of a male to fertilise females, but personality explains a large portion of variance in reproductive success among males. Non-docile rams show higher reproductive success than docile males early in life, but do not survive as long as docile males. As a result, docile males have the greatest reproductive success after seven years of age.

In bighorn sheep, boldness does not affect reproductive success early in life, but bold males are more successful than shy males later in life (Réale *et al.* 2009). The high heritability of these two personality traits suggests the existence of specialists in this species. In western bluebirds, male reproductive strategies vary according to aggressiveness (Duckworth & Badyaev 2007). Highly aggressive males disperse and colonise new populations, where they show a high success in territory acquisition and mating. On the other hand, non-aggressive male bluebirds exhibit high levels of parental care, which allows them to raise more offspring than aggressive males (Duckworth 2006). The latter results may explain why western bluebird populations vary in their degree of aggressiveness along their current range of expansion in Montana, and the ability of western bluebirds to displace mountain bluebird *Sialia currucoides* populations (Duckworth & Badyaev 2007).

Personality differences and mating behaviour have also been studied in females. Forstmeier (2007) found that female zebra finches differed consistently in the propensity to engage in extra-pair copulations (EPC). By measuring sexual responsiveness in young unpaired females, and by testing their tendency to engage in EPC later in life, Forstmeier showed that most variation among females was caused by individual differences, whereas the attractiveness of a female's partner had no effect on her rate of EPC. It is conceivable that this weak relationship may be caused by the fact that individual females vary in the way they adjust their propensity to engage in extra-pair mating to the quality of the potential extra-pair male, with some females showing highly consistent fidelity, some females showing a high rate of EPC independent of the quality of the male presented, whereas other females vary their tendency for EPC with the attractiveness of the male.

In a recent study of great tits, paternity analyses shows that females with extreme personalities (either fast or slow) are more likely to have extra-pair offspring in their nests when they are paired with a social mate of similar extreme personality (van Oers *et al.* 2008). Pairing of similar extreme individuals has been shown to produce offspring with a lower fitness (Dingemanse *et al.* 2004). Therefore, female great tits of extreme personality might seek extra-pair mates of dissimilar personality, and these adaptive mate-choice decisions might thus allow them to produce offspring of intermediate personality type. Here, both types of bird appear to be generalists, as they engage in EPCs only when mated with certain types of social mate.

Much work remains to be done on the link between personality and mating strategies. The existence of personality differences in a population and its potential role in mating strategies, and the possibility that personality differences also correspond to different degrees of specialisation, would imply that fixed mating strategies and conditional mating strategies coexist in natural populations. However, it has been assumed that these two strategies would be evolutionarily incompatible (Andersson 1994), and that conditional mating strategies would be observed in most cases (Gross 1996). Plaistow *et al.* (2004) have shown that pure strategies (i.e. genetically determined, or specialists) and conditional strategies (i.e. generalists) could coexist in some restricted conditions, and that mixed strategies are also possible. They found that costs of (or limits to) plasticity, and a strong mating skew, can prevent conditional strategies from invading a population consisting of individuals with fixed strategies.

16.5.6 Personality and group living

Many animals live in groups, and living in groups is associated with benefits (e.g. better predator detection and dilution effects, and/or higher chance of finding food) and costs (e.g. increased competition for resources, aggression or lack of synchronisation with the rest of the group: Chapter 9, Danchin & Giraldeau 2008, Giraldeau 2008). Within a group some individuals may be able to cheat and not cooperate while benefiting from the cooperation of others, some may provide some information, and others may exploit the information provided by others (Giraldeau & Dubois 2008). Such social alternatives permit the coexistence of individuals with different degrees of specialisation for these behaviours.

What do we know about the link between personality, group living and cooperation? First, animals differ in their sociability (Réale *et al.* 2007), and in the way they are attracted and depend on the presence of other group members. Sociability has been studied mainly in domestic animals (cattle, Müller & Schrader 2005; Japanese quail *Coturnix japonica*, Faure & Mills 1998; sheep, Sibbald & Hooper 2004) and captive animals (spotted hyenas *Crocuta crocuta*, Gosling 1998; greylag geese *Anser anser*, Kralj-Fišer *et al.* 2007). This can be explained by the fact that social isolation experiments are easier to perform with captive animals than in the wild. For example, Faure and Mills (1998) measured sociability by separating an individual quail from the group and measuring the distance the quail would cover on a treadmill to join the group. Nevertheless, it is possible to measure sociability in the field. For example, Kralj-Fišer *et al.* (2007) measured the average number of neighbouring geese resting in close proximity to a focal individual. Alternatively, it might be possible to use indices from social network theory (Chapter 9; Krause *et al.* 2007) as measures of social personality traits.

Depending on their personality, individuals may be constrained in their activities by the activities of other individuals in the group. For example, individuals with different levels of activity may have to adjust their activity according to the activity of other individuals in order to maintain the group cohesion. The benefits and the costs for an individual to join a group may depend on an individual's own personality and on the personality of individuals in the group. Highly aggressive and less aggressive individuals may pay different costs associated with increased density in their group. An animal may also benefit from joining a group with bolder individuals by being able to reach areas that it could never reach alone. As far as

we know no study has looked at the different costs and benefits of living in groups for individuals with different personalities.

There is now some evidence that personality traits of an individual can be affected by the personalities of individuals in the group. For example, young perch *Perca fluviatilis* adjust their boldness and exploration relative to the boldness and exploratory tendencies of other individuals in the group (Magnhagen & Staffan 2005, Magnhagen 2007). Ward *et al.* (2004) showed that in three-spined sticklebacks bold individuals generally lead groups and have a lower tendency to shoal than shy ones. They hypothesised that natural selection might favour the mix of shy and bold individuals, because the bold individuals, who are generally at the front of the group, would benefit from increased food intake but suffer from increased predation risk. The situation can be more complex, as depending on their personality individuals may show different antipredator responses and therefore run different risks (Quinn & Creswell 2005).

Group composition in terms of personalities may influence how well a group behaves in a particular condition, which can affect the fitness of individuals. For example Sih and Waters (2005) showed that experimental groups of water striders *Aquarius remigis* consisting of extremely aggressive males decrease the mating success of the whole group because of the harassment of females by a single hyper-aggressive male within the group. The coexistence of different behavioural types and the importance of the mix of behavioural types for the fitness of individuals within a group have been largely studied in the context of social foraging. In groups of animals, individuals can use two different tactics, one which consists of searching actively for food patches (producing) and one which consists of exploiting the food patches and stealing the food discovered by producers (scrounging). The maintenance of both producing and scrounging tactics in a group has been thoroughly studied (Giraldeau 2008). Scroungers do better than producers in a group with a lot of producers, but producers have an advantage over scroungers when the group is mainly composed of scroungers. The group can reach a stable equilibrium frequency when both tactics provide equal payoffs (Giraldeau 2008).

It is tempting to consider that producing and scrounging tactics could be related to personality, although no study has taken this approach as yet. In wild Carib grackles *Quiscalus lugubris*, individuals can switch reversibly from one tactic to the other, although birds vary in the proportion of time they spend playing one tactic or the other (Fig. 16.4; Morand-Ferron *et al.* 2007). Theoretical models show the possible coexistence of producer and scrounger specialists, and of generalists that switch from one tactic to the other and contribute to restoring equilibrium frequencies (Giraldeau & Dubois 2008, Dubois, Morand-Ferron and Giraldeau unpublished). This situation represents a nice example of how evolution could have led to a mix of personality specialists and generalists within the same population.

Finally, one of the most potentially fruitful and unexplored areas for the study of personality in a social context is the role of personality differences in cooperative breeding. Arnold *et al.* (2005) looked at the coexistence of breeding roles in groups of noisy miners *Manorina melanocephala*, a cooperatively

breeding bird from Australia. They found that some helpers specialised in chick feeding whereas others were defending the chicks against predators. They suggested that personality differences could explain this division of labour within a group, but did not provide any evidence for such a link. Furthermore, Arnold and colleagues mentioned the existence of specialised mobbers and specialised provisioners, while other noisy miners behaved more as generalists. Bergmüller and Taborsky (2007) reported a similar division of labour in the cooperatively breeding Lake Tanganyika cichlid *Neolamprologus pulcher*. In that species, some helpers invest more time in territory defence while others spend more time in territory maintenance. Interestingly, the former were more aggressive and explorative than the latter.

These two studies raise questions that, if addressed, would evaluate how integrating information on personality differences could inform research on cooperative breeding. For example, does personality explain the variation in life-history strategies among helpers, and the decision to leave the parents' territory? Does parental personality affect such a decision? Do parents manipulate the proportion of helpers of

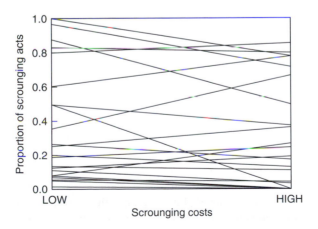

Figure 16.4 Individual reaction norm for the proportion of scrounging as a function of increasing costs of scrounging in Carib grackles *Quiscalus lugubris*. Carib grackles can be victims of food stealing when they dunk a hard food item into a puddle. By changing the shape of the puddle, Morand-Ferron *et al.* could limit access to the puddle by potential scroungers and affect scrounging cost. There was no difference in the ranking of individuals according to their proportion of scrounging acts between the low and high scrounging costs. After Morand-Ferron *et al.* (2007).

different personalities in order to ensure a balanced division of labour? Do personality differences play a key role in the affinities between parents and helpers in a cooperatively breeding group?

16.6 Conclusions and future directions

The future seems bright for studies on individual personality differences and their social context. There is evidence for consistent individual differences in social behaviour in several instances such as offspring solicitation and parental care, the propensity to disperse from the natal area, the establishment of a dominance rank, mating strategies, group living anti-predator or foraging strategies, and cooperative breeding. Furthermore, studies have shown how these individual differences are related to variation in boldness, aggressiveness, activity, exploration and sociability. These suggest that the fate of an individual at each stage of its life history may be affected by its personality. Despite these studies, not much has been done on the fate of particular personality types in different social contexts and on the way in which social interactions affect the development and evolution of personality. Finally, with this review we hope to stimulate research on proximate and ultimate reasons for the coexistence of individuals with varying degrees of specialisation for the social behaviour studied. This could only be done by marking individuals of a population, carrying out personality tests on each of these individuals, and following them at different stages of their lives. An additional promising direction lies in the use of personality-trait measurements in studies of social behaviour based on experimental breeding designs and animal models.

Acknowledgements

We would like to thank John Quinn and two other anonymous reviewers for their comments and suggestions, which improved our manuscript. We also thank the Groupe de Recherche en Écologie Comportementale et Animale at the Université du Québec à Montréal (UQAM) for comments and discussions on a previous draft of the paper. NJD was supported by the Netherlands Organisation for Scientific Research (Grant 863.05.002). DR was supported by the Natural Sciences and Engineering Research Council of Canada.

Suggested readings

Biro, P. A. & Stamps, J. A. (2008) Are animal personality traits linked to life-history productivity? *Trends in Ecology and Evolution*, **23**, 361–368.

Réale, D., Reader, S. M., Sol, D., McDougall, P. T. & Dingemanse, N. J. (2007) Integrating animal temperament within ecology and evolution. *Biological Reviews of the Cambridge Philosophical Society*, **82**, 291–318.

Sih, A., Bell, A. M., Johnson, J. C. & Ziemba, R. E. (2004) Behavioral syndromes: an integrative overview. *Quarterly Review of Biology*, **79**, 241–277.

Wilson, D. S., Clark, A. B., Coleman, K. & Dearstyne, T. (1994) Shyness and boldness in humans and other animals. *Trends in Ecology and Evolution*, **9**, 442–446.

References

Adkins-Regan, E. (2005) *Hormones and Animal Social Behavior*. Princeton, NJ: Princeton University Press.

Agrawal, A. F., Brodie, E. D. & Brown J. (2001) Parent–offspring coadaptation and the dual genetic control of maternal care. *Science*, **292**, 1710–1712.

Albers, P. C. H., Timmermans, P. J. A. & Vossen, J. M. H. (1999) Evidence for the existence of mothering styles in Guinea pigs (*Cavia aperea f. porcellus*). *Behaviour*, **136**, 469–479.

Andersson, M. B. (1994) *Sexual Selection*. Princeton, NJ: Princeton University Press.

Armitage, K. B. (1986) Individuality, social behavior, and reproductive success in yellow-bellied marmots. *Ecology*, **67**, 1186–1193.

Arnold, K. E., Owens, I. P. F. & Goldizen, A. W. (2005) Division of labour within cooperatively breeding groups. *Behaviour*, **142**, 1577–1590.

Arnold, K. E., Ramsay, S. L., Donaldson, C. & Adam, A. (2007) Parental prey selection affects risk-taking behaviour and spatial learning in avian offspring. *Proceedings of the Royal Society B*, **274**, 2563–2569.

Bardi, M. & Huffman, M. A. (2002) Effects of maternal style on infant behavior in Japanese macaques (*Macaca fuscata*). *Developmental Psychobiology*, **41**, 364–372.

Beckman, D. W., Enns, R. M., Speidel, S. E., Brigham, B. W. & Garrick, D. J. (2007) Maternal effects on docility in Limousin cattle. *Journal of Animal Science*, **85**, 650–657.

Bell, A. M. (2005) Behavioural differences between individuals and two populations of stickleback (*Gasterosteus aculeatus*). *Journal of Evolutionary Biology*, **18**, 464–473.

Bell, A. M. & Sih, A. (2007) Exposure to predation generates personality in threespined sticklebacks (*Gasterosteus aculeatus*). *Ecology Letters*, **10**, 828–834.

Benus, R. F. & Rondig, M. (1996) Patterns of maternal effort in mouse lines bidirectionally selected for aggression. *Animal Behaviour*, **51**, 67–75.

Bergmüller, R. & Taborsky, M. (2007) Adaptive behavioural syndromes due to strategic niche specialisation. *BMC Ecology*, **7**, 12.

Bergstrom, C. T. & Godfrey-Smith, P. (1998) On the evolution of behavioral heterogeneity in individuals and populations. *Biology and Philosophy*, **13**, 205–231.

Berman, C. M. (1990) Consistency in maternal behavior within families of free-ranging rhesus monkeys: an extension of the concept of maternal style. *American Journal of Primatology*, **22**, 159–169.

Bester-Meredith, J. K. & Marler, C. A. (2001) Vasopressin and aggression in cross-fostered California mice (*Peromyscus californicus*) and white-footed mice (*Peromyscus leucopus*). *Hormones and Behavior*, **40**, 51–64.

Biro, P. A. & Stamps, J. A. (2008) Are animal personality traits linked to life-history productivity? *Trends in Ecology and Evolution*, **23**, 361–368.

Biro, P. A., Abrahams, M. V., Post, J. R. & Parkinson, E. A. (2004) Predators select against high growth rates and risk-taking behaviour in domestic trout populations. *Proceedings of the Royal Society B*, **271**, 2233–2237.

Boissy, A., Bouix, J., Orgeur, P. *et al.* (2005) Genetic analysis of emotional reactivity in sheep: effects of the genotypes of the lambs and of their dams. *Genetics, Selection, Evolution*, **37**, 381–401.

Bolnick, D. I., Svanbäck, R., Fordyce, J. A. *et al.* (2003) The ecology of individuals: incidence and implications of individual specialization. *American Naturalist*, **161**, 1–28.

Boon, A. K., Réale, D. & Boutin, S. (2007) The interaction between personality, offspring fitness, and food abundance in North American red squirrels. *Ecology Letters*, **10**, 1094–1104.

Both, C., Dingemanse, N. J., Drent, P. J. & Tinbergen, J. M. (2005) Pairs of extreme avian personalities have highest reproductive success. *Journal of Animal Ecology*, **74**, 667–674.

Brockmann, J. A. (2001) The evolution of alternative strategies and tactics. *Advances in the Study of Behavior*, **30**, 1–51.

Cameron N. M., Parent C., Champagne F. A. *et al.* (2005) The programming of individual differences in defensive responses and reproductive strategies in the rat through variations in maternal. *Neuroscience and Biobehavioural Reviews*, **29**, 843–886.

Carere, C., Welink, D., Drent, P. J., Koolhaas, J. M. & Groothuis, T. G. G. (2001) Effect of social defeat in a territorial bird (*Parus major*) selected for different coping styles. *Physiology and Behavior*, **73**, 427–433.

Carere, C., Groothuis, T. G. G., Moestl, E., Daan, S. & Koolhaas, J. M. (2003) Fecal corticosteroids in a territorial bird selected for different personalities: daily rhythm and the response to social stress. *Hormones and Behavior*, **43**, 540–548.

Carere, C., Drent, P. J., Koolhaas, J. M. & Groothuis, T. G. G. (2005a) Epigenetic effects on personality traits: early food provisioning and sibling competition. *Behaviour*, **142**, 1329–1355.

Carere, C., Drent, P. J., Privitera, L., Koolhaas, J. M. & Groothuis, T. G. G. (2005b) Personalities in great tits, *Parus major*: stability and consistency. *Animal Behaviour*, **70**, 795–815.

Chase, I. D., Bartolomeo, C. & Dugatkin, L. A. (1994) Aggressive interactions and inter-contest interval: how long do winners keep winning? *Animal Behaviour*, **48**, 393–400.

Clark, A. B. & Ehlinger, T. J. (1987) Pattern and adaptation in individual behavioral differences. *Perspectives in Ethology*, **7**, 1–47.

Clobert, J., Danchin, E., Dhondt, A. A. & Nichols, J. D., eds. (2001) *Dispersal*. New York, NY: Oxford University Press.

Clutton-Brock, T. H. (1991) *The Evolution of Parental Care*. Princeton, NJ: Princeton University Press.

Cote, J. & Clobert, J. (2007) Social personalities influence natal dispersal in a lizard. *Proceedings of the Royal Society B*, **274**, 383–390.

Dall, S. R. X., Houston, A. I. & McNamara, J. M. (2004) The behavioural ecology of personality: consistent individual differences from an adaptive perspective. *Ecology Letters*, **7**, 734–739.

Danchin, E. & Giraldeau, L.-A. (2008) Animal aggregation: hypotheses and controversies. In: *Behavioural Ecology: an Evolutionary Perspective on Behaviour*, ed. E. Danchin, L.-A. Giraldeau & F. Cézilly. Oxford: Oxford University Press, pp. 503–545.

Danchin, E., Giraldeau, L.-A. & Cézilly, F., eds. (2008) *Behavioural Ecology: an Evolutionary Perspective on Behaviour.* Oxford: Oxford University Press.

D'Eath, R. B. & Burn, C. C. (2002) Individual differences in behaviour: a test of 'coping style' does not predict resident–intruder aggressiveness in pigs. *Behaviour,* **139,** 1175–1194.

De Witt, T. J. (1998) Costs and limits of phenotypic plasticity: tests with predator-induced morphology and life history in a freshwater snail. *Journal of Evolutionary Biology,* **11,** 465–480.

De Witt, T. J., Sih, A. & Wilson D. S. (1998) Costs and limits of phenotypic plasticity. *Trends in Ecology and Evolution,* **13,** 77–81.

Dingemanse, N. J. & de Goede, P. (2004) The relation between dominance and exploratory behavior is context-dependent in wild great tits. *Behavioral Ecology,* **15,** 1023–1030.

Dingemanse, N. J. & Réale, D. (2005) Natural selection and animal personality. *Behaviour,* **142,** 1159–1184.

Dingemanse, N. J., Both, C., Drent, P. J., van Oers, K. & van Noordwijk, A. J. (2002) Repeatability and heritability of exploratory behaviour in great tits from the wild. *Animal Behaviour,* **64,** 929–937.

Dingemanse, N. J., Both, C., van Noordwijk, A. J., Rutten, A. L. & Drent, P. J. (2003) Natal dispersal and personalities in great tits (*Parus major*). *Proceedings of the Royal Society B,* **270,** 741–747.

Dingemanse, N. J., Both, C., Drent, P. J. & Tinbergen, J. M. (2004) Fitness consequences of avian personalities in a fluctuating environment. *Proceedings of the Royal Society B,* **271,** 847–852.

Dingemanse, N. J., Wright, J., Kazem, A. J. N. *et al.* (2007) Behavioural syndromes differ predictably between 12 populations of stickleback. *Journal of Animal Ecology,* **76,** 1128–1138.

Dingemanse, N.J., van der Plas, F., Wright, J. *et al.* (2009) Individual experience and evolutionary history of predation affect expression of heritable variation in fish personality and morphology. *Proceedings of the Royal Society B,* **276,** 1285–1293.

Drent, P. J. & Marchetti, C. (1999) Individuality, exploration and foraging in hand raised juvenile great tits. In: *Proceedings of the 22nd International Ornithological Congress,* ed. N. J. Adams & R. H. Slotow. Johannesburg: Birdlife South Africa, pp. 896–914.

Drews, C. (1993) The concept and definition of dominance in animal behaviour. *Behaviour,* **125,** 283–311.

Duckworth, R. A. (2006) Behavioral correlations across breeding contexts provide a mechanism for a cost of aggression. *Behavioral Ecology,* **17,** 1011–1019.

Duckworth, R. A. & Badyaev, A. V. (2007) Coupling of dispersal and aggression facilitates the rapid range expansion of a passerine bird. *Proceedings of the National Academy of Sciences of the USA,* **104,** 15017–15022.

Dugatkin, L. A. (1997) Winner and loser effects and the structure of dominance hierarchies. *Behavioral Ecology,* **8,** 583–587.

Dwyer C. M. & Lawrence A. B. (1998) Variability in the expression of maternal behaviour in primiparous sheep: effects of genotype and litter. *Applied Animal Behaviour Sciences,* **58,** 311–330.

Fairbanks, L. A. (1996) Individual differences in maternal style: causes and consequences for mothers and offspring. *Advances in the Study of Behavior,* **25,** 579–611.

Fairbanks, L. A. & McGuire, M. T. (1993) Maternal protectiveness and response to the unfamiliar in vervet monkeys. *American Journal of Primatology,* **30,** 119–129.

Falconer, D. S. & Mackay, T. F. C. (1996) *Introduction to Quantitative Genetics.* New York, NY: Longman.

Faure, J.-M., Mills, A. (1998) Improving the adaptablity of animals by selection. In: *Genetics and the Behavior of Domestic Animals,* ed. T. Grandin. San Diego, CA: Academic Press, pp. 235–264.

Forstmeier, W. (2007) Do individual females differ intrinsically in their propensity to engage extra-pair copulations? *PLoS ONE,* **2** (9), e952.

Forstmeier, W., Coltman, D. W. & Birkhead, T. R. (2004) Maternal effects influence the sexual behavior of sons and daughters in the zebra finch. *Evolution,* **58,** 2574–2583.

Francis, D. D., Diorio, J., Liu, D. & Meaney, M. J. (1999) Nongenomic transmission across generations in maternal behavior and stress responses in the rat. *Science,* **286,** 1155–1158.

Fraser, D. F., Gilliam, J. F., Daley, M. J., Le, A. N. & Skalski, G. T. (2001) Explaining leptokurtik movement distributions: intrapopulation variation in boldness and exploration. *Amercian Naturalist,* **158,** 124–135.

Giraldeau, L.-A. (1984) Group foraging: the skill pool effect and frequency-dependent learning. *American Naturalist,* **124,** 72–79.

Giraldeau, L.-A. (2008) Social foraging. In: *Behavioural Ecology: an Evolutionary Perspective on Behaviour,* ed. E. Danchin, L.-A. Giraldeau & F. Cézilly. Oxford: Oxford University Press, pp. 257–283.

Giraldeau, L.-A. & Dubois, F. (2008) Social foraging and the study of exploitative behavior. *Advances in the Study of Behavior*, **38**, 59–104.

Gosling, S. D. (1998) Personality dimension in spotted hyenas (*Crocuta crocuta*). *Journal of Comparative Psychology*, **112**, 107–118.

Gosling, S. D. (2001) From mice to men: what can we learn about personality from animal research? *Psychological Bulletin*, **137**, 45–86.

Grandison, K. (2005) Genetic background of maternal behaviour and its relation to offspring survival. *Livestock Production Science*, **93**, 43–50.

Groothuis, T. G. G. & Carere, C. (2005) Avian personalities: characterization and epigenesis. *Neuroscience Biobehavioural Review*, **29**, 137–150.

Groothuis, T. G. G., Muller, W., von Engelhardt, N., Carere, C. & Eising, C. (2005) Maternal hormones as a tool to adjust offspring phenotype in avian species. *Neuroscience and Biobehavioral Reviews*, **29**, 329–352.

Groothuis, T. G. G., Carere, C., Lipar, J., Drent, P. J. & Schwabl, H. (2008) Selection on personality in a songbird affects maternal hormone levels tuned to its effect on timing of reproduction. *Biology Letters*, **4**, 465–467.

Gross, M. R. (1996) Alternative reproductive strategies and tactics: diversity within sexes. *Trends in Ecology and Evolution*. **11**, 92–98.

Hamilton, W. D. & May, R. M. (1977) Dispersal in stable habitats. *Nature*, **269**, 578–581.

Hansson, B., Bensch, S. & Hasselquist, D. (2003) Heritability of dispersal in the great reed warbler. *Ecology Letters*, **6**, 290–294.

Hemelrijk, C. K. & Wiantia, J. (2005) Individual variation by self-organisation. *Neuroscience and Biobehavioural Reviews*, **29**, 125–136.

Huntingford, F. A. (1976) The relationship between antipredator behaviour and aggression among conspecifics in the three-spined stickleback, *Gasterosteus aculeatus*. *Animal Behaviour*, **24**, 245–260.

Johnson, M. L. & Gaines, M. S. (1990) Evolution of dispersal: theoretical models and empirical tests using birds and mammals. *Annual Review of Ecology and Systematics*, **21**, 449–480.

Kent, J. W. & Rankin, M. A. (2001) Heritability and physiological correlates of migratory tendency in the grasshopper *Melanoplus sanguinipes*. *Physiological Entomology*, **26**, 371–380.

Kölliker, M. (2005) Ontogeny in the family. *Behaviour Genetics*, **35**, 7–18.

Kölliker, M. & Richner, H. (2001) Parent–offspring conflict and the genetics of offspring solicitation and parental response. *Animal Behaviour*, **62**, 395–407.

Koolhaas, J. M., Korte, S. M., de Boer, S. F. *et al.* (1999) Coping styles in animals: current status in behavior and stress-physiology. *Neuroscience and Biobehavioral Reviews*, **23**, 925–935.

Krackow, S. (2003) Motivational and heritable determinants of dispersal latency in wild male house mice (*Mus musculus musculus*). *Ethology*, **109**, 671–689.

Kralj-Fišer, S., Scheiber, I. B. R., Blejec, A., Moestl, E., Kotrschal, K. (2007) Individualities in a flock of free-roaming greylag geese: behavioral and physiological consistency over time and across situations. *Hormones and Behavior*, **51**, 239–248.

Krause, J., Croft, D. P. & James R. (2007) Social network theory in the behavioural sciences: potential applications. *Behavioral Ecology and Sociobiology*, **62**, 15–27.

Krebs, J. & Davies, N. B. (1997) The evolution of behavioural ecology. In *Behavioural Ecology: an Evolutionary Approach*, 4th edn, ed. J. R. Krebs and N. B. Davies. Oxford: Blackwell, pp. 3–14.

Leimar, O. (2005) The evolution of phenotypic polymorphism: randomized strategies versus evolutionary branching. *American Naturalist*, **165**, 669–681.

Lessells, C. & Boag, P. T. (1987) Unrepeatable repeatabilities: a common mistake. *Auk*, **104**, 116–121.

Lock, J. E., Smiseth, P. T. & Moore A. J. (2004) Selection, inheritance, and the evolution of parent–offspring interactions. *American Naturalist*, **164**, 13–24.

Lynch, M. & Walsh, B. (1998) *Genetics and Analysis of Quantitative Traits*, Sunderland, MA: Sinauer Associates.

Maestripieri, D. (2003) Similarities in affiliation and aggression between cross-fostered Rhesus macaque females and their biological mothers. *Developmental Psychobiology*, **43**, 321–327.

Magnhagen, C. (2007) Social influence on the correlation between behaviours in young-of-the-year perch. *Behavioral Ecology and Sociobiology*, **61**, 525–531.

Magnhagen, C. & Staffan, F. (2005) Is boldness affected by group composition in young-of-the-year perch (*Perca fluviatilis*)? *Behavioral Ecology and Sociobiology*, **57**, 295–303.

Mangel, M. & Stamps J. (2001) Trade-offs between growth and mortality and the maintenance of individual variation in growth. *Evolutionary Ecology Research*, **3**, 583–593.

Martin, J. M. & Réale, D. (2008) Temperament, risk assessment and habituation to novelty in eastern chipmunks, Tamias striatus. *Animal Behaviour*, **75**, 309–318.

Maynard Smith, J. (1982) *Evolution and the Theory of Games*. Cambridge: Cambridge University Press.

McElreath, R. & Strimling, P. (2006) How noisy information and individual asymmetries can make 'personality' an adaptation: a simple model. *Animal Behaviour*, **72**, 1135–1139.

Meaney, M. J. (2001) Maternal care, gene expression, and the transmission of individual differences in stress reactivity across generations. *Annual Review of Neuroscience*, **24**, 1161–1192.

Morand-Ferron, J., Lefebvre, L. & Giraldeau, L.-A. (2007) Wild carib grackles play a producer–scrounger game. *Behavioral Ecology*, **18**, 916–921.

Müller, L. & Schrader, R. (2005) Behavioural consistency during social separation and personality in dairy cows. *Behaviour*, **142**, 1289–1306.

Nettle, D. (2005) An evolutionary approach to the extraversion continuum. *Evolution and Human Behaviour*, **26**, 363–373.

Nussey, D. H., Wilson, A. J. & Brommer, J. E. (2007) The evolutionary ecology of individual phenotypic plasticity in wild populations. *Journal of Evolutionary Biology*, **20**, 831–844.

Oliveira, R. F., Taborsky M. & Brockmann, H. J. (2008) *Alternative Reproductive Strategies*. Cambridge: Cambridge University Press.

Pasinelli, G. & Walters, J. R. (2002) Social and environmental factors affect natal dispersal and philopatry of male red-cockaded woodpeckers. *Ecology*, **83**, 2229–2239.

Pasinelli, G., Schiegg, K. & Walters, J. R. (2004) Genetic and environmental influences on natal dispersal distance in a resident bird species. *American Naturalist*, **164**, 660–669.

Penke, L., Dennissen, J. J. A. & Miller, G. F. (2007) The evolutionary genetics of personality. *European Journal of Personality*, **21**, 549–587.

Peripato, A. C. & Cheverud, J. M. (2002) Genetic influence on maternal care. *American Naturalist*, **160**, S173–185.

Pervin, L. A., Cervone, D. & Oliver, P. J. (2005) *Personality: Theory and Research*, 9th edn. Hoboken, NJ: Wiley.

Plaistow, S. J., Johnstone, R. A., Colegrave, N. & Spencer, M. (2004) Evolution of alternative mating tactics: conditional versus mixed strategies. *Behavioral Ecology*, **15**, 534–542.

Quinn, J. L. & Creswell, W. (2005) Personality, anti-predation behaviour and behavioural plasticity in the chaffinch *Fringilla coelebs*. *Behaviour*, **142**, 1377–1402.

Réale, D., Gallant, B. Y., Lelbanc, M. & Festa-Bianchet, M. (2000) Consistency of temperament in bighorn ewes and correlates with behaviour and life history. *Animal Behaviour*, **60**, 589–597.

Réale, D., Reader, S. M., Sol, D., McDougall, P. T. & Dingemanse, N. J. (2007) Integrating animal temperament within ecology and evolution. *Biological Reviews of the Cambridge Philosophical Society*, **82**, 291–318.

Réale, D., Martin, J., Coltman, D. W., Poissant, J. & Festa-Bianchet, M. (2009) Male personality, life-history strategies, and reproductive success in a promiscuous mammal. *Journal of Evolutionary Biology*, **22**, 1599–1607.

Roff, D. A. (1997) *Evolutionary Quantitative Genetics*. New York, NY: Chapman and Hall.

Roff, D. A. & Fairbairn, D. J. (2007) The evolution of trade-offs: where are we? *Journal of Evolutionary Biology*, **20**, 443–447.

Saastamoinen, M. (2008) Heritability of dispersal rate and other life history traits in the Glanville fritillary butterfly. *Heredity*, **100**, 39–46.

Schino, G., Speranza, L. & Troisi, A. (2001) Early maternal rejection and later social anxiety in juvenile and adult Japanese macaques. *Developmental Psychobiology*, **38**, 186–190.

Schlichting, C. D. & Pigliucci, M. (1998) *Phenotypic Plasticity: a Reaction Norm Perspective*. Sunderland, MA: Sinauer Associates.

Sibbald, A. M. & Hooper, R. J. (2004) Sociability and the willingness of individual sheep to move away from their companions in order to graze. *Applied Animal Behaviour Science*, **86**, 51–62.

Sih, A. & Watters, J. (2005) The mix matters: behavioural types and group dynamics in water striders. *Behaviour*, **142**, 1417–1431.

Sih, A., Kats, L. B. & Maurer, E. F. (2003) Behavioural correlation across situations and the evolution of antipredator behaviour in a sunfish–salamander system. *Animal Behaviour*, **65**, 29–44.

Sih, A., Bell, A. M., Johnson, J. C. & Ziemba, R. E. (2004) Behavioral syndromes: an integrative overview. *Quarterly Review of Biology*, **79**, 241–277.

Sinervo, B. & Clobert, J. (2003) Morphs, dispersal behavior, genetic similarity, and the evolution of cooperation. *Science*, **300**, 1949–1951.

Sinervo, B. & Lively, C. M. (1996) The rock–paper–scissors game and the evolution of alternative mating strategies. *Nature*, **380**, 240–243.

Sinn, D. L., Gosling, S. D. & Moltschaniwskyj, N. A. (2008) Development of shy/bold behaviour in squid: context-specific phenotypes associated with developmental plasticity. *Animal Behaviour*, **75**, 433–442.

Stamps, J. A. (2007) Growth–mortality tradeoffs and 'personality traits' in animals. *Ecology Letters*, **10**, 355–363.

Stead, J. D. H., Clinton, S., Neal C. *et al.* (2006) Selective breeding for divergence in novelty-seeking traits: heritability and enrichment in spontaneous anxiety-related behaviors. *Behavior Genetics*, **36**, 697–712.

Strandberg, E. Jacobsson, J. & Saetre P. (2005) Direct genetic, maternal and litter effects on behaviour in German shepherd dogs in Sweden. *Livestock Production Science*, **93**, 33–42.

Trivers, R. L. (1972) Parental investment and sexual selection. In: *Sexual Selection and the Descent of Man, 1871–1971*, ed. B. Campbell. Chicago, IL: Aldine, pp. 136–179.

Trivers, R. L. (1974) Parent–offspring conflict. *American Zoologist*, **14**, 249–264.

van Oers, K., Drent. P. J., De Jong, G., Van Noordwijk, A. J. (2004) Additive and nonadditive genetic variation in avian personality traits. *Heredity*, **93**, 496–503.

van Oers, K., Drent, P. J., Dingemanse, N. J. & Kempenaers, B. (2008) Personality is associated with extrapair paternity in great tits, *Parus major. Animal Behaviour*, **76**, 555–563.

van Tienderen, P. H. (1991) Evolution of generalist and specialists in spatially heterogeneous environments. *Evolution*, **45**, 1317–1331.

Verbeek, M. E. M. (1998) Bold or cautious: behavioural characteristics and dominance in great tits. Unpublished PhD thesis, University of Wageningen.

Verbeek, M. E. M., de Goede, P., Drent, P. J. & Wiepkema, P. R. (1999) Individual behavioural characteristics and dominance in aviary groups of great tits. *Behaviour*, **136**, 23–48.

Ward, A. J. W., Thomas, P., Hart, P. J. B. & Krause, J. (2004) Correlates of boldness in three-spined sticklebacks

(*Gasterosteus acualeatus*). *Behavioral Ecology and Sociobiology*, **55**, 561–568.

Waser, P. M. & Jones, W. T. (1989) Heritability of dispersal in banner-tailed kangaroo rats, *Dipodomys spectabilis*. *Animal Behaviour*, **37**, 987–991.

West-Eberhard, M. J. (2003) *Developmental Plasticity and Evolution*. Oxford: Oxford University Press.

Wheelwright, N. T. & Mauck, R. A. (1998) Philopatry, natal dispersal, and inbreeding avoidance in an island population of Savannah Sparrows. *Ecology*, **79**, 755–767.

Whitlock, M. C. (2001) Dispersal and the genetic properties of metapopulations. In: *Dispersal*, ed. J. Clobert, E. Danchin, A. A. Dhondt & J. D. Nichols. New York, NY: Oxford University Press, pp. 273–298.

Wigger, A., Loerscher, P., Weissenbacher, P. Holsboer, F. & Landgraf, R. (2001) Cross-fostering and cross-breeding of HAB and LAB rats: a genetic rat model of anxiety. *Behaviour Genetics*, **31**, 371–382.

Wilson, A. J., Gélin, U. Perron, M.-C. & Réale, D. (2009) Indirect genetic effects and the evolution of aggression in a vertebrate system. *Proceedings of the Royal Society B*, **276**, 533–541.

Wilson, D. S. & Yoshimura, J. (1994) On the coexistence of specialists and generalists. *American Naturalist*, **144**, 692–707.

Wilson, D. S., Clark, A. B., Coleman, K. & Dearstyne, T. (1994) Shyness and boldness in humans and other animals. *Trends in Ecology and Evolution*, **9**, 442–446.

Wolf, M., van Doorn, G. S., Leimar, O. & Weissing, F. J. (2007) Life-history trade-offs favour the evolution of animal personalities. *Nature*, **447**, 581–584.

Wolf, M., van Doorn, G. S. & Weissing, F. J. (2008) Evolutionary emergence of responsive and unresponsive personalities. *Proceedings of the National Academy of Sciences of the USA*, **105**, 15825–15830.

Behavioural ecology, why do I love thee? Let me count the reasons

Paul W. Sherman

Behavioural ecology is the study of how behaviour is influenced by natural selection in relation to ecological conditions. It is a relatively new field – about 40 years old – to which I have been an enthusiastic contributor for 30 years. During this time behavioural ecology has grown in popularity, empirical richness and theoretical sophistication. Around the world, behavioural ecologists are employed in universities, conservation organisations and government agencies; they have been elected to national academies of sciences, and received prestigious prizes (Crafoord, Cosmos, Kyoto); at least a dozen scientific journals publish articles on behavioural ecology; and the biennial meeting of the International Behavioral Ecology Society regularly draws more than 1000 participants.

Why is behavioural ecology so appealing? For me, a curious naturalist, it is the challenge of asking new questions, the fun of addressing them using the theoretical framework pioneered by Darwin and embellished by Williams, Hamilton, Maynard Smith, Trivers and Dawkins and the empirical approaches pioneered by Tinbergen, Lack and Goodall, as well as the deep satisfaction of cracking an unsolved puzzle – at least occasionally. For example, in my case, why do bank swallows breed colonially, why do Belding's ground squirrels give alarm calls and how do they recognise half-sisters, why do wood ducks lay multiple parasitic eggs,

why do queens of many social insects mate so frequently, why do naked mole-rats live like eusocial insects, and how have bdelloid rotifers survived and speciated without sex for 40 million years?

Attempting to resolve these issues essentially involves 'falling in love' with each study organism and question. For example, in my current study of the social behaviour of Washington ground squirrels (pictured), the first challenges were practical: locating populations in undisturbed habitats, capturing the animals, obtaining DNA samples, and marking them individually for recognition (hair dye) and long-term identification (eartags). Then there was the 'head work' of developing alternative hypotheses about the possible functions of various social and reproductive behaviours and deriving critical predictions from each. Next came the real fun – observing the ground squirrels behave, discovering the uniqueness of their individual personalities, documenting variations in cooperation and competition among animals differing in kinship, age and microhabitat, quantifying the effects of such variations on fitness, and devising and conducting strong inference tests of alternative hypotheses for behavioural differences among individuals. And now there is the warm anticipation of returning each spring, to greet 'old friends' and meet new ones, to study how particular individuals will respond to that season's biotic and

Social Behaviour: Genes, Ecology and Evolution, ed. Tamás Székely, Allen J. Moore and Jan Komdeur. Published by Cambridge University Press. © Cambridge University Press 2010.

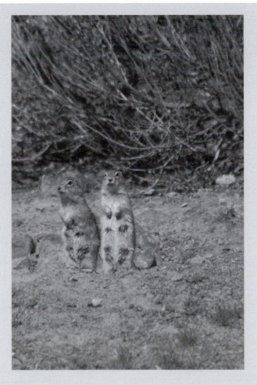

A cooperatively breeding pair of female Washington ground squirrels *Urocitellus washingtoni* (sisters) at the entrance to their shared burrow. Photo: Janet Shellman Sherman.

abiotic challenges (and our experiments), and to use that information to resolve the original questions.

Scientific fields often grow most rapidly at their intersections with other fields. Therefore, one of the most exciting new developments for behavioural ecology is that it has begun to influence and be influenced by multiple, traditionally human-oriented disciplines, including psychology, anthropology, economics, medicine, genetics and conservation biology. There are several reasons for these intersections. First, there is growing acceptance that natural selection is the only evolutionary force that results in adaptation. As a result, the cornerstone principles of behavioural ecology, such as sexual selection, kin selection, honesty and deceit, and the analytical approaches of optimality and game theory, are immediately applicable to human affairs.

Second, there is the growing appreciation that behaviours do not have to be inborn (innate) to be adaptive. Rather, behaviours result from developmental programmes that always are influenced by both genes and environments. Natural selection has favoured the sensory capabilities, brain structures and decision rules ('Darwinian algorithms') that enable individuals to experience relevant aspects of their biotic and abiotic environments and learn what to do – and what not to do – to reproduce successfully. So, although behaviours are genetically influenced, they are not genetically determined. In turn, this means that Darwinism is not incompatible with human free will or with differences in individuals' personalities.

Third, there is a growing consensus – to which I am delighted to have contributed (Sherman 1988) – that questions of the general form 'Why does individual *A* perform behaviour *X*?' can be answered from four different, complementary perspectives, or 'levels of analysis'. Two provide 'proximate' (immediate-cause) explanations and the other two provide 'ultimate' (long-term) explanations, the former focusing on how a behaviour *develops* in an individual (i.e. its ontogeny) and on its underlying *mechanisms* (physiological and cognitive), and the latter focusing on how the behaviour affects individuals' *fitnesses* (reproduction) and on its *history* through evolutionary time. For example, mothers care for their children because: hormones influence maternal behaviours (a physiological mechanism), mothers love their children (a cognitive mechanism), women learn mothering behaviour from their own mothers (an ontogeny), raising children enhances fitness (effect on reproduction), and maternal behaviour is ancient and ubiquitous among mammals (evolutionary history). These are complementary explanations, not alternatives, and complete understanding requires explanations at all levels of analysis. In regard to personalities (see Chapter 16), differences arise due to variations in individuals' ontogenies and physiological and cognitive mechanisms; personality differences are maintained evolutionarily by context-dependent fitness variations in the different biotic (e.g. conspecific density, predator pressure) and abiotic (weather conditions, food availability) microenvironments inhabited by members of each species.

Recently, I have been contributing to the intersection of behavioural ecology and medicine, by using Darwinian principles to understand the occurrence of allergies (Sherman *et al.* 2008), morning sickness (Flaxman & Sherman 2008), lactose intolerance (Bloom & Sherman 2005), cooking with painfully hot spices (Sherman 2007) and senescence (Blanco & Sherman 2005). Whereas medical researchers traditionally investigate the mechanisms underlying annoying symptoms and attempt to design more effective ways to ameliorate them, from a Darwinian perspective the questions are why they occur (their reproductive consequences) and whether it is advisable to work with or against them. These two approaches are complementary, because they are on different levels of analysis.

The promise of Darwinian medicine is that it will lead to better-informed medical practices because, in deciding whether to suppress a symptom, it is useful to know if it is or is not adaptive. For example, we recently showed that allergies can help protect against certain types of cancers (Sherman *et al.* 2008). Thus, allergies may be adaptations rather than immune-system disorders and, if so, the advisability of routinely suppressing them requires reconsideration. A non-adaptive example involves eating habits. Our love of fat evolved in antecedent environments where fat was nutritious in the small quantities that were available. Today the abundance of fat in diets of industrialised countries often leads to overindulgence, resulting in obesity and poor health. Although we are 'evolutionarily trapped' (Schlaepfer *et al.* 2002) in our physiological cravings for fat, recognising why we love something that may be bad for us can help individuals to reduce their fat intake and thereby enhance survival in fat-rich modern environments.

Growing acceptance of the fundamental concepts of behavioural ecology by traditionally anthropocentric fields has opened exciting possibilities for interdisciplinary research and teaching, for funding and job opportunities, and for addressing societal problems. Results of my studies, and those of like-minded colleagues, already have spawned innovative collaborations and resulted in practical applications. At least four new sub-disciplines have recently sprung up – evolutionary psychology, Darwinian anthropology, evolutionary genetics and Darwinian medicine – each with its own textbooks, websites, college courses and coverage in the popular press. Thus behavioural ecology is growing rapidly at its seams, and the field is poised for further increases in scope and importance in the twenty-first century.

I encourage you to consider joining the behavioural ecology 'team', and contributing to the excitement of further developing this field. If you choose to do so, you may find six principles that have guided my research useful in your own:

- *Hypothesis conception requires Darwinism*, because it is the only scientific theory for the evolution and maintenance of adaptation.
- *Hypothesis development requires levels of analysis*, in order to distinguish hypotheses that truly are alternatives (on the same analytical level) from hypotheses that are complementary (on different levels).
- *Hypothesis testing requires strong inference*, because attempting to falsify alternative hypotheses via experimentation and observation is the most efficient way to achieve scientific understanding.
- *Understanding adaptations requires field studies*, because the fit between organisms and their environments must be assessed under the appropriate (normal) circumstances.
- *Field work requires perseverance*, because studies must continue for multiple years to encompass the range of environmental variations experienced by the animals – and, unfortunately, in some field seasons nothing seems to go right.

- *There are no uninteresting organisms*, which will be obvious once you mark individuals, watch them behave, and then apply the first five principles to analyse what they are doing and why they are doing it (its reproductive consequences).

References

Blanco, M. A. & Sherman, P. W. (2005) Maximum longevities of chemically protected and non-protected fishes, reptiles, and amphibians support evolutionary hypotheses of aging. *Mechanisms of Ageing and Development*, **126**, 794–803.

Bloom, G. & Sherman, P. W. (2005) Dairying barriers affect the distribution of lactose malabsorption. *Evolution and Human Behavior*, **26**, 301–312.

Flaxman, S. M. & Sherman, P. W. (2008) Morning sickness: adaptive cause or nonadaptive consequence of embryo viability? *American Naturalist*, **172**, 54–62.

Schlaepfer, M. A., Runge, M. C. & Sherman, P. W. (2002) Ecological and evolutionary traps. *Trends in Ecology and Evolution*, **17**, 474–480.

Sherman, P. W. (1988) The levels of analysis. *Animal Behaviour*, **36**, 616–619.

Sherman, P. W. (2007) Why we cook with spices: preventative Darwinian medicine. Lecture 25 in *Evolution and Medicine*, ed. R. M. Nesse. London: Henry Stewart Talks Ltd (available by subscription at www.hstalks.com/evomed).

Sherman, P. W., Holland, E. & Shellman Sherman, J. S. (2008) Allergies: their role in cancer prevention. *Quarterly Review of Biology*, **83**, 339–362.

17

Molecular and genetic influences on the neural substrate of social cognition in humans

Louise Gallagher and David Skuse

Overview

Human social behaviour is wonderfully complex, and influenced by manifold effects including genetic, environmental and cultural factors (Chapter 15). Here we focus on one aspect of human social behaviour: social cognition. Human social cognition, or the ability to process social information thus influencing human social behaviour, is a broad and complex concept, as yet not defined unambiguously. The aim of this chapter is to introduce the basic neural processes underlying human social cognition, and the genetic and molecular influences that may shape behavioural variation between individuals. To this end, we describe the neural circuits in the brain underlying social cognition, particularly with reference to self-knowledge and the concept of theory of mind – the ability to think about things from the perspective of another. Cellular aspects of social cognition, although still unclear, are explored in relation to the putative role of mirror neurons. The neurobiology of attachment underlying social relationships aids the discussion of the molecular underpinnings of social cognition with particular reference to neuropeptides: oxytocin and vasopressin. Oxytocin and vasopressin are nonapeptides that have been increasingly identified as playing a pivotal role in social cognition. Animal studies have highlighted the role of these peptides in social roles as diverse as parenting behaviour, social recognition and affiliative behaviours (Chapter 11). Here we discuss the evidence implicating these neuropeptides in humans. Moreover, it is increasingly recognised in animal studies that the processes of social cognition are supported by reward circuitry, underpinned by the dopaminergic neurotransmitter system in the brain. Reward processes appear to reinforce bonds, both parental and for mating purposes, and possibly also the rewarding aspects of human social interactions, trust and altruism. Also significant are the potential effects of mood and anxiety, mediated through the serotonergic system. Although the plasticity of human brain is well established, our understanding of how heritable and environmental influences might influence social cognition in humans is at an early stage. We discuss how genetic variation is increasingly implicated, and postulate mechanisms that may underlie gene–environment interactions.

Social Behaviour: Genes, Ecology and Evolution, ed. Tamás Székely, Allen J. Moore and Jan Komdeur. Published by Cambridge University Press. © Cambridge University Press 2010.

17.1 Introduction

Humans possess the ability to process huge quantities of social information, and interact in complex ways with others. Social cognition comprises a set of skills that enable us to understand the thoughts and intentions of others. These enable us to take another person's perspective, to develop self-knowledge, to predict another's behaviour accurately from our social perceptions, and to understand what motivates other people in their social interactions, even if these do not directly involve us. These skills map onto schemas that are encoded in an associative network in memory orchestrated to ensure normal, skilled social adaptation (Frith & Frith 2007).

The process by which we acquire social cognitive competence evolves with development and is modified in response to the environment. To begin with, infants cannot easily differentiate between themselves and other people, but they rapidly become aware that their actions have an impact on the physical and social world around them. In due course, they develop social understanding, language and imitation. Recent research suggests these skills may be learned in part by means of a mirror neural system that enables us to map our own actions onto our perceptions of other people's actions. Of course, to be able to do this successfully, we need to have an associated control system that allows for the differentiation between what we perceive in others and our own behaviour (Keysers & Perrett 2004).

A fully functioning social brain entails the development of a coordinated network of human cortical brain regions, the original components of which

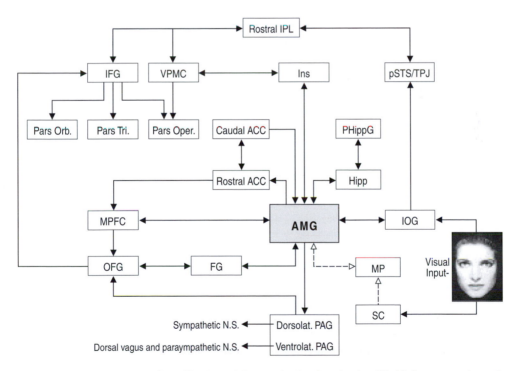

Figure 17.1 Neural interconnectivity of social brain. Facial processing involves the visual limbic face-responsive pathway to the fusiform gyrus (FG) and the visual prefrontal face-responsive pathway to the orbitofrontal cortex (OFC) (Fairhall & Ishai 2007). Damage to the OFC impairs face and voice expression recognition (Rolls 2007). Face-responsive neurons in the OFC (Rolls *et al.* 2006) link to mesolimbic reward circuits (Fig. 17.2) which contribute to social reinforcement (Young & Wang 2004). This system offers the potential for modulating social behaviour, as in the rewarding impact on a child's behaviour of a parent's expressed pleasure. From Skuse & Gallagher (2009). For abbreviations, see Table 17.1.

were outlined by Brothers *et al.* (1990). Illustrated in Figure 17.1, these include the amygdala, orbito-frontal cortex and parts of the temporal cortex (the temporoparietal junction, posterior superior temporal sulcus and the temporal poles). Recent research has added regions comprising the medial prefrontal cortex, the adjacent paracingulate cortex and the

mirror system (Rizzolatti & Craighero 2004; Box 17.1). Genetic, molecular and hormonal factors all impact on this network, influencing behavioural functions. The concepts underlying these influences have been discussed in Chapters 1, 2 and 3. Here we investigate genetic and neuropeptidergic mechanisms that influence the functioning of the social brain.

Box 17.1 Mirror neurons and their roles in humans

The discovery of mirror neurons is considered one of the most exciting and important findings in the field of neuroscience in recent times. They were described first by Rizzolati and colleagues, who observed that some neurons in the inferior frontal lobe and inferior parietal lobule (IPL) in monkeys had a similar reaction both when an action was conducted and when it was observed. Subsequently, Keysers and colleagues demonstrated that a mirror-neuron system in humans and monkeys fired in response to the sound of an action.

In humans the IPL and part of the frontal lobe (ventral premotor cortex and the posterior part of the inferior frontal gyrus, IFG) have been demonstrated on functional neuroimaging to be activated when performing or observing an action (Rizzolatti & Craighero 2004). These regions are proposed to be a mirror-neuron system in humans (Iacoboni *et al.* 1999). This system is implicated in monitoring other people's actions and emotions during social interactions (Iacoboni & Dapretto 2006, Gallese *et al.* 2007). The mechanism through which this occurs appears to be the mapping of the visual description of an action onto the corresponding motor cortex.

The anterior and posterior mirror systems may underpin different aspects of social cognition such as understanding others' action and intention, and social communication (Gallese *et al.* 2007). For example, witnessing others being touched activates our secondary somatosensory cortex 'as if' we had ourselves been touched (Keysers *et al.* 2004). Other people's facial expressions can evoke in us similar feelings; for example, the insula plays a critical role in our empathic response to seeing another person pull a disgusted facial expression (Jabbi *et al.* 2007). Our ability accurately to interpret facial expressions involves the observation and interpretation of movement. The motor aspects of expressions are processed in the posterior superior temporal sulcus (pSTS) and the temporoparietal junction (TPJ). These regions are specialised for detecting biological motion (Thompson *et al.* 2005) and could be associated with mirror neurons both posteriorly in the inferior parietal lobule (IPL) (Iacoboni & Dapretto 2006) and in the anterior ventral premotor cortex (VPMC). The VPMC is closely linked to the pars opercularis (Pars Oper.) of the inferior frontal gyrus (IFG), and both are concerned with emotion recognition along with the pars triangularis (Pars Tri.) and the pars orbitalis (Pars Orb.) (Fig. 17.1). It appears that the response of empathy, mediated by connections between the insula (Ins) and amygdala (AMG), may require concurrent activation of the mirror-neuron system (Singer 2007).

17.2 Neural circuits of the social brain

The neural interconnectivity of the social cognition is outlined schematically in Figure 17.1, and the location and function of the constituent parts are given in Table 17.1. The relationship of circuitry is decribed to social cognitive constructs such as theory of mind (section 17.2.1), and social behaviour in the form of attachment (section 17.2.2).

The amygdalae play a central role, and interact with specialised neural mechanisms responsible for processing social perceptions (Adolphs & Spezio 2006). Social information is presented mainly in the visual domain in primates (Insel & Fernald 2004). Key among these perceptions is the ability to interpret and recall information from faces, which is processed in parallel pathways. High-resolution visual information undergoes initial processing in the inferior occipital gyrus (IOG). There is a parallel pathway which runs through the superior colliculus (SC) and the medial pulvinar nucleus of the thalamus (MP). This rapidly processes degraded input (a very low-resolution representation) before it reaches the amygdala, and seems to be specialised for detecting faces making direct eye contact (Skuse 2006). Via a feedback loop, faces of particular interest are thereby highlighted: the amygdala alerts the IOG to focus attention upon salient details in order to ascertain rapidly whether someone is making eye contact with us, and whether that is a potential threat. Evidence from animal studies suggests that connectivity between amygdala and hippocampal/perihippocampal centres (Hipp/PHippG) is involved in contextual ascertainment of the arousing stimulus (Malin & McGaugh 2006). Direct eye-to-eye contact is not always threatening, of course, but it is arousing: it facilitates social bonding, and may lead to sexual encounters in the appropriate circumstances.

17.2.1 Self-knowledge and theory of mind

The concepts of self-knowledge and theory of mind neatly illustrate the complexity of human social cognition in terms of the underlying neural circuitry. Integration of information about actions and outcomes, including self-knowledge, person knowledge and mentalising (the ability to put oneself in the mind of another), occurs in the anterior region of the rostral medial prefrontal cortex, which some have termed a theory-of-mind area (Amodio & Frith 2006). The medial prefrontal cortex (MPFC), the temporoparietal junction (TPJ) and the temporal poles are activated when we think about other people's mental states (Amodio & Frith 2006). This aids our ability to interpret false beliefs, to avoid deception and to follow the course of real-time social interactions. We also activate these circuits when we judge people's dispositions and attitudes to us or others, and when we make moral judgements about other people's behaviour.

17.2.2 Neurobiology of attachment

The modulation and inhibition of defensive behaviour occurs via connections from the amygdala to the periaqueductal grey matter (PAG) and thence to the autonomic nervous system. Activation of the ventrolateral PAG is associated with a passive response, including immobility and cardiac slowing. Porges (2007) and Zeki (2007) proposed that mutual inhibition of socially adaptive defensive behaviours makes mother–infant attachment possible. The PAG contains a high density of both oxytocin and vasopressin receptors, which facilitate maternal behaviour and pair bonding. Caring for offspring stimulates the orbitofrontal cortex (OFC), which responds to sensations that are perceived as pleasurable. Taken together, these characteristics strongly suggest that social bonding is facilitated by interactions between dopaminergic reward systems that project to the OFC and the neuropeptides oxytocin and vasopressin (see also Chapter 11).

The amygdala is central to the neural circuitry underlying social cognition. It plays a key role in systems that associate social stimuli (auditory, visual, olfactory) with value (Dolan 2007), it directs our unconscious responses during social encounters (Frith & Frith 2007), and it arouses us to potential threats from our environment. The amygdala's reciprocal connections with the primary visual processing area in the inferior occipital gyrus facilitates the rapid analysis of socially salient information.

Table 17.1. Constituents of neural pathway, as shown in Figure 17.1, and associated functions

Abbreviation	Full name	Location	Function
AMG	Amygdala	Group of neurons in medial temporal lobes	Emotion processing/memory
Caudal ACC	Caudal part of anterior cingulate cortex	Anterior part of cortical region surrounding the central corpus callosum	Cognitive functions associated with reward, decision making, empathy and emotion. Autonomic effects: regulation of heart rate and blood pressure
Dorsal vagus	Dorsal vagal complex	Motor nucleus located in the floor of the fourth ventricle	Gives rise to parasympathetic fibres of the vagal nerve
Parasympathetic N.S.	Parasympathetic nervous system	Division of autonomic nervous system, peripheral nervous system	Regulation of innervation of visceral organs
Dorsolat. PAG	Dorsolateral periaqueductal grey matter	Midbrain grey matter surrounding cerebral aqueduct	Modulation response to pain, defensive behaviour and reproductive behaviour
FG	Frontal gyrus	Cortical regions located in the frontal lobes of the brain, consisting of inferior, middle and superior gyri	Broadly implicated in emotions and personality
Hipp	Hippocampus	Medial temporal brain	Forms part of the limbic system and is involved in short-term memory and spatial navigation
IFG	Inferior frontal gyrus	Inferior part of frontal lobe, subdivided into Pars opercularis, Pars triangularis and Pars orbitalis	See Pars Oper. and Pars Tri.
IOG	Inferior occipital gyrus	Located on the lower lateral part of the occipital lobe	Receives visual information for initial processing
Ins	Insula	Within the lateral sulcus between the temporal lobe and the inferior parietal cortex	Considered part of the limbic cortex. Involved in body representation and subjective emotional experience. Potentially involved in mapping visceral states associated with emotional experience
MPFC	Medial prefrontal cortex	Prefrontal cortex is the anterior part of the frontal lobes, of which the MPFC is a constituent part	Involved in planning complex cognitive behaviours, personality and moderating social behaviour. The term *executive function* refers to processes that influence abstract thinking, cognitive flexibility and planning
MP	Medial pulvinar nucleus of the thalamus	One of the thalamic nuclei. The thalamus is located in the diencephalon, which is located between the brainstem and cerebrum	The functions of the thalamus are complex. The MP has rich connections with the cingulate cortex, prefrontal cortex and posterior parietal cortex

OFC	Orbitofrontal cortex	Located in the frontal cortex above the eyes	Involved in cognitive processes such as decision making
Pars Oper.	Pars opercularis	Part of the inferior frontal gyrus	Together with pars triangularis forms Broca's area, involved in language production and processing. Reduced activity reported in children with autism when viewing emotional faces
Pars Orb.	Pars orbitalis	Part of inferior frontal gyrus	
Pars Tri.	Pars triangularis	Part of inferior frontal gyrus.	Together with pars opercularis forms Broca's area, that part of the brain involved in language production and processing. Implicated in semantic processing of language and in processing of reading written words, particularly where the sounds deviate from the written form
PHippG	Parahippocampal gyrus	Grey-matter cortical region surrounding the hippocampus	Memory encoding and retrieval
pSTS	Posterior superior temporal sulcus	One of the boundaries of the superior temporal gyrus	Implicated in the detection of biological motion between two objects. Suggestion that increased activation on fMRI is associated with increased traits of altruism
TPJ	Temporoparietal junction	Point where temporal and parietal lobes meet	Implicated in processes underlying self-awareness and theory of mind
Rostral ACC	Rostral part of anterior cingulate cortex	Anterior cingulate cortex	Executive function
Rostral IPL	Rostral inferior parietal lobule	Inferior part of parietal lobe	Functionally heterogenous. Target for SC, hippocampus and cerebellum. Involved in aspects of sensory processing and sensorimotor integration
SC	Superior colliculus	Situated below the thalamus in the midbrain	Receives visual, auditory and somatosensory inputs. Involved in rapid processing of visual input
Sympathetic N.S.	Sympathetic nervous system	Part of the peripheral nervous system	Visceral homeostasis in the body. Mediates fight-or-flight phenomenon
Ventrolat PAG	Ventrolateral periaqueductal grey matter	Midbrain grey matter located around the cerebral aqueduct in the midbrain	Role in descending modulation of pain and defensive behaviour
VPMC	Ventral premotor cortex	Area of motor cortex in frontal lobe. Contains mirror neurons	Implicated in sensory guidance of movement and the control of proximal and trunk muscles

Neural circuits of the social brain activated by facial emotions, tone of voice or olfactory cues include the hippocampus, and are therefore linked to recognition memory. This mechanism allows us to contextualise our perceptions and hence find answers to questions such as Do I know this person? Do I like them? Do I trust them?

The biological basis of social cognition is based upon interactions between functionally relevant anatomic areas and neurochemical pathways. Here we review aspects of the molecular basis of social cognition and the putative influence of genetic variation on social cognition in humans.

17.3 The molecular basis of social cognition: role of oxytocin and vasopressin

Oxytocin (OT) and vasopressin (AVP) are nonapeptides with both central and peripheral actions that have been implicated in the molecular basis of social cognition in animal studies, and increasingly a role for these in human social cognition has been suggested. The OT and AVP proteins differ in structure by just two amino acids. The genes encoding the two proteins occur on chromosome 20, and are thought to have arisen from a gene duplication event; the ancestral gene is estimated to be about 500 million years old (Gimpl & Fahrenholz 2001). The presence of nonapeptides similar to oxytocin and vasopressin across diverse species, and their relative similarity, suggests they have been conserved during evolution.

Both have widespread receptor-mediated effects on behaviour and physiology (Landgraf & Neumann 2004). Oestrogens modulate both the synthesis of and receptors for oxytocin, while androgens act similarly on vasopressin (although some species-specific differences exist), and therefore these neuropeptides have an effect upon sexually dimorphic social behaviours (Ferris 2005).

17.3.1 Oxytocin

Oxytocin (OT) is produced in the magnocellular neurosecretory cells located in the supraoptic and paraventricular nuclei of the hypothalamus and in the parvocellular neurons of the paraventricular nuclei. Projections from the former link to the posterior pituitary, from where oxytocin is released into the general circulation. From the latter there are centrally acting projections to limbic-system (hippocampus, amygdala, striatum, hypothalamus, nucleus accumbens) and mid- and hind-brain nuclei (Campbell 2008). Peripheral oxytocin does not cross the blood–brain barrier easily, although it is observed in human cerebrospinal fluid (CSF) just minutes after intranasal administration (Born *et al.* 2002). Peripherally oxytocin acts as a hormone, while centrally it acts as a neuromodulator via a G-protein-coupled receptor (Box 17.2). Only a single type of oxytocin receptor (OTR) has been identified. It can be found in many different tissues in the body, but its distribution is highly variable, both within and between species (Lim & Young 2006).

Box 17.2 Essential terminology

G-protein-coupled receptor – A molecule bound to the inside surface of the cell membrane which acts as a second-messenger protein. It acts to increase or decrease the levels of cyclic AMP, a second messenger within the cell. G-proteins may thus be excitatory or inhibitory.

Cyclic AMP (cAMP) – A second messenger involved in intracellular signal transduction. Binds to protein kinase regulatory units to activate protein kinase.

Protein kinase A – Family of enzymes involved in cell metabolism. Activity dependent on cyclic AMP. Involved in activation of reward system in the nucleus accumbens.

> **Epigenetic mechanisms** – Changes in gene expression caused by factors other than the DNA sequence (see Chapters 1 and 2). Changes persist within the cell and during cell division which can result in the change being transmitted to offspring. Explains how environmental influence might cause changes in an organism which are then transmitted in a heritable manner.
>
> **CpG islands** – Genomic regions containing high numbers of CG repeats. Often located in the promotors of genes. If unmethylated, the gene is expressed, but methylation of the CpG island leads to inhibition of gene expression. They are relatively rare, and are likely to occur in the promotors of genes where there is selective pressure to enable regulation of specific genes.

The potential for environmental influences on the functioning of oxytocin and related proteins exists. CpG islands (Box 17.2) upstream of the transcription start site of the oxytocin receptor gene (*OXTR*) suggest it may be susceptible to epigenetic regulation (Box 17.2) through methylation (see Chapter 1); this modification appears to influence the pattern of tissue expression (Carter 2007). By this, or other means, lifelong expression differences may be influenced by experience, such as the quality of early maternal care (Meaney & Szyf 2005).

Synthesis of oxytocin and transcription of the OTR are influenced by exposure to oestrogen (Carter 2007). Oestrogen acts through its receptors ERα and ERβ; ERβ is expressed in the hypothalamic neurons that synthesise oxytocin, whereas ERα is required for synthesis of OTRs in the amygdala (Broad *et al.* 2006). Oxytocin influences maternal behaviour and pair-bond formation, mainly in females (Chapter 11), and can also facilitate social recognition, including the perception of social threat. It also modulates social motivation and sexual behaviour. Here we focus on maternal behaviour, pair bonding, social recognition and response to threat.

Maternal behaviour and pair bonding

In mammals, females typically form strong bonds with their infants, and their female–female relationships are also affiliative, especially among matrilineal kin who assist with child care (Keverne & Curley 2004). The underlying molecular biology of this process has been studied largely in rodent models.

During pregnancy, oxytocin receptors and dopamine D2 receptors are synthesised in the nucleus accumbens of the mother (Fig. 17.2), and there is a surge of oxytocin release at parturition (Liu & Wang 2003). The involvement of dopaminergic reward pathways suggests that oxytocin and dopamine receptors may interact to facilitate recognition of, and bonding to, the offspring. As discussed in Chapter 11, similar pathways could play a role in the formation of selective partner bonds in adulthood, as found in the monogamous female prairie vole *Microtus ochrogaster*, where the key stimuli comprise a pulsatile release of oxytocin associated with olfactory signals from the male (Williams *et al.* 1992). As yet there is no confirmation that similar processes exist in monogamous primates, where the development of social ties is more complex, and the perceptual cues from a potential partner comprise a set of sensory stumuli that are not primarily olfactory.

Oxytocin, social recognition and the response to threat

Complex social behaviours are critically dependent upon the normal functioning of the amygdala and, as discussed, the amygdala plays a central role in threat detection (Adolphs 2003, Porges 2007). Amygdala activation in response to a potential threat is mediated via excitatory pathways that connect the central amygdala nucleus to the midbrain, and thence to the autonomic nervous system (Kirsch *et al.* 2005) (Fig. 17.1). Excessive amygdala activation during social encounters raises anxiety, leading to social withdrawal (Stein

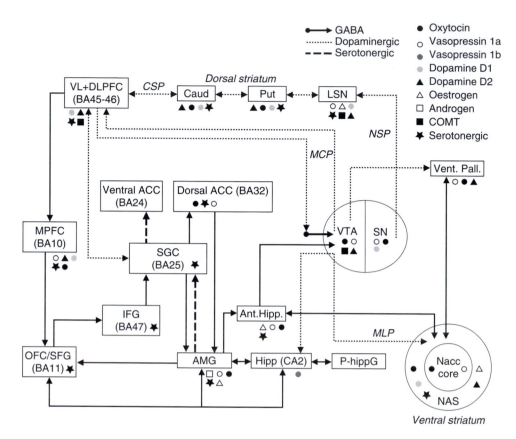

Figure 17.2 Neural circuits underlying social brain and associated neurotransmitter systems. From Skuse and Gallagher (2009). ACC, anterior cingulate cortex; AMG, amygdala; Ant. Hyp. anterior hypothalamus; BA, Brodmann area; Caud., caudate; CSP, corticostriatal pathway; Hipp. hippocampus; IFG, inferior frontal gyrus; LSN, lateral septal nucleus; MCP, mesocortical pathway; MLP, mesolimbic pathway; MPFC, mesial prefrontal cortex; Nacc core, nucleus accumbens core; NAS, nucleus accumbens shell; NSP, nigrostriatal pathway; OFC/SFG, orbitofrontal cortex/superior frontal gyrus; P-hippG, parahippocampal gyrus; Put., putamen; SGC, subgenual cortex; SN, substantia nigra; Vent. Pall., ventral pallidum; VL + DLPFC, ventrolateral and dorsolateral prefrontal cortex; VTA, ventral tegmental area.

et al. 2002). In humans, such activation is potently increased by direct eye contact (Whalen *et al.* 2004; Adolphs *et al.* 2005). Oxytocin adminstration in normal individuals decreases amygdala activation to context-dependent social threats (Kirsch *et al.* 2005), including eye contact (Guastella *et al.* 2008). Oxytocin therefore serves to reduce social fear and anxiety (Heinrichs *et al.* 2003) by changing the relative balance of parasympathetic to sympathetic nervous system (calming versus arousing) activity mediated by pathways that lead from the central

amygdala nucleus to the periaqueductal grey matter, the reticular formation and the nucleus accumbens (Huber *et al.* 2005) (Fig. 17.1). Oxytocin administration in humans potentiates interpersonal trust (Kirsch *et al.* 2005, Kosfeld *et al.* 2005). Baumgartner and colleagues demonstrated this through a study involving an economic game of trust, administration of oxytocin by inhalation and functional neuroimaging (Baumgartner *et al.* 2008). A control group who received placebo rather than oxytocin were found to have diminished trusting behaviour compared with the oxytocin group. The oxytocin group had reduced activation of the amygdala, midbrain regions and the dorsal striatum. It appeared that the oxytocin group had less difficulty overcoming concern about betrayal (betrayal aversion). The authors proposed that it was specifically the reduced activation in the amygdala and brainstem effector sites that enhanced the ability to trust.

Oxytocin and animal models

Reports on the functions of oxytocin in human social behaviour are consistent with reports from animal models. These show enhanced negative reactivity to social encounters associated with knockout of both oxytocin and its receptor (Ferguson *et al.* 2000, Takayanagi *et al.* 2005). In contrast, the exogenous administration of oxytocin reduces social anxiety in both sexes, and negative responses in knockouts are ameliorated by oxytocin infusion (Lim *et al.* 2005). In both sexes, oxytocin knockout mice have seriously impaired recognition memory for conspecifics (Ferguson *et al.* 2000, 2001), but their recognition ability can be rescued by infusing oxytocin into the medial amygdala. Recognition memory appears to be modulated by oestrogen receptor (α and β) expression, pointing to potential sexual dimorphism in the substrates of (olfactory) social recognition (Choleris *et al.* 2003).

Oxytocin and autism

Human disorder occasionally has the potential to inform us about mechanisms underlying human behaviour. Autism is a behavioural disorder with an onset in childhood associated with impairments in communication and social interaction, and with restricted and repetitive behaviour patterns. Children with autism may vary in terms of cognitive ability: some are quite profoundly learning disabled while others have normal intellectual ability. However, social deficits are observed in children with autism regardless of the level of intellectual functioning.

Given the role for oxytocin in social behaviour, abnormalities in oxytocin regulation have been hypothesised to contribute to susceptibility to autism,

and a number of lines of evidence have leant support to this hypothesis. Plasma oxytocin levels have been found to be reduced in some individuals with autism (Modahl *et al.* 1998). A further study of adult males with autism reported that oxytocin, compared with placebo, improved their comprehension of another person's vocal emotional tone (Hollander *et al.* 2007). Autism affects four times as many males as females, and higher levels of testosterone have been hypothesised as contributing to male vulnerability to the disorder (Baron-Cohen 2002). Oestrogen affects the synthesis of oxytocin (Nomura 2002) and enhances activity of the oxytocin receptor (OTR) (Gimpl & Fahrenholz 2001); thus higher levels of oxytocin (particularly in females) might be protective within the neural circuitry of social cognition. Hypothetically, the gender imbalance observed in autism could be mediated through the influence of sex steroids, oestrogen and testosterone, on oxytocin and vasopressin activity (by synthesis or receptor sensitivity).

Other mechanisms influencing oxytocin release

A potential role for immune-mediated regulation of oxytocin release has been suggested by recent investigations of a mouse knockout of the *CD38* gene (*CD38*-/-), encoding a glycoprotein implicated in humoral immune responses (Jin *et al.* 2007). The *CD38*-/- mouse demonstrates reduced social recognition and poorer maternal nurturing behaviour than the wild type, and this impairment is associated with reduced plasma oxytocin. These deficits were ameliorated by both oxytocin infusion and lentiviral vector-mediated delivery of *CD38* to the hypothalamus. Further investigations by the authors revealed that *CD38* seems to facilitate oxytocin release. The findings established a role for *CD38* in neuropeptide release. They implied it could play a role in the regulation of maternal and social behaviours, and indicated a potential immune-mediated influence on oxytocin release.

17.3.2 Vasopressin

Vasopressin (AVP) synthesis occurs in the hypothalamus, but it is released into general circulation from the pituitary. Vasopressin acts as a hormone regulating water balance in the periphery, but it has neuropeptidergic actions in the central nervous system (CNS). Androgen-dependent synthesis occurs in parvocellular neurons within the paraventricular nuclei, the bed nucleus of the stria terminalis, the medial amygdala and suprachiasmatic nucleus (De Vries & Panzica 2006, Bales *et al.* 2007). Vasopressin expression is modulated by as yet unidentified genes on the X- or Y-chromosomes (Gatewood *et al.* 2006). Three distinct vasopressin receptor subtypes have been described. The V1aR receptor is expressed widely in the brain, as well as in the liver, kidney and peripheral vasculature. The V1bR receptor is expressed in the brain and also peripherally (kidney, thymus, heart, lung, spleen, uterus and breast). The AVPR2 receptor is expressed primarily in the kidneys.

Behavioural effects of vasopressin have been described in males. They include the promotion of both aggression and affiliation, as well as other aspects of social interaction including parental care (Chapter 11). Vasopressin enhances social recognition, non-spatial learning and memory, and the emotional response to stress (Caldwell *et al.* 2008). Here we focus on aggression and affiliative behaviour and social recognition as it is more pertinent to the discussion of social cognition.

Aggression and affiliative behaviour

Activation of the V1aR vasopressin receptor increases male anxiety and facilitates aggression in animal models (Storm & Tecott 2005). The degree of behavioural response depends upon early social experience. Aggressive behaviour in females is not normally observed in response to vasopressin. The behavioural differences in response to vasopressin in males and females are thought to be consequential to a neonatal surge in oxytocin, which has sexually dimorphic effects on the later expression of vasopressin receptors (Bales *et al.* 2007). There is cross-receptor reactivity between oxytocin and vasopressin in early life. The oxytocin surge leads to increased vasopressin receptor binding in the ventral pallidum, the lateral septum and cingulate cortex in males. In contrast,

in females it leads to reduced vasopressin receptor binding in the equivalent sites. Thus some sexually dimorphic behaviours in adult males could reflect the synergistic interaction between vasopressin receptor sensitivity to androgens, and to vasopressin, as a consequence of neonatal oxytocin exposure. On the other hand, males with a higher density of V1aR receptors in the lateral septum (Figs. 17.1, 17.2) are more likely to provide paternal behaviour, and the same receptors also play a role in stimulating maternal care (Caldwell *et al.* 2008). The administration of vasopressin intranasally to normal males increases the subjective impression of threat to neutral social stimuli (Thompson *et al.* 2006) and, by implication, the risk of an aggressive response. Females are less vulnerable to manipulation of vasopressin receptors in the lateral septum (Bielsky *et al.* 2005).

Social recognition

Animal knockouts of *Avpr1a* are associated with impairment of social memory, reduced anxiety-like behaviour and selective social amnesia in male knockouts. Consequences can be corrected by re-expressing the gene (Bielsky *et al.* 2004). Overexpression of the *Avpr1a* gene in the lateral septum of males facilitates social memory formation and hence social recognition. The effect of vasopressin on social memory appears to be specific to the lateral septum (Bielsky *et al.* 2005), where there is the highest density of V1aR binding in the human and animal brain (Loup *et al.* 1991).

Vasopressin–dopaminergic interactions

Vasopressin facilitates affiliation and social attachment by modulating neural processes underlying reward and motivation. The process involves dopamine in the nucleus accumbens, which plays a major role in the regulation of pair-bond formation (Hammock & Young 2006). Oxytocin and vasopressin also shape the neural representation of the partner by building a profile through olfactory cues, which remains stable (Zeki 2007). For rodents, at least, the odour of the partner comes to be associated with a pleasurable and rewarding encounter. Bonding based on sensory stimuli also works in the visual domain, as has been shown in sheep (Broad *et al.* 2006). Zeki (2007) suggests that human adaptations of the same essential mechanisms underlie romantic and maternal love. Falling in love requires us not only to activate neural circuits that facilitate attachment but also to deactivate defensive circuits: physical proximity to strangers would normally trigger aversive reactions.

17.4 Serotonergic influences on social cognition

Social cognition is not solely the function of innate influences such as personality (Chapter 16); the influences of current state, e.g. mood and level of anxiety, have also been shown to impact on social cognitive functions. Mood and anxiety states are susceptible to changes in the brain's serotonergic system. The serotonergic system is the largest efferent system in the brain. It has wide-ranging functions, from behavioural inhibition, appetite, aggression, mood, social affiliation and sleep to sensory gating (Azmitia 1999). In the limbic brain, serotonergic innervation modulates emotional expression, and a direct influence of serotonin on social cognition, independent of mood and anxiety, is increasingly apparent. For example, in depressed individuals medications increasing the bioavailability of serotonin in the brain (selective serotonin reuptake inhibitors, SSRIs) are associated with improvement in social behaviour independent of their effects on mood or other core symptoms of depression. In primate studies, experimentally elevated serotonin has been shown to decrease aggression and increase cooperativeness and social potency. Contrastingly, reduction in serotonin leads to aggression and deterioration of cooperativeness (Carver & Miller 2006). Hence there is a suggestion from studies in both animals and humans that increased serotonin activity positively influences social interaction and cooperation, while decreases in serotonin activity appear to have the opposite effect.

Evidence from neuropsychological studies has shown that serotonergic activity influences emotional facial processing, and treatment with SSRIs (infusion of citalopram) improves the ability of formerly depressed people to detect happiness and fear (Harmer *et al.* 2003). In contrast, there was decreased recognition of fearful, disgusted and surprised facial expressions in normal volunteers following seven days' administration of citalopram (Harmer *et al.* 2004). There is a suggestion from these findings that an optimal level of serotonergic activity is required for normal social recognition, while abnormally low levels are associated with increased sensitivity to negative emotional expressions and elevated levels decrease sensitivity to negative expressions.

Until recently, the effects of serotonin on social cognition have been attributed to changes in mood. However, as discussed above, recent studies have shown that direct effects on cognition might occur independently of mood. Brain neuroimaging studies have detected differential activation and structure in regions implicated in social cognition in association with genetic variation in the serotonin transporter protein (Canli & Lesch 2007; see section 17.6.3).

17.4.1 Serotonergic interaction with vasopressin and oxytocin

If serotonin influences human social cognition directly, then it might be hypothesised that there is an interaction with the neuropeptides oxytocin and vasopressin. Indeed, an association exists between these neuropeptides and the serotonergic system through the hypothalamic–pituitary–adrenal (HPA) axis. Functions of the paraventricular nucleus of the hypothalamus are regulated by serotonin, and serotonin receptor subtypes influence release of oxytocin and vasopressin (Ho *et al.* 2007). The effects of elevated levels of serotonin on oxytocin and vasopressin have been demonstrated in animal models of elevated serotonin levels during development (developmental hyperserotonaemia). Animals exposed to elevated serotonin have reduced oxytocin expression, and loss of oxytocin-containing cells in the paraventricular nucleus associated with reduced maternal bonding and socially explorative behaviours (McNamara *et al.* 2008). How this fits with the evidence discussed in the preceding section is not clear, but the link is perhaps related to the hypothesis that there is an optimal level of serotonergic functioning. Thus during development excess serotonin may be as detrimental as too little, although the molecular basis of this remains to be elucidated.

Interactions between the serotonergic and vasopressin systems are not well understood (Caldwell *et al.* 2008). Serotonin desensitises the vasopressin receptor, which could reduce affiliative behaviour in adult males (Veenema *et al.* 2006). V1aR and 5-HT1B receptors (a subtype of serotonin receptor) have been shown to co-localise in the anterior hypothalamus, indicating putative serotonergic synapses on vasopressin neurons and therefore the potential for serotonin to influence behavioural aggression mediated by vasopressin (Ferris 2005).

17.4.2 Serotonin and reward

Effects of serotonin on reward circuitry have been observed in animal studies. Given the relationships between reward circuitry, social cognition and behaviour, it is plausible that serotonin may influence both reward and social cognition through the same brain circuitry. Systemic serotonergic depletion in rats results in a preference for small more immediate rewards, although it is possible that this observation may be related to reduced impulse control (Denk *et al.* 2005). Rhesus monkeys *Macaca mulatta* possessing a variant in the promoter of the serotonin transporter gene associated with reduced transcription (and consequently reduced serotonergic functioning) were found to be impaired on tasks involving reward contingencies. In particular, they failed to inhibit responses to an existing stimulus when presented with the opportunity to explore a new stimulus (Izquierdo *et al.* 2007). Here again, it might also be hypothesised that impulse control is the greater influencing factor.

Human reward circuitry is influenced by activity of the serotonergic system, also apparently as a result of impulse control. Decreases in serotonin are associated with impulsive choices (i.e. the choice of a smaller sooner reinforcer over a larger later one) (Wogar

et al. 1993, Bizot *et al.* 1999, Mobini *et al.* 2000), and increases are associated with decreased impulsive choices (Poulos *et al.* 1996, Bizot *et al.* 1999), although the literature on this is not consistent (reviewed by Cardinal 2006). As highlighted here, the influence of serotonin on the reward system appears complex. Subgroups of regions within corticobasal ganglia networks seem to be recruited for reward prediction at different times (Tanaka *et al.* 2004), and these subregions appear to be differentially regulated by serotonergic pathways both temporally (Doya 2002) and in relation to the bioavailability of serotonin (Tanaka *et al.* 2007). Thus we can conclude that the relationships between serotonin and reward are influenced by changes in impulse control. However, there seems to be little evidence suggesting a broader influence of serotonin on social cognition mediated through reward circuitry.

17.5 The dopaminergic system and social cognition

A clearer picture is emerging of the role of another major neurotransmitter system, the dopaminergic system, in social cognition. Dopamine is an important neurotransmitter in the brain, and dopaminergic neurons are located in a number of brain regions known as mesolimbic, mesocortical, nigrostriatal and tuberoinfundibular. The mesolimbic system, connecting the ventral tegmental area (VTA) and the nucleus accumbens, is known as the dopaminergic reward system (Fig. 17.2), and it has been specifically implicated in processes underlying reward. The mesocortical system connects the ventral tegmental area to the frontal cortex, and is therefore closely associated with the pathways that form the dopaminergic reward system.

Psychological reward is a process that reinforces behaviour, and the reward system in the brain in animals and humans appears to reward behaviour by inducing pleasurable effects. The misuse of alcohol and drugs is associated with activity in the reward system (Nestler 2005). Here we focus on the reward system in regulating social behaviour.

Activity in dopaminergic reward pathways is associated with a range of socially affiliative behaviours including oral reward (Prinssen *et al.* 1994) and parenting behaviour (Keer & Stern 1999), and in the formation, expression and maintenance of monogamous pair bonds in rodents (Young *et al.* 2005). Studies of humans with generalised social phobia have demonstrated alterations in dopamine functioning particularly in the striatum (Matthew *et al.* 2001). Here we are particularly concerned with the role of dopamine in the formation of social preferences during pair bonding, which has been the subject of most of the relevant research.

17.5.1 Dopaminergic influences on reward and affiliative behaviours

The ventral and dorsal striatum are subcortical structures that are critically involved in reward-related learning (Delgado 2007). Both contain vasopressin and oxytocin receptors, as well as dopamine receptors. There are five types of dopamine receptors in the brain (D1–5). D1 and D5 are grouped as the D1-like family and are excitatory, whereas D2, D3 and D4 are grouped as the D2-like family and are inhibitory. Activation of the D1-like family is coupled to an excitatory G-protein inreasing the production of cAMP intracellularly (see Box 17.2). The D2-like family of receptors are coupled with an inhibitory G-protein inhibiting the production of cAMP.

Dopamine has been implicated in the motivational aspects of reward seeking: lesions of the nucleus accumbens shell (NAS) are associated with reduced reward-seeking behaviour (Ishiwari *et al.* 2004). Oxytocin interacts with dopamine in the NAS, located in the ventral striatum and the VTA, which is a central part of the reward circuitry (Fig. 17.2) and which projects to the nucleus accumbens. Vasopressin interacts in the NAS, the lateral septal nucleus (LSN) and other areas of the dorsal striatum. Studies in voles have demonstrated that activation of dopamine receptors D1 and D2 in the NAS differentially influence mating and the formation and maintenance of pair bonds. D2 receptors are particularly implicated in pair-bond formation (Curtis *et al.* 2006).

As outlined above, D1 and D2 receptors have potentially opposite effects on second messengers at a cellular level. Activation of D2 receptors has been shown to facilitate pair-bond formation in prairie voles. Further exploration of the cellular mechanisms has revealed that decreased cAMP signalling mediates the formation of pair bonds in prairie voles, while activation of protein kinase A through increased cAMP signalling prevents partner preference (Aragona *et al.* 2003, Aragona & Wang 2007). There is some evidence that oxytocin is coupled to inhibitory G-proteins (Burns *et al.* 2001) and thus also downregulates the intracellular cAMP cascade. Blockade of OTRs in the nucleus accumbens is also associated with impaired partner preference formation (Young *et al.* 2001); thus Curtis *et al.* (2006) have suggested that oxytocin and dopamine act synergistically in the nucleus accumbens during pair-bond formation.

Further evidence suggests that the ventral and dorsal striatum have potentially dissociable roles in modulating social behaviour (Balleine *et al.* 2007). The dopaminergic circuit in the ventral striatum is engaged in predictions about whether a course of action may result in a future reward. In contrast, the dorsal striatum monitors the outcome of actions to optimise future choices that could lead to a reward (Delgado 2007). Investigations using functional neuroimaging have also suggested that reward circuitry is implicated in more complex social interactions such as cooperation and revenge. The notion of reciprocal altruism refers to the tendency to behave altruistically towards another person in the full expectation that they will reciprocate our positive action at some point in the future. Mutual cooperation can be rewarding, and evokes activity in several regions that contain oxytocin and/or vasopressin receptors (Rilling *et al.* 2002). Altruistic punishment, i.e. punishment of those who do not reciprocate our good deeds (de Quervain *et al.* 2004), is also associated with activation of dopaminergic reward circuits. Reflecting on this basic system of social reward for good deeds, and satisfaction at seeing transgressors get their just deserts, is itself so rewarding to us that its portrayal (in terms of real and fictional accounts of variable complexity) pervades popular culture.

17.6 The influence of genetic variation on social cognition

A reductionist view of genetic influences on human behaviour is to hypothesise that variation within genes influencing the molecular systems implicated in the behaviour directly influences the behaviour. The influences on human behaviour are far more complex, as it is rarely influenced by a single locus, and is subject to the influence of environment. However, in an effort to explore possible genetic contributions to behaviour, genetic variation is frequently investigated as a starting point in relation to how it might contribute to disease or behaviour. Investigations of genes involved in any of the systems discussed here have been reported on in a heterogeneous literature, and therefore it is difficult to tie the evidence together in a meaningful way in relation to social cognition. Hopefully the discussion that follows serves to introduce the reader to the concepts of genetic susceptibility and risk for diseases and behaviour.

17.6.1 Oxytocin-related genes

Genetic studies in complex disease may be based both on a-priori and on hypothesis-free approaches. A priori, a role for genes related to oxytocin in causing autism susceptibility has been suggested from the animal literature discussed above. Studies of the gene encoding the oxytocin receptor, *OXTR*, located at chromosome 3p26.2, reported association with variants in the gene and autism in Chinese and North American populations (Wu *et al.* 2005, Jacob *et al.* 2007). Association with autism has been reported in a high-functioning cluster of Irish individuals with autism (Tansey *et al.* 2008). However, hypothesis-free approaches using genome-wide investigations have also yielded some evidence for the involvement of oxytocin-related genes in autism. Pooled analysis of data derived from two family-based autism samples using genome-wide linkage approaches

found the best evidence for linkage on the short arm of chromosome 3 (3p24–26) which harbours *OXTR* (Ylisaukko-oja *et al.* 2006). A recent report of de-novo copy-number variations associated with autism (Sebat *et al.* 2007) noted a high-functioning autistic individual had deleted one copy of the oxytocin gene *OXT* at 20p13.

17.6.2 Vasopressin-related genes

Based on the same premise, vasopressin-related genes have been investigated in autism. Preliminary evidence from three studies suggests a role for polymorphisms in the *Avpr1a* gene in autism susceptibility (Kim *et al.* 2002, Wassink *et al.* 2004, Yirmiya *et al.* 2006). Deficits in social recognition are found in autistic probands, and in their first-degree relatives, to a far greater extent than would be predicted by chance (D. Seigal *et al.* unpublished). The *Avpr1b* receptor has also been implicated in the formation of social memories (Caldwell *et al.* 2008), but knowledge about this receptor is still relatively patchy. There is prominent *Avpr1b* expression in the hippocampal field CA2 pyramidal neurons (Fig. 17.2), which facilitates the contexualisation, via memory, of novel social encounters (Young *et al.* 2006).

17.6.3 Serotonin-related genes

The serotonergic system is ubiquitous, and serotonergic genes have been widely investigated in relation to human behaviour and mental-health disorders. Two genes that have been widely studied are the gene encoding the serotonin transporter protein (5-HTT), and the gene encoding tryptophan dehydroxylase (TPH2), an enzyme involved in serotonin synthesis. Genetic variation in the genes encoding for the serotonin transporter and tryptophan dehydroxylase affect expression and function of the proteins, and have been implicated in influencing social cognition (Wendland *et al.* 2006). Attempts to link genotype directly to brain function have adopted functional neuroimaging approaches specifically investigating effects of genotype on social cognition.

17.6.4 Serotonin transporter variants and social cognition

Polymorphic variation in the serotonin transporter gene (*SLC6A4*) includes a 44 bp insertion (or deletion) in the promoter. The basal activity of the long promoter allele (*l*) is three times higher than that of the short promoter allele (*s*), while *s* allele carrier status is associated with reduced transcription of the gene. Since the function of the protein product of the *SLC6A4* gene is to clear serotonin from the synapse, reduced transcription in *s* allele carriers should be associated with increased availability of serotonin in the synapse. However, rs25531, a functional SNP in the long promotor allele of the transporter, has further effects on the transcription of the gene. This A/G variant is located in the *l* allele of the promotor variant. The A allele is associated with higher levels of transcription than the G allele.

The *s* allele has been reported to be associated with higher levels of neuroticism and susceptibility to depression (Munafo *et al.* 2005), although effect sizes are reported to be small (Flint *et al.* 2008). Brain imaging studies have highlighted the relationship between *s* allele carriers and greater activation to emotional than neutral stimuli in the limbic system. The *s* and *l* alleles have been implicated in emotional regulation. Physiological influence of the variants in the prefrontal cortex and amygdala have been reported. Greater right amygdala neuronal activity in response to faces showing threatening expressions (anger/fear) has been detected in individuals with one or two copies of the *s* allele, compared with those who are homozygous for the *l* allele (Hariri *et al.* 2002). The right posterior fusiform gyrus also showed greater activity in the *s* allele groups, indicating that there could be excitatory feedback from the amygdala to these visual object-processing regions, potentially leading to improved recognition and refined behavioural responses to cues such as faces showing negative emotions. A hyper-responsive amygdala has been proposed as a consequence of *s* allele carrier status (Pezawas *et al.* 2005), associated with reduced grey matter in the perigenual anterior cingulate cortex (pACC) and amygdala. The pACC is richly innervated by serotonin, with the greatest density of serotonergic terminals within the human cortex, and it is a major target for projections from the amygdala. Individuals who are homozygous for the *l* allele, and thus have more efficient transporter protein function, showed strong functional interactions between these regions during facial processing tasks. Thus a feedback circuit between the pACC and amygdala potentially is involved in extinguishing negative affect evoked by a stimulus (e.g. negative emotional valence). The efficiency of this circuitry is diminished in people homozygous or heterozygous for the *s* allele. Inadequate regulation of amygdala arousal, aggregated over lifetime experiences, could result in different susceptibilities to depression or anxiety depending on the intensity and negative quality of those experiences (Hariri *et al.* 2005).

Another perspective is that carriers of the *s* allele could have elevated baseline levels of arousal – a tonic activation model (Canli & Lesch 2007), associated with persistent hypervigilance, perhaps because these individuals engage in the act of scanning the environment, which is itself arousing. Canli and Lesch (2007) identified increased activation in the amygdala and hippocampus at rest in *s* allele carriers that correlated with self-reported life events using functional neuroimaging, possibly highlighting potential effects of environmental interaction with genotype in influencing outcome for *s* allele carriers. Supporting the hypothesis is the evidence that life events also appeared to correlate with functional connectivity of the amygdala as a function of genotype. Perhaps epigenetic interactions between stressful life events and genotype upregulate resting activation in key regions and impact on the structure of emotional circuitry, possibly contributing to susceptibility to depression (Canli & Lesch 2007).

Differences in variation in the serotonin transporter across phylogeny also appear to influence social behaviour. Species of macaques with tolerant societies and higher levels of conciliatory behaviours are monomorphic at the promotor variant, whereas intolerant, hierarchical societies (e.g. rhesus monkeys) are polymorphic at this locus (Wendland *et al.* 2006).

Moreover, gene–environment investigations in rhesus monkeys have demonstrated interaction between early adverse life experience and the rhesus promotor genotype which correlates with negative outcomes in attentional and emotional processes, stress reactivity and alcohol dependance (Suomi 2005).

17.6.5 Tryptophan dehydroxylase 2 (*TPH2*)

TPH2 encodes the enzyme tryptophan dehydroxylase, a rate-limiting enzyme in serotonin synthesis in the brain. Functional neuroimaging approaches based on genotype have also been employed to investigate the link between genotype and function. A functional variant (rs4570625, or SNP G-703T, i.e. a variant causing a functional change in the corresponding protein) in *TPH2* is associated with increased amygdala response to viewing negative emotional faces (Brown *et al.* 2005). The same variant has also been associated with increased amygdala response to any stimulus regardless of emotional valence (Canli *et al.* 2005). Additive effects of variants in both *TPH2* and *SLC6A4* have been reported: carriers who had both the *s* allele of the promotor polymorphism of *SLC6A4* and the T allele of the G-703T SNP in *TPH2* had the greatest degree of neural activation in response to emotionally arousing stimuli (based on event-related potentials) (Herrmann *et al.* 2007). A dosage effect for the variants is noted, with individuals without the *s* allele or the *T* allele showing the least amount of activation, and those who were heterozygotes for the *s* and *T* alleles showing intermediate effects. Interestingly, these observations were particularly robust in the striatum (putamen), which, as discussed above, is involved in processes underlying reward and in response to aversive stimuli.

17.6.6 Genetic regulation of dopamine flux

While allelic variation in dopaminergic-system genes has not been widely investigated in relation to social cognition, the catechol-*O*-methyltransferase (*COMT*) gene, which encodes an enzyme of the same name and which is involved in the degradation of catecholamines (Tunbridge *et al.* 2006), is one of the most widely studied genes in relation to human cognition and brain function. The *COMT* gene is located on chromosome 22q11.2. The enzyme occurs on intracellular membranes of post-synaptic neurons, and is believed to play a critical role in the modulation of dopamine in the prefrontal cortex with widespread effects upon cortical dopamine flux via mesocortical and corticostriatal pathways (Meyer-Lindenberg *et al.* 2005). *COMT* activity influences performance on cognitive tasks related to prefrontal cortical functions, and potentially also on aspects of social cognition.

The *COMT* gene contains a common (~50%) single nucleotide polymorphism that has a major impact on the enzyme's efficiency (G → A; leading to a valine-to-methionine substitution at codon 158, referred to as Val158Met). The allelic variants are codominant. Homozygotes for the *Met* allele, the protein product of which is relatively inefficient at deaminating dopamine, have about one-third less prefrontal *COMT* activity and corresponding higher levels of dopamine compared with homozygotes for the *Val* allele, with associated effects on working memory and executive function tasks dependent on prefrontal function (Chen *et al.* 2004, Tunbridge *et al.* 2007).

Met carriers have higher levels of circulating dopamine in the prefrontal cortex. They show increased activation in limbic circuitry on functional neuroimaging elicited by unpleasant stimuli, i.e. negative emotional faces (Tessitore 2002). The amygdala response is potentiated because the excess dopamine is thought to attenuate the inhibitory input from the prefrontal cortex to the amygdala, and because there is enhanced excitatory input to the amygdala from the sensory cortices. Drabant *et al.* (2006) reported a dose-dependent increase of hippocampal and venterolateral prefrontal cortex activation in *Met* allele carriers when viewing faces with negative emotional valence. This was associated with increased functional coupling between amygdala and orbitofrontal cortex in *Met* homozygotes, the magnitude of which was inversely correlated with the personality characteristic novelty seeking (i.e. the opposite to novelty seeking was considered an index of temperamental inflexibility) (Drabant *et al.* 2006). They suggested that inherited variation in dopamine neurotransmission related to *Met* carrier status is associated with heightened reactivity and connectivity in the corticolimbic circuitry, which may reflect genetic predisposition to inflexible processing of affective stimuli.

COMT has also been implicated in activities of the social brain, such as theory of mind and social functioning (Bassett *et al.* 2007). In a study of individuals with 22q11 deletion syndrome, *Met* allele carriers performed poorly on three frontal cognitive tasks, including theory of mind, trails and olfactory identification. Severe social-cognitive deficits of an autistic type that are associated with 22q11.2 deletion syndrome have only recently been reported (Vorstman *et al.* 2006). The contributory role played by haploinsufficiency for *COMT* in this disorder as a result of the deletion is not yet known.

17.7 Conclusions and future directions

A well-described coordinated neural network as outlined above underlies social cognition in humans. Gradually, the genetic and neuropeptidergic processes that influence and regulate it are being elucidated. These cognitive processes are highly complex, and the biological substrate of their activity is likely to be subject to environmental modifications. Evidence from animal studies has emphasised that neural processes underlying affiliation and cooperation, coupled with reward, are critical influences on social behaviour. The normal functioning of the social cognition network is linked to central actions of the neuropeptides oxytocin and vasopressin. The transcription of these neuropeptides is regulated in part by sex steroids, and they may have sexually dimorphic effects on social behaviour as a consequence. Preliminary evidence suggests that susceptibility to disorders of social interaction such as autism could be associated with functional variation in the genes encoding these neuropeptides or their receptors. Dopaminergic circuitry in the striatum and orbitofrontal cortex serves to support social cognition by promoting trust and

the rewarding aspects of affiliation. There is some evidence that oxytocin and dopamine may act synergistically in the neural processes that underlie affiliation, possibly through the activation of inhibitory proteins involved in second-messenger cascades, guanine nucleotide binding proteins (G-proteins) leading to downregulation of the intracellular cyclic AMP cascade. Dopamine flux also influences inhibitory inputs to the amygdala from the prefrontal and sensory cortices, and is influenced by genetic variation in *COMT*, and some studies suggest that this is associated with increased reactivity in emotional circuitry.

The serotonergic system has been studied largely in relation to the regulation of mood and anxiety. Because it innervates those parts of the brain crucial to social cognition, and appears to regulate the release of oxytocin and vasopressin in the paraventricular nucleus of the hypothalamus, functional variants in genes involved in the transport and receptors for serotonin could influence the functioning of the social brain. Recent evidence suggests the development of these systems could be particularly susceptible to influences from early environmental circumstances of upbringing.

In part we are reliant on literature emanating from animal studies to inform our understanding of human social cognition, as there are weaknesses in the approaches utilised to investigate social cognition in humans. It is difficult to find the ideal neuropsychological paradigms to investigate complex cognitive functions, and it could be argued that the paradigms used are by necessity overly simplistic. Imaging genetics investigations such as those highlighted here are difficult to interpret, particularly with respect to effect size of genotype on the traits being measured. It is also difficult to find a study design that takes account of the environment without the inclusion of significant confounders. Future methodological and analytical approaches in imaging, e.g. diffusion tensor imaging helping to link brain structure to function, are likely to provide a powerful way to investigate the neural basis of brain functions, including social cognition.

Advances in behavioural genetics are likely to emerge from a range of whole-genome approaches such as whole-genome association studies and the investigation of structural rearrangements of the genome such as copy-number variation assisting in the identification of genes that influence cognition and behaviour. However, given that similar investigations in other complex traits only explain a small proportion of the heritability, the contributions of the genetic variants discussed here to behavioural effects are likely to have relatively small effects. Importantly, throughout development and in response to experience, gene expression is switched on and off, adding further complexity to the relationships between genotypes and behavioural outcomes. A variety of other mechanisms, that have not been discussed in detail here, are also likely to be at play, and these require a good deal more investigation. Focus on other neurotransmitter systems, e.g. glutamate and GABA, will be informative. A potential influence of neurotrophic factors, e.g. brain-derived neurotrophic factor, also needs to be considered specifically in relation to the influence of environmental factors on social cognition. Sexually dimorphic influences that account for gender differences are driven by differential exposure to the sex hormones, and a potential mechanism for neuroimmune influences has also come to light (Bartz & McInnes 2007). Future studies investigating the genetic influences on social cognition will need to examine gene–environment interactions, gene–gene interactions and epigenetic factors, and will have to address the persistent difficulty in linking genotype to function and behaviour.

Acknowledgements

During the preparation of this chapter LG was supported by the Health Research Board, Ireland, and Autism Speaks; DS was supported by the Wellcome Trust, the Nancy Lurie Marks Family Foundation, the Simons Foundation and the European Commission (Framework 6).

Suggested readings

Gallinat, J., Bauer, M. & Heinz, A. (2008) Genes and neuroimaging: advances in psychiatric research. *Neurodegenerative Diseases*, **5**, 277–285.

Plomin, R., DeFries, J. C., Craig, I. & McGuffin, P. (2003) *Behavioral Genetics in the Postgenomic Era*. Washington, DC: American Psychological Association.

Rutter, M. (2006) *Genes and Behavior: Nature–Nurture Interplay Explained*. Oxford: Blackwell.

References

Adolphs, R. (2003) Is the human amygdala specialized for processing social information? *Annals of the New York Academy of Sciences*, **985**, 326–340.

Adolphs, R. & Spezio, M. (2006) Role of the amygdala in processing visual social stimuli. *Progress in Brain Research*, **156**, 363–378.

Adolphs, R., Gosselin, F., Buchanan, T. W. *et al.* (2005) A mechanism for impaired fear recognition after amygdala damage. *Nature*, **433**, 68–72.

Amodio, D. M. & Frith, C. D. (2006) Meeting of minds: the medial frontal cortex and social cognition. *Nature Reviews Neuroscience*, **7**, 268–277.

Aragona, B. J. & Wang, Z. (2007) Opposing regulation of pair bond formation by cAMP signaling within the nucleus accumbens shell. *Journal of Neuroscience*, **27**, 13352–13356.

Aragona, B. J., Liu, Y., Curtis, J.T., Stephan, F.K. & Wang, Z. (2003) A critical role for nucleus accumbens dopamine in partner-preference formation in male prairie voles. *Journal of Neuroscience*, **23**, 3483–3490.

Azmitia, E. C. (1999) Serotonin neurons, neuroplasticity, and homeostasis of neural tissue. *Neuropsychopharmacology*, **21** (2 Suppl), 33–45S.

Bales, K. L., Plotsky, P. M., Young, L. J. *et al.* (2007) Neonatal oxytocin manipulations have long-lasting, sexually dimorphic effects on vasopressin receptors. *Neuroscience*, **144**, 38–45.

Balleine, B. W., Delgado, M. R. & Hikosaka, O. (2007) The role of the dorsal striatum in reward and decision-making. *Journal of Neuroscience*, **27**, 8161–8165.

Baron-Cohen, S. (2002) The extreme male brain theory of autism. *Trends in Cognitive Sciences*, **6**, 248–254.

Bartz, J. A. & McInnes, L. A. (2007) CD38 regulates oxytocin secretion and complex social behavior. *BioEssays*, **29**, 837–841.

Bassett, A. S., Caluseriu, O., Weksberg, R., Young, D. A. & Chow, E. W. (2007) Catechol-O-methyl transferase and expression of schizophrenia in 73 adults with 22q11 deletion syndrome. *Biological Psychiatry*, **61**, 1135–1140.

Baumgartner, T., Heinrichs, M., Vonlanthen, A., Fischbacher, U. & Fehr, E. (2008) Oxytocin shapes the neural circuitry of trust and trust adaptation in humans. *Neuron*, **58**, 639–650.

Bielsky, I. F., Hu, S. B., Szegda, K. L., Westphal, H. & Young, L. J. (2004) Profound impairment in social recognition and reduction in anxiety-like behavior in vasopressin V1a receptor knockout mice. *Neuropsychopharmacology*, **29**, 483–493.

Bielsky, I. F., Hu, S. B., Ren, X., Terwilliger, E. F. & Young, L. J. (2005) The V1a vasopressin receptor is necessary and sufficient for normal social recognition: a gene replacement study. *Neuron*, **47**, 503–513.

Bizot, J., Le Bihan, C., Puech, A. J., Hamon, M. & Thiebot, M. (1999) Serotonin and tolerance to delay of reward in rats. *Psychopharmacology (Berlin)*, **146**, 400–412.

Born, J., Lange, T., Ker, W. *et al.* (2002) Sniffing neuropeptides: a transnasal approach to the human brain. *Nature Neuroscience*, **5**, 514–516.

Broad, K. D., Curley, J. P. & Keverne, E. B. (2006) Mother–infant bonding and the evolution of mammalian social relationships. *Philosophical Transactions of the Royal Society B*, **361**, 2199–2214.

Brothers, L., Ring, B. & Kling, A. (1990) Response of neurons in the macaque amygdala to complex social stimuli. *Behavioural Brain Research*, **41**, 199–213.

Brown, S. M., Peet, E., Manuck, S. B. *et al.* (2005) A regulatory variant of the human tryptophan hydroxylase-2 gene biases amygdala reactivity. *Molecular Psychiatry*, **10**, 884–888, 805.

Burns, P. D., Mendes, J. O., Yemm, R. S., *et al.* (2001) Cellular mechanisms by which oxytocin mediates ovine endometrial prostaglandin Fα synthesis: role of g(i) proteins and mitogen-activated protein kinases. *Biology of Reproduction*, **65**, 1150–1155.

Caldwell, H. K., Lee, H. J., Macbeth, A. H. & Young, W. S. (2008) Vasopressin: behavioral roles of an original neuropeptide. *Progress in Neurobiology*, **84**, 1–24.

Campbell, A. (2008) Attachment, aggression and affiliation: the role of oxytocin in female social behavior. *Biological Psychology*, **77**, 1–10.

Canli, T. & Lesch, K. P. (2007) Long story short: the serotonin transporter in emotion regulation and social cognition. *Nature Neuroscience*, **10**, 1103–1109.

Canli, T., Congdon, E., Gutknecht, L., Constable, R. T. & Lesch, K. P. (2005) Amygdala responsiveness is modulated by tryptophan hydroxylase-2 gene variation. *Journal of Neural Transmission*, **112**, 1479–1485.

Cardinal, R. (2006) Neural systems implicated in delayed and probabilistic reinforcement. *Neural Networks*, **19**, 1277–1301.

Carter, C. S. (2007) Sex differences in oxytocin and vasopressin: implications for autism spectrum disorders? *Behavioural Brain Research*, **176**, 170–186.

Carver, C. S. & Miller, C. J. (2006) Relations of serotonin function to personality: current views and a key methodological issue. *Psychiatry Research*, **144**, 1–15.

Chen, J., Lipska, B. K., Halim, N. *et al.* (2004) Functional analysis of genetic variation in catechol-O-methyltransferase (COMT): effects on mRNA, protein, and enzyme activity in postmortem human brain. *American Journal of Human Genetics*, **75**, 807–821.

Choleris, E., Gustafsson, J. A., Korach, K. S. *et al.* (2003) An estrogen-dependent four-gene micronet regulating social recognition: a study with oxytocin and estrogen receptor-alpha and -beta knockout mice. *Proceedings of the National Academy of Sciences of the USA*, **100**, 6192–6197.

Curtis, J. T., Liu, Y., Aragona, B. J. & Wang, Z. (2006) Dopamine and monogamy. *Brain Research*, **1126**, 76–90.

Delgado, M. R. (2007) Reward-related responses in the human striatum. *Annals of the New York Academy of Sciences*, **1104**, 70–88.

Denk, F., Walton, M. E., Jennings, K. A. *et al.* (2005) Differential involvement of serotonin and dopamine systems in cost–benefit decisions about delay or effort. *Psychopharmacology (Berlin)*, **179**, 587–596.

de Quervain, D. J., Fischbacher, U., Treyer, V. *et al.* (2004) The neural basis of altruistic punishment. *Science*, **305**, 1254–1258.

De Vries, G. J. & Panzica, G. C. (2006) Sexual differentiation of central vasopressin and vasotocin systems in vertebrates: different mechanisms, similar endpoints. *Neuroscience*, **138**, 947–955.

Dolan, R. J. (2007) The human amygdala and orbital prefrontal cortex in behavioural regulation. *Philosophical Transactions of the Royal Society B*, **362**, 787–799.

Doya, K. (2002) Metalearning and neuromodulation. *Neural Networks*, **15**, 495–506.

Drabant, E. M., Hariri, A. R. Meyer-Lindenberg, A. *et al.* (2006) Catechol *O*-methyltransferase val[158]met genotype and neural mechanisms related to affective arousal and regulation. *Archives of General Psychiatry*, **63**, 1396–1406.

Fairhall, S. L. & Ishai, A. (2007) Effective connectivity within the distributed cortical network for face perception. *Cerebral Cortex*, **17**, 2400–2406.

Ferguson, J. N., Young, L. J., Hearn, E. F. *et al.* (2000) Social amnesia in mice lacking the oxytocin gene. *Nature Genetics*, **25**, 284–288.

Ferguson, J. N., Aldag, J. M., Insel, T. R. & Young, L. J. (2001) Oxytocin in the medial amygdala is essential for social recognition in the mouse. *Journal of Neuroscience*, **21**, 8278–8285.

Ferris, C. F. (2005) Vasopressin/oxytocin and aggression. *Novartis Foundation Symposium*, **268**, 190–198; discussion 198–200, 242–253.

Flint, J., Shifman, S., Munafo, M. & Mott, R.. (2008) Genetic variants in major depression. *Novartis Foundation Symposium*, **289**, 23–32.

Frith, C. D. & Frith, U. (2007) Social cognition in humans. *Current Biology*, **17**, R724–732.

Gallese, V., Eagle, M. N. & Migone, P. (2007) Intentional attunement: mirror neurons and the neural underpinnings of interpersonal relations. *Journal of the American Psychoanalytic Association*, **55**, 131–176.

Gatewood, J. D., Wills, A., Shetty, S. *et al.* (2006) Sex chromosome complement and gonadal sex influence aggressive and parental behaviors in mice. *Journal of Neuroscience*, **26**, 2335–2342.

Gimpl, G. & Fahrenholz, F. (2001) The oxytocin receptor system: structure, function, and regulation. *Physiological Reviews*, **81**, 629–683.

Guastella, A. J., Mitchell, P. B. & Dadds, M. R. (2008) Oxytocin increases gaze to the eye region of human faces. *Biological Psychiatry*, **63**, 3–5.

Hammock, E. A. & Young, L. J. (2006) Oxytocin, vasopressin and pair bonding: implications for autism. *Philosophical Transactions of the Royal Society B*, **361**, 2187–2198.

Hariri, A. R., Mattay, V. S. Tessitore, A. *et al.* (2002) Serotonin transporter genetic variation and the response of the human amygdala. *Science*, **297**, 400–403.

Hariri, A. R., Drabant, E. M., Munoz, K. E. *et al.* (2005) A susceptibility gene for affective disorders and the response of the human amygdala. *Archives of General Psychiatry*, **62**, 146–152.

Harmer, C. J., Bhagwagar, Z., Perrett, D. I. *et al.* (2003) Acute SSRI administration affects the processing of social cues in healthy volunteers. *Neuropsychopharmacology*, **28**, 148–152.

Harmer, C. J., Shelley, N. C., Cowen, P. J. & Goodwin, G. M. (2004) Increased positive versus negative affective perception and memory in healthy volunteers following selective serotonin and norepinephrine reuptake inhibition. *American Journal of Psychiatry*, **161**, 1256–1263.

Heinrichs, M., Baumgartner, T., Kirschbaum, C. & Ehlert, U. (2003) Social support and oxytocin interact to suppress cortisol and subjective responses to psychosocial stress. *Biological Psychiatry*, **54**, 1389–1398.

Herrmann, M., Huter, T., Müller, F. *et al.* (2007) Additive effects of serotonin transporter and tryptophan hydroxylase-2 gene variation on emotional processing. *Cerebral Cortex*, **5**, 1160–1163.

Ho, S. S., Chow, B. K. & Yung, W. H. (2007) Serotonin increases the excitability of the hypothalamic paraventricular nucleus magnocellular neurons. *European Journal of Neuroscience*, **25**, 2991–3000.

Hollander, E., Bartz, J., Chaplin, W. *et al.* (2007) Oxytocin increases retention of social cognition in autism. *Biological Psychiatry*, **61**, 498–503.

Huber, D., Veinante, P. & Stoop, R. (2005) Vasopressin and oxytocin excite distinct neuronal populations in the central amygdala. *Science*, **308**, 245–248.

Iacoboni, M. & Dapretto, M. (2006) The mirror neuron system and the consequences of its dysfunction. *Nature Reviews Neuroscience*, **7**, 942–951.

Iacoboni, M., Woods, R. P., Brass, M. *et al.* (1999) Cortical mechanisms of human imitation. *Science*, **286**, 2526–2528.

Insel, T. R. & Fernald, R. D. (2004) How the brain processes social information: searching for the social brain. *Annual Review of Neuroscience*, **27**, 697–722.

Ishiwari, K., Weber, S. M., Mingote, S., Correa, M. & Salamone, J. D. (2004) Accumbens dopamine and the regulation of effort in food-seeking behavior: modulation of work output by different ratio or force requirements. *Behavioural Brain Research*, **151**, 83–91.

Izquierdo, A., Newman, T. K., Higley, J. D. & Murray, E. A. (2007) Genetic modulation of cognitive flexibility and socioemotional behavior in rhesus monkeys. *Proceedings of the National Academy of Sciences of the USA*, **104**, 14128–14133.

Jabbi, M., Swart, M. & Keysers, C. (2007) Empathy for positive and negative emotions in the gustatory cortex. *NeuroImage*, **34**, 1744–1753.

Jacob, S., Brune, C. W., Carter, C. S. *et al.* (2007) Association of the oxytocin receptor gene (OXTR) in Caucasian children and adolescents with autism. *Neuroscience Letters*, **417**, 6–9.

Jin, D., Liu, H. X., Hirai, H. *et al.* (2007) CD38 is critical for social behaviour by regulating oxytocin secretion. *Nature*, **446**, 41–45.

Keer, S. E. & Stern, J. M. (1999) Dopamine receptor blockade in the nucleus accumbens inhibits maternal retrieval and licking, but enhances nursing behavior in lactating rats. *Physiology and Behavior*, **67**, 659–669.

Keverne, E. B. & Curley, J. P. (2004) Vasopressin, oxytocin and social behaviour. *Current Opinion in Neurobiology*, **14**, 777–783.

Keysers, C. & Perrett, D. I. (2004) Demystifying social cognition: a Hebbian perspective. *Trends in Cognitive Sciences*, **8**, 501–507.

Keysers, C., Wicker, B., Gazzola, V. *et al.* (2004) A touching sight: SII/PV activation during the observation and experience of touch. *Neuron*, **42**, 335–346.

Kim, S. J., Young, L. J., Gonen, D. *et al.* (2002) Transmission disequilibrium testing of arginine vasopressin receptor 1A (AVPR1A) polymorphisms in autism. *Molecular Psychiatry*, **7**, 503–507.

Kirsch, P., Esslinger, C., Chen, Q. *et al.* (2005) Oxytocin modulates neural circuitry for social cognition and fear in humans. *Journal of Neuroscience*, **25**, 11489–11493.

Kosfeld, M., Heinrichs, M., Zak, P. J., Fischbacher, U. & Fehr, E. (2005) Oxytocin increases trust in humans. *Nature*, **435**, 673–676.

Landgraf, R. & Neumann, I. D. (2004) Vasopressin and oxytocin release within the brain: a dynamic concept of multiple and variable modes of neuropeptide communication. *Frontiers in Neuroendocrinology*, **25**, 150–176.

Lim, M. M. & Young, L. J. (2006) Neuropeptidergic regulation of affiliative behavior and social bonding in animals. *Hormones and Behavior*, **50**, 506–517.

Lim, M. M., Bielsky, I. F. & Young, L. J. (2005) Neuropeptides and the social brain: potential rodent models of autism. *International Journal of Developmental Neuroscience*, **23**, 235–243.

Liu, Y. & Wang, Z. (2003) Nucleus accumbens oxytocin and dopamine interact to regulate pair bond formation in female prairie voles. *Neuroscience*, **121**, 537–544.

Loup, F., Tribollet, E., Dubois-Dauphin, M. & Dreifuss, J. J. (1991) Localization of high-affinity binding sites for oxytocin and vasopressin in the human brain: an autoradiographic study. *Brain Research*, **555**, 220–232.

Malin, E. L. & McGaugh, J. L. (2006) Differential involvement of the hippocampus, anterior cingulate cortex, and basolateral amygdala in memory for context and footshock. *Proceedings of the National Academy of Sciences of the USA*, **103**, 1959–1963.

Matthew, S. J., Coplan J. D. & Gorman, J. M. (2001) Neurobiological mechanisms of social anxiety disorder. *American Journal of Psychiatry*, **158**, 1558–1567.

McNamara, I. M., Borella, A. W., Bialowas, L. A. & Whitaker-Azmitia, P. M. (2008) Further studies in the developmental hyperserotonemia model (DHS) of autism: social, behavioral and peptide changes. *Brain Research*, **1189**, 203–214.

Meaney, M. J. & Szyf, M. (2005) Maternal care as a model for experience-dependent chromatin plasticity? *Trends in Neuroscience*, **28**, 456–463.

Meyer-Lindenberg, A., Kohn, P. D., Kolachana, B. *et al.* (2005) Midbrain dopamine and prefrontal function in humans: interaction and modulation by COMT genotype. *Nature Neuroscience*, **8**, 594–596.

Mobini, S., Chiang, T. J., Ho, M. Y., Bradshaw, C. M. & Szabadi, E. (2000) Effects of central 5-hydroxytryptamine depletion on sensitivity to delayed and probabilistic reinforcement. *Psychopharmacology (Berlin)*, **152**, 390–397.

Modahl, C., Green, L., Fein, D. *et al.* (1998) Plasma oxytocin levels in autistic children. *Biological Psychiatry*, **43**, 270–277.

Munafo, M. R., Clark, T. & Flint, J. (2005) Does measurement instrument moderate the association between the serotonin transporter gene and anxiety-related personality traits? A meta-analysis. *Molecular Psychiatry*, **10**, 415–419.

Nestler, E. (2005) Is there a common molecular pathway for addiction? *Nature Neuroscience*, **8**, 1445–9.

Nomura, M., McKenna, E., Korach, K. S., Pfaff, D. W. & Ogawa, S. (2002) Estrogen receptor-beta regulates transcript levels for oxytocin and arginine vasopressin in the hypothalamic paraventricular nucleus of male mice. *Brain Research, Molecular Brain Research*, **109**, 84–94.

Pezawas, L., Meyer-Lindenberg, A., Drabant, E. *et al.* (2005) 5-HTTLPR polymorphism impacts human cingulate-amygdala interactions: a genetic susceptibility mechanism for depression. *Nature Neuroscience*, **8**, 828–834.

Porges, S. W. (2007) The polyvagal perspective. *Biological Psychology*, **74**, 116–143.

Poulos, C., Parker, J. L. & Le, A. D. (1996) Dexfenfluramine and 8-OH-DPAT modulate impulsivity in a delay-of-reward paradigm: implications for a correspondence with alcohol consumption. *Behavioural Pharmacology*, **17**, 395–399.

Prinssen, E. P., Balestra, W., Bemelmans, F. F. & Cools, A. R. (1994) Evidence for a role of the shell of the nucleus accumbens in oral behaviour of freely moving rats. *Journal of Neuroscience*, **14**, 1555–1562.

Rilling, J., Gutman, D., Zeh, T. *et al.* (2002) A neural basis for social cooperation. *Neuron*, **35**, 395–405.

Rizzolatti, G. & Craighero, L. (2004) The mirror-neuron system. *Annual Review of Neuroscience*, **27**, 169–192.

Rolls, E. T. (2007) The representation of information about faces in the temporal and frontal lobes. *Neuropsychologia*, **45**, 124–143.

Rolls, E. T., Critchley, H. D., Browning, A. S. & Inoue, K. (2006) Face-selective and auditory neurons in the primate orbitofrontal cortex. *Experimental Brain Research*, **170**, 74–87.

Sebat, J., Lakshmi, B., Malhotra, D. *et al.* (2007) Strong association of de novo copy number mutations with autism. *Science*, **316**, 445–449.

Singer, T. (2007) The neuronal basis of empathy and fairness. *Novartis Foundation Symposium*, **278**, 20–30; discussion 30–40, 89–96, 216–221.

Skuse, D. (2006) Genetic influences on the neural basis of social cognition. *Philosophical Transactions of the Royal Society B*, **361**, 2129–2141.

Skuse, D. H. & Gallagher, L. (2009) Dopaminergic-neuropeptide interactions in the social brain. *Trends in Cognitive Sciences*, **13**, 27–35.

Stein, M. B., Goldin, P. R., Sareen, J., Zorrilla, L. T. & Brown, G. G. (2002) Increased amygdala activation to angry and contemptuous faces in generalized social phobia. *Archives of General Psychiatry*, **59**, 1027–1034.

Storm, E. E. & Tecott, L. H. (2005) Social circuits: peptidergic regulation of mammalian social behavior. *Neuron*, **47**, 483–486.

Suomi, S. J. (2005) Aggression and social behaviour in rhesus monkeys. *Novartis Foundation Symposium*, **268**, 216–222.

Takayanagi, Y., Yoshida, M., Bielsky I. F. *et al.* (2005) Pervasive social deficits, but normal parturition, in oxytocin receptor-deficient mice. *Proceedings of the National Academy of Sciences of the USA*, **102**, 16096–16101.

Tanaka, S., Doya, K., Okada, G. *et al.* (2004) Prediction of immediate and future rewards differentially recruits cortico-basal ganglia loops. *Nature Neuroscience*, **7**, 887–893.

Tanaka, S., Schweighofer, N, Asahi, S. *et al.* (2007) Serotonin differentially regulates short- and long-term prediction of rewards in the ventral and dorsal striatum. *PLoS ONE*, **2** (12), e1333.

Tansey, K., Anney, R., Cochrane, L. E., Gil, M. & Gallagher, L. (2008) Further evidence supporting oxytocin receptor in an Irish sample. International Meeting for Autism Research (IMFAR), London.

Tessitore, A., Hariri, A. R., Fera, F. *et al.* (2002) Dopamine modulates the response of the human amygdala: a study in Parkinson's disease. *Journal of Neuroscience*, **22**, 9099–9103.

Thompson, J. C., Clarke, M., Stewart, T. & Puce, A. (2005) Configural processing of biological motion in human superior temporal sulcus. *Journal of Neuroscience*, **25**, 9059–9066.

Thompson, R. R., George, K., Walton, J. C., Orr, S. P. & Benson, J. (2006) Sex-specific influences of vasopressin on human social communication. *Proceedings of the National Academy of Sciences of the USA*, **103**, 7889–7894.

Tunbridge, E. M., Harrison, P. J. & Weinberger, D. R. (2006) Catechol-o-methyltransferase, cognition, and psychosis: Val158Met and beyond. *Biological Psychiatry*, **60**, 141–151.

Tunbridge, E. M., Weickert, C. S., Kleinman, J. E. *et al.* (2007) Catechol-o-methyltransferase enzyme activity and protein expression in human prefrontal cortex across the postnatal lifespan. *Cerebral Cortex*, **17**, 1206–1212.

Veenema, A. H., Blume, A., Niederle, D., Buwalda, B. & Neumann, I. D. (2006) Effects of early life stress on adult male aggression and hypothalamic vasopressin and serotonin. *European Journal of Neuroscience*, **24**, 1711–1720.

Vorstman, J. A., Jalali, G. R., Rappaport, E. F. *et al.* (2006) MLPA: a rapid, reliable, and sensitive method for detection and analysis of abnormalities of 22q. *Human Mutation*, **27**, 814–821.

Wassink, T. H., Piven, J., Vieland, V. J. *et al.* (2004) Examination of AVPR1a as an autism susceptibility gene. *Molecular Psychiatry*, **9**, 968–972.

Wendland, J. R., Lesch, K. P., Newman, T. K. *et al.* (2006) Differential functional variability of serotonin transporter and monoamine oxidase a genes in macaque species displaying contrasting levels of aggression-related behavior. *Behavior Genetics*, **36**, 163–172.

Whalen, P. J., Kagan, J., Cook, R. G. *et al.* (2004) Human amygdala responsivity to masked fearful eye whites. *Science*, **306**, 2061.

Williams, J. R., Catania, K. C. & Carter, C. S. (1992) Development of partner preferences in female prairie voles (*Microtus ochrogaster*): the role of social and sexual experience. *Hormones and Behavior*, **26**, 339–349.

Wogar, M., Bradshaw, C. M. & Szabadi, E. (1993) Effect of lesions of the ascending 5-hydroxytryptaminergic pathways on choice between delayed reinforcers. *Psychopharmacology (Berlin)*, **111**, 239–243.

Wu, S., Jia, M., Ruan, Y. *et al.* (2005) Positive association of the oxytocin receptor gene (OXTR) with autism in the Chinese Han population. *Biological Psychiatry*, **58**, 74–77.

Yirmiya, N., Rosenberg, C., Levi, S. *et al.* (2006) Association between the arginine vasopressin 1a receptor (AVPR1a) gene and autism in a family-based study: mediation by socialization skills. *Molecular Psychiatry*, **11**, 488–494.

Ylisaukko-Oja T., Alarcon, M., Cantor, R. M. *et al.* (2006) Search for autism loci by combined analysis of autism genetic resource exchange and Finnish families. *Annals of Neurology*, **59**, 145–155.

Young, L. J. & Wang, Z. (2004) The neurobiology of pair bonding. *Nature Neuroscience*, **7**, 1048–1054.

Young, L. J., Lim, M. M., Gingrich, B. & Insel, T. R. (2001) Cellular mechanisms of social attachment. *Hormones and Behavior*, **40**, 133–138.

Young, L. J., Murphy Young, A. Z. & Hammock, E. A. (2005) Anatomy and neurochemistry of the pair bond. *Journal of Comparative Neurology*, **493**, 51–57.

Young, W. S., Li, J., Wersinger, S. R. & Palkovits, M. (2006) The vasopressin 1b receptor is prominent in the hippocampal area CA2 where it is unaffected by restraint stress or adrenalectomy. *Neuroscience*, **143**, 1031–1039.

Zeki, S. (2007) The neurobiology of love. *FEBS Letters*, **581**, 2575–2759.

Anonymous (and other) social experience and the evolution of cooperation by reciprocity

Michael Taborsky

Animals behave according to their previous social experience. This has been demonstrated in a wide range of species all across the animal kingdom (Rutte *et al.* 2006). Remarkably, this response to previous social interactions is not confined to experience with known individuals. It appears to be a much simpler trait than we might assume from our own intuition. If an animal fights with *any* conspecific, it will behave differently in future encounters, depending on whether it won or lost. These renowned winner and loser effects are among the most predictable traits in animal interactions (see Chapter 14). In humans, we term the psychological mechanism involved 'self-confidence'. But, most interestingly, animals respond contingently upon social experience also in a sociopositive context. If they received help, they are more likely to help others as well, even if donors and receivers are completely unknown to each other. This generalised form of reciprocity has been demonstrated in humans and Norway rats so far (Bartlett & DeSteno 2006, Rutte & Taborsky 2007), but we assume it to be a general phenomenon, just like the ubiquitous winner and loser effects.

In the early 1970s, after Hamilton's (1964) and Trivers' (1971) revelations on kin selection and reciprocity as key mechanisms of altruistic behaviour and advanced sociality, we were tempted to believe that the major riddles in this field had been solved. The vast literature that emerged on the evolutionary mechanisms of altruism and (eu)sociality since then, at both theoretical and empirical levels, proved us dead wrong. Benefits of cooperation between kin were shown to be levelled out easily by competition among relatives (Taylor 1992, Wilson *et al.* 1992, Queller 1994), and reciprocal altruism turned out to be a concept with intellectual beauty but notoriously unrealistic assumptions as far as organisms under natural conditions are concerned. Nevertheless, cooperation is widespread in nature, and this demands to be explained. Not for nothing Charles Darwin regarded the abandonment of reproduction for the benefit of others as the crux of his theory of natural selection.

Despite enormous effort, the role of reciprocity as a mechanism of cooperation in nature has remained an enigma. Overall, existing evidence suggests that direct reciprocity is hardly involved when animals cooperate, and indirect reciprocity seems to be far beyond the scope of animals other than humans, due to its great cognitive demands. In contrast, the cognitive demands of generalised reciprocity are negligible. An animal needs to remember only if it received help by any conspecific on a past occasion to decide whether it should be helpful or not. How

Social Behaviour: Genes, Ecology and Evolution, ed. Tamás Székely, Allen J. Moore and Jan Komdeur. Published by Cambridge University Press. © Cambridge University Press 2010.

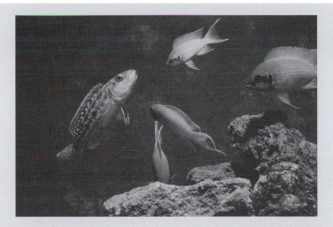

Two large helpers of the Lake Tanganyika cichlid *Neolamprologus pulcher* attack an intruding predator (*Lepidiolamprologus elongatus*; leftmost, dotted fish) above the breeding shelter. This defence behaviour for the benefit of smaller group members is payment of the helpers for being allowed to stay in the territory of dominant breeders, which is reciprocal trading of different commodities. The breeders are to the right (male) and bottom (female, partly visible) of the picture. Photo: Michael Taborsky.

can this be stable against cheating – individuals enjoying the benefits of cooperation but not paying its costs?

Theoretical models and computer simulations revealed various ways in which generalised reciprocity can generate evolutionarily stable levels of cooperation in a group or population. For instance, in very small groups it can establish cooperation virtually as reliably as direct reciprocity (Pfeiffer *et al.* 2005), but the latter is much more demanding and confined to specific conditions. In large but viscous populations, where interactions between individuals are not completely random, it can cause cooperation just as among a group of relatives (Rankin & Taborsky 2009). If the decisions to stay in a group and to cooperate through generalised reciprocity evolve independently, stable levels of cooperation and assortment between more and less cooperative individuals may result (Hamilton & Taborsky 2005).

So is generalised reciprocity responsible for cooperation among animals in nature? We know that it works in rats and humans, but we do not know yet how widespread it is, especially under natural conditions. If similar mechanisms, both at the ultimate and proximate levels, are responsible for winner and loser effects, this may be a very common phenomenon, indeed. To unravel its underlying mechanisms and importance in nature is one of the challenges I envisage for my future research. Simple mechanisms causing complex behaviour have always been the focus of my work. I believe in rule-of-thumb solutions. Animals are not selected to optimise responses to very specific situations, because the costs to acquire the appropriate information – both in the direct and in the evolutionary sense – are too high. Rather, animals are selected to get it *generally* right, and simple mechanisms such as winner and loser effects, and generalised reciprocity, do just this.

I have always been intrigued by the mechanisms underlying behavioural decisions, and particularly so in the social context, i.e. when interests of individuals differ. Most challenging, in my view, is the occurrence of cooperation and altruism, whereas egoism and exploitation is the default solution to competition that we should expect, treading in Darwin's footsteps. Why is cooperation so frequent between reproductive competitors, even if they are not related, and how does this work?

Fish are an excellent group to study this because of their enormous behavioural variation and complexity (Taborsky 1994, 2008a), and they also provide unique possibilities for an experimental approach, both in the field and in the lab (e.g. Taborsky 1984, 1985, Heg *et al.* 2004). Our research on cooperatively breeding fish has revealed that the importance of reciprocity had been vastly underestimated, mainly because of unrealistic assumptions about what is traded. In the past, research focused on potential cases where favours would be returned the like. It seems much more likely that the commodities traded between social partners differ, i.e. not a bone for a bone and a scratch for a scratch; rather, a reproductive opportunity is traded for help in defence (Taborsky *et al.* 1987, Martin & Taborsky 1997), or access to resources for participation in brood care (i.e. pay-to-stay: Taborsky 1984, 1985, Bergmüller & Taborsky 2005). This is probably where reciprocity has its greatest potential in nature.

My message here is that if we are not bedazzled by imagining 'what should be' and elegant theoretical paradigms that rest on sometimes unrealistic assumptions, but rather take into account what animals do and can do, we will understand the evolutionary mechanisms of cooperation much quicker. Empiricists tend to keep an eye on what theoreticians predict. Indeed, this is how science should work: theory – hypothesis – test (Taborsky 2008b). However, this should not be a view through a one-way mirror, theoreticians should also keep an eye on empirical results. We must learn better to learn from each other. Ironically, cooperation between theoreticians and empiricists is badly needed to unravel the mechanisms of cooperation.

References

Bartlett, M. Y. & DeSteno, D. (2006) Gratitude and pro-social behavior. *Psychological Science*, **17**, 319–325.

Bergmuller, R. & Taborsky, M. (2005) Experimental manipulation of helping in a cooperative breeder: helpers 'pay to stay' by pre-emptive appeasement. *Animal Behaviour*, **69**, 19–28.

Hamilton, I. M. & Taborsky, M. (2005) Contingent movement and cooperation evolve under generalized reciprocity. *Proceedings of the Royal Society B*, **272**, 2259–2267.

Hamilton, W. D. (1964) The genetical evolution of social behaviour, I & II. *Journal of Theoretical Biology*, **7**, 1–52.

Heg, D., Bachar, Z., Brouwer, L. & Taborsky, M. (2004) Predation risk is an ecological constraint for helper dispersal in a cooperatively breeding cichlid. *Proceedings of the Royal Society B*, **271**, 2367–2374.

Martin, E. & Taborsky, M. (1997) Alternative male mating tactics in a cichlid, *Pelvicachromis pulcher*: a comparison of reproductive effort and success. *Behavioral Ecology and Sociobiology*, **41**, 311–319.

Pfeiffer, T., Rutte, C., Killingback, T., Taborsky, M. & Bonhoeffer, S. (2005) Evolution of cooperation by generalized reciprocity. *Proceedings of the Royal Society B*, **272**, 1115–1120.

Queller, D. C. (1994) Genetic relatedness in viscous populations. *Evolutionary Ecology*, **8**, 70–73.

Rankin, D. J. & Taborsky, M. (2009) Assortment and the evolution of generalized reciprocity. *Evolution*, **63**, 1913–1922.

Rutte, C. & Taborsky, M. (2007) Generalized reciprocity in rats. *PLoS Biology*, **5** (7), 1421–1425.

Rutte, C., Taborsky, M. & Brinkhof, M. W. G. (2006) What sets the odds of winning and losing? *Trends in Ecology and Evolution*, **21**, 16–21.

Taborsky, M. (1984) Broodcare helpers in the cichlid fish *Lamprologus brichardi*: their costs and benefits. *Animal Behaviour*, **32**, 1236–1252.

Taborsky, M. (1985) Breeder-helper conflict in a cichlid fish with broodcare helpers: an experimental analysis. *Behaviour*, **95**, 45–75.

Taborsky, M., Hudde, B. & Wirtz, P. (1987) Reproductive behaviour and ecology of *Symphodus* (*Crenilabrus*) *ocellatus*, a European wrasse with four types of male behaviour. *Behaviour*, **102**, 82–118.

Taborsky, M. (1994) Sneakers, satellites and helpers: parasitic and cooperative behavior in fish reproduction. *Advances in the Study of Behavior*, **23**, 1–100.

Taborsky, M. (2008a) Alternative reproductive tactics in fish. In: *Alternative Reproductive Tactics: an Integrative Approach*, ed. R. F. Oliveira, M. Taborsky & H. J. Brockmann. Cambridge: Cambridge University Press, pp. 251–299.

Taborsky, M. (2008b) The use of theory in behavioural research. *Ethology*, **114**, 1–6.

Taylor, P. D. (1992) Altruism in viscous populations: an inclusive fitness model. *Evolutionary Ecology* **6**, 352–356.

Trivers, R. L. (1971) The evolution of reciprocal altruism. *Quarterly Review of Biology*, **46**, 35–57.

Wilson, D. S., Pollock, G. B. & Dugatkin, L. A. (1992) Can altruism evolve in purely viscous populations? *Evolutionary Ecology*, **6**, 331–341.

18

Population density, social behaviour and sex allocation

Suzanne H. Alonzo and Ben C. Sheldon

Overview

Evolution and ecology naturally intersect through birth, death and dispersal rates as they determine both population dynamics and individual fitness. However, we still understand very little about the connections between population dynamics, the evolution of individual behaviour patterns and the resulting social interactions. In this chapter, we first review how density affects individuals and discuss various ways in which population density is expected to influence social behaviour, using local competition for resources, reproductive cooperation and mating systems as illustrative examples. Following a brief introduction to evolutionary theory on sex allocation, we consider a few empirical examples from social insects, hermaphroditic fish, breeding birds and group-living mammals to demonstrate some of the observed patterns of sex allocation and the effect of density and social behaviour on these patterns. We then explore how sex allocation in hermaphrodites and sex ratios in cooperatively breeding animals can be used to demonstrate the links between sex allocation, sex ratio and social behaviours, as well as the difficulty and importance of understanding links between ecological and evolutionary dynamics generally. We finish the chapter with a discussion of directions for future empirical and theoretical research.

18.1 Introduction

Social behaviour takes diverse and fascinating forms in a wide variety of taxa, as the chapters in this book demonstrate. In this chapter, we examine the links between population density, social behaviour and sex allocation as an illustrative example of the general connection between individual-level processes and population patterns. Sex allocation refers to the way in which parental reproductive value, or other resources (such as time or energy), are divided into the production of sons and daughters in species with separate sexes, or to male and female reproduction (production of sperm and eggs) in hermaphrodites. There is a rich body of theory, and associated empirical work, dealing with the circumstances that favour the departures from equal allocation into males and females (Shaw & Mohler 1953, Charnov 1982). Whereas population density is inherently a population-level phenomenon,

Social Behaviour: Genes, Ecology and Evolution, ed. Tamás Székely, Allen J. Moore and Jan Komdeur. Published by Cambridge University Press. © Cambridge University Press 2010.

it results from the reproduction, survival and movement of individuals. These individual processes are often the outcome of social interactions, where population density affects the evolution and expression of individual behaviour, for example by influencing the frequency of encounters and the intensity of competition between individuals (Chapters 4 and 6). If we define a social behaviour as any direct behavioural interaction between individuals, then it becomes clear that social interactions provide an intuitive link between individual and population processes. Here, we focus our discussion on interactions within species. Yet social behaviour will also be influenced by other species through the abundance of prey, interspecific competition and the prevalence of disease and other natural enemies.

The links between population density, social behaviour and sex allocation demonstrate the connection between evolutionary and ecological dynamics (Fig. 18.1). Extensive theoretical and empirical research on behaviour has shown that ecological conditions (such as the abundance of food or risk of predation) affect the evolution and expression of traits (such as foraging and mating behaviour: see Chapters 9–12). Research also clearly demonstrates that individual behaviour affects population dynamics and thus local density. We know therefore that ecological conditions affect evolutionary dynamics, and that evolved traits affect ecology (see also Chapter 4). However, relatively little is known about how the feedback loops between ecological and evolutionary dynamics affect social

behaviour. For example, local population density will influence social interactions by affecting competition, mating opportunities and the potential for cooperation (Fig. 18.2 left and middle). However, social behaviours also affect population dynamics through their effect on reproduction, survival and dispersal (Fig. 18.2 top and left). Thus population growth rate and ecological conditions affect density, and density influences selection on social behaviours (such as group living or territoriality), which themselves feed back to influence density. In addition, sex allocation affects the number of females in the population and thus population growth rate, but also responds to local density and competition for resources (Fig. 18.2 right). Finally, dispersal affects not only density but also relatedness among individuals in a social group, which may together affect the evolution of social behaviours and sex allocation (Fig. 18.2 bottom). In reality, these dynamics are tightly coupled, such that one does not simply cause the other. Instead, multiple feedback loops exist where density affects selection on social behaviour, which influences sex allocation, which then affects density and behaviour (Figs. 18.1, 18.2). The study of social behaviour thus provides a challenging opportunity to examine the links between evolutionary and ecological dynamics.

In this chapter we first examine the effect of density on individuals, and how social behaviour is both affected by, and in turn affects, density. Following an overview of sex-allocation theory, we consider how sex allocation may be affected by population density

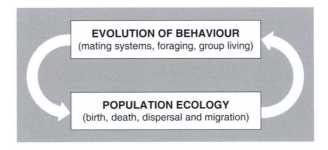

Figure 18.1 Ecological and evolutionary dynamics interact and form feedback loops. Whereas much is known about how ecological conditions affect behaviour, and how behaviours affect population ecology, little is known about how evolutionary and ecological dynamics interact to simultaneously generate observed patterns.

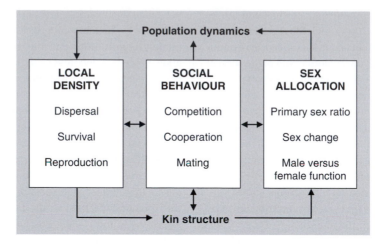

Figure 18.2 There are many interactions between density, social behaviour and sex where both population dynamics and kin structure influence and are influenced by selection on individuals and population-level patterns. See text for details.

and social structure. We then consider sex allocation in hermaphrodites, and sex ratios in cooperatively breeding animals, as illustrative examples, and finish the chapter with a discussion of directions for future empirical and theoretical research.

18.2 Density links individuals and populations

Animals and plants distribute themselves across environments, either through passive dispersal (e.g. in winds and currents) or by active movement and subsequent habitat choice. In either case, environmental heterogeneity in the processes causing passive dispersal, or in the suitability of habitats for animals to settle in, often creates spatial variation in density of individuals. This is further augmented by temporal variation in density, due both to variation over the course of reproductive and annual cycles and to longer-period variation (e.g. climatic effects on population size, masting in food plants, population cycles in prey, directional changes due to human modification of environments: see Turchin 2005 for a general review). Hence, population density is variable at many levels, from short-term local effects (e.g. transient changes over the course of seconds in the

number of animals exploiting a patch of food) up to long-term broad-scale effects (e.g. large-scale long-term synchrony in the population dynamics of many boreal vertebrates, which may have periodicity of several generations, and show synchrony over distances of thousands of kilometres: e.g. Stenseth *et al.* 1999).

The focus above suggests that inferences about the effect of density on behaviours will depend on the temporal and spatial scale at which density is measured, and will vary among individuals within the same population. Population density can obviously only be estimated once one has information about a sample of individuals in some defined area. Yet individuals are not likely to experience the same population density, either because they were sampled at different times within a population cycle, or because they came from different parts of an organism's range or from different habitats in which the local density varies. For example, in group-living, territorial organisms, the size of the social group may be the aspect of population density that has the largest effect on individual behaviour and expected fitness (rather than the density of individuals at a larger spatial scale: e.g. Brouwer *et al.* 2006). The effect of density on individuals is generally mediated through social interactions, which will also vary spatially and temporally. For example, the effect of population density (measured as distribution of competitors per unit area) on the behaviour of territorial male reef fish may be stronger when mating opportunities are scarce or on parts of the reef that attract fewer females (e.g. Warner 2002).

The extent to which an individual measure of population density is relevant, or can be replaced by a population-specific measure, is likely to depend on the biological details of the processes under study. For example, in territorial animals, such as altricial birds rearing offspring, the constraints imposed by central-place foraging mean that the scale of competition that is relevant for density-dependent effects is likely to be rather small for that stage of the reproductive cycle. Later, if those offspring disperse to find breeding sites of their own, the relevant scale at which density should be measured, if one is interested in the direct effects of population density on the probability of settling on a territory, is likely to be much larger, and will be a function of the dispersal distance. Studies that have explored the operation of density dependence within populations often find that the scale depends on the process considered (e.g. Wilkin *et al.* 2006).

18.3 Interactions between density, dispersal and social behaviour

Density affects, and is affected by, social interactions in a myriad ways well beyond the scope of what can be covered here. We describe some of the ways in which density and social behaviour interact, and then illustrate these interactions with examples. At a basic level, population density affects the frequency of individual encounters and thus the potential for social interactions. Increased density also generally increases competition. As a result, density has the potential to affect any behavioural interaction from foraging and hunting to mating and parental care. When individuals compete, the frequency and intensity of antagonistic interactions over limiting resources will often increase with density. However, competition for limited reproductive sites can also favour cooperative breeding by reducing the potential for individuals to disperse and reproduce independently (e.g. Komdeur 1992). Mating systems

are also affected by local density, with high density increasing competition for mates while also increasing the potential for individuals to defend and compare among multiple mates (e.g. Emlen & Oring 1977). Hence the effect of density on social behaviours is complex, and increasing density can either enhance antagonism or favour cooperation, depending on the specific situation. At present, no general theory exists that can predict the expected effect of population density on whether cooperation or conflict arises among individuals.

Density influences behaviour, and social interactions affect density through patterns of dispersal, survival and reproductive rates (Fig. 18.2). Antagonistic interactions typically increase dispersion, and thus decrease density. For example, territoriality causes individuals to be overdispersed in space, all else being equal. By contrast, local density typically increases when individuals cooperate with respect to breeding, hunting and predator defence. Dispersal is influenced by the social system, but also itself influences the social behaviour of species through its effect on local density and population structure (see also Chapter 12). Organisms with low dispersal distances and rates may occur in groups of related individuals, which allows for the evolution of cooperation through kin selection but also enhances direct competition among relatives (Hamilton 1963). High dispersal rates typically lead to low relatedness among individuals in a location and can be associated with both high and low population density, depending on habitat selection and population dynamics. In general, density, dispersal and habitat selection will depend on the intensity of competition for resources and the extent to which social interactions are antagonistic versus cooperative within a given species.

We now examine specific examples that illustrate how social interactions affect, and are affected by, density and dispersal. In many marine organisms dispersal distance is high, and most individuals will not interact frequently with close relatives. However, this does not mean that marine organisms do not live in social groups at high density or exhibit complex behavioural interactions. For example, in the clown anemonefish *Amphiprion percula*, larvae disperse widely but settle on their host anemones with con-specifics, leading to groups of unrelated individuals living together, with as many as six individuals living on one anemone (Buston *et al.* 2007). Size-dependent dominance hierarchies form on each anemone host, where typically only the largest individuals repro-duce (Buston 2003a). However, all individuals bene-fit from the shared defence of their anemone, which provides essential refuge from predation, and non-reproductive subordinates typically grow and replace the dominant reproductive individuals when they die (Buston 2004). High densities of fish can lead to conflict during reproduction and settlement affect-ing survival, dispersal and reproduction, and thus influencing future population density (Buston 2003a, 2003b). However, evidence also exists that the body size and dominance hierarchies can stabilise social interactions within a group (Buston 2003a), despite the inherent evolutionary conflict between individ-uals over reproduction.

In many birds and mammals dispersal is sex-biased, leading to social groups with individuals of one sex being closely related, whereas the other sex is unrelated (Greenwood 1980, Clobert *et al.* 2001). Sex-specific differences in dispersal affect both local population density and patterns of relatedness among individuals. In the Belding's ground squirrel *Spermophilus beldingi*, females tend to remain near their natal site, are often closely related, and prod-uce alarm calls that increase the survival of their female relatives (Sherman 1977). In contrast, males do not produce alarm calls and often disperse far from the natal sites, presumably to avoid inbreed-ing and decrease competition for mates (Holekamp & Sherman 1989). However, dispersal, survival and reproduction also increase with individual body condition and respond to local density (Holekamp & Sherman 1989). In this species, male-biased dispersal leads to female relatives living in close proximity at high density. The evolution of female alarm calls has likely been favoured through kin selection due to the enhanced survival of relatives, and through the dir-ect benefits of exhibiting alarm calls at high density to decrease individual predation risk. However, selec-tion on dispersal (which affects both local density

and the potential for kin selection) is influenced by the costs and benefits of social interactions and local density (see Chapter 12). In the Belding's ground squirrel, patterns of dispersal affect local population density and social interactions among females, while these social interactions may further favour high density and limited dispersal of females.

One of the best examples of population density affecting social behaviour comes from long-term studies of Seychelles warblers *Acrocephalus sechellen-sis*. The Seychelles warbler is restricted to a few small islands in the Indian Ocean, where it often lives in extended family groups composed of a pair of adults and a variable number of their offspring from previ-ous breeding attempts. Birds defend reproductive ter-ritories that differ in the abundance of important food resources (Komdeur 1992). These reproductive sites can be limiting at high density, in which case some of the offspring, frequently daughters, remain in their natal territory and help their parents raise the next brood (Komdeur 2003). In an elegant experiment, birds were transplanted to islands with unoccupied territories (as part of a reintroduction plan following habitat restoration) where the behaviour, density and dispersal of the birds were observed following the transplant (Komdeur 1992, 2003). Immediately fol-lowing the transplant, when birds were at low dens-ities and when many high-quality territories were available, surviving offspring dispersed from their natal territory and attempted to breed independ-ently, and no helping behaviour was observed. As the density of birds increased on the island, offspring from high-quality territories (with more abundant food) began to stay at their natal territory to help raise young even though low-quality territories (with lim-ited food) were available. Subsequent research has shown that a few helpers on a high-quality territory increase the total reproductive success of the group, while individuals that remain on low-quality terri-tories actually increase competition for food such that the reproductive success of the group decreases (Komdeur 2003). This species therefore exhibits a strong effect of density on dispersal, cooperative breeding and competition for territories and food resources. However, the abundance of food resources interacts with density to influence patterns of dispersal, competition and cooperative breeding (which in turn affects group reproductive success and local density). It is worth noting that the powerful inferences drawn in these specific examples come from conducting careful experiments (mainly in the wild) combined with detailed, often lifetime, observations of individuals to determine patterns of density, social behaviour and fitness.

18.4 Sex allocation as an example linking density and social behaviour

18.4.1 A brief overview of the foundations of sex-allocation theory

It has long been noted that in most species with separate sexes (males and females), we observe approximately equal primary sex ratios (the proportion of sons versus daughters produced before any mortality occurs). The explanation for the ubiquity of equal primary sex ratios has traditionally been attributed to Fisher (1930). However, as detailed by Edwards (1998), the important elements of the idea were actually outlined by Darwin in the first edition of *The Descent of Man and Selection in Relation to Sex* in 1871 (subsequently removed from later editions and replaced with the famous statement that 'the whole problem is so intricate that it is safer to leave its solution for the future': Darwin 1874 p. 399), and a formal mathematical proof was provided by Düsing in 1884, almost half a century before Fisher (discussed in Edwards 1998). The central point of the argument, whoever it is attributed to, is based on the realisation that, because each individual (in a diploid sexual species) has exactly one mother and one father, then the total reproductive success of males and females must be equal. As a consequence, the individual expected fitness of sons and daughter will be negatively frequency-dependent. When males are rarer than females, females will have lower average fitness than males, as although all females may be fertilised by a male, the average male will fertilise more eggs than the average female produces. By contrast, if males are common and females

rare, the average male will have lower reproductive success than the average female. The evolutionarily stable sex ratio (assuming equal costs of males and females) occurs where equal proportions of sons and daughters are produced, because otherwise individuals of the less common sex would have greater relative fitness (see also Chapter 4).

This can be proven mathematically in many ways. For example, consider the following mathematical representation of Fisher's (1930) argument (Maynard Smith 1982). Let s represent the sex ratio (proportion of individuals that are male) where N is the total number of offspring produced per female. The expected fitness (measured as the number of grand-offspring) of an individual producing sex ratio s in a population of individuals that produce a sex ratio s' will be

$$w(s,s') = N\left[N(1-s) + Ns\left(\frac{1-s'}{s'}\right)\right]$$
$$= N^2(1-s) + N^2 s\left(\frac{1-s'}{s'}\right)$$

(18.1)

where $N^2(1-s)$ gives the number of grand-offspring produced by $N(1-s)$ daughters and $N^2 s((1-s')/s')$ gives the number of grand-offspring produced by Ns sons, assuming male fertilisation success is determined by the ratio of females to males in the population (given by $(1-s')/s'$). The evolutionarily stable sex ratio occurs at the sex ratio s^* for which there is no other sex ratio s that could have higher fitness when the rest of the population adopts s^* (Maynard Smith 1982). Mathematically this is found by differentiating the fitness function $w(s,s^*)$ with respect to s, setting $\partial w(s,s^*)/\partial s$ equal to zero and solving for s^* when $s = s^*$ (Maynard Smith 1982) which gives

$$\frac{\partial w(s,s^*)}{\partial s}\bigg|_{s=s^*} = -N^2 + N^2 \frac{(1-s^*)}{s^*} = 0$$

(18.2)

which can be rearranged to show that $s^* = 1 - s^*$ or $s^* = 1/2$, which implies that the stable sex ratio is equal sons and daughters. Note that this argument holds even if mortality is not equal between sons and daughters (Fisher 1930). Also, Fisher couched his model in terms of investment in the two sexes, and this provides a general model, in which the evolutionarily stable strategy (ESS) is for equality in the investment ratio of the two sexes.

Based on the above, one might not expect to find any deviations from an equal investment ratio in the two sexes. However, biased offspring sex ratios are not infrequently observed at the population level (e.g. Hamilton 1967, Godfray & Werren 1996, West *et al.* 2005). Furthermore, because Fisher's model is one that predicts the ESS, which is a population-level phenomenon, it has rather little to say about the way that individuals invest in the two sexes. For example, unless population size is very small, there is no difference between a population in which all females invest exactly equally in males and females, and one in which half invest everything in males and half invest everything in females (Charnov 1982).

There are many potential explanations for deviations from the basic Fisherian model, which can all be expressed in terms of breaking of implicit assumptions of the model. For example, when sex is inherited in a non-Mendelian fashion, or when mating is non-random within kin-structured populations, then spectacular deviations from an equal sex allocation ratio may arise. In this sense, Fisher's argument provides a useful null model with which to explore the evolution of deviations from equal investment ratios.

A general way to express the class of explanations for deviations from ideal Fisherian equal sex allocation is based upon the idea that the costs and benefits associated with producing male and female offspring are not necessarily equal for all individuals, or perhaps, in general, for all replicating entities (this phrasing captures, for example, the way that selection acts on sex allocation from the perspective of sex-linked drive genes: Hamilton 1967). Many developments in sex-ratio theory demonstrate that differences in the net benefit from sons versus daughters can favour biased sex ratios (e.g. Hamilton 1967, Charnov 1982, Pen & Weissing 2000, Alonzo & Sinervo, 2007, Wild & West 2007). For example, Hamilton (1967) recognised that differences between the sexes in the effects of local mate competition among related individuals affect the net benefit of producing sons and daughters in structured populations, whereas Trivers and Willard (1973) argued that when the net benefit of producing

sons and daughters is condition-dependent, individuals may have different sex-ratio optima.

The argument that sex allocation biases are expected when individuals experience a net fitness gain by biasing their allocation to one sex over the other is captured by the Shaw–Mohler equation (Shaw & Mohler 1953). Imagine that an individual can allocate energy (or other resources) between sons and daughters. Then, a biased sex ratio (or change in sex allocation more generally) will be favoured whenever individual fitness is increased by an adjustment in investment such that

$$\frac{\Delta m}{M} + \frac{\Delta f}{F} > 0 \qquad (18.3)$$

where Δm and Δf represent the change in fitness through sons and daughters based on the deviation in sex allocation (or changes in allocation to male versus female reproduction in hermaphrodites), and M and F represent the average fitness of males and females in the population. If an individual experiences a net fitness gain (i.e. the left-hand side of the equation is greater than zero) then a change in sex allocation is predicted to be favoured by selection. This argument is especially important for understanding sex allocation in hermaphrodites, as is discussed in more detail below.

It is important to remember that Fisher's theory only relates to the investment ratio at the end of parental care. Differences in male and female survival (perhaps due to sex-specific dispersal or reproductive patterns) can easily cause deviations from unity in the adult sex ratio overall, or in the operational sex ratio (defined as the ratio of sexually receptive males to receptive females: Emlen & Oring 1977), but these differences of themselves have no consequence for the sex-allocation decisions of the parent, provided that they cannot be anticipated by parental behaviour.

18.4.2 Sex allocation from populations to individuals

A particularly instructive example of sex-allocation theory, which has been studied extensively both empirically and theoretically, and which captures the way that individual and population-level phenomena can blend into each other, concerns the effect of local mate competition on the sex ratio. Hamilton pointed out, in his classic 1967 paper entitled 'Extraordinary sex ratios' that, when populations were highly structured, with the result that competition for matings occurred between male relatives, this caused selection for a sex ratio biased strongly towards females. In effect, because competition between brothers for matings is wasted from the point of view of the female, the fact that the reproductive output of her daughters is limited by the rate at which they can produce eggs becomes much more important than in outbreeding populations. Hamilton showed that, when N females laid eggs in a patch, and when mating was restricted to patches, the ESS sex ratio was a simple function of the number of females, being equal to $(N - 1)/2N$. There are spectacular examples of strongly biased sex ratios that seem compatible with Hamilton's model, such as the mite *Acarophenox tribolii* in which a female's sons copulate with their sisters inside their mother: because competition does not get much more local than this, the observation that the sex ratio is biased as much as 14 to 1 in favour of females is not surprising (Hamilton 1967). In addition to explaining such fascinating and – from a human perspective – bizarre biology, applications of local mate competition have produced key tests of general principles in evolutionary biology, such as Herre's demonstration that the precision of sex-ratio adaptation in fig wasps depends on the selective regime they experience (Herre 1987). Local mate-competition theory has also been applied to predict important population characteristics, such as the rate of outcrossing in malaria parasites (see West *et al.* 2000 for a general review, and Reece *et al.* 2008 for empirical evidence).

Hamilton's basic model is thus very powerful, even if it is simple, with only one variable entering the equation to predict the ESS. His model can be considered to be a more general sex-ratio model than Fisher's, with respect to the effects of population size. Fisher's model applies to ideal populations, i.e. those in which, among other things, an infinite number of individuals mate at random. From Hamilton's equation, when N is large, the ESS sex ratio tends towards 0.5; Hamilton's model also tells us what happens when population size becomes small, and, as a result, mating becomes increasingly non-random, and hence competition between males for matings becomes increasingly between brothers. One reason why Fisher's theory is considered important in the history of evolutionary biology is that it demonstrates that selection at the level of groups may be overwhelmed by selection at the level of individuals: although the sex ratio that would maximise population growth rate is one that is strongly female-biased, this is vulnerable to invasion by strategies that produce more males. Hamilton's treatment of local mate competition shows us that both individual and group-level selection can converge, but this only happens when groups become very small – effectively the same as individuals.

18.5 Empirical examples connecting density, social behaviour and sex allocation

18.5.1 From individual allocation to population patterns in hermaphrodites

In species with separate sexes an equal sex ratio is the most common expected and observed pattern, but this need not be the case either theoretically or empirically in hermaphroditic species (Charnov 1982, Allsop & West 2004). In simultaneous hermaphrodites (species where individuals simultaneously produce both male and female gametes, such as many snails and marine flatworms), individuals often allocate more of their gonad mass to the production of eggs, especially at low densities (e.g. Johnston *et al.* 1998). Density directly affects the frequency of individual encounters and thus the potential for mating opportunities (Fig. 18.2). At one extreme, some simultaneous hermaphrodites rarely encounter conspecifics, and are thus capable of self-fertilisation. In the latter case, sex-allocation theory would predict that individuals should only produce sufficient sperm to fertilise their own eggs, otherwise their own sperm will be in competition (as in the case of competition among siblings described above). However, when density is high, mating opportunities may increase. If individuals mate with (and receive sperm from) multiple individuals, then the risk and intensity of sperm competition will be high. Sperm-allocation theory then predicts that individuals should increase their allocation to sperm production compared to the situation where individuals usually self-fertilise or mate with a single individual (all else being equal: Parker 1998). Hence, in simultaneous hermaphrodites, population density can influence sex allocation through the effect of density on the frequency of self-fertilisation and multiple mating.

Sequential hermaphrodites (species that change sex over their lifetime) typically exhibit a population-level sex-ratio bias towards the sex that occurs first (Charnov 1982, Allsop & West 2004). However, extensive within- and between-species variation in these patterns exists (Allsop & West 2004), and much research has focused on documenting the predicted patterns and understanding the many deviations from those expectations.

The most influential theory for understanding sex allocation in sequential hermaphrodites has been the size-advantage model (Ghiselin 1969, Warner 1975, Charnov 1982). This theory makes predictions about the direction and timing of sex change (Fig. 18.3). First, it predicts that if the expected reproductive success of one sex increases more than the other sex with size (or related traits such as age or dominance), individuals should switch from the sex that has the reproductive advantage when small to the sex that has the reproductive advantage when large. Individuals are predicted to change sex at the size (or level of other trait) at which the residual reproductive value of the second sex exceeds the first (Fig. 18.3). In sex-changing species in which males defend females, territories or resources (and large males have greater reproductive success than small males), we tend to observe that species change from female to male as they grow larger (as in the bluehead wrasse discussed below). In contrast, in sequential hermaphrodites where male reproductive success is relatively unaffected by size relative to the increase in female fecundity with size, we tend to observe that species change from male to female (which is observed in the clown anemonefish described above).

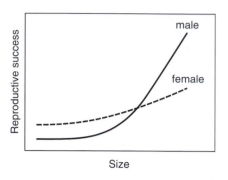

Figure 18.3 The size-advantage model. Each line represents expected male or female reproductive success as a function of individual size. Sex change is predicted to occur at the size where the lines intersect. Protogynous sex change (female to male) is expected if male reproductive success (e.g. solid line) increases more rapidly with size than female fitness (e.g. dashed line). In contrast, protandrous sex change (male to female) would be predicted if females were represented by the solid line and males by the dashed line (adapted from Ghiselin 1969).

One of the best-studied species exhibiting sex change is the bluehead wrasse *Thalassoma bifasciatum*, in which some individuals change sex from female to male, whereas other individuals mature as small males and remain male. Large males exhibit different colour and behaviour patterns (termed terminal-phase or TP males) than either females or small males (initial-phase or IP males and females: Warner 2002). Large TP males defend spawning territories and court females but do not provide parental care of offspring (Warner 2002). Smaller (IP) males either spawn parasitically with a territorial male and female or join groups of other small males and spawn within a group. Given the advantage of being a territorial male when large, the direction of sex change (from female to male) is consistent with the size-advantage model (Warner 2002). However, this does not explain why other individuals start life as male and remain male as they grow larger. These males do, however, exhibit a striking stage change from IP male to TP male, with associated physical and behavioural changes (Warner 2002).

Density-dependent variation in the frequency, reproductive success and behaviour of IP males exists among populations. However, no evidence for local genetic structure among population exists (Haney *et al.* 2007), and larvae can be dispersed widely during a pelagic larval stage (Swearer *et al.* 1999). At sites with high population density, IP males are common and defend the best mating sites as a group, thus achieving high mating success (Warner 2002). However, at low density, large TP males tend to dominate territories and group spawning is much less common. Instead, small males spawn as sneakers with much lower mating success. At extremely high densities, territoriality does not occur, and all fish spawn in large groups (of more than 10 000 fish). Recent evidence exists that local population density affects the primary sex ratio (e.g. how many larvae at a site develop into initial-phase males versus initial females at a site: Munday *et al.* 2006). Hence local density, produced largely by externally determined patterns of settlement (Swearer *et al.* 1999), affects the social system, reproductive patterns and primary sex ratio observed in this species.

Sex change in this species is also socially controlled (Warner & Swearer 1991). When a large TP male dies or is removed experimentally, the next largest IP individual typically takes over his territory, and if female changes sex (Warner & Swearer 1991). Sex change occurs rapidly, with individuals producing male-typical behaviour within minutes, changing colour pattern within days and producing viable sperm in about a week (Warner & Swearer 1991). Although social dominance is the external trigger for sex change, gonadectomy has shown that behavioural change from IP female to TP male can occur in the absence of a gonad (Godwin *et al.* 1996), and that behaviour, social interactions and patterns of sex change can all be altered by neuropeptides (e.g. Semsar & Godwin 2003)

Sex allocation in hermaphrodites is of broad general interest to evolutionary biologists; it also has important implications for population dynamics. Population growth is typically assumed to be determined by female rather than male biomass, and thus (all else being equal) allocation to female function in hermaphrodites should also influence population dynamics (e.g. Alonzo & Mangel 2004).

A number of commercially exploited marine species are sequential hermaphrodites, making it important to understand the effect of sex change on population dynamics (Alonzo & Mangel 2004). In California sheephead *Semicossyphus pulcher*, large individuals are preferentially removed by the fishery, and recent evidence exists that this stock has been heavily fished, reducing male biomass in the population (Alonzo *et al.* 2008). If size at sex change is fixed, this could lead to large, sudden, effects of fishing on population dynamics so that traditional management measures underestimate the effect of fishing on stock populations (Alonzo & Mangel 2004). Yet the effect of rapid changes in density on patterns of sex allocation are not known. Evidence exists that fishing mortality can alter life-history patterns such as age at maturity (e.g. Munch *et al.* 2005). However, we know little about how human-induced evolution of sex allocation will affect management and conservation. Changes to the mating system and population structure are also likely when large individuals are preferentially removed, and this can have unknown effects on sex allocation and population dynamics, especially as we do not know the cues or mechanisms that govern sex allocation in most organisms. A greater understanding of the interaction between density, social behaviour and sex allocation will not only allow us to explore the evolutionary and ecological dynamics linking populations and individual processes but will also aid in our conservation and management of many commercially exploited species.

18.5.2 Competitive and cooperative interactions between relatives and sex allocation

Above, we outlined core ideas involved in the effects of local mate competition on sex allocation. Local mate competition is a special case of a general set of effects on sex ratio, which can be viewed as resulting from sex-biased social interactions between relatives that are either competitive or cooperative in nature. These are generally termed local resource competition and local resource enhancement, respectively,

Table 18.1. Classification of sex-biased interactions between relatives that influence optimal sex-allocation behaviour, with empirical examples discussed in the text.

		Type of interaction between relatives	
		Positive	Negative
Generational interaction	Within	Coalitions of male lions (Packer & Pusey 1987)	Local mate competition (Hamilton 1967)
	Between	Repayment by helpers at the nest (Komdeur et al. 1997)[a]	Competition between female possums (Johnson et al. 2001)

[a] Komdeur et al. (1997) can also provide an example of negative, intergenerational interactions selecting on the sex ratio.

and can occur due to interactions either between or within generations (e.g. local mate competition is an example of a competitive sex-biased interaction occurring within a generation; see Table 18.1 for a summary, with associated empirical examples, which are discussed below). These effects can be thought of as lying at either end of a continuum from positive through to negative interactions between individuals of the same sex, and there are some striking examples of these processes known, particularly from vertebrates. In many cases, the operation of these effects depends critically upon an effect of density, or on the operation of processes that are density-dependent. We review some of these cases below.

Whereas local mate competition involves competitive interactions between males from the same generation, sex-biased competitive interactions may arise between generations when one sex shows limited dispersal. An illuminating example of this is the work by Johnson et al. (2001) on local resource competition in common brushtail possums *Trichosurus vulpecula*. In this species, as in many mammals, females show strong natal philopatry whereas males disperse when they reach sexual maturity. Since daughters remain close to their mother, the potential exists for competition between mothers and their daughters over access to any limiting resource. The key limiting resource in this example concerns access to dens in trees. When these are in short supply, the effect of having daughters will be to elevate competition between mother and daughters, reducing the expected fitness return from female offspring (this could be argued as resulting

both from negative effects of the daughters on their mother, and from negative effects of the mother and of other daughters on any given daughter). Johnson et al. (2001) showed that, across eight populations of possums, areas with high food density could support high-density possum populations, and that the offspring sex ratio was inversely related to the per capita availability of dens: more sons were produced when the competition was more intense.

Thus far, we have only discussed competitive interactions, but there are cases in which there might be positive (i.e. cooperative) interactions between same-sex relatives. An interesting example of this process, and its consequences for sex allocation, occurring within generations, was provided by Packer and Pusey's (1987) study of the sex-ratio distribution in litters of African lions *Panthera leo*. Female lions are the core members of social groups, known as prides; males generally enjoy much briefer tenure of a pride, and while they have tenure they are selected to maximise their reproductive output. Packer and Pusey (1987) showed that the success of a male lion in gaining tenure, in maintaining tenure in the face of challenges from other males, and in terms of the size of pride in which he gained tenure, were all steeply increasing functions of the number of male cubs born in the same year in the male's natal pride. In contrast, the fitness of a female was unrelated to the number of females in her cohort. These functions suggest that male fitness, relative to female fitness, would be increased if males were more often born together with male siblings. Packer and Pusey showed that this prediction was indeed borne out by the data, with three- and four-cub litters being disproportionately often composed of an excess of males.

We close this selection of empirical examples with one of the most striking examples of adaptive sex-ratio variation in a vertebrate, that of sex allocation in response to helper number and territory quality in the Seychelles warbler (e.g. Komdeur 2003). This example illustrates that positive and negative sex-biased interactions can occur within the same species, even within the same population. In the Seychelles warbler, extended family groups are composed of a pair of adults and a variable number of their offspring from previous breeding attempts. Many of these offspring assist their parents in rearing more young, but most of this helping behaviour is provided by females. This provides the opportunity for female offspring to repay part of the cost of their rearing to the parents, and suggests that parents might be selected to produce an overall bias in their offspring towards females. However, the effect of helpers on the fitness of their parents depends on the quality of the territory on which they live, and this has important consequences for the way that selection acts on the sex ratio. In short, when territory quality (measured as food abundance) is high, then there is sufficient food for both helpers and the production of more offspring; when territory quality is low, helpers deplete food and thus make it harder for parents to rear their own offspring successfully. Komdeur and colleagues have shown that female warblers exhibit remarkably strong shifts in the sex ratio of their offspring in response to territory quality, with a shift from 80% male offspring on lower-quality territories to < 20% males on the highest-quality territories (Komdeur 2003). In effect, as territory quality changes across the population, helpers shift from being helpful to being unhelpful, an effect mediated by an interaction between group size and food abundance. Comparative analyses across helping species of vertebrates show that the same effect can be seen across species, with stronger sex-ratio biases towards the helping sex in species where helpers are most helpful (Griffin et al. 2005).

18.6 Conclusions and future directions

In this chapter we have discussed some of the linkages between individuals and populations mediated through social behaviour, concentrating specifically on the links between population density and sex allocation. We summarise numerous areas of linkage between these areas, and conclude with challenges and suggestions for further work.

A common difficulty in this field is in moving beyond the observation of patterns to understanding their causal and functional significance. For example, many studies of sex-ratio variation, in this field of sex allocation as well as in others, draw strong inferences about the adaptive value of sex-ratio strategies without sufficient information on the effect of sex allocation on individual fitness. Studies are often observational, rather than experimental, and this presents the usual problems with respect to assuming causality. The minority of studies that are experimental in nature generally take the form of manipulating variable X, where X is assumed to be selecting for changes in the sex ratio, and then observing whether or not the sex ratio changes in response (under an assumption of phenotypic plasticity). Although this provides good evidence that any relationship between X and the sex ratio is causal, it provides little relevant evidence to test the hypothesis that the sex-ratio change in response to X is adaptive (i.e. increases fitness relative to other patterns). There are many other potential causes of changes in the sex ratio, such as sex-biased mortality, pathology, and non-selected physiological artefacts. It is perhaps surprising that an area often heralded as providing exceptional support for adaptive theories of animal behaviour (e.g. West et al. 2000) consists of so few direct tests of whether the observed patterns of sex allocation are actually adaptive (though see Reece et al. 2008 for a fascinating recent exception). These sorts of experiments are challenging to carry out (as they require both phenotypic variation in sex allocation and information on the long-term fitness effects of these patterns). One alternative approach may be to test the predictions of the hypotheses using phylogenetic comparative methods (Chapter 5; Griffin et al. 2005).

Sex allocation illustrates some other general problems that are common to many fields in evolutionary and behavioural ecology. In many cases, theoretical developments have proceeded to the extent that there are highly complex theoretical predictions about the interacting effects of different selection pressures in different environments. For instance, a recent model of sex ratios by Wild and West (2007), combining the effects of local resource competition and conditional sex allocation, constitutes an intimidating landscape (a veritable 'Wild West') for those seeking simple, easily testable empirical predictions. Of course, our ultimate aim is to try to understand how to apply these models to real-world systems, which are surely just as complex, if not more so, but we are hampered by our lack of ability to measure key variables. For example, the extent to which sex-biased interactions are competitive or cooperative is key for understanding the relative fitness of male and female offspring, but it may be difficult to establish even something as simple as the sign of the effect. One approach is to use theory to predict adaptive rules of thumb for species in which sufficient long-term data are available so that models can be parameterised, and in which experiments can allow rigorous tests of the theory (e.g. Alonzo & Sinervo 2007).

We wish to conclude by suggesting that, while further progress will require some hard work, the prospects are not universally gloomy. Sometimes, simple theory provides a remarkably accurate and powerful tool for understanding remarkable biological details. For example, Hamilton's sex-ratio models to account for local mate competition are simple but have great explanatory power (Hamilton 1967, Herre 1987). Similarly, the size-advantage model (though not without flaws) can explain much of the observed within-species patterns of sequential sex change. In addition, the lack of experimental work examining the fitness effects of sex allocation (mentioned above) does not seem, at least to us, to be due to insurmountable difficulties with the experiments; we hope that many such experiments will be performed in the near future. In fact, one very exciting area of research on sex allocation, and more

generally sex determination, is the intersection of proximate and ultimate explanations to explain not only how and why animals deviate from equal sex allocation, but also the degree to which the underlying mechanisms evolve both within and between species.

Acknowledgements

We thank our many colleagues who have helped shape our thoughts on this subject, especially Erem Kazancioglu, Marc Mangel, Robert Warner and Stuart West. We also acknowledge two anonymous reviewers for constructive comments on an earlier draft of this chapter. SHA was supported by funds from the Royal Society of London, the National Science Foundation and Yale University.

Suggested readings

Charnov, E. L. (1982) *The Theory of Sex Allocation*. Princeton, NJ: Princeton University Press.

Hamilton, W. D. (1967) Extraordinary sex ratios. *Science*, **156**, 477–487.

Komdeur, J. (2003) Daughters on request: about helpers and egg sexes in the Seychelles warbler. *Proceedings of the Royal Society B*, **270**, 3–11.

Trivers, E. L. & Willard, D. E. (1973) Natural selection of parental ability to vary the sex ratio of offspring. *Science*, **179**, 90–92.

West, S. A. (2009) *Sex Allocation*. Princeton, NJ: Princeton University Press.

West, S. A., Shuker, D. M. & Sheldon, B. C. (2005) Sex-ratio adjustment when relatives interact: a test of constraints on adaptation. *Evolution*, **59**, 1211–1228.

References

Allsop, D. J. & West, S. A. (2004) Sex-ratio evolution in sex changing animals. *Evolution*, **58**, 1019–1027.

Alonzo, S. H. & Mangel, M. (2004) The effects of size-selective fisheries on the stock dynamics of and sperm limitation in sex changing fish: California sheephead (*Semicossyphus pulcher*) as an illustrative example. *Fishery Bulletin*, **102**, 1–13.

Alonzo, S. H. & Sinervo, B. (2007) The effect of sexually antagonistic selection on adaptive sex ratio allocation. *Evolutionary Ecology Research*, **9**, 1097–1117.

Alonzo, S. H., Ish, T., Key, M., MacCall, A. & Mangel, M. (2008) The importance of incorporating protogynous sex change into stock assessments. *Bulletin of Marine Science*, **83**, 163–179.

Brouwer, L., Richardson, D. S., Eikenaar, C. & Komdeur, J. (2006). The role of group size and environmental factors on survival in a cooperatively breeding tropical passerine. *Journal of Animal Ecology*, **75**, 1321–1329.

Buston, P. M. (2003a) Social hierarchies: size and growth modification in clownfish. *Nature*, **424**, 145–146.

Buston, P. M. (2003b) Forcible eviction and prevention of recruitment in the clown anemonefish. *Behavioral Ecology*, **14**, 576–582.

Buston, P. M. (2004) Territory inheritance in clownfish. *Proceedings of the Royal Society Series B*, **271**, S252–254.

Buston, P. M., Bogdanowicz, S. M., Wong, A. & Harrison, R. G. (2007) Are clownfish groups composed of close relatives? An analysis of microsatellite DNA variation in *Amphiprion percula*. *Molecular Ecology*, **16**, 3671–3678.

Charnov, E. L. (1982) *The Theory of Sex Allocation,* Princeton, NJ: Princeton University Press.

Clobert, J., Danchin, E., Dhondt, A. A. & Nichol, J. D. (2001) *Dispersal.* Oxford: Oxford University Press.

Darwin, C. (1871) *The Descent of Man, and Selection in Relation to Sex.* London: John Murray.

Darwin, C. (1874) *The Descent of Man and Selection in Relation to Sex*, 2nd edn. London: John Murray.

Düsing, C. (1884) *Die Regulierung des Geschlechtsverhältnisses bei der Vermehrung der Menschen, Tiere und Pflanzen.* Jena: Gustav Fischer Verlag.

Edwards, A. W. F. (1998) Natural selection and the sex ratio: Fisher's sources. *American Naturalist*, **151**, 564–569.

Emlen, S. T. & Oring, L. W. (1977) Ecology, sexual selection, and the evolution of mating systems. *Science*, **197**, 215–223.

Fisher, R. A. (1930) *The Genetical Theory of Natural Selection.* Oxford: Clarendon Press.

Ghiselin, M. T. (1969) The evolution of hermaphroditism among animals. *Quarterly Review of Biology*, **44**, 189–208.

Godfray, H. C. J. & Werren, J. H. (1996) Recent developments in sex ratio studies. *Trends in Ecology and Evolution*, **11**, 59–63.

Godwin, J., Crews, D. & Warner, R. R. (1996) Behavioural sex change in the absence of gonads in a coral reef fish. *Proceedings of the Royal Society B*, **263**, 1683–1688.

Greenwood, P. J. (1980) Mating systems, philopatry and dispersal in birds and mammals. *Animal Behaviour*, **28**, 1140–1162.

Griffin, A. S., Sheldon, B. C. & West, S. A. (2005) Cooperative breeders adjust offspring sex ratios to produce helpful helpers. *American Naturalist*, **166**, 628–632.

Hamilton, W. D. (1963) The evolution of altruistic behavior. *American Naturalist*, **97**, 354–356.

Hamilton, W. D. (1967) Extraordinary sex ratios. *Science*, **156**, 477–487.

Haney, R. A., Silliman, B. R. & Rand, D. M. (2007) A multi-locus assessment of connectivity and historical demography in the bluehead wrasse (*Thalassoma bifasciatum*). *Heredity*, **98**, 294–302.

Herre, E. A. (1987) Optimality, plasticity and selective regime in fig wasps. *Nature*, **329**, 627–629.

Holekamp, K. E. & Sherman, P. W. (1989) Why male ground squirrels disperse. *American Scientist*, **77**, 232–239.

Johnson, C. N., Clinchy, M., Taylor, A. C. *et al.* (2001) Adjustment of offspring sex ratios in relation to availability of resources for philopatric offspring in the common brushtail possum. *Proceedings of the Royal Society B*, **268**, 2001–2005.

Johnston, M. O., Das, B. & Hoeh, W. R. (1998) Negative correlation between male allocation and rate of self-fertilization in a hermaphroditic animal. *Proceedings of the National Academy of Sciences of the USA*, **95**, 617–620.

Komdeur, J. (1992) Importance of habitat saturation and territory quality for evolution of cooperative breeding in the Seychelles warbler. *Nature*, **358**, 493–495.

Komdeur, J. (2003) Daughters on request: about helpers and egg sexes in the Seychelles warbler. *Proceedings of the Royal Society B*, **270**, 3–11.

Komdeur, J., Daan, S., Tinbergen, J. & Mateman, C. (1997) Extreme adaptive modification in sex ratio of the Seychelles warbler's eggs. *Nature*, **385**, 522–525.

Maynard Smith, J. (1982) *Evolution and the Theory of Games.* Cambridge: Cambridge University Press.

Munch, S. B., Walsh, M. R. & Conover, D. O. (2005) Harvest selection, genetic correlations, and evolutionary changes in recruitment: one less thing to worry about? *Canadian Journal of Fisheries and Aquatic Sciences*, **62**, 802–810.

Munday, P. L., White, J. W. & Warner, R. R. (2006) A social basis for the development of primary males in a sex-changing fish. *Proceedings of the Royal Society B*, **273**, 2845–2851.

Packer, C. & Pusey, A. E (1987) Intrasexual cooperation and the sex ratio in African lions. *American Naturalist*, **130**, 636–642.

Parker, G. A. (1998) Sperm competition and the evolution of ejaculates: towards a theory base. In: *Sperm Competition and Sexual Selection*, ed. T. R. Birkhead and A. P. Møller, London: Academic Press, pp. 3–54.

Pen, I. & Weissing, F. J. (2000) Sex-ratio optimization with helpers at the nest. *Proceedings of the Royal Society B*, **267**, 539–543.

Reece, S. E., Drew, D. R. & Gardner, A. (2008). Sex ratio adjustment and kin discrimination in malaria parasites. *Nature*, **453**, 609–614.

Semsar, K. & Godwin, J. (2003) Social influences on the arginine vasotocin system are independent of gonads in a sex-changing fish. *Journal of Neuroscience*, **23**, 4386–4393.

Shaw, R. F. & Mohler, J. D. (1953) The selective significance of the sex ratio. *American Naturalist*, **837**, 337–342.

Sherman, P. W. (1977) Nepotism and evolution of alarm calls. *Science*, **197**, 1246–1253.

Stenseth, N. C., Chan, K.S., Tong, H. *et al.* (1999) Common dynamic structure of Canada lynx populations within three climatic regions. *Science*, **285**, 1071–1073.

Swearer, S. E., Caselle, J. E., Lea, D. W. & Warner, R. R. (1999) Larval retention and recruitment in an island population of a coral-reef fish. *Nature*, **402**, 799–802.

Trivers, E. L. & Willard, D. E. (1973) Natural selection of parental ability to vary the sex ratio of offspring. *Science*, **179**, 90–92.

Turchin, P. (2005) *Complex Population Dynamics*. Princeton, NJ: Princeton University Press.

Warner, R. R. (1975) The adaptive significance of sequential hermaphroditism in animals. *American Naturalist*, **109**, 61–82.

Warner, R. R. (2002) Synthesis: environment, mating systems, and life-history allocations in the bluehead wrasse. In: *Model Systems in Behavioral Ecology*, ed. L. A. Dugatkin. Princeton, NJ: Princeton University Press, pp. 227–244.

Warner, R. R. & Swearer, S. E. (1991) Social control of sex change in the bluehead wrasse, *Thalassoma bifasciatum* (Pisces, Labridae). *Biological Bulletin*, **181**, 199–204.

West, S. A., Herre, E. A. & Sheldon, B. C. (2000) The benefits of allocating sex. *Science* **290**, 288–290.

West, S. A., Shuker, D. M. & Sheldon, B. C. (2005) Sex-ratio adjustment when relatives interact: a test of constraints on adaptation. *Evolution*, **59**, 1211–1228.

Wild, G. & West, S. A. (2007) A sex allocation theory for vertebrates: combining local resource competition and condition-dependent allocation. *American Naturalist*, **170**, E112–128.

Wilkin, T. A., Garant, D., Gosler, A. G. & Sheldon, B. C. (2006). Density effects on life-history traits in a wild population of the great tit (*Parus major*): analyses of long-term data with GIS techniques. *Journal of Animal Ecology*, **75**, 604–615.

Social theory based on natural selection

Robert Trivers

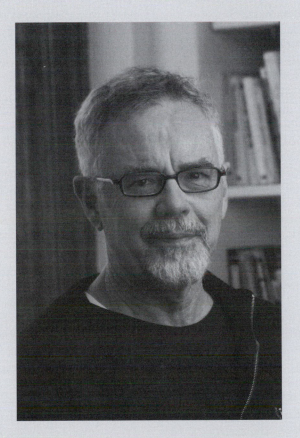

Robert Trivers. Photo: R. Trivers.

I went into evolutionary biology because I became convinced in 1965 that the foundation for psychology and social theory more generally should, and could, be based on the theory of natural selection.

In 1964, a senior-year course at Harvard in psychology convinced me that that discipline was nowhere near putting itself together as a unified science, and that their approach was, in fact, hopeless

Social Behaviour: Genes, Ecology and Evolution, ed. Tamás Székely, Allen J. Moore and Jan Komdeur. Published by Cambridge University Press. © Cambridge University Press 2010.

at the outset, a series of competing guesses about what was important in human development, none based on any underlying knowledge. Within a year, while writing and illustrating children's books on animal behaviour, I was exposed to animal behaviour (chiefly gulls and baboons), and the logic based on natural selection for interpreting their behaviour. It was at once obvious that this was the logic missing from psychology, and that rooting psychology in biology not only gave it a firm foundation in pre-existing knowledge but also greatly expanded the available evidence, even if you were only interested in humans. I had never had a course before in biology or chemistry, but it seemed worthwhile learning at least the former because of the importance of building a secure scientific foundation for social theory. I spent a year learning biology and began graduate work at age 25.

I then threw myself into a series of interrelated topics – reciprocal altruism, parental investment and sexual selection, parent–offspring conflict, adaptive control of variation in the primary sex ratio, and the evolution of the social insects. I had meant to complete this work with a paper on the logic of self-deception and (separately) the logic of female choice. The first one was never written and the second appeared 10 years later but was so poorly presented that it was completely overlooked (Seger and Trivers 1986).

After reviewing 'social evolution' for undergraduates (Trivers 1985), I turned to genetics and the problem of within-individual genetic conflict, a topic I naively thought I could handle in 3–5 years before returning to the logic of self-deception. Fully 15 years of work later – not just by myself but also by Austin Burt – we produced a review of what turned out to be an enormous subject (in eukaryotes alone: Burt & Trivers 2006), a subject that has grown every week since then. At the end, Austin and I used to joke that we were quite mad to have undertaken this task since neither of us was a geneticist. In effect,

we had to teach ourselves the underlying discipline before we could write our book. (Of course, we did the two things together.)

More recently I have returned full-time to the topic of self-deception, and I have recently finished a book on 'Deceit and self-deception'. There is now almost enough evidence from a great range of sources – e.g. neurophysiology, evolutionary theory, social psychology, immunology, and the study of everyday life – to put together a detailed theory of the evolution of human self-deception. Once again, this is an intrinsically important subject, worth the trouble of mastering the various sub-disciplines.

In summary, in three different cases I have been primarily motivated by the intrinsic importance of the subject itself and have been willing to master what needs to be mastered in order to do the relevant work. For the first subject, that choice has been immensely rewarding. I learned evolutionary biology sufficiently deeply to make some useful contributions to social theory based on natural selection. These have generated very large literatures, which have, of course, deepened my own understanding along with that of many others. In the second case, time will tell whether the synthesis Austin Burt and I produced will be worth the time and effort put into it. Regarding self-deception, the material I have taught myself is much less detailed and difficult than genetics, and I have no question of the importance of getting the logic of self-deception on a firm scientific footing.

References

Burt, A. & Trivers, R. L. (2006) *Genes in Conflict: the Biology of Selfish Genetic Elements*. Cambridge, MA: Harvard University Press.

Seger, J. & Trivers, R. (1986) Asymmetry in the evolution of female mating preferences. *Nature*, **319**, 771–773.

Trivers, R. (1985) *Social Evolution*. Menlo Park, CA: Benjamin/Cummings.

19

Social behaviour and speciation

Gerald S. Wilkinson and Leanna M. Birge

Overview

Speciation results from the evolution of traits that inhibit reproduction between populations. This chapter discusses theoretical and empirical studies that relate to how social behaviour influences those reproductive barriers. Behaviour can influence prezygotic isolation by causing non-random mating or non-random fertilisation. Learning can affect mate recognition through cultural transmission of mate advertisement signals and sexual imprinting. Behaviour can also contribute to reproductive isolation if hybrids are discriminated against as mates or if female re-mating influences fertilisation success.

A general theory of speciation does not exist, but a variety of models have been developed to describe how selection can favour speciation in particular situations. Theory suggests that sexual selection, in particular, should be a diversifying force. However, among vertebrates sexual selection by female choice has favoured expression of condition-dependent traits, which are typically not reliable for species recognition. Better examples of sexually selected traits functioning in both mate-choice and species-recognition contexts can be found among some insects, such as crickets. The best examples of sexual selection influencing speciation in vertebrates come from cases of sexual imprinting in birds where offspring learn species-recognition cues in the nest.

Sexual selection can also operate after mating by sperm competition or cryptic female choice. Either or both of these mechanisms likely contribute to conspecific sperm precedence, which may result in reproductive isolation after mating. Sexually antagonistic coevolution has the potential to drive speciation in systems with sexual conflict. However, evidence demonstrating that sexual conflict causes reproductive isolation is currently equivocal in cases involving traits that influence mating or fertilisation success.

Few studies have attempted to determine the genetic basis of prezygotic isolation in comparison to postzygotic isolation. However, among the exceptions are studies in which one or two physically linked genetic factors influence both mate preference and a recognition cue. New methods for genomic mapping in non-model organisms promise to add considerable insight into how genes influence prezygotic reproductive isolation.

Social Behaviour: Genes, Ecology and Evolution, ed. Tamás Székely, Allen J. Moore and Jan Komdeur. Published by Cambridge University Press. © Cambridge University Press 2010.

A variety of claims have been made that social behaviour accelerates speciation rates in, for example, mammals, birds and social insects. In general, these claims have not been supported by comparative studies. With regard to sexual selection, this may be because extinction rates are also accelerated. Focused research on groups of closely related species that exhibit different mating systems should help to clarify which processes are involved in the initial stages of speciation.

19.1 Introduction

A hallmark of sexual organisms is that populations of reproductive individuals typically exhibit categorical, rather than continuous, differences in morphological and behavioural traits, particularly those related to mating (Maynard Smith & Szathmáry 1995). Whereas the existence of these differences has been used to identify and organise species since Linnaeus first published *Systema Naturae* in 1735, the process and temporal sequence by which a single population diverges over time into two distinct forms, i.e. speciation, remains hotly debated and is arguably the most active area of investigation in evolutionary biology today. An important part of this process involves mate (and gamete) selection. In this sense, behavioural processes that influence mating and fertilisation are key pieces to the puzzle of speciation, and they are the focus of this chapter.

The biological species concept (Dobzhansky 1937, Mayr 1942) defines a species as a group of interbreeding populations that is reproductively isolated from other such groups. Although conceptually simple, this definition can be difficult to apply because breeding opportunities between species pairs may not exist, and in some cases traditional species with morphological differences do not show complete isolation. These issues have led to alternative definitions and considerable debate (e.g. Mallet 1995, Harrison 1998, Shaw 1998). Nevertheless, the biological species concept provides the best framework for considering how social behaviour may influence the speciation process.

A key element of the biological species concept is that speciation requires reproductive isolation. Reproductive isolation describes the outcome of interactions between individuals from two populations and results whenever the temporal sequence associated with the formation and development of a zygote is interrupted. An *isolating mechanism* (Dobzhansky 1937), or *barrier to reproduction*, refers to reproductive failure that occurs at one or more of the following four life-cycle stages: (1) mating, (2) gamete union, (3) hybrid development or (4) hybrid reproduction. Failure at the first two of these steps is prezygotic isolation (either pre-mating or post-mating), whereas failure at the last two is postzygotic isolation (either hybrid inviability or infertility).

In this chapter our goal is to summarise and evaluate the ways in which social behaviour may be involved in the speciation process. In most situations, speciation occurs on timescales that cannot be observed in a lifetime. Thus, inferences about process must rely on phenotypic or genetic differences that can be detected between extant taxa and used to evaluate alternative models. For this reason, we briefly summarise relevant theory, when available, and then consider how selection on behaviour could influence reproductive isolation before or after mating. For example, social behaviour can impact the speciation process if non-random mating occurs, either indirectly through changes in host preference or directly through changes in mate preference. Learning can impact mate recognition through cultural transmission of mate advertisement signals (ten Cate 2000) and sexual imprinting (Bateson 1978). Social behaviour can also contribute to post-mating, prezygotic isolation to the extent that female re-mating influences fertilisation success (Jennions & Petrie 2000, Birkhead & Billard 2007). After reviewing each of these possibilities in turn, we then discuss examples and methods that could be used to determine the number of genetic changes required to cause sexual isolation. We end by considering several ideas for how social behaviour might influence speciation rate.

19.2 Speciation theory

A general theory of speciation does not yet exist (Gavrilets 2004, Turelli *et al.* 2001), and may be difficult to construct given the diversity of ways populations can become isolated. However, a large number of speciation models have been developed for particular geographic situations, which are referred to as *modes* of speciation (Box 19.1), and different selection scenarios. Rather than attempt to summarise those models, we refer the interested reader to Gavrilets (2004) for a comprehensive discussion. Here we use the scheme proposed by Kirkpatrick and Ravigne (2002) to highlight where social behaviour is important in five essential features that can be found in all models of prezygotic isolation. This deconstruction applies only when selection, rather than drift or mutation, is invoked to cause speciation.

Box 19.1 Modes of speciation

The structure of diverging populations in space is typically referred to as the *mode* of speciation.

Allopatric speciation is considered to be the most common mode of speciation (Mayr 1942, 1963). It occurs after a *vicariant* event, e.g. a river, glacier or island, divides the distribution of a species and creates geographically isolated populations. Subsequent adaptation to local environmental conditions or drift then results in genetic divergence over time. Speciation is verified when two previously isolated populations restore contact but remain distinct.

Peripatric speciation is a type of allopatric speciation that occurs when small peripheral populations are isolated from a parent population. This process is frequently invoked to explain the origin of island endemics after a colonisation event. The radiation of *Drosophila* in Hawaii (Hollocher & Williamson 1996) and in the Caribbean (Paulay & Meyer 2002) provides compelling examples.

Sympatric speciation, in contrast, occurs when disruptive selection within a single parent population results in daughter populations that are reproductively isolated from each other in the same geographic area (Via 2001). Host switching is one mechanism by which sympatric speciation can occur. For example, the apple-feeding race of the apple maggot fly *Rhagoletis pomonella* is believed to have evolved from the hawthorn-feeding race after apples were introduced into North America. Each race now shows restricted host preferences, and consequently they are reproductively isolated from each other (Bush 1969, Feder *et al.* 1994, 2003). Pea aphids *Acyrthosiphon pisum* that feed on clover or alfalfa provide a second example of host switching at an earlier stage of differentiation (Via 1999, Hawthorne & Via 2001).

Parapatric speciation refers to intermediate situations in which gene flow occurs between neighbouring populations but not between distant populations. This is most dramatically illustrated by what has been referred to as a *ring species*. Greenish warblers *Phylloscopus trochiloides* are forest-dwelling birds that inhabit mountains surrounding deserts in Asia. In central Siberia, two distinct variants coexist with narrowly overlapping distributions. These forms differ in plumage colour and song. Males of each type do not recognise the song of the other form as a competitor, resulting in reproductive isolation. However, the two forms are connected by a series of populations that exhibit geographic variation in morphological and behavioural traits (Irwin 2000, Irwin *et al.* 2001). Genetic evidence indicates that gene flow occurs between all but the most distant populations in the ring (Irwin *et al.* 2005).

The first element of any speciation model is a source of disruptive selection that favours reproduction among different genetic combinations. Disruptive selection prevents gene flow from homogenising the genomes of two incipient species. For example, local adaptation to spatially varying habitats is a common form of disruptive selection, and frequency-dependent natural selection is another. Behaviour might be involved in mediating these processes, e.g. through habitat choice, although such decisions do not require social interactions and so we will not consider them further. However, disruptive selection can also result from sexual selection if populations diverge in female preferences and male traits. We discuss these possibilities in the following two sections.

The second element is the presence of an isolating mechanism. Alternative possibilities for prezygotic isolation include assortative mating, where mating pairs exhibit similar values of a single trait such as body or bill size, and mating preferences, where members of one sex (usually females) prefer members of the opposite sex that exhibit particular display traits. Kirkpatrick and Ravigne (2002) argue that the mode of speciation can be viewed as a mechanism that either enforces (allopatry), or does not enforce (sympatry) assortative mating. While we agree that this is a useful way to think about model assumptions, it is important to recognise that males and females can differ in mate preferences, which might generate mating asymmetries and patterns of gene flow that differ from that expected under simple allopatry or sympatry.

The third element is a way to connect disruptive selection to the isolating mechanism. This can occur by direct selection, e.g. when assortatively mating parents produce more progeny, or by indirect selection, e.g. when genes that affect the isolating mechanism are associated (by linkage disequilibrium or pleiotropy) with genes that are the target of sexual selection. For example, hybrids that suffer reduced mating success would be a case of indirect selection mediated by sexual selection (Liou & Price 1994, Servedio 2000, 2004). Selection for assortative mating to reduce gamete loss after secondary contact of isolated populations

is known as *reinforcement* (Howard 1993, Servedio & Noor 2003, Coyne & Orr 2004).

Direct selection is often more efficient than indirect selection, because the strength of indirect selection depends on the genetic correlation between selection and the prezygotic isolating mechanism (Kirkpatrick & Barton 1997). Genetic correlations would not be expected to be high unless there is very strong selection against hybrids, a situation that would only occur in regions of species overlap, such as in hybrid zones. When genetic linkage in this context is caused by pleiotropy, this is referred to as *genetic coupling* (Hoy *et al.* 1977).

The fourth element involves the type of assumption made about the genetic basis of the isolating mechanism. Felsenstein (1981) first recognised that isolation can occur either when two different alleles spread to fixation in two different populations, or when a single allele goes to fixation in both populations. For example, an allele that causes individuals to mate with others of the same size is a single-allele model, whereas mating preferences for two different male forms represents a two-allele model. Single-allele models require an initial difference between populations, and then function to maintain that difference, whereas two-allele models produce tension between selection and gene flow. For this reason, isolation by a one-allele mechanism may evolve more quickly.

The final element is whether or not populations differ at the outset. Most models of speciation have been developed to describe how either sympatric speciation or reinforcement could occur. In many cases, the outcome depends not only on the genetic and ecological assumptions but also on the initial conditions. The situations that do or do not favour fusion of two genetically distinct populations have, therefore, not yet led to general conclusions, particularly with respect to behaviour.

In the next two sections of the chapter we focus on alternative ways in which reproductive isolation, either before or after mating, could be influenced by social behaviour. The five steps outlined above should be kept in mind, because we will discuss both theory and data that pertain to each of these elements.

19.3 Pre-mating isolation

How species acquire distinctive recognition cues has a history of debate. Patterson (1985) argued that pre-mating reproductive isolation arises as a consequence of the evolution of a specific mate-recognition system that involves cooperative coadaptation between males and females in a population, but rejected the possibility that there might be species-recognition cues. In contrast, Mayr (1942) argued that mating barriers arise between populations after secondary contact as a consequence of reinforcement and are subsequently maintained by stabilising selection for distinctive courtship behaviours (e.g. Kyriacou & Hall 1982, Butlin et al. 1985, Gerhardt 1991). If species recognition causes reproductive isolation, then cases of reproductive character displacement should be common, i.e. male mating signals should be similar in allopatry but different in sympatry. In contrast, reproductive character displacement is generally thought to be uncommon (Howard 1993, West-Eberhard 1983), although some notable cases have been found (Noor 1995, Higgie et al. 2000, Higgie & Blows 2007). The rarity of reproductive character displacement led West Eberhard (1983) to conclude that most cases of prezygotic reproductive isolation are likely the result of sexual selection, a conclusion that has been endorsed by others (e.g. Ryan & Rand 1993, Panhuis et al. 2001). However, the extent to which divergence in mating signals causes, rather than evolves after, reproductive isolation is unclear. Understanding the mechanisms of sexual selection helps to appreciate the reasons for this uncertainty.

19.3.1 Sexual selection

Sexual selection is a potentially powerful diversifying force because non-random mating increases the chance that genes influencing traits and preferences will become associated (Chapter 10). As Lande (1981) and Kirkpatrick (1982) have shown, linkage disequilibrium between genes that influence expression of a male ornament and a female preference for it can give rise to a runaway process, as Fisher (1930) envisioned. In the absence of selection on females, a runaway

process ends either in extinction or in a neutral line of equilibrium where sexual selection is balanced by natural selection on males, and therefore any combination of trait or preference can be stable. Theoretically, populations that are displaced off an equilibrium line by a chance event will evolve back to the line, but to a different location dictated by the genetic regression of trait on preference. Thus, episodic fluctuations in population size could cause populations to end up at different locations along the equilibrium line. These populations would then possess distinctive male traits and female preferences and might, therefore, be reproductively isolated (Lande 1981).

While a Fisherian runaway process can generate rapid change in male traits and female preferences, the evolutionary outcome of a neutral line of equilibrium depends on the assumption that selection does not act on females either positively or negatively. If females benefit directly from mating, then preferences should converge to maximise female fecundity (Kirkpatrick & Ryan 1991). The strength of selection on preferences for direct benefits is expected to be stronger than for indirect benefits, i.e. benefits attributable to genes inherited by offspring (Kirkpatrick & Barton 1997). Whether preferences for male genetic quality should give rise to disruptive selection in isolated populations then depends on how genetic variation for quality is maintained. If females choose males based on a random process, such as recurrent deleterious mutations (Pomiankowski et al. 1991), then isolated populations would only be expected to diverge by drift. However, if females prefer males that are resistant to pathogens, and pathogen resistance is coevolving with pathogen virulence independently in isolated populations, then trait and preference could be under disruptive selection in isolated populations. Female preference for genetic compatibility could also lead to disruptive selection in isolated populations, particularly if the nature of the compatibility depends on some form of genomic conflict (Haig & Bergstrom 1995, Zeh & Zeh 1996, Tregenza & Wedell 2000), such as meiotic drive (Lande & Wilkinson 1999).

If speciation is driven by sexual selection operating through either a runaway or good-genes process, then the male traits that females prefer within a population should also be the traits that are used for mate recognition between populations. Evidence for this prediction is not easy to find (Arnegard & Kondrashov 2004). A common observation is that female vertebrates exhibit directional preferences, such as best-of-*n* (Janetos 1980), for increased levels of display by males (Ryan & Keddy-Hector 1992, Andersson 1994, Alexander *et al.* 1997). Louder calls, faster displays (Gibson & Bradbury 1985), increased levels of pigmentation (Griffith *et al.* 1999, Hill *et al.* 2002) and greater diversity of syllables in a song repertoire (Searcy 1992, Hasselquist *et al.* 1996) provide a few examples in which females prefer extreme male traits. In all cases, the preferred male trait is condition-dependent, i.e. trait expression varies among males depending on their condition. Condition-dependent trait expression provides a reliable mechanism for advertising genetic quality (Grafen 1990, Rowe & Houle 1996) but not for indicating species identity, because individuals are often phenotypically variable within a population. Not surprisingly, extreme male display traits are rarely used for mate recognition in vertebrates (Ptacek 2000).

There are, however, examples in which sexual selection for mating signals in insects appear to be involved in recent speciation events, perhaps because insects are more likely to rely on threshold mating preferences (Alexander *et al.* 1997). For example, male field crickets of the species *Gryllus texensis* and *G. rubens* exhibit different pulse rates, but are otherwise indistinguishable (Gray & Cade 2000). Females exhibit preferences for conspecific song, and female preference exhibits a significant, although weak, genetic correlation with male song. Character displacement does not occur in sympatric populations, and hybrids are readily produced in the laboratory. Thus, reproductive isolation is plausibly attributed to differences in male advertisement signals, although, as the authors note, conspecific sperm precedence provides an untested competing hypothesis. Similar evidence for speciation as a consequence of sexual selection on male courtship song has also been obtained for *Laupala* crickets (Shaw 1996, Shaw *et al.* 2007), and *Chrysoperla* lacewings (Wells & Henry 1992).

Sexual selection on traits that influence mating success need not always lead to behavioural isolation in insects, particularly in species with multimodal displays. For example, *Drosophila heteroneura* and *D. sylvestris* are two closely related species of picture-winged flies that co-occur on the island of Hawaii, but differ in appearance in that male *D. heteroneura* have broad heads whereas male *D. sylvestris* do not. Female *D. heteroneura* exhibit preferences for broad-headed conspecific males yet do not use head width when discriminating conspecific from reciprocal F_1 males (Boake *et al.* 1997). These results suggest that behavioural isolation between these two species depends on other cues, perhaps olfactory or tactile, that are used earlier in the courtship sequence and may or may not be subject to within-species sexual selection (Price & Boake 1995, Boake 2002). We have reached similar conclusions for diopsid stalk-eyed flies, where females from sexually dimorphic species prefer males with longer eye stalks (Wilkinson *et al.* 1998), but populations that exhibit behavioural isolation (Christianson *et al.* 2005) do not differ in relative head shape (Swallow *et al.* 2005), although they do differ in sperm length and female sperm storage-organ size (E. Rose and G. Wilkinson, unpublished data).

Sexual selection could also cause pre-mating reproductive isolation if male–male interactions generate disruptive selection for alternative mating strategies (Gray & McKinnon 2007), as has been described for side-blotched lizards *Uta stansburiana* (Calsbeek *et al.* 2002) and lazuli buntings *Passerina amoena* (Greene *et al.* 2000). Disruptive selection can also occur when two isolated populations come together to form hybrids that then successfully reproduce to form a new species. This process is best known in plants, such as sunflowers in the genus *Helianthus* (Rieseberg 2006, Rieseberg & Willis 2007), but has also recently been reported in some animals. For example, based on patterns of inheritance of wing colour markings, *Heliconius heurippa* appears to be a hybrid butterfly species that was created by the union of *H. cydno* and *H. melpomene* (Mavarez *et al.* 2006). In this case, sexual selection is not driving speciation, but instead is acting to reinforce speciation, because hybrid butterflies prefer to mate with each other rather than with the parental species. Speciation by hybridisation has also been proposed for the swordtail fish *Xiphophorus clemenciae* and for some African cichlid fishes in the *Haplochromis nyererei* complex (Seehausen 2004, Salzburger *et al.* 2002, Meyer *et al.* 2006).

19.3.2 Sexual conflict

Sexual conflict occurs whenever male and female reproductive opportunities differ (Chapter 10; Parker 1979, 2006). One example occurs when there is a cost to females of mating. If the source of the cost is under female control, then females would be expected to minimise their cost (Kirkpatrick 1996). In contrast, if male displays exploit or manipulate female perceptual responses, then males will be under selection to be more persistent and females will be under selection to resist to the extent that females benefit. This process has long been thought to lead to a sexual arms race within species (Trivers 1972, Dawkins & Krebs 1979, Parker 1979), and more recently has been viewed as a form of antagonistic coevolution that may drive speciation (Rice 1998).

Several lines of evidence have been used to argue that antagonistic coevolution between male and female reproductive traits should facilitate reproductive isolation (Arnqvist & Rowe 2005). First, models of sexual conflict in which there is a greater cost to females than males of producing hybrids (Parker & Partridge 1998), or in which females exhibit less mate compatibility than do males (Gavrilets 2000, Gavrilets & Waxman 2002), have shown that sexual conflict can lead to an arms race between males and females that results in reproductive isolation both in allopatry and in sympatry. Second, females seem likely to be able to evade male courtship efforts in more ways than they can track male traits, as expected by both runaway and good-genes models of sexual selection. Furthermore, if females exhibit perceptual biases in multiple signal modalities, multiple male display traits should evolve (Johnstone 1995, Andersson *et al.* 2002). In general, sexual conflict is expected to produce a variety of trait-combination outcomes because males and females have divergent interests. In contrast, fewer trait-combination outcomes are likely when males and females have convergent interests.

Despite these reasons to expect sexually antagonistic coevolution to drive speciation, evidence that sexual conflict causes reproductive isolation is equivocal. The strongest support comes from an experimental evolution study of the dung fly *Sepsis cynipsea*, where sexual conflict was created by varying fly density (either 500 or 50 flies/line), and contrasted with lines maintained by pair-mating. After 35 generations in these mating regimes females from both sexual-conflict treatments were less willing to mate with males from different than from same lines (Martin & Hosken 2003), indicative of incipient reproductive isolation. However, the analysis of these data has been questioned (Bacigalupe *et al.* 2007). Furthermore, two similar experiments on *Drosophila* failed to detect such an effect. After 41 generations of elevated sexual conflict, no decrease in female mating frequency was observed between replicate lines of *D. melanogaster* (Wigby & Chapman 2006). Similarly, after 50 generations female *D. pseudoobscura* actually mated more frequently with males from different sexual-conflict lines than they did with males from their own selection lines – the opposite of the predicted outcome (Bacigalupe *et al.* 2007). In both *Drosophila* studies female resistance to mating increased within the sexual-conflict lines (Wigby & Chapman 2004, Crudgington *et al.* 2005), indicating that the experimental treatment was effective. While it is possible that sexual conflict in *Drosophila* is mediated more by post-mating than pre-mating effects, given that males pass accessory gland proteins to females during mating and these proteins can influence sperm precedence (Clark *et al.* 1995), female re-mating and oviposition rate (Wolfner 2002), these studies cast significant doubt on the role of sexual conflict in causing rapid evolution of pre-mating sexual isolation in *Drosophila*.

In the wild the best example of sexual conflict potentially influencing speciation occurs in water striders, where male claspers and female structures to resist mating exhibit correlated evolution (Arnqvist & Rowe 2002a, 2002b). Unfortunately, by themselves these results do not reveal if the clasping structures evolved before or after reproductive isolation appeared.

Additional studies of sexual conflict and sexually antagonistic coevolution are clearly warranted, especially with regard to post-mating effects (see below), although it must be recognised that sexual conflict can also act to oppose speciation depending on which sex controls reproduction (Parker 2006). If females control mating and fertilisation, population divergence should persist or increase, and speciation is favoured. However, if males control mating, gene flow should be common and operate against speciation. A detailed understanding of how mating is influenced by male and female behaviour is, therefore, essential to inferring the underlying evolutionary process driving speciation (Rowe & Day 2006).

19.3.3 Cultural transmission and sexual imprinting

The ability to acquire mate-recognition traits, such as song (see Chapter 3), by learning has long been viewed as an important mechanism that can contribute to reproductive isolation in birds (Martens 1996, Price 1998, Edwards *et al.* 2005). Models of speciation involving song learning reveal that the ability of males to copy songs of others in allopatry can accelerate the speciation process (Lachlan & Servedio 2004). The reason for this effect is that males with a disadvantageous genotype for singing a particular type of song are nevertheless able to produce the preferred song type if they can learn. Similarly, females with rare preference alleles will mate with the common song type if they learn which males to mate with. In both cases, the difficulty associated with increasing the frequency of a novel allele in an isolated population by drift or directional sexual selection is lessened. Thus, in the short term learning will decrease phenotypic diversity within populations, but over the long term phenotypic diversity between populations will be increased. Song learning is predicted to hinder speciation when male song traits and female song preferences are inherited independently and females only mate once. The Lachlan–Servedio model assumes that

songs are learned from unrelated adults in the population (i.e. transmission is oblique). This assumption is clearly false in some cases: e.g. males learn their songs from their fathers in Darwin's finches *Geospiza* spp. (Grant & Grant 1996). Vertical transmission creates an opportunity for mate recognition signals to be acquired by offspring early in life from their parents, a process referred to as sexual imprinting (ten Cate & Bateson 1988, Weary *et al.* 1993, Owens *et al.* 1999a).

Theoretically, sexual imprinting could involve offspring learning species-recognition signals produced by mothers, fathers or unrelated individuals (Irwin & Price 1999). Models of these alternatives reveal that maternal imprinting, where females copy their mother's mate preferences, is most similar to phenotype matching (Hauber & Sherman 2001). This can lead to traits and preferences becoming associated, which favours speciation. Maternal imprinting occurs in many bird species (Kruijt *et al.* 1982, ten Cate & Vos 1999, Witte *et al.* 2000) as well as some mammal species (Kendrick *et al.* 1998). In contrast, when females imprint on their fathers or obliquely on unrelated individuals, genetic associations between trait and preference are weak and unlikely to cause sufficient assortative mating for reproductive isolation (Laland 1994, Aoki *et al.* 2001, Verzijden *et al.* 2005). Paternal imprinting is expected to differ from maternal imprinting if mating success varies among males, thereby reducing the degree to which assortative mating can occur. Mate-choice copying, such as that reported for guppies *Poecilia reticulata* (Dugatkin & Godin 1992), provides an example of oblique transmission of mating preferences. Guppies exhibit a high degree of variation in male colour patterns, but despite evidence for genetic variation in female preferences (Brooks 2002), that variation has not led to reproductive isolation between populations.

The African indigobirds *Vidua* spp. are brood parasites that exhibit heterospecific sexual imprinting (Payne *et al.* 1998, 2000), and they provide a compelling example of sympatric speciation in birds (Fig. 19.1; Edwards *et al.* 2005). Male indigobirds mimic the songs of their hosts, which include several estrildid finch species in the genus *Lagonosticta*, which they learn as nestlings. Females use those songs to choose

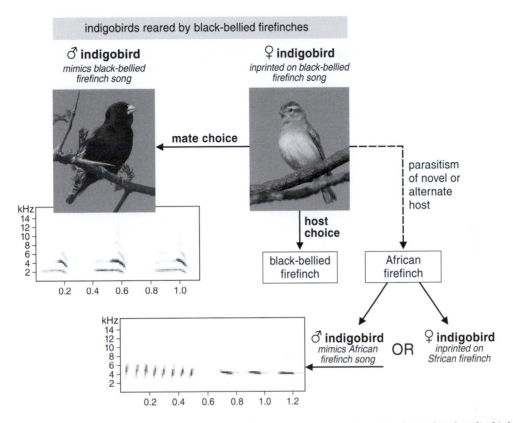

Figure 19.1 Sexual imprinting provides a mechanism for rapid speciation when new hosts are colonised. Male indigobirds mimic the songs of their hosts, whereas females use song cues to choose both their mates and the nests they parasitise (Payne *et al.* 1998, 2000). Rarely, females lay in the nest of a novel or alternative host (i.e. one already associated with another indigobird species). The resulting offspring imprint on the novel host and are therefore reproductively isolated from their parent population (Balakrishnan & Sorenson 2006). Minimal differentiation in neutral genetic markers among the indigobird species within each geographic region support a model of rapid sympatric speciation by host shift (Sorenson *et al.* 2003, Sefc *et al.* 2005)

their mates and to locate nests to parasitise. These behavioural traits ensure that a population of brood parasites remains closely associated with a host species. Furthermore, if a female parasitises the nest of a different species, her offspring will imprint on the songs produced by males of that species. Thus, host switching potentially results in reproductive isolation. Phylogenetic evidence confirms that indigobirds have speciated much more rapidly than their finch hosts (Sorenson *et al.* 2003). A remarkable aspect of this system is that the brood-parasite chicks mimic the gape patterns of their host species (Payne 2005).

Thus, in addition to imprinting, rapid morphological evolution appears to occur among nestling gape patterns of *Vidua* species.

19.4 Prezygotic isolation after mating

The possibility that sexual selection operates after mating on traits that can influence reproductive isolation has been gaining recognition (e.g. Birkhead & Billard 2007). Part of the reason for this recognition is the growing realisation that multiple mating by females is common (Jennions & Petrie 2000), which creates opportunities for postcopulatory sexual selection. In addition, in a growing number of cases the outcome of competition among sperm from heterospecific and conspecific males often favours the conspecific male. The degree to which females mate with more than one male provides, therefore, another way in which behaviour can influence speciation.

Recently, Coyne and Orr (2004) distinguished two types of post-mating, prezygotic barriers: competitive and non-competitive fertilisation barriers. Non-competitive barriers involve factors that cause heterospecific gametes to fail to fertilise ova (see Coyne & Orr 2004 for review). Competitive barriers refer to mechanisms by which conspecific gametes outcompete heterospecific gametes in fertilisation contests. This process is referred to as conspecific

sperm precedence, and it has been reported in a variety of animals (Katakura 1986, Hewitt *et al.* 1989, Bella *et al.* 1992, Wade *et al.* 1994, Price 1997, Howard 1999, Dixon *et al.* 2003, Geyer & Palumbi 2005, Ludlow & Magurran 2006, Mendelson *et al.* 2007, Rugman-Jones & Eady 2007). The appearance of conspecific sperm precedence among isolated populations (Fig. 19.2) or incipient species (e.g. Chang 2004) suggests that it can evolve rapidly and could create one of the first barriers to fertilisation (Howard 1999, Coyne & Orr 2004).

The mechanisms responsible for conspecific sperm precedence are not yet well understood in any species, but almost certainly result from postcopulatory sexual selection operating by sperm competition or gamete choice. Gamete choice by females, often referred to as cryptic female choice (Eberhard 1996), involves

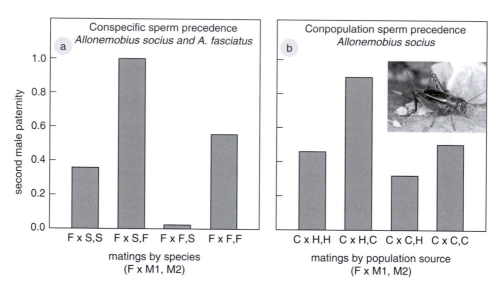

Figure 19.2 Sperm precedence between incipient species provides a mechanism for post-mating, prezygotic reproductive isolation. (a) Reciprocal crosses between allopatric populations of striped ground crickets *Allonemobius socius* (S) and *A. fasciatus* (F) reveals that conspecific males have a fertilisation advantage over heterospecific males (Gregory & Howard 1994). This graph shows the proportion of offspring sired by the second male. Treatments are labelled according to the species of the female followed by the species of the first and second male. (b) In similar reciprocal crosses between allopatric populations, *A. socius* exhibits conpopulation sperm precedence (L. Birge, unpublished data). Treatment labels indicate female population of origin (conpopulation (C) or heteropopulation (H)) followed by source of each male. Thus, fertilisation barriers at the population and species level maintain reproductive isolation. Mating does not appear to be costly in this system, as female fecundity increases with mating opportunities in *A. socius* as a consequence of female consumption of male haemolymph (Fedorka & Mousseau 2002).

situations in which there is differential selection by the female reproductive tract or egg for specific types of sperm. Because postcopulatory contests between males occur among ejaculates within females, female behaviour, morphology, and physiology, as well as the number and type of sperm produced by each male, can influence male success in these contests (reviewed in Eberhard 1996).

When females re-mate, sperm are under selection to avoid competition and outcompete other sperm (Parker 1970). If there is variation among populations in female reproductive traits or in the types of sperm strategies used by males, the evolutionary trajectories of male traits may follow different directions in different populations (e.g. Pitnick *et al.* 2003). Moreover, because of the variety of strategies that may evolve, males that are successful in one population may not be successful in another (Dixon *et al.* 2003, Attia & Tregenza 2004, Chang 2004). Thus, sperm competition can result in reproductive barriers between populations that act after copulation but before fertilisation.

If, as seems likely, the female reproductive system influences which sperm succeed at fertilisation, postcopulatory sexual selection can operate in different ways depending on whether copulation has positive, negative or neutral effects on females. Positive effects often occur in systems where there is nuptial feeding, i.e. the male passes nutrients to females during mating (although see Sakaluk *et al.* 2006). In contrast, negative fitness effects lead to sexual conflict, which, as noted above, have been argued to provide an explanation for why populations may diverge in postcopulatory traits. In situations where the act of mating has little or no fitness consequences for females, selection could act directly on the type of sperm chosen. We consider these options below as possible explanations for the patterns of conspecific sperm precedence that have been observed.

19.4.1 Sexual conflict after mating

Finding evidence that antagonistic coevolution operates on postcopulatory traits has proven difficult, because early in the process of divergence it is unclear

which males will have a fertilisation advantage (Chapman *et al.* 2003, Rowe *et al.* 2003). One possibility is that males from a different population (heteropopulation) have an advantage because females are not adapted to resist them. This outcome should retard speciation, because gene flow is enhanced. For example, in the house fly *Musca domestica* (Andres & Arnqvist 2001) female oviposition rates are highest when they are mated to heteropopulation males, and in the yellow dung fly *Scathophaga stercoraria* (Hosken *et al.* 2002) females preferentially mate with heteropopulation males.

Alternatively, males from the same population as females (conpopulation males) may have an advantage because they are better adapted to female defences. Such conpopulation sperm precedence reduces gene flow and should drive speciation. For example, reciprocal crosses between populations of the bean weevil *Callosobruchus maculatus* reveal that conpopulation males induce longer refractory periods in females than heteropopulation males (Brown & Eady 2001). Futhermore, conspecific males have a fertilisation advantage when *C. subinnotatus* females are mated to both conspecific and *C. maculatus* males (Rugman-Jones & Eady 2007). Similarly, conpopulation male guppies have a fertilisation advantage over heteropopulation males when females are inseminated with a mixture of sperm obtained from males captured in allopatric river systems (Ludlow & Magurran 2006).

The degree to which the preceding examples provide evidence for sexually antagonistic coevolution can be debated, because in most cases the fitness costs to females of mating are not known. Comparative studies have also yielded conflicting evidence regarding sexual conflict and speciation. For example, the rate of speciation was higher in insects where females mate multiple times as compared to related taxa where single mating occurs, as expected if sexual conflict has driven speciation (Arnqvist *et al.* 2000). However, subsequent studies using different methods and larger samples of other insects and spiders (Gage *et al.* 2002, Eberhard 2004) have failed to find evidence indicating that sexual conflict influences speciation.

19.4.2 Sexually selected sperm

Sexual selection has been hypothesised to operate on sperm in ways analogous to how it operates on males. In the sexy-sperm hypothesis multiple mating by females creates a situation in which eggs are fertilised by the most competitive sperm and sperm competitive ability is inherited by sons (Sivinski 1984, Curtsinger 1991, Keller & Reeve 1995, Simmons & Kotiaho 2007). This process could also operate on accessory gland proteins if better fertilisers produce more competitive accessory gland proteins (Cordero 1995, Eberhard & Cordero 1995). The sexy-sperm hypothesis predicts that fertilisation success varies among males and is paternally heritable (Pizzari & Birkhead 2002, Simmons 2003). Furthermore, female genotype is not expected to influence which male genotypes will be superior fertilisers (Birkhead & Billard 2007). For this process to influence speciation, conpopulation males would be expected to have an advantage over heterospecific males because their sperm are better adapted to female reproductive tracts.

In the good-sperm hypothesis multiple mating by females ensures that ova are fertilised by males of superior genetic quality. This hypothesis predicts that fertilisation success should correlate with offspring genetic quality (Harvey & May 1989, Simmons & Kotiaho 2007, Birkhead & Billard 2007). For example, yellow dung fly males that were superior at sperm competition produced offspring with faster development time independent of female genotype (Hosken *et al.* 2003). For this process to influence speciation, sperm from conpopulation males would also be expected to have an advantage over sperm from heterospecific males, but it should in addition produce better offspring.

The overall importance of the sexy-sperm and good-sperm hypotheses for explaining cases of postcopulatory, prezygotic reproductive isolation is currently unknown (see Birkhead & Billard 2007). Nevertheless, the possibility that competitive barriers to fertilisation evolve rapidly and influence speciation (Civetta & Singh 1998, Panhuis *et al.* 2006) continues to motivate research in this area. From the perspective of social behaviour, if postcopulatory reproductive isolation is important, then females should re-mate more often in areas of sympatry, where the possibility of producing hybrid offspring exists, than in areas of allopatry. To our knowledge, this prediction has yet to be tested.

19.5 Genetic basis of prezygotic barriers

In an influential series of papers, Coyne and Orr (1989, 1997, 1998) summarised a large number of studies in which the degree of prezygotic or postzygotic isolation varies as a function of genetic distance (as measured by allozymes) among species pairs of *Drosophila*. They found several notable patterns. In particular, prezygotic isolation typically evolves faster than postzygotic isolation. Furthermore, prezygotic isolation evolves faster among sympatric taxa than among allopatric taxa (Fig. 19.3), as expected if there has been reinforcement. Despite this evidence for the importance of behavioural traits in rapid speciation, the vast majority of genetic studies of speciation have focused on postzygotic effects, e.g. hybrid sterility and inviability, predominantly in *Drosophila* (Coyne & Orr 2004, Orr *et al.* 2007), and a few in other animals, such as house mice *Mus musculus* (Payseur & Place 2007) and marine copepods (Burton *et al.* 2006). In comparison, relatively little is known about the genetic basis of traits involved in pre-mating isolation. Below, we discuss some of the reasons for this discrepancy, describe a few exceptions to this claim, and then summarise new methods that should make it possible to greatly expand this list in the near future.

Identifying genes that are important for sexual isolation is challenging for several reasons. First, once populations become isolated, they will begin diverging at many loci across the genome. The rate of divergence at each locus depends on selection, recombination and population size (which might vary within the genome, e.g. autosomes vs. sex chromosomes vs. cytoplasmic factors), so determining which changes have behavioural consequences is critical and determining the order in which changes have occurred is difficult. Furthermore, estimates of

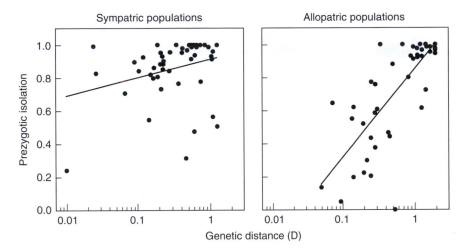

Figure 19.3 Prezygotic isolation, as measured by the ability of males to transfer sperm, evolves more rapidly among closely related, as measured by Nei's genetic distance, species of *Drosophila* that have sympatric rather than allopatric distributions. Each point represents a pair of species. See Coyne & Orr (1989, 1997, 1998) for details.

the number of genetic factors involved in isolating any particular pair of species (e.g. Coyne & Orr 1998) could be due either to differences in divergence times or to differences in selection and recombination, or both.

A second issue relates to how species recognition occurs. For example, two species may differ in aspects of courtship song, e.g. *Drosophila heteroneura* and *D. sylvestris* (Boake & Poulsen 1997), but if song only occurs after mate attraction by a pheromone, then genes that influence song variation may be unimportant for sexual isolation. Thus, it is critical that the signal that is involved in mate recognition is identified for study.

Finally, understanding the genetic basis of premating isolation potentially involves studying the genetic basis of mate-recognition signals that are produced by either or both sexes as well as the preference exhibited by each sex for conspecific versus heterospecific signals. Simple experiments that do not attempt to separate signal production from reception can be used to determine the presence of sexual isolation, but typically cannot be used to identify the genetic basis of the traits that are evolving. One exception to this assertion would be when there is a one-allele

mechanism of sexual isolation (e.g. Ortiz-Barrientos & Noor 2005).

When there are divergent recognition signals and corresponding preferences, a critical question is how genes for divergent traits and divergent preferences become and remain associated. Two genetic alternatives are possible. One scenario is that the gene influencing the species-recognition signal has pleiotropic effects on the preference for that signal, i.e. there is *genetic coupling* of trait and preference (Hoy *et al.* 1977). The alternative is that genes for the recognition signal and preference are independent, and allelic associations at these loci are maintained by selection.

Whereas the genetic-coupling hypothesis has long been viewed with scepticism (Butlin & Ritchie 1989, Boake 1991, Simmons *et al.* 2001, Simmons 2004), several recent studies provide intriguing evidence consistent with either coupling or close physical linkage of genes that influence a recognition cue and mate preference. The neotropical butterflies *Heliconius cydno* and *H. pachinus* differ in forewing band colour. Recent fine-scale genetic mapping experiments reveal that the genes for forewing colour and for male preference for that colour both map to a small

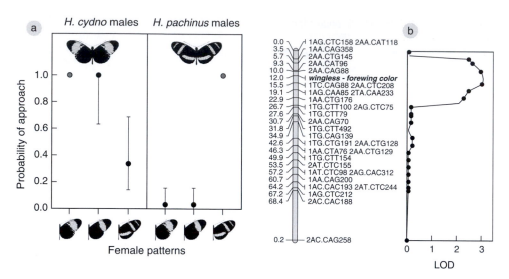

Figure 19.4 Mate preference and mate-recognition cue map to the same genetic region in *Heliconius* butterflies (Kronforst *et al.* 2006b), which provides evidence in support of the genetic-coupling hypothesis. (a) *Heliconius cydno* and *H. pachinus* males recognise conspecific females based on wing colour. This graph shows the probability that a male of each species will approach female wings with either parental or F$_1$ hybrid colour patterns. (b) Composite interval mapping indicates that male mate preference maps to a small autosomal region that includes *wingless*, a gene that is involved in controlling forewing colour in these butterflies.

region on an autosome that contains the gene *wingless* (Fig. 19.4; Kronforst *et al.* 2006a). The authors propose that this gene simultaneously influences wing colour and mate preference by influencing the production of pigments that are found in both wing scales and ommatidia. This scenario provides, therefore, a mechanism by which selection on either wing coloration or on preference for wing coloration would drive the other character. Correlated evolution of this type would facilitate the evolution of the remarkable mimicry complexes that are exhibited by *Heliconius* butterflies (Kronforst *et al.* 2006b, 2007). In *D. melanogaster* a mutation in the *desaturase 1* gene influences both signal production and discrimination, apparently as a consequence of pleiotropic effects of this gene (Marcillac *et al.* 2008). Finally, genetic linkage between mate-recognition signals and preferences has recently been reported for pied flycatchers *Ficedula hypoleuca* (Saether *et al.* 2007).

The alternative to genetic coupling is that independent loci influence mate recognition signals and

preferences. Most evidence from *Drosophila* (Coyne & Orr 1998), particularly that from recently diverged species, is consistent with this view. For example, by testing flies that resulted from backcrosses to either of two parental species, *D. santomea* or *D. yakuba*, Moehring *et al.* (2006) found that the QTL associated with male copulation occurrence or latency were different than those for females, which suggests that the two sexes use different cues for mating and that at least a few genes are important for species discrimination. Similar results have been reported for *D. simulans* and *D. sechellia*, which differ in cuticular hydrocarbons that are used by females for mate recognition (Gleason *et al.* 2005).

With the availability of relatively inexpensive genetic markers, such as amplified fragment length polymorphisms (Mueller & Wolfenbarger 1999), it is now possible to scan the genome of any organism to locate regions potentially important for speciation. Several methods have been proposed (Noor & Feder 2006) and more will likely follow. One approach uses variation in F_{st} at multiple loci to indicate regions of the genome that are adapted to different locations (Beaumont 2005), and is based on the premise that genomic regions near a polymorphic site under positive or negative selection will show deviations from random segregation due to hitchhiking (Maynard Smith & Haigh 1974). Genome scans are attractive because variation in population history can be controlled, and they can be applied without phenotype information because they rely on identifying parts of the genome that exhibit non-random segregation (Vasemagi & Primmer 2005).

An alternative approach for locating genomic regions involved in reproductive isolation is to perform admixture mapping. In effect, this is a form of QTL mapping in which a variety of backcross and other intercrosses are taken from a hybrid zone and used for the mapping population. Genomic heterogeneity among hybrid individuals then reveals regions undergoing strong selection, particularly when compared to populations in allopatry. In the larch bud moth *Zeiraphera improbana*, such analyses have revealed evidence of selection in hybrid populations (Emelianov *et al.* 2004). In those species where microarray technology is available (e.g. Gresham *et al.* 2006), precise localisation of genomic regions involved in reproductive isolation is now possible, as has been demonstrated for races of the mosquito *Anopheles gambiae* (Turner *et al.* 2005).

Association studies (also referred to as linkage disequilibrium mapping) test if a certain genotype (or multilocus haplotype) is associated more frequently with a phenotypic trait than expected by chance using the non-random occurrence of alleles at linked loci, i.e. linkage disequilibrium (LD). The extent of LD depends on many biological and demographic factors, including recombination rate, population history, selection and mating system. As a result, the extent of linkage disequilibrium varies across species, populations and genomic regions (Jorde 2000). Thus, high LD in an organism allows for genome scans with relatively few evenly spaced markers, but fine-scale mapping will be very difficult. In contrast, low LD means that the hitchhiking regions will be small and genomic scans will require many markers

to be informative. A hybrid approach is to survey markers near candidate genes for association. One method partitions a haplotype tree into two or more clades, and then estimates the phenotypic association related to the specific substitution(s) in the tree (Templeton *et al.* 2005). Analyses that incorporate an evolutionary framework should be especially useful for candidate gene association studies of behaviour in non-model organisms.

19.6 Social behaviour and speciation rate

Several hypotheses have been proposed to link variation in social behaviour to the likelihood that new species will evolve (see also Chapter 5). In an influential paper, Bush *et al.* (1977) proposed that speciation rate in vertebrates varies with social organisation. The basis of their argument was that species with harem mating systems, particularly mammals such as horses and primates, are likely to have smaller effective population sizes, which allows chromosomal rearrangements to go to fixation more quickly. In support of this idea the authors reported a correlation between the rate of karyotypic change (due to change in chromosome or arm number) and the rate of speciation as measured by estimates of the number of extant and extinct species per lineage among orders of mammals and other vertebrate groups. Bush *et al.* (1977) suggested that this correlation could result either from *stasipatric* speciation (White 1968), where a chromosomal rearrangement goes to fixation in an isolated population and then forms a postmating reproductive isolating mechanism, or from creation of a coadapted gene complex that resists recombination.

The social organisation/speciation hypothesis motivated a considerable amount of research on the amount of standing genetic variation in populations of different species. An extensive review of that literature indicates that while considerable variation in genetic structure exists among species of social mammals, the amount of gene flow that is typically present in most taxa is more than enough to cast doubt on the drift-induced speciation idea (Storz

1999). Higher rates of karyotypic change and speciation in mammals, as compared to ectothermic vertebrates, has more recently been attributed to differences in genome organisation (Bernardi 1993, Bernardi *et al.* 1997). Correlations between chromosomal change and species diversity have also been reported for some lizards and snakes (Olmo 2005), casting further doubt on any role for social organisation in speciation. The role of chromosomal rearrangements in speciation has, however, experienced a resurgence of interest.

Recent theory (Kirkpatrick & Barton 2006) reveals that new inversions, which capture locally adapted alleles, can increase in frequency under a variety of conditions. Such inversions can then contribute to reproductive isolation via postzygotic isolation (Navarro & Barton 2003, Noor *et al.* 2001), or by prezygotic isolation when the inversions contain loci that affect pre-mating behaviours. High rates of chromosomal rearrangement have recently been associated with rapid speciation in lycaenid butterflies, murid rodents and gerbils (Pialek *et al.* 2001, Dobigny *et al.* 2002, Veyrunes *et al.* 2006, Kandul *et al.* 2007). The extent to which social behaviour contributes to any of these cases remains to be determined.

A very different hypothesis for how social behaviour affects speciation rate has recently been proposed for birds. In a large phylogenetic analysis of parental care in birds, Cockburn (2003) found that cooperative breeding is often the ancestral trait (see also Ekman & Ericson 2006), and predominantly cooperative genera are species-poor compared to their pair-breeding counterparts. Cooperatively breeding species tend to be sedentary residents, while pair-breeding species are more likely to be migratory and inhabit oceanic islands. In support of these results, high annual dispersal has recently been identified as the best predictor of phylogenetic diversification in birds (Phillimore *et al.* 2006). Sociality does not appear to accelerate speciation in other taxa, either. Social carnivores have higher extinction rates than solitary carnivores (Munoz-Duran 2002), and social insects, including termites, ants, eusocial bees and eusocial wasps, tend to have higher rates of outbreeding and slower rates of evolution than vertebrates (Wilson

1992). Thus, rather than accelerate speciation, sociality may constrain speciation.

As noted previously, the most commonly invoked behavioural cause for high rates of speciation is sexual selection (Dominey 1984, Ringo 1997, Price 1998, Edwards *et al.* 2005). While several comparative analyses of birds using degree of sexual dimorphism (Barraclough *et al.* 1995, Barraclough *et al.* 1998, Møller & Cuervo 1998, Owens *et al.* 1999b) or mating system (Mitra *et al.* 1996) to predict species richness have supported this claim, more recent studies using sexual size dimorphism, sexual dichromatism, or relative testis size and improved methods have failed to find any relationship to taxonomic diversity in birds, mammals or fishes (Gage *et al.* 2002, Morrow *et al.* 2003, Ritchie *et al.* 2005). One possible reason for failing to detect such a correlation is that sexual selection may also accelerate extinction rates (Morrow & Pitcher 2003). Resolution of this issue likely will require focused studies on groups of organisms where traits that are known to influence reproductive isolation can be measured and their evolutionary rates compared (e.g. Mendelson & Shaw 2005).

19.7 Conclusions and future directions

The process of speciation is arguably one of the most active areas of research in evolutionary biology. Considerable interest focuses on understanding how sexual selection, acting both before and after mating, may either accelerate or retard the speciation process. In addition, unravelling the temporal sequence of events that has led to divergence in traits that affect fertilisation success is critical for identifying the factors that cause, rather than correlate with, reproductive isolation. Despite intense interest in this topic, clear examples of sexual selection driving speciation are not widespread. One of the most dramatic examples of rapid speciation in birds involves sexual imprinting. This observation suggests that more study of cases where cultural transmission is involved in mate recognition is warranted.

A related challenge remains to assess the general importance of sexual conflict in driving speciation.

While studies from a variety of taxa suggest that rapid amino-acid sequence divergence of sex-related proteins is likely caused by sexually antagonistic coevolution, the relationship between such protein change and reproductive isolation remains poorly understood in most taxa. Given that sexual conflict also has the potential to increase gene flow and oppose speciation whenever males control mating decisions, resolution of this issue will depend critically on understanding how mating is influenced by male and female behaviour.

The development of new and increasingly less expensive technologies for identifying genetic variants on a genome-wide scale can be predicted to advance understanding of the genetic basis of prezygotic reproductive isolation in a variety of organisms. Because most genetic studies of speciation to date have focused on postzygotic isolation in *Drosophila*, at this point it is difficult to know if general patterns will be uncovered. Certainly, additional fine-scale genetic mapping experiments should reveal if recognition cues and mate preferences share a common genetic basis or exhibit close genetic linkage in butterflies or any other taxa. Perhaps more interesting, though, will be genome scans that reveal previously uncharacterised regions that have undergone recent divergence. Such discovery-based study has the potential to identify new candidate genes whose role in speciation and possibly mate recognition can then be explored through experimental and association studies. By studying groups of closely related species, the temporal sequence of genetic events that have resulted in reproductive isolation can also be deduced. While such insights undoubtedly will require effort, revealing the origin of species has never been more attainable.

Acknowledgements

We are grateful to Mike Sorenson, Marcus Kronforst and H. Allen Orr for sharing data or images that were used in the figures, Emily Rose and two anonymous reviewers for constructive comments on the manuscript, and the National Science Foundation for support from grants DEB-0343617, DEB-0444886 and DEB-0611534 to GSW.

Suggested readings

Coyne, J. A. & Orr, H. A. (2004) *Speciation*. Sunderland, MA: Sinauer Associates.

Etges, W. J. & Noor, M. A. F. (2002) *Genetics of Mate Choice: from Sexual Selection to Sexual Isolation*. New York, NY: Kluwer.

Gavrilets, S. (2004) *Fitness Landscapes and the Origin of Species,* Princeton, NJ: Princeton University Press.

Ptacek, M. B. (2000) The role of mating preferences in shaping interspecific divergence in mating signals in vertebrates. *Behavioural Processes*, **51**, 111–134.

West-Eberhard, M. J. (1983) Sexual selection, social competition, and speciation. *Quarterly Review of Biology*, **58**, 155–183.

References

Alexander, R. D., Marshall, D. C. & Cooley, J. R. (1997) Evolutionary perspectives on insect mating. In: *The Evolution of Mating Systems in Insects and Arachnids*, ed. J. C. Choe & B. J. Crespi. Cambridge: Cambridge University Press, pp. 4–31.

Andersson, M. (1994) *Sexual Selection*. Princeton, NJ: Princeton University Press.

Andersson, S., Pryke, S. R., Ornborg, J., Lawes, M. J. & Andersson, M. (2002) Multiple receivers, multiple ornaments, and a trade-off between agonistic and epigamic signaling in a widowbird. *American Naturalist*, **160**, 683–691.

Andres, J. A. & Arnqvist, G. (2001) Genetic divergence of the seminal signal–receptor system in houseflies: the footprints of sexually antagonistic coevolution? *Proceedings of the Royal Society of London Series B-Biological Sciences*, **268**, 399–405.

Aoki, K., Feldman, M. W. & Kerr, B. (2001) Models of sexual selection on a quantitative genetic trait when preference is acquired by sexual imprinting. *Evolution*, **55**, 25–32.

Arnegard, M. E. & Kondrashov, A. S. (2004) Sympatric speciation by sexual selection alone is unlikely. *Evolution*, **58**, 222–237.

Arnqvist, G. & Rowe, L. (2002a) Antagonistic coevolution between the sexes in a group of insects. *Nature*, **415**, 787–789.

Arnqvist, G. & Rowe, L. (2002b) Correlated evolution of male and female morphologies in water striders. *Evolution*, **56**, 936–947.

Arnqvist, G. & Rowe, L. (2005) *Sexual Conflict*. Princeton, NJ: Princeton University Press.

Arnqvist, G., Edvardsson, M., Friberg, U. & Nilsson, T. (2000) Sexual conflict promotes speciation in insects. *Proceedings of the National Academy of Sciences of the USA*, **97**, 10460–10464.

Attia, F. A. & Tregenza, T. (2004) Divergence revealed by population crosses in the red flour beetle *Tribolium castaneum*. *Evoutionary Ecology Research*, **6**, 927–935.

Bacigalupe, L. D., Crudgington, H. S., Hunter, F., Moore, A. J. & Snook, R. R. (2007) Sexual conflict does not drive reproductive isolation in experimental populations of *Drosophila pseudoobscura*. *Journal of Evolutionary Biology*, **20**, 1763–1771.

Balakrishnan, C. N. & Sorenson, M. D. (2006) Song discrimination suggests premating isolation among sympatric indigobird species and host races. *Behavioral Ecology*, **17**, 473–478.

Barraclough, T. G., Harvey, P. H. & Nee, S. (1995) Sexual selection and taxonomic diversity in passerine birds. *Proceedings of the Royal Society B*, **259**, 211–215.

Barraclough, T. G., Vogler, A. P. & Harvey, P. H. (1998) Revealing the factors that promote speciation. *Philosophical Transactions of the Royal Society B*, **353**, 241–249.

Bateson, P. (1978) Sexual imprinting and optimal outbreeding. *Nature*, **273**, 659–660.

Beaumont, M. A. (2005) Adaptation and speciation: what can Fst tell us? *Trends in Ecology and Evolution*, **20**, 435–440.

Bella, J. L., Butlin, R. K., Ferris, C. & Hewitt, G. M. (1992) Asymmetrical homogamy and unequal sex-ratio from reciprocal mating-order crosses between *Chorthippus parallelus* subspecies. *Heredity*, **68**, 345–352.

Bernardi, G. (1993) Genome organization and species formation in vertebrates. *Journal of Molecular Evolution*, **37**, 331–337.

Bernardi, G., Hughes, S. & Mouchiroud, D. (1997) The major compositional transitions in the vertebrate genome. *Journal of Molecular Evolution*, **44**, S44–51.

Birkhead, T. R. & Billard, P. (2007) Reproductive isolation in birds: postcopulatory, prezygotic barriers. *Trends in Ecology and Evolution*, **22**, 266–272.

Boake, C. R. B. (1991) Coevolution of senders and receivers of sexual signals – genetic coupling and genetic correlations. *Trends in Ecology and Evolution*, **6**, 225–227.

Boake, C. R. B. (2002) Sexual signaling and speciation: a microevolutionary perspective. *Genetica*, **116**, 205–214.

Boake, C. R. B. & Poulsen, T. (1997) Correlates versus predictors of courtship success: courtship song in *Drosophila silvestris* and *D. heteroneura*. *Animal Behaviour*, **54**, 699–704.

Boake, C. R. B., Deangelis, M. P. & Andreadis, D. K. (1997) Is sexual selection and species recognition a continuum? Mating behavior of the stalk-eyed fly *Drosophila heteroneura*. *Proceedings of the National Academy of Sciences of the USA*, **94**, 12442–12445.

Brooks, R. (2002) Variation in female mate choice within guppy populations: population divergence, multiple ornaments and the maintenance of polymorphism. *Genetica*, **116**, 343–358.

Brown, D. V. & Eady, P. E. (2001) Functional incompatibility between the fertilization systems of two allopatric populations of *Callosobruchus maculatus* (Coleoptera: Bruchidae). *Evolution*, **55**, 2257–2262.

Burton, R. S., Ellison, C. K. & Harrison, J. S. (2006) The sorry state of F-2 hybrids: consequences of rapid mitochondrial DNA evolution in allopatric populations. *American Naturalist*, **168**, S14–S24.

Bush, G. L. (1969) Sympatric host race formation and speciation in frugivorous flies of genus *Rhagoletis* (Diptera, Tephritidae). *Evolution*, **23**, 237–251.

Bush, G. L., Case, S. M., Wilson, A. C. & Patton, J. L. (1977) Rapid speciation and chromosomal evolution in mammals. *Proceedings of the National Academy of Sciences of the USA*, **74**, 3942–3946.

Butlin, R. K. & Ritchie, M. G. (1989) Genetic coupling in mate recognition systems: what is the evidence? *Biological Journal of the Linnean Society*, **37**, 237–246.

Butlin, R. K., Hewitt, G. M. & Webb, S. F. (1985) Sexual selection for intermediate optimum in *Chorthippus brunneus* (Orthoptera: Acrididae). *Animal Behaviour*, **33**, 1281–1292.

Calsbeek, R., Alonzo, S. H., Zamudio, K. & Sinervo, B. (2002) Sexual selection and alternative mating behaviours generate demographic stochasticity in small populations. *Proceedings of the Royal Society B*, **269**, 157–164.

Chang, A. S. (2004) Conspecific sperm precedence in sister species of *Drosophila* with overlapping ranges. *Evolution*, **58**, 781–789.

Chapman, T., Arnqvist, G., Bangham, J. & Rowe, L. (2003) Sexual conflict. *Trends in Ecology and Evolution*, **18**, 41–47.

Christianson, S. J., Swallow, J. G. & Wilkinson, G. S. (2005) Rapid evolution of postzygotic reproductive isolation in stalk-eyed flies. *Evolution*, **59**, 849–857.

Civetta, A. & Singh, R. S. (1998) Sex and speciation: genetic architecture and evolutionary potential of sexual versus nonsexual traits in the sibling species of the *Drosophila melanogaster* complex. *Evolution*, **52**, 1080–1092.

Clark, A. G., Aguade, M., Prout, T., Harshman, L. G. & Langley, C. H. (1995) Variation in sperm displacement and its association with accessory-gland protein loci in *Drosophila melanogaster*. *Genetics*, **139**, 189–201.

Cockburn, A. (2003) Cooperative breeding in oscine passerines: does sociality inhibit speciation? *Proceedings of the Royal Society B*, **270**, 2207–2214.

Cordero, A. (1995) Ejaculate substances that affect female insect reproductive physiology and behavior: honest or arbitrary? *Journal of Theoretical Biology*, **192**, 453–461.

Coyne, J. A. & Orr, H. A. (1989) Patterns of speciation in *Drosophila*. *Evolution*, **43**, 362–381.

Coyne, J. A. & Orr, H. A. (1997) 'Patterns of speciation in *Drosophila*' revisited. *Evolution*, **51**, 295–303.

Coyne, J. A. & Orr, H. A. (1998) The evolutionary genetics of speciation. *Philosophical Transactions of the Royal Society B*, **353**, 287–305.

Coyne, J. A. & Orr, H. A. (2004) *Speciation*. Sunderland, MA: Sinauer Associates.

Crudgington, H. S., Beckerman, A. P., Brustle, L., Green, K. & Snook, R. R. (2005) Experimental removal and elevation of sexual selection: does sexual selection generate manipulative males and resistant females? *American Naturalist*, **165**, S72–87.

Curtsinger, J. W. (1991) Sperm competition and the evolution of multiple mating. *American Naturalist*, **138**, 93–102.

Dawkins, R. & Krebs, J. R. (1979) Arms races between and within species. *Proceedings of the Royal Society B*, **295**, 489–511.

Dixon, S. M., Coyne, J. A. & Noor, M. A. F. (2003) The evolution of conspecific sperm precedence in *Drosophila*. *Molecular Ecology*, **12**, 2028–2037.

Dobigny, G., Aniskin, V. & Volobouev, V. (2002) Explosive chromosome evolution and speciation in the gerbil genus *Taterillus* (Rodentia, Gerbillinae): a case of two new cryptic species. *Cytogenetic and Genome Research*, **96**, 117–124.

Dobzhansky, T. (1937) *Genetics and the Origin of Species*. New York, NY: Columbia University Press.

Dominey, W. J. (1984) Effects of sexual selection and life histories on speciation: species flocks in African cichlids and Hawaiian *Drosophila*. In: *Evolution of Fish Species Flocks*, ed. A. A. Echelle & I. Kornfield. Orono, ME: University of Maine Press, pp. 231–249.

Dugatkin, L. A. & Godin, J. G. J. (1992) Reversal of female mate choice by copying in the guppy (*Poecilia reticulata*). *Proceedings of the Royal Society B*, **249**, 179–184.

Eberhard, W. G. (1996) *Female Control: Sexual Selection and Cryptic Female Choice*, Princeton, NJ: Princeton University Press.

Eberhard, W. G. (2004) Male–female conflict and genitalia: failure to confirm predictions in insects and spiders. *Biological Reviews*, **79**, 121–186.

Eberhard, W. G. & Cordero, A. (1995) Sexual selection by cryptic female choice on male seminal products: a bridge between sexual selection and reproductive physiology. *Trends in Ecology and Evolution*, **10**, 493–496.

Edwards, S. V., Kingan, S. B., Calkins, J. D. *et al.* (2005) Speciation in birds: genes, geography, and sexual selection. *Proceedings of the National Academy of Sciences of the USA*, **102**, 6550–6557.

Ekman, J. & Ericson, P. G. P. (2006) Out of Gondwanaland: the evolutionary history of cooperative breeding and social behaviour among crows, magpies, jays and allies. *Proceedings of the Royal Society B*, **273**, 1117–1125.

Emelianov, I., Marec, F. & Mallet, J. (2004) Genomic evidence for divergence with gene flow in host races of the larch budmoth. *Proceedings of the Royal Society of London Series B-Biological Sciences*, **271**, 97–105.

Feder, J. L., Opp, S. B., Wlazlo, B. *et al.* (1994) Host fidelity is an effective premating barrier between sympatric races of the apple maggot fly. *Proceedings of the National Academy of Sciences of the USA*, **91**, 7990–7994.

Feder, J. L., Berlocher, S. H., Roethele, J. B. *et al.* (2003) Allopatric genetic origins for sympatric host-plant shifts and race formation in *Rhagoletis*. *Proceedings of the National Academy of Sciences of the USA*, **100**, 10314–10319.

Fedorka, K. M. & Mousseau, T. A. (2002) Nuptial gifts and the evolution of male body size. *Evolution*, **56**, 590–596.

Felsenstein, J. (1981) Skepticism towards Santa Rosalia, or why are there so few kinds of animals? *Evolution*, **35**, 124–138.

Fisher, R. A. (1930) *The Genetical Theory of Natural Selection*. Oxford: Clarendon Press.

Gage, M. J. G., Parker, G. A., Nylin, S. & Wiklund, C. (2002) Sexual selection and speciation in mammals, butterflies and spiders. *Proceedings of the Royal Society B*, **269**, 2309–2316.

Gavrilets, S. (2000) Rapid evolution of reproductive barriers driven by sexual conflict. *Nature*, **403**, 886–889.

Gavrilets, S. (2004) *Fitness Landscapes and the Origin of Species.* Princeton, NJ: Princeton University Press.

Gavrilets, S. & Waxman, D. (2002) Sympatric speciation by sexual conflict. *Proceedings of the National Academy of Sciences of the USA*, **99**, 10533–10538.

Gerhardt, H. C. (1991) Female mate choice in treefrogs: static and dynamic acoustic criteria. *Animal Behaviour*, **42**, 615–635.

Geyer, L. B. & Palumbi, S. R. (2005) Conspecific sperm precedence in two species of tropical sea urchins. *Evolution*, **59**, 97–105.

Gibson, R. M. & Bradbury, J. W. (1985) Sexual selection in lekking sage grouse: phenotypic correlates of male mating success. *Behavioral Ecology and Sociobiology*, **18**, 117–123.

Gleason, J. M., Jallon, J. M., Rouault, J. D. & Ritchie, M. G. (2005) Quantitative trait loci for cuticular hydrocarbons associated with sexual isolation between *Drosophila simulans* and *D. sechellia. Genetics*, **171**, 1789–1798.

Grafen, A. (1990) Biological signals as handicaps. *Journal of Theoretical Biology*, **144**, 517–546.

Grant, B. R. & Grant, P. R. (1996) Cultural inheritance of song and its role in the evolution of Darwin's finches. *Evolution*, **50**, 2471–2487.

Gray, D. A. & Cade, W. H. (2000) Sexual selection and speciation in field crickets. *Proceedings of the National Academy of Sciences of the USA*, **97**, 14449–14454.

Gray, S. M. & Mckinnon, J. S. (2007) Linking color polymorphism maintenance and speciation. *Trends in Ecology and Evolution*, **22**, 71–79.

Greene, E., Lyon, B. E., Muehter, V. R., Ratcliffe, L., Oliver, S. J. & Boag, P. T. (2000) Disruptive sexual selection for plumage coloration in a passerine bird. *Nature*, **407**, 1000–1003.

Gregory, P. G. & Howard, D. J. (1994) A post-insemination barrier to fertilization isolates two closely related ground crickets. *Evolution*, **48**, 705–710.

Gresham, D., Ruderfer, D. M., Pratt, S. C. *et al.* (2006) Genome-wide detection of polymorphisms at nucleotide resolution with a single DNA microarray. *Science*, **311**, 1932–1936.

Griffith, S. C., Owens, I. P. F. & Burke, T. (1999) Environmental determination of a sexually selected trait. *Nature*, **400**, 358–360.

Haig, D. & Bergstrom, C. T. (1995) Multiple mating, sperm competition and meiotic drive. *Journal of Evolutionary Biology*, **8**, 265–282.

Harrison, R. G. (1998) Linking evolutionary pattern and process: the relevance of species concepts for the study of speciation. In: *Endless Forms: Species and Speciation*, ed.

D. J. Howard & S. H. Berlocher. Oxford: Oxford University Press, pp. 19–31.

Harvey, P. H. & May, R. M. (1989) Out for the sperm count. *Nature*, **337**, 508–509.

Hasselquist, D., Bensch, S. & von Schantz, T. (1996) Correlation between male song repertoire, extra-pair paternity and offspring survival in the great reed warbler. *Nature*, **381**, 229–232.

Hauber, M. E. & Sherman, P. W. (2001) Self-referent phenotype matching: theoretical considerations and empirical evidence. *Trends in Neurosciences*, **24**, 609–616.

Hawthorne, D. H. & Via, S. (2001) Genetic linkage facilitates ecological specialization and reproductive isolation in pea aphids. *Nature*, **412**, 904–907.

Hewitt, G. M., Mason, P. & Nichols, R. A. (1989) Sperm precedence and homogamy across a hybrid zone in the alpine grasshopper *Podisma pedestris. Heredity*, **62**, 343–353.

Higgie, M. & Blows, M. W. (2007) Are traits that experience reinforcement also under sexual selection? *American Naturalist*, **170**, 409–420.

Higgie, M., Chenoweth, S. & Blows, M. W. (2000) Natural selection and the reinforcement of mate recognition. *Science*, **290**, 519–521.

Hill, G. E., Inouye, C. Y. & Montgomerie, R. (2002) Dietary carotenoids predict plumage coloration in wild house finches. *Proceedings of the Royal Society B*, **269**, 1119–1124.

Hollocher, H. & Williamson, M. (1996) Island hopping in *Drosophila*: patterns and processes. *Philosophical Transactions of the Royal Society B*, **351**, 735–743.

Hosken, D. J., Blanckenhorn, W. U. & Garner, T. W. J. (2002) Heteropopulation males have a fertilization advantage during sperm competition in the yellow dung fly (*Scathophaga stercoraria*). *Proceedings of the Royal Society B*, **269**, 1701–1707.

Hosken, D. J., Garner, T. W. J., Tregenza, T., Wedell, N. & Ward, P. I. (2003) Superior sperm competitors sire higher-quality young. *Proceedings of the Royal Society B*, **270**, 1933–1938.

Howard, D. J. (1993) *Reinforcement: Origin, Dynamics, and Fate of an Evolutionary Hypothesis.* Oxford: Oxford University Press.

Howard, D. J. (1999) Conspecific sperm and pollen precedence and speciation. *Annual Review of Ecology and Systematics*, **30**, 109–132.

Hoy, R. R., Hahn, J. & Paul, R. C. (1977) Hybrid cricket auditory behavior: evidence for genetic coupling in animal communication. *Science*, **195**, 82–84.

Irwin, D. E. (2000) Song variation in an avian ring species. *Evolution*, **54**, 998–1010.

Irwin, D. E. & Price, T. (1999) Sexual imprinting, learning and speciation. *Heredity*, **82**, 347–354.

Irwin, D. E., Bensch, S. & Price, T. D. (2001) Speciation in a ring. *Nature*, **409**, 333–337.

Irwin, D. E., Bensch, S., Irwin, J. H. & Price, T. D. (2005) Speciation by distance in a ring species. *Science*, **307**, 414–416.

Janetos, A. C. (1980) Strategies of female mate choice: a theoretical analysis. *Behavioral Ecology and Sociobiology*, **7**, 107–112.

Jennions, M. D. & Petrie, M. (2000) Why do females mate multiply? A review of the genetic benefits. *Biological Reviews*, **75**, 21.

Johnstone, R. A. (1995) Honest advertisement of multiple qualities using multiple signals. *Journal of Theoretical Biology*, **177**, 87–94.

Jorde, L. B. (2000) Linkage disequilibrium and the search for complex disease genes. *Genome Research*, **10**, 1435–1444.

Kandul, N. R., Lukhtanov, V. A. & Pierce, N. E. (2007) Karyotypic diversity and speciation in *Agrodiaetus* butterflies. *Evolution*, **61**, 546–559.

Katakura, H. (1986) Evidence for the incapacitation of heterospecific sperm in the female genital tract in a pair of closely related ladybirds (Insecta, Coleoptera, Coccinellidae). *Zoological Science*, **3**, 115–121.

Keller, L. & Reeve, H. K. (1995) Why do females mate with multiple males? The sexually selected sperm hypothesis. *Advances in the Study of Behavior*, **24**, 291–315.

Kendrick, K. M., Hinton, M. R., Atkins, K., Haupt, M. A. & Skinner, J. D. (1998) Mothers determine sexual preferences. *Nature*, **395**, 229–230.

Kirkpatrick, M. (1982) Sexual selection and the evolution of female choice. *Evolution*, **36**, 1–12.

Kirkpatrick, M. (1996) Good genes and direct selection in the evolution of mating preferences. *Evolution*, **50**, 2125–2140.

Kirkpatrick, M. & Barton, N. H. (1997) The strength of indirect selection on female mating preferences. *Proceedings of the National Academy of Sciences of the USA*, **94**, 1282–1286.

Kirkpatrick, M. & Barton, N. (2006) Chromosome inversions, local adaptation and speciation. *Genetics*, **173**, 419–434.

Kirkpatrick, M. & Ravigne, V. (2002) Speciation by natural and sexual selection: models and experiments. *American Naturalist*, **159**, S22–35.

Kirkpatrick, M. & Ryan, M. J. (1991) The evolution of mating preferences and the paradox of the lek. *Nature*, **350**, 33–38.

Kronforst, M. R., Young, L. G., Kapan, D. D. *et al.* (2006a) Linkage of butterfly mate preference and wing color preference cue at the genomic location of wingless. *Proceedings of the National Academy of Sciences of the USA*, **103**, 6575–6580.

Kronforst, M. R., Kapan, D. D. & Gilbert, L. E. (2006b) Parallel genetic architecture of parallel adaptive radiations in mimetic *Heliconius* butterflies. *Genetics*, **174**, 535–539.

Kronforst, M. R., Young, L. G. & Gilbert, L. E. (2007) Reinforcement of mate preference among hybridizing *Heliconius* butterflies. *Journal of Evolutionary Biology*, **20**, 278–285.

Kruijt, J. P., Bossema, I. & Lammers, G. J. (1982) Effects of early experience and male activity on mate choice in mallard females (*Anas platyrhynchos*). *Behaviour*, **80**, 32–43.

Kyriacou, C. P. & Hall, J. C. (1982) The function of courtship song rhythms in *Drosophila*. *Animal Behaviour*, **30**, 794–801.

Lachlan, R. F. & Servedio, M. R. (2004) Song learning accelerates allopatric speciation. *Evolution*, **58**, 2049–2063.

Laland, K. N. (1994) On the evolutionary consequences of sexual imprinting. *Evolution*, **48**, 477–489.

Lande, R. (1981) Models of speciation by sexual selection on polygenic traits. *Proceedings of the National Academy of Sciences of the USA*, **78**, 3721–3725.

Lande, R. & Wilkinson, G. S. (1999) Models of sex-ratio meiotic drive and sexual selection in stalk-eyed flies. *Genetical Research*, **74**, 245–253.

Liou, L. W. & Price, T. D. (1994) Speciation by reinforcement of premating isolation. *Evolution*, **48**, 1451–1459.

Ludlow, A. M. & Magurran, A. E. (2006) Gametic isolation in guppies (*Poecilia reticulata*). *Proceedings of the Royal Society B*, **273**, 2477.

Mallet, J. (1995) A species definition for the modern synthesis. *Trends in Ecology and Evolution*, **10**, 294–299.

Marcillac, F., Grosjean, Y. & Ferveur, J.-F. (2008) A single mutation alters production and discrimination of *Drosophila* sex pheromones. *Proceedings of the Royal Society B*, **272**, 303–309.

Martens, J. (1996) Vocalizations and speciation of Palearctic birds. In: *Ecology and Evolution of Acoustic Communication in Birds*, ed. D. E. Kroodsma & E. H. Miller. Ithaca, NY: Cornell University Press, pp. 221–240.

Martin, O. Y. & Hosken, D. J. (2003) The evolution of reproductive isolation through sexual conflict. *Nature*, **423**, 979–982.

Mavarez, J., Salazar, C. A., Bermingham, E. *et al.* (2006) Speciation by hybridization in *Heliconius* butterflies. *Nature*, **441**, 868–871.

Maynard Smith, J. & Haigh, J. (1974) The hitchhiking effect of a favorable gene. *Genetical Research*, **23**, 23–35.

Maynard Smith, J. & Szathmáry, E. (1995) *The Major Transitions in Evolution*. New York, NY: W. H. Freeman.

Mayr, E. (1942) *Systematics and the Origin of Species*. New York, NY: Columbia University Press.

Mayr, E. (1963) *Animal Speciation and Evolution*. Cambridge, MA, Harvard University Press.

Mendelson, T. C. & Shaw, K. L. (2005) Rapid speciation in an arthropod. *Nature*, **433**, 375–376.

Mendelson, T. C., Imhoff, V. E. & Venditti, J. J. (2007) The accumulation of reproductive barriers during speciation: postmating barriers in two behaviorally isolated species of darters (Percidae : Etheostoma). *Evolution*, **61**, 2596–2606.

Meyer, A., Salzburger, W. & Schartl, M. (2006) Hybrid origin of a swordtail species (Teleostei : *Xiphophorus clemenciae*) driven by sexual selection. *Molecular Ecology*, **15**, 721–730.

Mitra, S., Landel, H. & Pruett Jones, S. (1996) Species richness covaries with mating system in birds. *Auk*, **113**, 544–551.

Moehring, A. J., Llopart, A., Elwyn, S., Coyne, J. A. & Mackay, T. F. C. (2006) The genetic basis of prezygotic reproductive isolation between *Drosophila santomea* and *D. yakuba* due to mating preference. *Genetics*, **173**, 215–223.

Møller, A. P. & Cuervo, J. J. (1998) Speciation and feather ornamentation in birds. *Evolution*, **52**, 859–869.

Morrow, E. H. & Pitcher, T. E. (2003) Sexual selection and the risk of extinction in birds. *Proceedings of the Royal Society B*, **270**, 1793–1799.

Morrow, E. H., Pitcher, T. E. & Arnqvist, G. (2003) No evidence that sexual selection is an 'engine of speciation' in birds. *Ecology Letters*, **6**, 228–234.

Mueller, U. G. & Wolfenbarger, L. L. (1999) AFLP genotyping and fingerprinting. *Trends in Ecology and Evolution*, **14**, 389–394.

Munoz-Duran, J. (2002) Correlates of speciation and extinction rates in the Carnivora. *Evolutionary Ecology Research*, **4**, 963–991.

Navarro, A. & Barton, N. H. (2003) Accumulating postzygotic isolation genes in parapatry: a new twist on chromosomal speciation. *Evolution*, **57**, 447–459.

Noor, M. A. F. (1995) Speciation driven by natural selection in *Drosophila*. *Nature*, **375**, 674–675.

Noor, M. A. F. & Feder, J. L. (2006) Speciation genetics: evolving approaches. *Nature Reviews Genetics*, **7**, 851–861.

Noor, M. A. F., Grams, K. L., Bertucci, L. A. & Reiland, J. (2001) Chromosomal inversions and the reproductive isolation of species. *Proceedings of the National Academy of Sciences of the USA*, **98**, 12084–12088.

Olmo, E. (2005) Rate of chromosome changes and speciation in reptiles. *Genetica*, **125**, 185–203.

Orr, H. A., Masly, J. P. & Phadnis, N. (2007) Speciation in *Drosophila*: from phenotypes to molecules. *Journal of Heredity*, **98**, 103–110.

Ortiz-Barrientos, D. & Noor, M. A. F. (2005) Evidence for a one-allele assortative mating locus. *Science*, **310**, 1467.

Owens, I. P. F., Rowe, C. & Thomas, A. L. R. (1999a) Sexual selection, speciation and imprinting: separating the sheep from the goats. *Trends in Ecology and Evolution*, **14**, 131–132.

Owens, I. P. F., Bennett, P. M. & Harvey, P. H. (1999b) Species richness among birds: body size, life history, sexual selection or ecology? *Proceedings of the Royal Society B*, **266**, 933–939.

Panhuis, T. M., Butlin, R., Zuk, M. & Tregenza, T. (2001) Sexual selection and speciation. *Trends in Ecology and Evolution*, **16**, 364–371.

Panhuis, T. M., Clark, N. L. & Swanson, W. J. (2006) Rapid evolution of reproductive proteins in abalone and *Drosophila*. *Philosophical Transactions of the Royal Society B*, **361**, 261–268.

Parker, G. A. (1970) Sperm competition and its evolutionary consequences in the insects. *Biological Reviews*, **45**, 525–567.

Parker, G. A. (1979) Sexual selection and sexual conflict. In: *Sexual Selection and Reproductive Competition in Insects*, ed. M. S. Blum & N. A. Blum. New York, NY: Academic Press, pp. 123–166.

Parker, G. A. (2006) Sexual conflict over mating and fertilization: an overview. *Philosophical Transactions of the Royal Society B*, **361**, 235–259.

Parker, G. A. & Partridge, L. (1998) Sexual conflict and speciation. *Philosophical Transactions of the Royal Society B*, **353**, 261–274.

Paterson, H. E. H. (1985) The recognition concept of species. In: *Species and Speciation*, ed. E. S. Vrba. Pretoria: Transvaal Museum, pp. 21–29.

Paulay, G. & Meyer, C. (2002) Diversification in the tropical Pacific: comparisons between marine and terrestrial systems and the importance of founder speciation. *Integrative and Comparative Biology*, **42**, 922–934.

Payne, R. B. (2005) Nestling mouth markings and colors of Old World finches Estrildidae: mimicry and coevolution of nesting finches and their *Vidua* brood parasites.

Miscellaneous Publications of the Museum of Zoology, University of Michigan, **194**, 1–45.

Payne, R. B., Payne, L. L. & Woods, J. L. (1998) Song learning in brood-parasitic indigobirds *Vidua chalybeata*: song mimicry of the host species. *Animal Behaviour*, **55**, 1537–1553.

Payne, R. B., Payne, L. L., Woods, J. L. & Sorenson, M. D. (2000) Imprinting and the origin of parasite-host species associations in brood-parasitic indigobirds, *Vidua chalybeata*. *Animal Behaviour*, **59**, 69–81.

Payseur, B. A. & Place, M. (2007) Searching the genomes of inbred mouse strains for incompatibilities that reproductively isolate their wild relatives. *Journal of Heredity*, **98**, 115–122.

Phillimore, A. B., Freckleton, R. P., Orme, C. D. L. & Owens, I. P. F. (2006) Ecology predicts large-scale patterns of phylogenetic diversification in birds. *American Naturalist*, **168**, 220–229.

Pialek, J., Hauffe, H. C., Rodriguez-Clark, K. M. & Searle, J. B. (2001) Raciation and speciation in house mice from the Alps: the role of chromosomes. *Molecular Ecology*, **10**, 613–625.

Pitnick, S., Miller, G. T., Schneider, K. & Markow, T. A. (2003) Ejaculate–female coevolution in *Drosophila mojavensis*. *Proceedings of the Royal Society B*, **270**, 1507.

Pizzari, T. & Birkhead, T. R. (2002) The sexually-selected sperm hypothesis: sex-biased inheritance and sexual antagonism. *Biological Reviews*, **77**, 183–209.

Pomiankowski, A., Iwasa, Y. & Nee, S. (1991) The evolution of costly male preferences. I. Fisher and biased mutation. *Evolution*, **45**, 1422–1430.

Price, C. S. C. (1997) Conspecific sperm precedence in *Drosophila*. *Nature*, **388**, 663–666.

Price, D. K. & Boake, C. R. B. (1995) Behavioral reproductive isolation in *Drosophila silvestris*, *D. heteroneura* and their F1 hybrids (Diptera: Drosophilidae). *Journal of Insect Behavior*, **8**, 595–616.

Price, T. (1998) Sexual selection and natural selection in bird speciation. *Philosophical Transactions of the Royal Society B*, **353**, 251–260.

Ptacek, M. B. (2000) The role of mating preferences in shaping interspecific divergence in mating signals in vertebrates. *Behavioural Processes*, **51**, 111–134.

Rice, W. R. (1998) Intergenomic conflict, interlocus antagonistic coevolution, and the evolution of reproductive isolation. In: *Endless Forms: Species and Speciation*, ed. D. J. Howard & S. H. Berlocher. Oxford: Oxford University Press, pp. 261–270.

Rieseberg, L. H. (2006) Hybrid speciation in wild sunflowers. *Annals of the Missouri Botanical Garden*, **93**, 34–48.

Rieseberg, L. H. & Willis, J. H. (2007) Plant speciation. *Science*, **317**, 910–914.

Ringo, J. M. (1997) Why 300 species of Hawaiian *Drosophila*? The sexual selection hypothesis. *Evolution*, **31**, 694–696.

Ritchie, M. G., Webb, S. A., Graves, J. A., Magurran, A. E. & Garcia, C. M. (2005) Patterns of speciation in endemic Mexican Goodeid fish: sexual conflict or early radiation? *Journal of Evolutionary Biology*, **18**, 922–929.

Rowe, L. & Day, T. (2006) Detecting sexual conflict and sexually antagonistic coevolution. *Philosophical Transactions of the Royal Society B*, **361**, 277–285.

Rowe, L. & Houle, D. (1996) The lek paradox and the capture of genetic variance by condition-dependent traits. *Proceedings of the Royal Society B*, **263**, 1415–1421.

Rowe, L., Cameron, E. & Day, T. (2003) Detecting sexually antagonistic coevolution with population crosses. *Proceedings of the Royal Society B*, **270**, 2009–2016.

Rugman-Jones, P. F. & Eady, P. E. (2007) Conspecific sperm precedence in *Callosobruchus subinnotatus* (Coleoptera : Bruchidae): mechanisms and consequences. *Proceedings of the Royal Society B*, **274**, 983.

Ryan, M. J. & Keddy-Hector, A. (1992) Directional patterns of female mate choice and the role of sensory biases. *American Naturalist*, **139**, s4–35.

Ryan, M. J. & Rand, A. S. (1993) Species recognition and sexual selection as a unitary problem in animal communication. *Evolution*, **47**, 647–657.

Saether, S. A., Saetre, G. P., Borge, T. *et al.* (2007) Sex chromosome-linked species recognition and evolution of reproductive isolation in flycatchers. *Science*, **318**, 95–97.

Sakaluk, S. K., Avery, R. L. & Weddle, C. B. (2006) Cryptic sexual conflict in gift-giving insects: chasing the chase-away. *American Naturalist*, **167**, 94–104.

Salzburger, W., Baric, S. & Sturmbauer, C. (2002) Speciation via introgressive hybridization in East African cichlids? *Molecular Ecology*, **11**, 619–625.

Searcy, W. A. (1992) Song repertoire and mate choice in birds. *American Zoologist*, **32**, 71–80.

Seehausen, O. (2004) Hybridization and adaptive radiation. *Trends in Ecology and Evolution*, **19**, 198–207.

Sefc, K. M., Payne, R. B. & Sorenson, M. D. (2005) Genetic continuity of brood-parasitic indigobird species. *Molecular Ecology*, **14**, 1407–1419.

Servedio, M. R. (2000) Reinforcement and the genetics of nonrandom mating. *Evolution*, **54**, 21–29.

Servedio, M. R. (2004) The what and why of research on reinforcement. *PLoS Biology*, **2** (12), e420.

Servedio, M. R. & Noor, M. A. F. (2003) The role of reinforcement in speciation: theory and data. *Annual Review of Ecology Evolution and Systematics*, **34**, 339–364.

Shaw, K. L. (1996) Polygenic inheritance of a behavioral phenotype: interspecific genetics of song in the Hawaiian cricket genus *Laupala*. *Evolution*, **50**, 256–266.

Shaw, K. L. (1998) Species and the diversity of natural groups. In: *Endless Forms: Species and Speciation*, ed. D. J. Howard & S. H. Berlocher. Oxford: Oxford University Press, pp. 44–56.

Shaw, K. L., Parsons, Y. M. & Lesnick, S. C. (2007) QTL analysis of a rapidly evolving speciation phenotype in the Hawaiian cricket *Laupala*. *Molecular Ecology*, **16**, 2879–2892.

Simmons, L. W. (2003) The evolution of polyandry: patterns of genotypic variation in female mating frequency, male fertilization success and a test of the sexy-sperm hypothesis. *Journal of Evolutionary Biology*, **16**, 624–635.

Simmons, L. W. (2004) Genotypic variation in calling song and female preferences of the field cricket *Teleogryllus oceanicus*. *Animal Behaviour*, **68**, 313–322.

Simmons, L. W. & Kotiaho, J. S. (2007) Quantitative genetic correlation between trait and preference supports a sexually selected sperm process. *Proceedings of the National Academy of Sciences of the USA*, **104**, 16604–16608.

Simmons, L. W., Zuk, M. & Rotenberry, J. T. (2001) Geographic variation in female preference functions and male songs of the field cricket *Teleogryllus oceanicus*. *Evolution*, **55**, 1386–1394.

Sivinski, J. (1984) Sperm in competition. In: *Sperm Competition and the Evolution of Animal Mating Systems*, ed. R. L. Smith. New York, NY: Academic Press, pp. 86–115.

Sorenson, M. D., Sefc, K. M. & Payne, R. B. (2003) Speciation by host switch in brood parasitic indigobirds. *Nature*, **424**, 928–931.

Storz, J. F. (1999) Genetic consequences of mammalian social structure. *Journal of Mammalogy*, **80**, 553–569.

Swallow, J. G., Wallace, L. E., Christianson, S. J., Johns, P. M. & Wilkinson, G. S. (2005) Genetic divergence does not predict change in ornament expression among populations of stalk-eyed flies. *Molecular Ecology*, **14**, 3787–3800.

Templeton, A. R., Maxwell, T., Posada, D. *et al.* (2005) Tree scanning: a method for using haplotype trees in phenotype/genotype association studies. *Genetics*, **169**, 441–453.

ten Cate, C. (2000) How learning mechanisms might affect evolutionary processes. *Trends in Ecology and Evolution*, **15**, 179–181.

ten Cate, C. & Bateson, P. (1988) Sexual selection: the evolution of conspicuous characteristics in birds by means of imprinting. *Evolution*, **42**, 1355–1358.

ten Cate, C. & Vos, D. R. (1999) Sexual imprinting and evolutionary processes in birds: a reassessment. *Advances in the Study of Behavior*, **28**, 1–31.

Tregenza, T. & Wedell, N. (2000) Genetic compatibility, mate choice and patterns of parentage: invited review. *Molecular Ecology*, **9**, 1013–1027.

Trivers, R. L. (1972). Parental investment and sexual selection. In: *Sexual Selection and the Descent of Man, 1871–1971*, ed. B. Campbell. Chicago, IL: Aldine, pp. 136–179.

Turelli, M., Barton, N. H. & Coyne, J. A. (2001) Theory and speciation. *Trends in Ecology and Evolution*, **16**, 330–343.

Turner, T. L., Hahn, M. W. & Nuzhdin, S. V. (2005) Genomic islands of speciation in *Anopheles gambiae*. *PLoS Biology*, **3** (9), e285.

Vasemagi, A. & Primmer, C. R. (2005) Challenges for identifying functionally important genetic variation: the promise of combining complementary research strategies. *Molecular Ecology*, **14**, 3623–3642.

Verzijden, M. N., Lachlan, R. F. & Servedio, M. R. (2005) Female mate-choice behavior and sympatric speciation. *Evolution*, **59**, 2097–2108.

Veyrunes, F., Dobigny, G., Yang, F. T. *et al.* (2006) Phylogenomics of the genus *Mus* (Rodentia; Muridae): extensive genome repatterning is not restricted to the house mouse. *Proceedings of the Royal Society B*, **273**, 2925–2934.

Via, S. (1999) Reproductive isolation between sympatric races of pea aphids. I. Gene flow restriction and habitat choice. *Evolution*, **53**, 1446–1457.

Via, S. (2001) Sympatric speciation in animals: the ugly duckling grows up. *Trends in Ecology and Evolution*, **16**, 381–390.

Wade, M. J., Patterson, H., Chang, N. W. & Johnson, N. A. (1994) Postcopulatory, prezygotic isolation in flour beetles. *Heredity*, **72**, 163–167.

Weary, D. M., Guilford, T. C. & Weisman, R. G. (1993) A product of discriminative learning may lead to female preferences for elaborate males. *Evolution*, **47**, 333–336.

Wells, M. L. M. & Henry, C. S. (1992) The role of courtship songs in reproductive isolation among populations of green lacewings of the genus *Chrysoperla* (Neuroptera: Chrysopidae). *Evolution*, **46**, 31–42.

West-Eberhard, M. J. (1983) Sexual selection, social competition, and speciation. *Quarterly Review of Biology*, **58**, 155–183.

White, M. J. D. (1968) Models of speciation. *Science*, **159**, 1065–1068.

Wigby, S. & Chapman, T. (2004) Female resistance to male harm evolves in response to manipulation of sexual conflict. *Evolution*, **58**, 1028–1037.

Wigby, S. & Chapman, T. (2006) No evidence that experimental manipulation of sexual conflict drives premating reproductive isolation in *Drosophila melanogaster*. *Journal of Evolutionary Biology*, **19**, 1033–1039.

Wilkinson, G. S., Kahler, H. & Baker, R. H. (1998) Evolution of female mating preferences in stalk-eyed flies. *Behavioral Ecology*, **9**, 525–533.

Wilson, E. O. (1992) The effects of complex social life on evolution and biodiversity. *Oikos*, **63**, 13–18.

Witte, K., Hirschler, U. & Curio, E. (2000) Sexual imprinting on a novel adornment influences mate preferences in the Javanese mannikin *Lonchura leucogastroides*. *Ethology*, **106**, 349–363.

Wolfner, M. F. (2002) The gifts that keep on giving: physiological functions and evolutionary dynamics of male seminal proteins in *Drosophila*. *Heredity*, **88**, 85–93.

Zeh, J. A. & Zeh, D. W. (1996) The evolution of polyandry, I. Intragenomic conflict and genetic incompatibility. *Proceedings of the Royal Society B*, **263**, 1711–1717.

PROFILE

Look to the ants

Edward O. Wilson

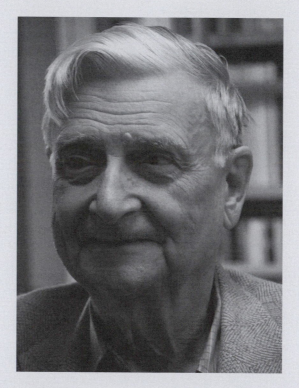

Edward Osborne Wilson. Photo: K. M. Horton.

When I was young I had a rather grim world view, which I developed while growing up in the impoverished state of Alabama during the Great Depression and World War II. Having decided to be an entomologist at any cost, I was under the impression that it was necessary to become an expert on a particular group of insects, and as soon as possible. So at the age of 16, after a passionate dalliance with butterflies, I turned to ants. It was a fortunate choice. Ants are among the most ubiquitous of all insects, they

Social Behaviour: Genes, Ecology and Evolution, ed. Tamás Székely, Allen J. Moore and Jan Komdeur. Published by Cambridge University Press. © Cambridge University Press 2010.

are social, and they are easy to culture and study in the laboratory. By the age of 17, as a freshman at the University of Alabama, I was already maintaining a colony of army ants *Neivamyrmex nigrescens* in the laboratory, where I made my first publishable observations on one of their symbionts, a minute limulodid beetle in the genus *Paralimulodes*.

This was easy! This was fun! Soon, as a senior at the University of Alabama, I took time off to work for the first time as a professional entomologist. By a remarkable stroke of luck, I had been one of the first two persons to record the arrival of the red imported fire ant *Solenopsis invicta* in the United States. That was the summer of 1942, I was 13, and the nest I found was fortuitously next to our house, located several blocks from the docks at Mobile, Alabama. The port was the point of entry of this remarkable species. I made a thorough study of its distribution in 1949, and of its natural history, and continued to use the species thereafter, especially in my later studies on pheromones.

These and other early studies of ants got me into the PhD programme at Harvard. Next I undertook postdoctoral expeditions to tropical America and the South Pacific. My interest at this time was primarily systematics and ecology, and my research resulted in a series of taxonomic monographs and the creation in 1963 of the theory of island biogeography. The latter, which was in collaboration with Robert H. MacArthur (MacArthur & Wilson 1967), has had a considerable impact on ecology and conservation science. But that is another story, to await another time.

Anyone who studies ants broadly, whatever their point of entry, will end up paying considerable attention to social behaviour. He or she is certain to become aware also of the immense diversity of species – 14 000 known in 2010 – and the vast range among them in patterns of social organisation. Very early, as an undergraduate and encouraged by William L. Brown, one of the first mentors who shaped my career, I took up comparative studies of the behaviour of North American dacetine ants. In 1957, using the Dacetini, we published one of the first studies in social insects that correlated the complexity of caste systems with foraging behaviour and prey choice. By this time I had become fascinated by the evolution of ant castes in general. I was inspired by Julian Huxley's earlier work on allometric growth, and took up the basic concept of the evolution of patterns of worker subcastes as generated by shifts in only two parameters of biology, their allometry and the size frequency of the worker population. This approach led to the discovery that size-frequency distributions also evolve as a consequence of colony-level natural selection. In 1953, working off this insight, I published a first account, based on measurements of many polymorphic species, of the evolution of ant castes.

It was obvious to me from this early experience that ants offer a superb opportunity to study the process of group selection in the moulding of social behaviour. Further, as first argued by Darwin in *The Descent of Man*, evolution is multilevel. In modern terms, the genes are the unit of heredity and selection, but the targets of selection are, at one level, the traits that affect the fitness of the individual and, at the second level, above the first, the traits arising from the properties of individuals that affect the fitness of the colony as a whole. The latter process, group selection, is the force that drives the origin and maintenance of altruism and the patterns of caste within colonies.

Working from this principle, I developed the theory of adaptive demography in 1968, and elaborated it in detail by adding colony life-cycle theory in *Caste and Ecology in the Social Insects*, with George F. Oster in 1978. In the early 1980s I extended the theory of adaptive demography to experiments on size-frequency determination in leafcutter ants of the genus *Atta*. By allometry and the negative feedback controls of size-frequency distributions, with the latter at least partially based on caste-specific pheromones, it may be possible to account fully for the evolution of castes in ants.

To study ants also leads one inexorably to pheromones. In the early 1950s, after hearing lectures at Harvard by Niko Tinbergen and Konrad Lorenz on the new discipline of ethology, I was fired by the idea of applying the concepts of sign stimuli and consummatory acts to the social insects. But where the early ethologists were focused on vertebrates, and hence hearing and sight, it was obvious that ants must achieve social order with smell and taste. I joined a small group of researchers pursuing the consequences of this intuition, and in 1959 I was the first to identify the glandular source of a trail substance (Dufour's gland of the imported fire ant). At this time we called the substances 'chemical releasers'; 'pheromone' came a bit later. By the early 1960s, natural products microanalysis had greatly advanced, to the point that micrograms could be identified, the amount present in the bodies of individual ants.

Within less than five years, it was possible for me, with William H. Bossert, to produce the first general theory of pheromone molecular evolution and the physical process of transmission. (For this and related work I was to receive the US National Medal of Science in 1976.)

By the late 1960s it was clear that we badly needed a synthesis of the rapidly growing knowledge of the biology of the eusocial insects – ants, bees, wasps and termites. I provided this in *The Insect Societies* (1971). In this work I also proposed the establishment of a new discipline, sociobiology, defined as the systematic study of the biological basis of all forms of social behaviour. The foundational discipline of sociobiology was (and has remained) population biology. In 1975 I followed this work with *Sociobiology*, in which I added other invertebrates as well as vertebrates. Because the latter included human beings, the book attracted far more attention than would otherwise have been the case. It also became the object of considerable personal animosity, for what in retrospect seem frivolous reasons based on political ideology and the devotion of most of the social sciences to the erroneous doctrine of the blank-slate human mind.

The sociobiology controversy helped to create widespread misperception of the word itself. For many, it came to mean the idea that human nature has a genetic basis (which, in fact, it does). For others, sociobiology came to mean the theory of the role of kinship in the origin of altruism and conflict, which in fact amounts to a particular form of theory addressing one topic of sociobiology. Psychologists tried to escape the confusion and political opposition by relabelling human sociobiology as evolutionary psychology.

In the past two decades, I have devoted more time to biodiversity (I introduced the term in 1988: Wilson & Peter 1988) and conservation biology (Wilson 1992). In 2003 I proposed the concept of the *Encyclopedia of Life*, an electronic register with a website for every species of organism on Earth and containing everything known about each species, available free on command to anyone, anywhere, any time. This idea has now caught on: it is institutionalised and growing at what appears to be an exponential rate.

Yet, in 2005 and continuing in 2009, I have also returned to sociobiology in a re-examination of the theory of the origin of altruism and eusociality. I became convinced that the standard theory, having produced very little new in the past four decades and even then not a great deal, is bankrupt. It has erroneously relied on top-down, mostly mathematical models meant to include all forms of social behaviour, but which from the start were so broad and abstract as to end up explaining very little of any heuristic value. In 2008, in an article in *BioScience*, and later the same year in an article with David S. Wilson in *American Scientist*, I used existing empirical information to suggest a new paradigm, based on what has actually happened in the social insects (Wilson 2008, Wilson & Wilson 2008). It points to close-pedigree kinship as inessential and a consequence rather than a cause of altruism and eusociality.

This suggestion of a radical revision of theory has fluttered the dovecotes among some theorists, and I may be wrong in what I have concluded. But I think it more likely that they are wrong, and in any case wish to make the case here and elsewhere that sociobiology, and in particular the study of social insects, is still wondrously wide open for future investigation.

References

MacArthur, R. H. & Wilson, E. O. (1967) *The Theory of Island Biogeography.* Princeton, NJ: Princeton University Press.

Oster, G. F. & Wilson, E. O. (1978) *Caste and Ecology in the Social Insects.* Princeton, NJ: Princeton University Press.

Wilson, D. S. & Wilson, E. O. (2008) Evolution 'for the good of the group.' *American Scientist*, **96**, 380–389.

Wilson, E. O. (1971) *The Insect Societies.* Cambridge, MA: Harvard University Press.

Wilson, E. O. (1975) *Sociobiology: the New Synthesis.* Cambridge, MA: Harvard University Press.

Wilson, E. O. (1992) *The Diversity of Life.* Cambridge, MA: Harvard University Press.

Wilson, E. O. (2008) One giant leap: how insects achieved altruism and colonial life. *BioScience*, **58**, 17–25.

Wilson, E. O. & Peter, F. M., eds. (1988) *Biodiversity.* Washington, DC: National Academy Press.

20

Social behaviour in conservation

Daniel T. Blumstein

Overview

This chapter develops links between social behaviour and demography, and illustrates how knowledge of social behaviour may be used to manage populations for conservation. The chapter is necessarily speculative, both because the 'formal' field of conservation behaviour is still only a decade old, and because explicit applications of social management are still relatively uncommon. I summarise case studies where social behaviour has been manipulated to manage populations, and suggest possible ways that behaviour could be used to manage populations. After defining effective population size, I list a number of ways that social behaviour may influence it, via genetic variation, survival and reproductive success. Reproductive skew emerges from unequal reproduction, which may be caused by (among other things) social stress, reproductive suppression and infanticide. Social aggregation may reduce natural mortality, and the observations that animals seek conspecifics may be used as a management tool to attract individuals to protected locations. But conspecific attraction and social aggregation may also predispose a population to be vulnerable to human exploitation. Social factors (including reproductive opportunities) may drive dispersal and movements between groups. Humans can influence the structure of social relationships in animals, and these manipulations may influence group stability. Knowledge of these and other mechanisms arms managers with tools to manipulate the habitat or relationships to favourably influence social behaviour and structure, and thereby better manage a population.

20.1 Introduction

Conservation behaviour applies behavioural principles to help conserve (or manage) animal populations (Blumstein & Fernández-Juricic 2004). The link between social behaviour and conservation works through demography. Many wildlife conservation problems are demographic, where a major objective is to increase (or maintain) a population's growth rate, or to increase its likelihood of persisting over time. Demography thus provides a unifying principle that links behaviour and conservation

Social Behaviour: Genes, Ecology and Evolution, ed. Tamás Székely, Allen J. Moore and Jan Komdeur. Published by Cambridge University Press. © Cambridge University Press 2010.

(Anthony & Blumstein 2000). The social structure, social interactions or social behaviour of a population or species may affect persistence via its effects on reproduction or survival. For instance, mating systems influence a population's genetic structure, and therefore population viability. Reproductive competition, a defining feature of highly social species, influences demography via reproductive suppression and infanticide, and these behaviours may influence sustainable harvesting levels in European brown bears *Ursus arctos*, African lions *Panthera leo*, and capybara *Hydrochoerus hydrochaeris*. A feature such as conspecific attraction may generate insights to attract animals to particular locations, but it may also make a species more vulnerable to exploitation. Grouping may reduce predation risk. Finally, because social structure and social behaviour are often adaptive responses to environmental variation, anthropogenic changes may have a profound influence on social behaviour, and consequently on demography and population viability. In this chapter I will describe these and other potential links between social behaviour and wildlife conservation, and provide examples to illustrate them.

What is best for individuals is not necessarily best for the population. This tension is no better illustrated than when we wish to understand how (and why) social behaviour influences demography, and thus population biology. Conservation biologists are obsessed with the number of individuals because they focus on population persistence. An important sub-discipline of conservation biology develops *population viability analyses* (PVA), where the goal is to estimate the likelihood of a population persisting over a given time (Soulé 1987, Beissinger 2002). The process requires decision makers to compile or estimate demographic parameters and to have a clear underlying demographic model (Beissinger & McCullough 2002). All else being equal, a large population is more likely to persist over a given amount of time than a small one.

Remarkably, many PVA models do not include relevant behavioural parameters (Derrickson *et al.* 1998). Whether and how behaviour may affect population persistence is an empirical question, but factors such as Allee effects (negative density dependence: Courchamp *et al.* 1999), conspecific attraction (Stamps 1988), reproductive suppression (Wasser & Barash 1983) and sexually selected infanticide (Ebensperger 1998) all are likely mechanisms through which behaviour influences population persistence. It is by developing explicit models of how these behaviours may influence demography that we will gain fundamental insights into the relationship between social behaviour and population persistence.

The relationship between behaviour and conservation should be explicitly experimental (Blumstein 2007). Wildlife managers are often reluctant to consider that behaviour may influence demography, or to consider potential behavioural interventions. This may be because they have not been formally trained in behaviour (for instance, to be a 'Wildlifer' certified by the US Wildlife Society, a course in behaviour is one of only many electives: www.wildlife.org/certification). Alternatively, it may be because they may believe that behaviour has a relatively small effect on population persistence. Thus, behavioural ecologists who wish to fundamentally influence wildlife conservation should be trained in adaptive management (Walters & Holling 1990, Johnson 1999), and should design their studies to measure the effect size of behaviour on population persistence (admittedly, this may require long-term studies and controlling for a variety of extrinsic and intrinsic factors that influence population persistence). If behaviour has a strong and compelling link to demographic processes, wildlife managers must seriously consider it – much as they already consider the relationship between genetic diversity and extinction risk (Frankham *et al.* 2002). (Remarkably, many decisions in conservation management are not based on adaptive management (Pullin *et al.* 2004, Sutherland *et al.* 2004, Blumstein 2007, Seddon *et al.* 2007). Thus, intrepid behavioural biologists who seek to integrate behaviour into conservation biology may face two sources of opposition: that against behaviour, and that against active adaptive management.)

The field of conservation behaviour is young (Buchholz 2007), and we are still at the stage of creating the toolkit for wildlife managers to deploy when they face a particular problem. The topics in this chapter should be viewed as ripe for exploration. Thus, this chapter is more a prospective review than a definitive summary. Students should realise that there is a lot to work on, and that they can make significant advances by integrating theoretical behavioural ecology with wildlife conservation biology.

20.2 The effect of social behaviour on effective population size (N_e), and its importance to conservation behaviour

20.2.1 Defining N_e

While the number of animals (N) in a population is a first approximation of endangerment, other factors may influence the likelihood of a population going extinct over time. One of these is the population's genetic variation. The effective population size (N_e) of a population better reflects the likelihood of extinction due to genetic homozygosity (Gilpin & Soulé 1986).

N_e is an estimate of the theoretical number of breeding individuals, assuming they behave in an ideal way. An ideal population has the following attributes: the population is split into subpopulations without migration between them, there are no overlapping generations, the number of breeding individuals is the same for all generations and subpopulations, individuals mate randomly, there is a random amount of self-fertilisation, there is no selection, and mutation is assumed to be unimportant (Falconer 1989). Clearly, these assumptions are not likely to be met in most populations of interest to conservation behaviourists. Regardless, low N_e may affect population viability by increasing homozygosity and decreasing the number of non-selected alleles. This loss of genetic variation may be compounded by an increase in linkage disequilibrium, which itself reduces the number of novel gene combinations.

N_e is influenced by factors that impinge on the ability of gametes to be passed to the next generation. Such factors include: exclusion of closely related mating, biased sex ratios, unequal generation sizes, unequal family sizes, inbreeding and overlapping generations (Falconer 1989).

We can see how behaviour may influence N_e by examining an equation to calculate N_e assuming no overlapping generations:

$$N_e = \frac{1}{\frac{1}{4N_m} + \frac{1}{4N_f}} \tag{20.1}$$

where N_e = the effective population size, N_m = the number of breeding males in the population, N_f = the number of breeding females in the population. Calculations of N_e explicitly acknowledge that not all individuals breed (e.g. Nunney 1993, Parker & Waite 1997).

Anthony and Blumstein (2000) suggested that behaviour influences N_e by influencing reproductive skew, the number of breeding individuals and the reproductive rate (Fig. 20.1). They suggested that by focusing on these pathways we could better integrate behaviour into PVA models. I will reiterate some of these suggestions as well as expand our previous discussion to include other social behaviours.

20.2.2 How mating systems may affect N_e

Mating systems influence N_e by determining which gametes will be passed on to the next generation (Anthony & Blumstein 2000). Contrast a genetically promiscuous duck, a harem-polygynous elephant seal *Mirounga* sp., and a genetically monogamous goose with biparental care. Parker and Waite (1997) illustrated (using a modification of the above equation) how mating system influences N_e. They assumed that the population size was 100 and there was a 50% failure rate. The promiscuous species (characterised by each male mating with each female) had an N_e of 67. The monogamous species (where each female mated only with a single male) had an N_e of 50. And the highly polygynous species (where males mated with multiple females but some males did not mate) had an N_e of 19. Interestingly, a highly polyandrous species (where females mated with multiple males but not all females mated) had an N_e of only 9.

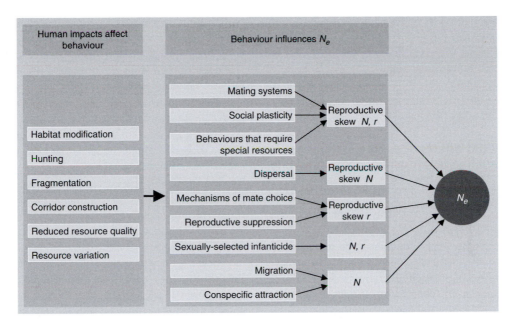

Figure 20.1 Conceptual links between behaviour and demography, and between anthropogenic impacts and behaviour. From Anthony & Blumstein (2000); used with permission.

Greene *et al.* (1998) explored the effects of mating system on the consequences of hunting. They incorporated breeding systems into demographic life-table analyses and subjected their populations to different types of hunting. The effect was profound: populations of monogamous breeders always grew at a slower rate than those of more polygynous breeders. This is because in monogamous systems both males and females are limited in their ability to obtain fertilisations. Hunting strategy (trophy or subsistence) interacted with mating system, but highly polygynous species were less susceptible to hunting-related mortality.

20.2.3 Managing N_e for conservation

A discussion of mate choice, while it may have an effect on N_e (Blumstein 1998), is beyond the scope of this review (see Chapter 10; Swaisgood & Schulte in press). However, mate choice can be manipulated experimentally, as the large literature on sexual selection demonstrates (Andersson 1994), and manipulating

mate choice has been used to address conservation problems (e.g. Fisher *et al.* 2003). For instance, male pygmy lorises *Nycticebus pygmaeus*, an endangered nocturnal primate that relies heavily on olfactory communication, could be made more attractive to females when females had olfactory experience with the males, and when the males' scent over-marked the scents of other males. Manipulating attractiveness is a conservation behaviour tool that can be used in other captive breeding situations.

Because the population sex ratio will influence N_e, and the adult sex ratios of endangered birds are often male-biased (Donald 2007), sex ratios may also need to be adjusted to manage N_e. In an elegant study of the endangered kakapo *Strigops habroptilus*, Robertson *et al.* (2006) capitalised on the evolutionary theory of sex allocation (Trivers & Willard 1973), which suggests that the offspring sex should be a function of maternal body condition. Kakapo managers wanted to ensure all females were in good condition, so they initially provided them ad lib food. This created an unexpected problem: clutches from these extremely well-fed females were highly male-biased! Robertson *et al.* (2006) then successfully shifted the offspring sex ratio by strategically manipulating breeding females' body condition. This technique could be employed in other captive breeding programmes where sex ratios became unnaturally biased towards one sex.

20.3 Other effects of mating systems on population structure and genetic variability

Patterns of reproduction in a group will influence the genetic properties of the subpopulation and population. Traditionally, population geneticists focused on three types of heterozygosity: variation within individuals, variation among individuals in the same subpopulation, and total population variation (Sugg *et al.* 1996). Sewall Wright (1969, 1978) developed fixation indices (F_{IS} – within subpopulations, F_{ST} – among subpopulations, and F_{IT} – within the entire population) that calculate an observed value of genetic variation compared to what would be expected in an ideal population (e.g. with random mating and no mutation or selection). These fixation indices can be used to estimate the degree of inbreeding and therefore the rate at which genetic variation is lost.

Species with social structure, however, violate a fundamental assumption of such models, namely that animals mate randomly within a subpopulation (Sugg *et al.* 1996, Dobson 1998). Does this make a difference in predicting the rate at which genetic variation is lost? Sugg *et al.* (1996), Dobson and Zinner (2003) and Dobson (2007) reviewed a series of studies that concluded it does. The key is that kinship relationships (coancestry), which develop from mating tactics and sex-specific dispersal strategies, develop more quickly than inbreeding in social groups. Historically, kinship and inbreeding were the only mechanisms proposed to account for genetic similarity. Yet the formal models developed to study gene dynamics describe how genetic variation changes as a function of social structure. And it is this genetic structure that it is essential to quantify if one is to properly calculate effective population sizes.

The argument is based on a formal model called the *breeding group model* (Chesser 1991a, 1991b, Chesser *et al.* 1993, Sugg & Chesser 1994). Sugg *et al.* (1996) evaluated the breeding group model by applying it to black-tailed prairie dogs *Cynomys ludovicianus*. These social rodents meet a key assumption of the model: populations are subdivided into groups comprised of kin. Several studies reported that the rate of female dispersal would influence the rate at which genetic variation was lost (Dobson *et al.* 1997, 1998, 2004). As female dispersal rates increased, heterozygosity was lost faster. This finding has a somewhat counterintuitive implication for a commonly used population recovery technique, translocation, which involves moving animals from one location to another to recover a locally extinct population (Kleiman 1989). By moving females from their original colonies to found new colonies, genetic variation was more quickly lost. The results from Dobson and colleagues suggest that it is essential to understand the effect of sociality on gene dynamics when designing management strategies to preserve genetic diversity (see also Chesser *et al.* 1996).

20.4 How relatedness among group members and reproductive skew influence reproduction and population size

Relatedness among group members is likely to influence cooperative and competitive social behaviour, and these are likely, in turn, to influence reproduction and population size. As one example, consider reproductive skew. Unequal sharing of reproduction (i.e. skew) within cooperative groups is a pervasive phenomenon. Vehrencamp (1983) was the first to explicitly propose that the ability to behaviourally create reproductive skew may play an important role in stabilising group cooperation. Her initial models of reproductive skew have been greatly elaborated to focus on the relative control of reproduction within groups by dominants and subordinates (e.g. Emlen 1982, Reeve & Ratnieks 1993, Reeve *et al.* 1998). Such 'transactional' skew models may explain shared reproduction because both dominants and subordinates can increase fitness by living in the groups relative to living alone (Nonacs 2001). Interestingly, transactional models predict that genetic relatedness can strongly influence skew, but this effect also depends on the environmental constraints on group and solitary living (Johnstone 2000, Nonacs 2001).

Because skew influences who breeds, anything that influences skew can affect gene dynamics, and therefore will effect N_e. Ecological constraints have long been known to be important factors explaining social-system variation (Crook 1970, Wilson 1975, Lott 1991) that may affect both social and non-social species. For instance, cooperatively breeding and reproductively suppressed Seychelles warblers *Acrocephalus sechellensis* that were translocated to an isolated island without resident warblers suddenly reproduced. As the small island began to saturate with breeding territories, newly born residents became reproductively suppressed (Komdeur 1992). Similarly, the removal of resident breeding male superb fairy-wrens *Malurus cyaneus* led to the immigration of males that were previously helping their parents raise young (Pruett-Jones & Lewis 1990). In both cases, the lack of available breeding vacancies was identified as an ecological constraint on breeding which consequently generated reproductive skew.

Patchy environments limit dispersal ability and form another possible constraint implicated in the origin of reproductive skew. For instance, in the family of rodents that includes the eusocial naked mole-rat *Heterocephalus glaber*, widely scattered food, arid habitats and hard soils are hypothesised to select for group living (Lacey & Sherman 1997, Lacey 2000). Interspecific variation in mole-rat group size is associated with food density and rainfall (Faulkes *et al.* 1997). However, such constraints are likely to be relatively rare compared to more dynamic variation in ecological factors, such as climate, that affect growing season.

Thus we should generally expect animals to engage in dynamic skew games that may have consequences for population persistence. Identifying the causes and consequences of skew within a species may provide strategies by which managers may increase the likelihood of a population persisting over time. In particular, reducing ecological constraints, and thereby reducing reproductive skew, should increase N_e.

20.5 How reproductive conflict may affect demography

Clearly, reproductive skew has demographic consequences. Skew results from competition among potential breeders, and we generally expect animals to compete for breeding opportunities. Here I discuss two mechanisms of reproductive conflict that may create reproductive skew and have profound effects on demography and population persistence: reproductive suppression and sexually selected infanticide.

20.5.1 Reproductive suppression

Complex sociality is characterised by a reduced probability that all individuals reproduce (Blumstein & Armitage 1998, Cahan *et al.* 2002). Often this is accomplished through reproductive suppression, whereby potentially fertile females do not breed (Solomon & French 1997), and such suppression is often a mechanism that leads to reproductive skew (see Chapter 14). If females living closely with others compete reproductively, then not all females breed or litter sizes are reduced. Reproductive suppression therefore reduces the population size and the effective population size by reducing the number of potentially reproductive females who are able to breed (Anthony & Blumstein 2000).

Habitat saturation may be a direct cause of reproductive suppression and alloparental helping (see Chapter 12). Some species, when faced with no chance to breed independently, engage in alloparental care, and therefore may obtain indirect fitness benefits. Such helping behaviour has been demonstrated to be a strategy whereby individuals make the 'best of a bad job' because, as discussed above, when individuals are translocated to a location with potentially available territories, they immediately begin breeding independently (e.g. Komdeur 1992). Thus, identifying species where habitat saturation suppresses independent reproduction gives us a tool to use should managers need to increase the number of breeders.

Alberts *et al.* (2002) experimentally removed dominant male Cuban iguanas *Cyclura nubila* from a population where they prevented subordinates from breeding. This removal led to formerly subordinate males taking over vacated territories and winning more fights. While the authors were unable to directly study the effect on reproductive success, such interventions might help increase the number of breeding individuals and thus, they argued, prevent the loss of genetic variation.

Mechanisms of suppression can be sophisticated, and they may also affect captive animals that, in theory, have sufficient resources to breed independently. One mechanism of suppression is via social stress (Wingfield & Sapolsky 2003). Such stress-induced sterility works through both the hypothalamic–pituitary–adrenal (HPA) and the hypothalamic–pituitary–gonadal (HPG) axes. Life-history theory leads us to expect that reproduction is traded off against growth and maintenance. Thus, when animals are particularly stressed, they should allocate energy away from reproduction and growth, and mobilise energy to facilitate escape. It is this reallocation of energy that leads to stress-induced sterility. If social animals, in which reproductive suppression is known or suspected to occur in the wild, fail to breed in captivity, then a strategy to increase reproduction might be to reduce the opportunity for social stress by moving animals apart. In some species social facilitation is required for breeding (Hearne *et al.* 1996, Swaisgood *et al.* 2006). It is therefore essential to conduct formal experiments to see whether stress-induced reproductive suppression is reduced by moving potential breeders apart, or whether grouping facilitates reproduction.

20.5.2 Sexually selected infanticide

In harem-polygynous species, sexually selected infanticide is seen when males kill the unrelated offspring of a female to whom they have just acquired access. Access may result from the previous male

dying (either naturally or via hunting), or it may be the outcome of a territorial take-over. Regardless, by killing unrelated young, the new male need not allocate time or energy to care for someone else's offspring and, by eliminating maternal care, he either reduces the time until the female can breed again or increases the likelihood of her breeding with him the next season. Infanticide mainly affects the population size by decreasing the survival rate of infants and reducing juvenile recruitment (Anthony & Blumstein 2000).

Such sexually selected infanticide has been reported in a variety of carnivores, including European brown bears, African lions, non-human primates and many rodents (see Sarah Hrdy's profile; Packer & Pusey 1984, Blumstein 2000, van Schaik & Janson 2000, Swenson 2003, Ebensperger & Blumstein 2007). It has a profound effect on demography because typically males are ignored when modelling population persistence. In populations or species that engage in sexually selected infanticide males (specifically fathers) suddenly become important for persistence, because their presence prevents other males from coming in and killing young.

Sustainable hunting models, in particular, can become more realistic when sexually selected infanticide is considered. For instance, brown bears in Scandinavia engage in sexually selected infanticide (strangely, North American brown bears, i.e. grizzlies, do not). Swenson *et al.* (1997) found that killing a single adult male would decrease the population growth rate by 3.4% and disrupt male social organisation for 1.5 years. However, models that explicitly examined the effects of killing male lions (another species that exhibits sexually selected infanticide) found that current hunting levels should not drive the population to extinction (Greene *et al.* 1998). A capybara harvest model that explicitly compared the effects of sexually selected infanticide by males and reproductive suppression on population size found that the effect size of infanticide was small compared to that of reproductive suppression (Maldonado-Chaparro & Blumstein 2008). Such behaviourally informed models are important tools for the managers of species that exhibit sexually selected infanticide, many of which exhibit declining populations.

20.6 Social aggregation reduces mortality

In some cases it is safer to be in a crowd than alone, and there are many ways that individuals may aggregate (see Chapter 9). For instance, animals may live in temporary or more stable social groupings, or they may breed in a colony site with many other conspecifics. Several models of predation hazard assessment note that per-capita risk declines as group size increases (Krause & Ruxton 2002). This may result from the confusion that multiple prey create when moving around, or it may result from the collective vigilance that emerges when animals are in groups. Regardless of the precise mechanism, for species that benefit from aggregation, predation rates may be density-dependent, and at lower densities there may be a greater risk of predation (e.g. Sandin & Pacala 2005).

The relationships between time allocation and group size are referred to as *group-size effects* (Bednekoff & Lima 1998). Importantly, group-size effects are not restricted to highly social species. Many species form transient foraging aggregations despite no long-lasting social bonds. Group-size effects are typically studied by looking at the relationship between group size and time allocation to foraging and anti-predator vigilance. The general assumption is that if group size provides safety, then we should expect to see that as group size increases, individuals allocate more time to foraging and less time to anti-predator vigilance. In most species, we assume that foraging and vigilance are mutually incompatible: thus time allocated to vigilance cannot be allocated to other beneficial activities, such as foraging.

There are a few difficulties with quantifying group-size effects. The first is that determining whether vigilance behaviour is directed to predators or conspecifics is difficult and not always possible. There have been some attempts in primates by looking at gaze direction (Treves 2000), but most studies are unable to precisely identify the target of vigilance. The second is that there are other reasons

why animals might forage more in larger groups. For instance, if feeding competition increases, then animals will forage more because of increased competition, rather than decreased risk. This is particularly a concern for species that engage in scramble competition on exploitable patches of food (Beauchamp 1998). However, if food is more or less abundant and not particularly patchy, then we should be able to infer that individuals benefit from aggregation if the time allocated to foraging increases as group size increases.

For such species, translocations or reintroductions may need to be carried out with complete social groups. Many translocations and reintroductions for conservation fail because recently introduced individuals end up being killed by predators (Beck *et al.* 1991, Short *et al.* 1992, Miller *et al.* 1994). This creates an ethical issue – animals die because of our actions (Bekoff 2002) – and a practical issue – the recovery may not work (Kleiman 1989). Doing anything to increase the survival of these animals is an important goal of much reintroduction and translocation research (Kleiman 1989, Seddon *et al.* 2007). Thus, by moving animals in social groups, predation rates may decline, and individuals may survive longer. The best evidence that social translocations may improve reintroduction success comes from a study of black-tailed prairie dogs (Shier 2005, Shier & Owings 2007a, 2007b). By moving intact social groups, individuals survived longer because the likelihood of predation was reduced.

20.7 Potential effects of conspecific attraction on survival and management

The presence of other conspecifics may provide compelling evidence that a particular location is suitable. There is a growing body of evidence that animals use conspecifics as cues when assessing habitat suitability and making habitat settlement decisions (Stamps 1988). This phenomenon has been used by conservation biologists to help attract individuals to a particular location (Schlossberg & Ward 2004).

For instance, on the Fort Hood military base in Texas, conservation biologists were trying to recover the endangered black-capped vireo *Vireo atricapilla*, a species that was negatively impacted by brown-headed cowbirds *Molothrus ater* (Ward & Schlossberg 2004). Cowbirds are brood parasites and lay their eggs in other species' nests. Cowbird nest parasitism is responsible for the decline of a number of species, including the black-capped vireo. On the base, cowbirds were eliminated and wildlife managers wanted to attract black-capped vireos to nest in areas where cowbirds were controlled. To do so, they played black-capped vireo song from 04:00 to 10:30 h during the nesting period. They found that in locations where song was played more vireos nested, and these nests were successful. Thus, by capitalising on conspecific attraction, conservation biologists were able to locally recover a population.

Social grouping (and conspecific attraction) may make a species more vulnerable to exploitation. Consider the large colonies of nesting seabirds and marine mammals that made them ripe for exploitation by sailors upon discovering the islands. And consider herding ungulates, such as the plains buffalo *Bison bison*, a species for which Richard Irving Dodge noted that in 1871, while riding through a 25-mile-long herd, 'the whole country seemed to be one mass of buffalo moving slowly northward' (Dodge 1877, p.120). This species was hunted almost to extinction. Or consider the extinct passenger pigeon *Ectopistes migratorius*, a species that lived in such large populations that 'flocks in the migratory period partially obscured the sun from view' (Anonymous 1910).

From the perspective of a hunter, hunting success may be higher on grouped than on solitary individuals. This is because in some situations there is a positive density-dependent relationship between population size and predatory success (Sih 1984). Such a relationship may arise from individuals forming search images, whereby hunting success increases with experience (which is correlated with population size), or because once a patch is located hunting success may increase. For any given predator–prey system, it is an empirical question whether there is positive or negative density dependence, and the specific nature of this relationship may inform conservation.

20.8 How social factors may influence dispersal and movement between groups

In many species, dispersal is influenced by social structure or group size. Residents may disperse if there are no breeding opportunities but remain if there are opportunities within the group. Such facultative dispersal increases the variation in the nature and types of interactions found.

In some cases, wildlife managers wish to eliminate individuals that may have a transmissible disease. However, the outcome of such culling may be an influx of immigrants, and these immigrants may have to form social relationships anew. Such a strategy of killing residents has proved counterproductive in at least two instances where residents were killed to reduce the spread of a disease.

Localised killing of resident European badgers *Meles meles* to eliminate outbreaks of bovine tuberculosis (TB) was found to be counterproductive because this led to the influx of immigrants (Woodroffe *et al.* 2006, Jenkins *et al.* 2007). Badgers can be carriers of TB, and for many years they were locally killed when infections were discovered. However, badger immigrants ranged widely and visited more setts (and communal latrines) than residents. This increased movement was counterproductive because it could increase the rate of transmission of TB between badgers, and potentially from badgers to livestock.

Such a result is generally expected (Smith 2001), and similar findings emerged from a study of brushtail possums *Trichosurus vulpecula* in New Zealand. Killing residents led to increased movement of males in controlled areas, which potentially exposed more possums (and livestock) to TB (Ramsey *et al.* 2002).

20.9 How phenotypic plasticity in social structure may predispose species to respond to anthropogenic activities

The social structure of many species is phenotypically plastic. Such intraspecific variation in social systems is thought to be adaptive (Lott 1991), but it raises the possibility that anthropogenic change can modify social structure. It could do so through at least two mechanisms: modifying the habitat, or modifying the nature of the social relationships.

20.9.1 Modifying the habitat may modify social structure

Modifying the habitat is easier to envision, because many models of social evolution are based on the link between the distribution and abundance of resources and the social system. For instance, the classic Emlen and Oring (1977) model of mating systems is based on the distribution of females being determined by the distribution of food, and the distribution of males being determined by the distribution of females. If females are clumped, and therefore defensible, polygyny may result. Thus, by modifying the distribution of critical resources, either intentionally (as part of a management intervention) or unintentionally (via anthropogenic changes), the mating system may vary. The genetic consequences of a variable mating system were discussed above, as were the consequences of variable group sizes. Thus, habitat modifications may influence survival and reproduction via their effects on mating systems.

20.9.2 Humans may change the nature of social relationships

To understand how human activity may affect the structure of groups, a very brief introduction to social network analysis is required. Social network analysis is a tool that can be used to study the structure of groups (Chapter 9; Croft et al. 2008). Social groups (and structure) emerge from interactions among individuals. In a network, individuals are nodes, and interactions between them form the links. By developing an association matrix of social interactions, it is possible to plot the social network, and to calculate a number of network statistics, both for individuals and for the overall group. These social network statistics formally describe attributes of sociality and, as such, provide a more comprehensive understanding of structure than simple measures like group size (Wey et al. 2008).

One insight from social network analysis is that all individuals in a group may not be equivalent. A network approach to studying sociality suggests that certain individuals may be 'key players' (Borgatti 2003). The removal of key players might have a disproportionate influence on social stability. For instance, in pig-tailed macaques *Macaca nemestrina*, adult males engage in third-party policing whereby they break up fights among females. By doing so, they have a stabilising influence on the rate of agonistic interactions among a group's females. Interestingly, their importance is even greater than would be predicted by a network analysis. Flack et al. (2006) created experimental groups, observed social interactions, and then graphed the resulting network. They then removed certain males from the simulated network, and recalculated network structure (this served as a control). Compared to this control, the network changed even more when males were experimentally removed from the social group.

In African elephants *Loxodonta africana*, female matriarchs possess knowledge that helps increase a group's per capita reproductive success (McComb et al. 2001). These large individuals are often targeted by hunters, and their removal may have disproportionate effects on group productivity. Importantly, their removal has long-term deleterious consequences for young males, who grow up without proper adult control/supervision and become a real problem when they become adolescents (Bradshaw et al. 2005).

Network analyses, and analyses of the pattern of social interactions, can be used to study the consequences of anthropogenic disturbance. For instance, social relationships can be influenced by tourism, as has been found in bottlenose dolphins *Tursiops* spp. (Lusseau 2003a). Specifically, Lusseau used Markov-chain analyses to quantify how behavioural patterns of dolphins were modified by ecotourists. He found that the presence of boats truncated dolphin social interactions. Such interactions are essential for structuring the social group of this fission–fusion species (Lusseau et al. 2005). Lusseau (2003b) also used insights about the scale-free nature of the structure of dolphin social networks to predict that the loss of individuals would not fragment the cohesiveness of a group.

20.10 Conclusions and future directions

This chapter has highlighted selected links between sociality and wildlife conservation. Because wildlife conservation biologists are often faced with relatively small populations, it is essential to understand behaviours that influence demography. I have illustrated how a variety of social behaviours may affect reproduction and mortality. I have also discussed how behaviour may influence gene dynamics, which itself may influence population persistence.

A criticism of conservation behaviour is that there are a lot of implications, but few applications in the form of practical examples of behavioural knowledge helping recovery (e.g. Caro 2007). While not entirely true, this is a valid concern, and conservation behaviourists should work to apply their knowledge to species recovery (Buchholz 2007, Swaisgood 2007). One impediment to application is that wildlife managers are often not trained in animal behaviour. It is by working closely with behavioural ecologists that they will learn how behavioural ecology may be helpful to them. Through such collaborations, they will see if this knowledge can help develop better population viability models, increase the likelihood that animals breed in captivity, and increase the success of population recovery tools such as translocation and reintroduction. Such studies should be designed in the context of adaptive management, whereby experiments are designed to see if a changed model, or a changed management option, has a significant and substantial outcome. If not, the extra costs associated with behaviourally based management may not be that useful. If so, then behavioural ecologists will have made a fundamentally important contribution to wildlife conservation.

Acknowledgements

I am grateful to Ron Swaisgood, Colleen Cassidy-St Claire and two anonymous reviewers for comments on previous versions of this chapter, to Steve Dobson for comments on the gene dynamics section, and to the editors for inviting me to crystallise these thoughts.

Suggested readings

Anthony, L. L. & Blumstein, D. T. (2000) Integrating behaviour into wildlife conservation: the multiple ways that behaviour can reduce N_e. *Biological Conservation*, **95**, 303–315.

Caro, T., ed. (1998) *Behavioral Ecology and Conservation Biology*. New York, NY: Oxford University Press.

Clemmons, J. R. & Buchholz, R., eds. (1997) *Behavioral Approaches to Conservation in the Wild*. Cambridge: Cambridge University Press.

Festa-Bianchet, M. & Apollonio, M., eds. (2003) *Animal Behavior and Wildlife Conservation*. Washington, DC: Island Press.

Gosling, L. M. & Sutherland, W. J., eds. (2000) *Behaviour and Conservation*. Cambridge: Cambridge University Press.

Several special issues of journals have been devoted to conservation behaviour, including the February 2007 issue of *Applied Animal Behaviour Science*.

References

Alberts, A. C., Lemm, J. M., Perry, A. M., Morici, L. A. & Phillips, J. A. (2002) Temporary alteration of local social structure in a threatened population of Cuban iguanas (*Cyclura nubila*). *Behavioral Ecology and Sociobiology*, **51**, 324–335.

Andersson, M. (1994) *Sexual Selection*. Princeton, NJ: Princeton University Press.

Anonymous (1910) Three hundred dollars reward. *New York Times*, 16 January 1910, SM7.

Anthony, L. L. & Blumstein, D. T. (2000) Integrating behaviour into wildlife conservation: the multiple ways that behaviour can reduce N_e. *Biological Conservation*, **95**, 303–315.

Beauchamp, G. (1998) The effect of group size on mean food intake rate in birds. *Biological Reviews*, **73**, 449–472.

Beck, B. B., Kleiman, D. G., Dietz, J. M. *et al.* (1991) Losses and reproduction in reintroduced golden lion tamarins *Leontopithecus rosalia*. *Dodo: Journal of the Jersey Wildlife Preservation Trust*, **27**, 50–61.

Bednekoff, P. A. & Lima, S. L. (1998) Randomness, chaos and confusion in the study of antipredator vigilance. *Trends in Ecology and Evolution*, **13**, 284–287.

Beissinger, S. R. (2002) Population viability analysis: past, present, future. In: *Population Viability Analysis*, ed. S. R. Beissinger & D. R. McCullough. Chicago, IL: University of Chicago Press, pp. 5–17.

Beissinger, S. R. & McCullough, D. R., eds. (2002) *Population Viability Analysis*. Chicago, IL: University of Chicago Press.

Bekoff, M. (2002) The importance of ethics in conservation biology: let's be ethicists not ostriches. *Endangered Species Update*, **19**, 23–26.

Blumstein, D. T. (1998) Female preferences and effective population size. *Animal Conservation*, **1**, 173–177.

Blumstein, D. T. (2000) The evolution of infanticide in rodents: a comparative analysis. In: *Infanticide by Males and its Implications*, ed. C. P. van Schaik & C. Janson. Cambridge: Cambridge University Press, pp. 178–197.

Blumstein, D. T. (2007) Darwinian decision making: putting the adaptive into adaptive management. *Conservation Biology*, **21**, 552–553.

Blumstein, D. T. & Armitage, K. B. (1998) Life history consequences of social complexity: a comparative study of ground-dwelling sciurids. *Behavioral Ecology*, **9**, 8–19.

Blumstein, D. T. & Fernández-Juricic, E. (2004) The emergence of conservation behavior. *Conservation Biology*, **18**, 1175–1177.

Borgatti, S. P. (2003) The key player problem. In: *Dynamic Social Network Modeling and Analysis: Workshop Summary and Papers*, ed. R. Brieiger, K. Carley & P. Pattison. Washington, DC: Committee on Human Factors, National Research Council, pp. 241–252.

Bradshaw, G. A., Schore, A. N., Brown, J. L., Poole, J. H. & Moss, C. J. (2005) Elephant breakdown. *Nature*, **433**, 807.

Buchholz, R. (2007) Behavioural biology: an effective and relevant conservation tool. *Trends in Ecology and Evolution*, **22**, 401–407.

Cahan, S. H., Blumstein, D. T., Sundström, L., Liebig, J. & Griffin, A. (2002) Social trajectories and the evolution of social behavior. *Oikos*, **96**, 206–216.

Caro, T. (2007) Behavior and conservation: a bridge too far? *Trends in Ecology and Evolution*, **22**, 394–400.

Chesser, R. K. (1991a) Gene diversity and female philopatry. *Genetics*, **127**, 437–447.

Chesser, R. K. (1991b) Influence of gene flow and breeding tactics on gene diversity within populations. *Genetics*, **129**, 573–583.

Chesser, R. K., Rhodes, O. E., Sugg, D. W. & Schnabel, A. (1993) Effective sizes for subdivided populations. *Genetics*, **135**, 1221–1232.

Chesser, R. K., Sugg, D. W., Rhodes, O. E. & Smith, M. H. (1996) Gene conservation. In: *Population Processes in Ecological Space and Time*, ed. O. E. Rhodes, R. H. Chesser & M. H. Smith. Chicago, IL: University of Chicago Press, pp. 237–252.

Courchamp, F., Clutton-Brock, T. & Grenfell, B. (1999) Inverse density dependence and the Allee effect. *Trends in Ecology and Evolution*, **14**, 405–410.

Croft, D. P., James, R. & Krause, J. (2008) *Exploring Animal Social Networks*. Princeton, NJ: Princeton University Press.

Crook, J. H. (1970) Social organization and the environment: aspects of contemporary social ethology. *Animal Behaviour*, **18**, 197–209.

Derrickson, S. R., Beissinger, S. R. & Synder, N. F. R. (1998) Directions in endangered species research. In: *Avian Conservation*, ed. J. M. Marzluff & R. Sallabanks. Washington, DC: Island Press, pp. 111–123.

Dobson, F. S. (1998) Social structure and gene dynamics in mammals. *Journal of Mammalogy*, **79**, 667–670.

Dobson, F. S. (2007) Gene dynamics and social behavior. In: *Rodent Societies: An Ecological and Evolutionary Perspective*, ed. J. O. Wolff & P. W. Sherman. Chicago, IL: University of Chicago Press, pp. 163–172.

Dobson, F. S. & Zinner, B. (2003) Social groups, genetic structure, and conservation. In: *Animal Behavior and Wildlife Conservation*, ed. M. Festa-Bianchet & M. Apollonio. Washington, DC: Island Press, pp. 211–228.

Dobson, F. S., Chesser, R. K., Hoogland, J. L., Sugg, D. W. & Foltz, D. W. (1997) Do black-tailed prairie dogs minimize inbreeding? *Evolution*, **51**, 970–978.

Dobson, F. S., Chesser, R. K., Hoogland, J. L., Sugg, D. W. & Foltz, D. W. (1998) Breeding groups and gene dynamics in a socially structured population of prairie dogs. *Journal of Mammalogy*, **79**, 671–680.

Dobson, F. S., Chesser, R. K., Hoogland, J. L., Sugg, D. W. & Foltz, D. W. (2004) The influence of social breeding groups on effective population size in black-tailed prairie dogs. *Journal of Mammalogy*, **85**, 58–66.

Dodge, R. I. (1877) *The Plains of the Great West and Their Inhabitants*. New York, NY: G. P. Putnam's Sons.

Donald, P. F. (2007) Adult sex ratios in wild bird populations. *Ibis*, **149**, 671–692.

Ebensperger, L. A. (1998) Strategies and counterstrategies to infanticide in mammals. *Biological Reviews*, **73**, 321–346.

Ebensperger, L. A. & Blumstein, D. T. (2007) Functions of non-parental infanticide in rodents. In: *Rodent Societies: an Ecological and Evolutionary Perspective*, ed. J. O. Wolff

& P. W. Sherman. Chicago, IL: University of Chicago Press, pp. 267–279.

Emlen, S. T. (1982) The evolution of helping. II. The role of behavioral conflict. *American Naturalist*, **119**, 40–53.

Emlen, S. T. & Oring, L. W. (1977) Ecology, sexual selection, and the evolution of mating systems. *Science*, **197**, 215–222.

Falconer, D. S. (1989) *Introduction to Quantitative Genetics*, 3rd edn. Hong Kong: Longman.

Faulkes, C. G., Bennett, N. C., Bruford, M. W. *et al.* (1997) Ecological constraints drive social evolution in the African mole-rats. *Proceedings of the Royal Society B*, **264**, 1619–1627.

Fisher, H. S., Swaisgood, R. R. & Fitch-Snyder, H. (2003) Odor familiarity and female preferences for males in a threatened primate, the pygmy loris, *Nycticebus pygmaeus*: applications for genetic management of small populations. *Naturwissenschaften*, **90**, 509–512.

Flack, J. C., Girvan, M., De Waal, F. B. M. & Krakauer, D. C. (2006) Policing stabilizes construction of social niches in primates. *Nature*, **439**, 426–429.

Frankham, R., Ballou, J. D. & Briscoe, D. A. (2002) *Introduction to Conservation Genetics*. Cambridge: Cambridge University Press.

Gilpin, M. E. & Soulé, M. E. (1986) Minimum viable populations: processes of species extinction. In: *Conservation Biology: the Science of Scarcity and Diversity*, ed. M. E. Soulé. Sunderland, MA: Sinauer Associates, pp. 19–34.

Greene, C., Umbanhowar, J., Mangel, M. & Caro, T. (1998) Animal breeding systems, hunter selectivity, and consumptive use in wildlife conservation. In: *Behavioral Ecology and Conservation Biology,* ed. T. Caro. New York, NY: Oxford University Press, pp. 271–305.

Hearne, G. W., Berghaier, R. W. & George, D. D. (1996) Evidence for social enhancement of reproduction in two *Eulemur* species. *Zoo Biology*, **15**, 1–12.

Jenkins, H. E., Woodroffe, R., Donnelly, C. A. *et al.* (2007) Effects of culling on spatial associations of *Mycobacterium bovis* infections in badgers and cattle. *Journal of Applied Ecology*, **44**, 897–908.

Johnson, B. L. (1999) The role of adaptive management as an operational approach for resource management agencies. *Conservation Ecology*, **3**, 8 [online] www.consecol.org/vol3/iss2/art8/.

Johnstone, R. A. (2000) Models of reproductive skew: a review and synthesis. *Ethology*, **106**, 5–26.

Kleiman, D. G. (1989) Reintroduction of captive mammals for conservation: guidelines for reintroducing endangered species into the wild. *BioScience*, **39**, 152–161.

Komdeur, J. (1992) Importance of habitat saturation and territory quality for evolution of cooperative breeding in the Seychelles warbler. *Nature*, **358**, 493–495.

Krause, J. & Ruxton, G. D. (2002) *Living in Groups*. Oxford: Oxford University Press.

Lacey, E. A. (2000) Spatial and social systems of subterranean rodents. In: *Life Underground: the Biology of Subterranean Rodents*, ed. E. A. Lacey, J. L. Patton & G. N. Cameron. Chicago, IL: University of Chicago Press, pp. 257–296.

Lacey, E. A. & Sherman, P. W. (1997) Cooperative breeding in naked mole rats: implications for vertebrate and invertebrate sociality. In: *Cooperative Breeding in Mammals,* ed. N. G. Solomon & J. A. French. Cambridge: Cambridge University Press, pp. 267–301.

Lott, D. F. (1991) *Intraspecific Variation in the Social Systems of Wild Vertebrates*. Cambridge: Cambridge University Press.

Lusseau, D. (2003a) Effects of tour boats on the behavior of bottlenose dolphins: using Markov chains to model anthropogenic impacts. *Conservation Biology*, **17**, 1785–1793.

Lusseau, D. (2003b) The emergent properties of a dolphin social network. *Biology Letters*, **270**, S186–188.

Lusseau, D., Wilson, B., Hammond, P. S. *et al.* (2005) Quantifying the influence of sociality on population structure in bottlenose dolphins. *Journal of Animal Ecology*, **75**, 14–24.

Maldonado-Chaparro, A. & Blumstein, D. T. (2008) Management implications of capybara (*Hydrochoerus hydrochaeris*) social behavior. *Biological Conservation*, **141**, 1945–1952.

McComb, K., Moss, C., Durant, S. M., Baker, L. & Sayialel, S. (2001) Matriarchs as repositories of social knowledge in African elephants. *Science*, **292**, 491–494.

Miller, B., Biggins, D., Hanebury, L. & Vargas, A. (1994) Reintroduction of the black-footed ferret (*Mustela nigripes*). In: *Creative Conservation: Interactive Management of Wild and Captive Animals*, ed. P. J. S. Olney, G. M. Mace & A. T. C. Feistner. London: Chapman and Hall, pp. 455–464.

Nonacs, P. (2001) A life-history approach to group living and social contracts between individuals. *Annales Zoologici Fennici*, **38**, 239–254.

Nunney, L. (1993) The influence of mating system and overlapping generations on effective population size. *Evolution*, **47**, 1329–1341.

Packer, C. & Pusey, A. E. (1984) Infanticide in carnivores. In: *Infanticide: Comparative and Evolutionary Perspectives*, ed. G. Hausfater & S. B. Hrdy. New York: Aldine, pp. 43–64.

Parker, P. G. & Waite, T. A. (1997) Mating systems, effective population size, and conservation of natural populations. In: *Behavioral Approaches to Conservation in the Wild,* ed. R. Buchholz and J. R. Clemmons. Cambridge: Cambridge University Press, pp. 243–261.

Pruett-Jones, S. G. & Lewis, M. J. (1990) Sex ratio and habitat limitation promote delayed dispersal in superb fairy-wrens. *Nature*, **348**, 541–542.

Pullin, A. S., Knight, T. M., Stone, D. A. & Charman, K. (2004) Do conservation managers use scientific evidence to support their decision-making? *Biological Conservation*, **119**, 245–252.

Ramsey, D., Spencer, N., Caley, P. *et al.* (2002) The effects of reducing population density on contact rates between brushtail possums: implications for transmission of bovine tuberculosis. *Journal of Applied Ecology*, **39**, 806–818.

Reeve, H. K. & Ratnieks, F. L. W. (1993) Queen–queen conflict in polygynous societies: mutual tolerance and reproductive skew. In: *Queen Number and Sociality in Insects,* ed. L. Keller. Oxford: Oxford University Press, pp. 45–85.

Reeve, H. K., Emlen, S. T. & Keller, L. (1998) Reproductive sharing in animal societies: reproductive incentives or incomplete control by dominant breeders? *Behavioral Ecology*, **9**, 267–278.

Robertson, B. C., Elliott, G. P., Eason, D. K., Clout, M. N. & Gemmell, N. J. (2006) Sex allocation theory aids species conservation. *Biology Letters*, **2**, 229–231.

Sandin, S. A. & Pacala, S. W. (2005) Fish aggregation results in inversely density-dependent predation on continuous coral reefs. *Ecology*, **86**, 1520–1530.

Schlossberg, S. R. & Ward, M. P. (2004) Using conspecific attraction to conserve endangered birds. *Endangered Species Update*, **21**, 132–138.

Seddon, P. J., Armstrong, D. P. & Maloney, R. F. (2007) Developing the science of reintroduction biology. *Conservation Biology*, **21**, 303–312.

Shier, D. M. (2005) Translocation are more successful when prairie dogs are moved as families. In *Conservation of the Black-tailed Prairie Dog*, ed. J. L. Hoogland. Washington, DC: Island Press, pp. 189–190.

Shier, D. M. & Owings, D. H (2007a) Social influences on predator training for conservation. *The Conservation Behaviorist*, **5**, 6–8.

Shier, D. M. & Owings, D. H. (2007b) Effects of social learning on predator training and postrelease survival in juvenile black-tailed prairie dogs, *Cynomys ludovicianus. Animal Behaviour*, **73**, 567–577.

Short, J., Bradshaw, S. D., Giles, J., Prince, R. I. T. & Wilson, G. R. (1992) Reintroduction of macropods (Marsupialia: Macropodoidea) in Australia: a review. *Biological Conservation*, **62**, 189–204.

Sih, A. (1984) Optimal behavior and density-dependent predation. *American Naturalist*, **123**, 314–326.

Smith, G. C. (2001) Models of *Mycobacterium bovis* in wildlife and cattle. *Tuberculosis*, **81**, 51–64.

Solomon, N. G. & French, J. A., eds. (1997) *Cooperative Breeding in Mammals.* Cambridge: Cambridge University Press.

Soulé, M. E., ed. (1987) *Viable Populations for Conservation.* Cambridge: Cambridge University Press.

Stamps, J. A. (1988) Conspecific attraction and aggregation in territorial species. *American Naturalist*, **131**, 329–347.

Sugg, D. W. & Chesser, R. K. (1994) Effective population sizes with multiple paternity. *Genetics*, **137**, 1147–1155.

Sugg, D. W., Chesser, R. K., Dobson, F. S. & Hoogland, J. L. (1996) Population genetics meets behavioral ecology. *Trends in Ecology and Evolution*, **11**, 338–343.

Sutherland, W. J., Pullin, A. S., Dolman, P. M. & Knight, T. M. (2004) The need for evidence-based conservation. *Trends in Ecology and Evolution*, **19**, 305–308.

Swaisgood, R. R. (2007) Current status and future directions of applied behavioral research for animal welfare and conservation. *Applied Animal Behaviour Science*, **102**, 139–162.

Swaisgood, R. R. & Schulte, B. A. (in press) Applying knowledge of mammalian social organization, mating systems and communication to management. In: *Wild Mammals in Captivity*, 2nd edn., ed. D. G. Kleiman, K. V. Thompson & C. K. Baer. Chicago, IL: University of Chicago Press.

Swaisgood, R. R., Dickman, D. M. & White, A. M. (2006) A captive population in crisis: testing hypotheses for reproductive failure in captive-born southern white rhinoceros females. *Biological Conservation*, **129**, 168–176.

Swenson, J. E. (2003) Implications of sexually selected infanticide for the hunting of large carnivores. In: *Animal Behavior and Wildlife Conservation*, ed. M. Festa-Bianchet & M. Apollonio. Washington, DC: Island Press, pp. 171–189.

Swenson, J. E., Sandegren, F., Söderberg, A. *et al.* (1997) Infanticide caused by hunting of male bears. *Nature*, **386**, 450–451.

Treves, A. (2000) Theory and method in studies of vigilance and aggregation. *Animal Behaviour*, **60**, 711–722.

Trivers, R. L. & Willard, D. E. (1973) Natural selection of parental ability to vary the sex ratio of offspring. *Science*, **179**, 90–92.

van Schaik, C. P. & Janson, C. H., eds. (2000) *Infanticide by Males and its Implications,* Cambridge: Cambridge University Press.

Vehrencamp, S. L. (1983) A model for the evolution of despotic versus egalitarian socieities. *Animal Behaviour*, **31**, 667–682.

Walters, C. J. & Holling, C. S. (1990) Large-scale management experiments and learning by doing. *Ecology*, **71**, 2060–2068.

Ward, M. P. & Schlossberg, S. R. (2004) Conspecific attraction and the conservation of territorial songbirds. *Conservation Biology*, **18**, 519–525.

Wasser, S. K. & Barash, D. P. (1983) Reproductive suppression among female mammals: implications for biomedicine and sexual selection theory. *Quarterly Review of Biology*, **58**, 513–538.

Wey, T., Blumstein, D. T., Shen, W. & Jordan, F. (2008) Social network analysis of animal behaviour: a promising tool for the study of sociality. *Animal Behaviour*, **75**, 333–344.

Wilson, E. O. (1975) *Sociobiology: the New Synthesis.* Cambridge, MA: Harvard University Press.

Wingfield, J. C. & Sapolsky, R. M. (2003) Reproduction and resistance to stress: when and how. *Journal of Neuroendocinology*, **15**, 711–724.

Woodroffe, R., Donnelly, C. A., Cox, D. R. *et al.* (2006) Effects of culling on badger (*Meles meles*) spatial organization: implications for the control of bovine tuberculosis. *Journal of Applied Ecology*, **43**, 1–10.

Wright, S. (1969) *Evolution and the Genetics of Populations. Vol. 2, The Theory of Gene Frequencies.* Chicago, IL: University of Chicago Press.

Wright, S. (1978) *Evolution and the Genetics of Populations. Vol. 4, Variability Within and Among Natural Populations.* Chicago, IL: University of Chicago Press.

The handicap principle and social behaviour

Amotz Zahavi

I have been watching birds since I was a child. H. Mendelssohn introduced me to the scientific aspect of ornithology. The book by Niko Tinbergen, *The Study of Instinct* (1951), convinced me that watching birds could be an intellectual challenge. I spent most of 1955 in Oxford with Tinbergen, a year that introduced me to ethology and to the study of behaviour at the gull colony in Ravenglass. In 1970, after working as an activist for conservation in the intervening years, I spent a few months at Oxford with David Lack, who convinced me that individual selection is the only mechanism by which to interpret adaptations.

My doctoral thesis was on the social behaviour of the white wagtail *Motacilla alba*. I was able to show by experiments how ecological conditions, especially food distribution, shape its social system. This study started my interest in studying the relationship between ecology and social systems (Ward & Zahavi 1973).

In 1972, my student and friend, Yoav Sagi, questioned the logic of Fisher's model of mate choice. This stimulated me to develop the handicap principle as an alternative to Fisher's model. The implications of the handicap principle dramatically changed my understanding of evolution. I soon realised that the handicap principle is a necessary component in the evolution of all signals (a signal is defined as a trait that has evolved in the signaller, in order to transfer information to receivers, to affect the behaviour of the receivers in a manner that is beneficial to the signaller). The receiver should respond only to reliable signals, and therefore evolves to respond only to signallers that handicap themselves in something that is related to the information presented by the signal, in a way that makes it harmful to them to make a false signal. This creates a logical connection between the pattern of the signal and the message encoded in it.

The investment in signals has to be differential, easier for the high-quality signaller and more difficult for the low-quality signaller. If the investment is reduced to the extent that all individuals can signal alike, the signal can no longer function to demonstrate differences between signallers, and is selected out by a process similar to inflation – unlike non-signal traits, which keep their value even if the investment required to have them is trivial. This suggests that the evolution of signals follows different rules than the evolution of all other traits. Consequently I modified Darwin's theory of sexual selection, suggesting that all signals, not only those relating to mate choice, are selected by a special mechanism involving waste, in contrast with all traits that are not signals, which are selected to be efficient (Zahavi 1981). I also suggested that the interaction between the two selection

Social Behaviour: Genes, Ecology and Evolution, ed. Tamás Székely, Allen J. Moore and Jan Komdeur. Published by Cambridge University Press. © Cambridge University Press 2010.

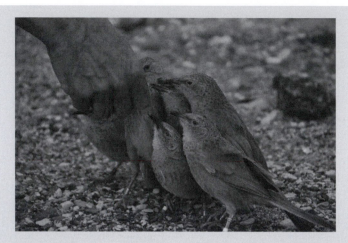

Arabian babblers *Turdoides squamiceps*. Photo: Yosi Fatael.

mechanisms can create novel traits that selection for efficiency alone could not achieve.

I started to interpret and understand the messages encoded in the colour patterns of birds, their vocalisations and movement displays, as well as their complex social displays, from the patterns of their signals. Gradually, I was able to point to the investment involved in patterns, such as lines and dots, that were assumed to display an individual's membership of a set (species, sex or age group), or considered to be indices that do not require investment. These implications of the handicap principle are presented in our book (Zahavi & Zahavi 1997).

Perhaps the most important implication of the handicap principle arose as a consequence of the data we collected on babblers *Turdoides squamiceps*, which compete with one another to serve their group. We interpreted their apparent altruism as a selfish investment in their claim for social prestige (Zahavi 2003). These findings stimulated me to explore the limitations of indirect selection models, and led me to conclude that all of them are vulnerable to exploitation by social parasites (Zahavi 1995, 2003), and consequently that they cannot play a role in the evolution of social behaviour. Hence, I started to explore whether it is possible to interpret other supposedly altruistic social systems

as arising from individual selection, and was able to explain even the 'apparent altruism' of the slime mould *Dictyostelium discoideum* as an example of individual selection (see also Chapter 13 and David Queller's profile).

I found that chemical signals are also loaded with handicaps, and that their patterns provide clues to the messages encoded in them. The same rules apply also to chemical signals within the multicellular organism, to ensure their reliability.

At present we (my wife and I) continue to spend half of our time watching the babblers in the field. I also spend much time reading about hormones and other signals in the multicellular body, and try with my students to reconstruct the evolution of hormones and to understand the relationship of their chemical structure to the information encoded in them. I also continue to participate in struggles for conservation, as I have been doing all my adult life.

I have no idea what might be the important issues in future studies of social behaviour, since there is much more in sociobiology than signals and their effects on social systems. However, I hope that once all the implications of the handicap principle are accepted, the interpretation of social systems and signalling will be greatly affected.

Perhaps it may help if I sum up the principles that have guided my research:

(1) Individual selection is the only selecting force in evolution, including that of microorganisms.

(2) Signals are selected by a different selection process than that of all other traits.

(3) The selection for reliability in signalling creates a logical connection between the pattern of a signal and the information encoded in it. This logical connection provides a clue to understanding the information encoded in the signal from its pattern.

(4) Patterns of signals that seem to be used alike by all individuals are standard patterns by which differences among signallers can be better displayed.

(5) I expect that most common characters have already arrived at an evolutionary equilibrium under the existing circumstances. Hence I question many of the interpretations based on cheating.

(6) I am cautious about formal models, because they are often too simple or wrong in their basic assumptions and hence may be misleading.

References

Tinbergen, N. (1951) *The Study of Instinct*. Oxford: Oxford University Press.

Ward, P. & Zahavi, A (1973) The importance of certain assemblages of birds as 'information-centres' for food-finding. *Ibis*, **115**, 517–534.

Zahavi, A. (1981) Natural selection, sexual selection and the selection of signals. In: *Evolution Today*, ed. G. G. E. Scudder & J. L. Reveal. Pittsburgh, PA: Carnegie-Melon University Press, pp. 133–138.

Zahavi, A. (1995) Altruism as a handicap: the limitations of kin selection and reciprocity. *Avian Biology*, **26**, 1–3.

Zahavi, A. (2003) Indirect selection and individual selection in sociobiology: my personal views on theories of social behaviour. *Animal Behaviour*, **65**, 859–863.

Zahavi, A. & Zahavi, A. (1997) *The Handicap Principle: a Missing Piece of Darwin's Puzzle*. Oxford: Oxford University Press.

21

Prospects for research in social behaviour: systems biology meets behaviour

Allen J. Moore, Tamás Székely and Jan Komdeur

Overview

The study of social behaviour, often called socio-biology, is entering a new phase. A growing focus on mechanisms has enriched the older, evolutionary, perspective of sociobiology. The chapters in this book provide an overview of some of the most influential examples of research adopting the multifaceted approaches used to understand social evolution. There are top-down examinations of the way selection influences behaviour and, therefore, its neural and genetic structure, and bottom-up examinations of the genetic, hormonal or neurobiological substrates of behaviour. We therefore have a detailed understanding of the social, ecological, physiological, neurological, hormonal and genetic factors leading to complex social behaviour, but little integration. Picking apart the components and influences on behaviour is a reductionist approach, and although this has provided considerable insights we argue that it is now time for a synthetic perspective. We argue that a complementary perspective that unifies the particulate knowledge we have gained is now possible, and in keeping with current fashion we label this a *systems biology approach* to studying behavioural complexity. In reality, this is not new but a re-emphasis of the original synthetic view of socio-biology. Systems biology is simply a focus on interactions among components, and it works towards developing a predictive framework for resulting emergent properties of a system. Systems biology depends on a detailed understanding of the component parts to a system, and we believe this will be increasingly available for social behaviour, given the availability of new and less expensive approaches to gaining mechanistic information. These three approaches (systems biology, top-down, bottom-up) will be complementary, and will lead to new ideas and understanding of how social behaviour evolves and structures complex interactions among animals.

21.1 Introduction

The study of the social behaviour of animals is conveniently called sociobiology (see Introduction), and this field of study has come a long way since J. P. Scott coined the term in 1946. The progress is impressive even if marked from 1975, the year of the landmark synthesis of social evolution produced by

E. O. Wilson. Since then, we have discovered an enormous amount about animal behaviour, and studies of social traits have benefited immensely from advances in disparate fields such as bioinformatics, biomedical sciences, statistical theory, economics and conservation biology. As this book attests, in spite of the controversies that plagued sociobiology in the late 1970s, and its predicted demise, the study of social behaviour is alive and flourishing.

21.2 Current research in social behaviour

We can give a brief caricature of sociobiology research from our own experiences as students who started as behavioural ecologists and then diverged. Research on social behaviour has the advantage of being grounded in the principles of evolutionary biology, generating hypotheses and providing a framework for virtually all modern studies. Books by Williams (1966), Wilson (1971, 1975), Dawkins (1976) and Krebs & Davies (1978, 1984, 1991, 1997) stimulated research on social behaviour, and focused on showing how evolution shaped behaviour or how behaviour could be used to test evolutionary principles. Ecology and behaviour were combined, and evolutionary biology and animal behaviour merged so that one was rarely described without the other.

Early behavioural ecologists focused almost exclusively on the adaptive value of behaviour, and were not overly concerned with a reductionist approach – that is, a consideration of the genetic, neurological, developmental and/or physiological mechanisms influencing behaviour. Details of genetic influences and actions were ignored, as genetic variation without constraints was simply assumed – a rationale labelled the *phenotypic gambit* (Grafen 1984). Although powerful, the phenotypic gambit is not as good at prediction as it is at explanation. Eventually, behavioural ecologists began to move towards and embrace a reductionist approach. Students interested in the evolution of behaviour realised that an understanding of mechanism adds to an understanding of evolution (Stamps 1991). Nowhere is this more evident than in recent studies of sexual selection and

maternal effects. Knowing that carotenoids influence colour leads to multiple hypotheses and new tests for why females might prefer bright males (e.g. Blount *et al.* 2003); realising that carotenoids may be passed by the mother to young in eggs only enhances our appreciation of how parents influence their offspring (e.g. Badyaev *et al.* 2006).

A reductionist approach, however, also has its limitations. Understanding genetic, hormonal, physiological, neurobiological or other inputs into behaviour can inform and enlighten, but the real benefits come when researchers combine approaches. New tools certainly help in this regard. Assaying hormones and studying other proximate influences on behaviour has never been easier. Genetic tools have moved from indirect assays of a few isozymes to high-throughput genetics describing entire genomes (Robinson *et al.* 2005, 2008). It therefore seems timely to us to begin to consider how we might unify the previous two top-down or bottom-up approaches to studying behaviour in a *systems biology framework* of social behaviour.

We suggest that developing a systems biology perspective will be critical to the development of our understanding of social behaviour. Systems biology is an approach defined by integration of component parts, with a focus on holism rather than reductionism. The value of systems biology is that it can be predictive, with a focus on interactions, and provide a predictive framework for the emergent properties that are likely to be associated with complex biological systems. Few traits are more complex than behaviour, but, as many chapters in this book attest, social behaviour can be treated like many other traits in terms of its evolution. As with systems biology of cells or enzyme pathways, however, knowing the constituents is insufficient. Knowing how the constituents work together to form a complex phenotype is the real challenge. It is the interactions and emergent properties of systems (and behaviour) that are interesting.

Although complex, the systems biology of behaviour is now within our reach. We are aided by the startling discovery that there is remarkable overlap in the genetic, physiological and neurological components that are combined to form very different behaviours. Who would have guessed that fruit flies and humans have roughly similar numbers of genes? But just as clearly, sequencing genomes alone will not explain how behaviours arise. There is still substantial distance from genome to complicated and complex phenotypes like behaviour. Yet the substrates for diverse behaviours in diverse organisms are often the same. An excellent example of this comes from studies of genetics of parental care and sociality in wasps (Toth *et al.* 2007). Caring wasps (workers or foundresses) have similar gene expression, and this differs from that of egg-laying (and non-caring) queens. Genes in the insulin pathway are involved, suggesting a role for the involvement of nutritional and reproductive pathways in the evolution of care and sociality. The insulin pathway is conserved from insects to mammals, and involved in metabolism, growth, reproduction and ageing (Wu & Brown 2006). The work on wasps, and other molecular genetic studies of social behaviour, suggests there will be great overlap in genetic influences (Robinson & Ben-Shahar 2002, Toth & Robinson 2007). The consequence is that studying one organism is not a luxury, or simply an exercise in natural history. We can expect overlap and insights emerging from seemingly entirely different studies. Generality is not a hope, it is a reality for behavioural evolution.

21.3 Systems biology of behaviour

What is our vision for a systems biology of behaviour? There are many ways to view and define systems biology. At the simplest level, systems biology, typically applied to the understanding of enzyme pathways, a cell, or the working of a simple organism (for instance, yeast), takes constituent parts and asks how they fit together to get a functioning whole. How do the individual pieces of information interact? Systems biology obviously has a long history in ecological research, but more recently systems biology has been used to define the integration of different '-omic' approaches. Systems biology asks 'given the data from multiple –omic approaches (genomics, transcriptomics, proteomics, metabalomics), can we define the way in which the system (cell) functions and the properties that arise?' For behaviour, we feel

we need to go beyond this most narrow definition of systems biology and ask 'given multiple data, from –omics to neurobiology to development to physiology to social systems, can we combine these data to reconstruct the complexity of a behavioural system?' Thus, we advocate the more holistic approach (integrating –omics with other data in studying behaviour) presented by Robinson *et al.* (2008).

Behaviour, especially social behaviour, is best viewed as a complex system with emergent properties arising from the interactions of component parts. Behaviours are rarely simple, single component traits. Consider a trait such as parenting: this can involve direct provisioning of the young, caring for and defending the home, and may even include one parent caring for the other parent (which then allows the first to care for the young). Thus, if we want to understand parenting, we need to understand not only the influences on single behaviours, but also the way in which the behaviours (and other factors) interact. A simple way to rephrase a systems approach is as follows: if we know the parts, can we put them together and get a complete working whole? For behaviour, this would mean understanding the genetic influences (including all of the above –omic approaches), the functional aspects (hormonal, neurobiological) and the ecological and social influences. This is a tall order, but students of social behaviour have long known that emergent properties are an aspect of behaviour that should not be neglected (Fewell 2003). However, neglecting one level can provide a very incomplete picture. As Robinson *et al.* (2008) point out, for example, there is considerable homology at the level of genes for organisms that are distinctly different in their social behaviour.

To develop this argument we provide a somewhat self-indulgent hypothetical example, and develop a scenario where systems biology might be productively applied to temporal kin recognition in burying beetles. We chose this example in part because of its familiarity (Oldekop *et al.* 2007), but also because it provides a tangible example where we can investigate how we might fuse mechanistic and evolutionary approaches and examine interactions at various levels. Our example also contains elements that are traditional subjects for students of behaviour: biological timing, parenting and kin recognition.

Parental attention often increases the fitness of offspring, leading to the evolution of parental care (Chapter 11; Clutton-Brock 1991). However, ensuring that care is provided to related rather than unrelated offspring is a critical parameter that influences many aspects of care, including which sex cares and where and when care might occur (Neff & Sherman 2002, Houston *et al.* 2005, Gray *et al.* 2007). Thus it is unsurprising that in many species mechanisms exist to ensure parental care is directed towards genetic offspring (Neff & Sherman 2002). The question is, however, what sort of mechanism is needed (or can evolve) so that parental care is appropriately expressed. Answering this requires that we know something about the requirements of the system, what existing mechanisms are available and how evolution might fine-tune the system to work. Identifying some potential components of a system should lead to predictions of where other components might be found, thus illustrating one benefit of the systems biology approach. Finally, we expect the system (and therefore its components) to be general.

Temporal kin recognition is a mechanism used by a wide variety of organisms to ensure that they care for their genetic offspring (Elwood 1994). Temporal kin recognition depends on recognising 'own' offspring by the timing of their arrival rather than some endogenous cue. Under this system, potential parents either care for or kill offspring. Related individuals are more likely to receive care, and unrelated to be killed. This is perhaps not 'recognition' per se, but if the arrival time of related offspring is predictable, then the killing of offspring that are around at the wrong time can evolve. Temporal kin recognition is taxonomically widespread, but perhaps best studied in mice, where a male kills offspring that are born earlier than expected based on the timing of his mating with the female (Perrigo *et al.* 1992, Elwood 1994).

Box 21.1 provides an example of how a systems biology approach might lead to understanding the emergent properties we describe as temporal kin recognition. There are undoubtedly unrecognised components in our example; neurobiological aspects of temporal kin recognition have been neglected so far, but given the work on neurobiology of circadian rhythms in *Drosophila* we at least have a starting point. Nevertheless, the burying-beetle example does suggest how adopting an integrative, holistic approach might help us better understand a complex behaviour such as temporal kin recognition.

Box 21.1 A systems biology approach to understanding temporal kin recognition in the burying beetle *Nicrophorus vespilloides*

Burying beetles are among the champion parents of the insect world, directly provisioning their young with predigested carrion (Fig. 21.1a; Eggert & Müller 1997; Scott 1998). Burying beetles such as *Nicrophorus vespilloides* normally kill and eat all insect larvae, only caring for larvae in the nest when their own offspring should be present (Müller & Eggert 1990, Eggert & Müller 1997, 2000). However, during this period, adult beetles will provide care to any larvae. The cue initiating the change appears to be access to a carcass, a resource that is both necessary and sufficient for reproduction by mated females (Eggert & Müller 1997, Scott 1998). The arrival time of larvae is predictable for parents. Females lay eggs 6–12 hours after arrival on the carcass (Eggert & Müller 2000). These eggs begin to hatch around two days later (Smiseth *et al.* 2006). Immediately upon hatching, larvae wander to the carcass, where they are fed by their parents. Disrupting circadian timing with light pulses at other points during breeding affects the timing of the shift from infanticide to parental care (Oldekop *et al.* 2007). Thus, the mechanism that influences timing

Box 21.1 Continued

remains sensitive to photic inputs. This suggests that a timing mechanism that can be reset or refined, such as the circadian system, is involved rather than kin recognition simply being dependent on counting from the discovery of a carcass, as has been suggested for mice (Perrigo *et al*. 1992).

How might such a mechanism work? It isn't a simple coopting without alteration of an existing mechanism, such as endogenous circadian rhythms or seasonal behaviour, as the beetles need to tell time for more than one day and less than a season. It therefore might help if we knew as much as possible about the different components involved. Luckily, there is considerable information available on the genetic aspects of biological timing, especially clocks, in many organisms (Takahashi *et al*. 2008), and hormonal control of insect behaviour (Trumbo 1997). Although there are no studies of clock genes in burying beetles, the genetic and functional components of the circadian clock have been elucidated for many organisms, and shown to be highly homologous (Dunlap 1999, Panda *et al*. 2002, Stanewsky 2003, Looby & Loudon 2005, Merrow *et al*. 2005). In contrast, much is known about the hormonal influences on care in burying beetles because of the work of Steve Trumbo and Michelle Scott in a related burying beetle. In *N. orbicollis*, juvenile hormone (JH, the 'master' hormone in insects) levels spike when burying beetle females are provided with a carcass (Trumbo *et al*. 1995, Trumbo 1997, Scott *et al*. 2001). JH levels rapidly decline, and then gradually rise to a peak around the time of parental care, remaining high throughout the parental-care period (Panaitof *et al*. 2004). This suggests that JH may be the trigger that starts the stopwatch, coordinating egg laying (see Scott *et al*. 2005) and the eventual acceptance of larvae and parental care. A similar though less dramatic spike of JH is seen in males when they first discover a carcass (Panaitof *et al*. 2004, Scott & Panaitof 2004). Levels of JH in males are more dependent on the presence of a mate or larvae (Panaitof *et al*. 2004, Scott & Panaitof 2004), supporting our hypothesis of social facilitation of temporal kin recognition in males. Regardless of the relationship between JH and the initiation of timekeeping associated with temporal kin recognition, however, the mechanism by which the timekeeping ends is not clear. It may be related to the decline in JH, but there must be a cue to initiate this decline.

The details of how nature might convert an oscillatory system, such as the circadian clock, into a stopwatch remain unclear and controversial. However, the possibility that there are shared mechanisms between circadian rhythms and temporal kin recognition, coupled with the detailed understanding of the hormonal changes associated with breeding and parental care in burying beetles, provides a tractable system for experimental investigation. Highly homologous clock genes can provide potential inroads into molecular tools, even though burying beetles are not one of the model organisms for molecular biology. At a minimum they suggest candidate genes that could be investigated with other gene-discovery techniques (Fitzpatrick *et al*. 2005, Toth & Robinson 2007).

At this point, all we know about burying beetles is that they have a complex adaptive behaviour we call temporal kin recognition. We know or can hypothesise some of the components: that the timing mechanism is influenced by photoperiod, that changes in levels of JH are associated with the switch to caring behaviour, and that social influences may be important at least for males. With knowledge of these factors, and given the prevalence of shared components coopted from other pathways shaping complex behaviour, we can begin to speculate on how various mechanisms might fit together and lead to emergent properties seen in this behaviour. In addition, because we have an understanding of the ecological factors, social influences and fitness consequences of temporal kin recognition, we have an evolutionary template for combining components. The richness of this systems biology approach to behaviour is that once we have described the system under specific conditions, we can begin to ask questions of plasticity, gender influences and evolvability.

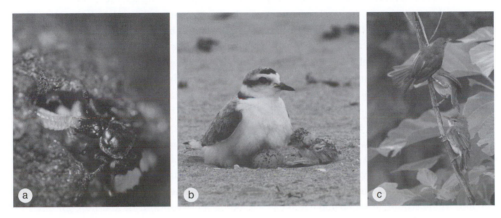

Figure 21.1 Cooperation and conflict in parental care of three organisms. (a) Burying beetle *Nicrophorus vespilloides*: family interactions are structured by both cooperation and conflict; parents feed larvae that beg, but offspring compete for feedings (photo by Allen J. Moore). (b) Snowy plover *Charadrius nivosus*: both parents cooperate during incubation of the eggs, but shortly after hatching one parent (either the male or the female) deserts the brood and leaves the burden of care to its mate (photo by Larry Wan). (c) Seychelles warbler *Acrocephalus sechellensis*: a bird that exhibits cooperative breeding, with parents assisted by non-breeding female helpers (photo by Danny Ellinger).

A systems biology approach to understanding social behaviour does not imply that higher-level investigations are unimportant. The ubiquity of shared mechanisms across species and groups suggests that phylogeny should play a role in systems biology of behaviour research as well. Furthermore, we would ultimately hope to find predictable relationships, and it may be that systems biology approaches further phylogenetic analyses. Is 'parental care' the same trait across groups? At what point are forms of parental care the same or different? We suggest that many of the components that influence parental care should be shared, whether we are examining disparate birds such as plovers (Fig. 21.1b) and Seychelles warblers (Fig. 21.1c), or parental care in birds and burying beetles. Perhaps a systems biology approach will allow us to identify the level of shared components necessary to better interpret phylogenetic comparisons of behaviour. If the interactions of the same components result in the same emergent properties across species or groups, then phylogenetic comparisons may be enhanced.

21.4 What have we learnt from the book?

Our advocacy of adopting a systems biology approach to the study of behaviour should not be read as a criticism of previous approaches, or a suggestion that these are somehow no longer needed. Indeed, this book demonstrates that regardless of the approach that is used to study social behaviour, the hallmark of behaviour is immense diversity. Animals exhibit weird and wonderful behaviours, and when researchers dissect behaviour they reveal unexpectedly complex networks of mechanisms. Furthermore, the areas of biology where an understanding of social behaviour is important are multiplying. This diversity in behaviour, study methodology, research paradigm and applications contributes to the fascination that sociobiology still holds.

Researchers interested in behaviour, including Darwin, Mayr, Fisher, Williams, Wilson, Trivers, Maynard Smith, Parker, Hamilton and many others, have a long tradition of informing evolutionary biology. More recently, we have seen an expansion of the areas on which research in social behaviour has an influence, including topics such as human health, epidemiology, biological conservation, pest control and developmental biology. Yet it is important to know how, when and where studies of social behaviour can be applied, and this requires an understanding of the common mechanisms, substrates and influences. While this sounds straightforward, it can be difficult. Finding homology in behaviour has never been trivial, and remains controversial (Rendall & DiFiore 2007).

Social behaviours are typically complex, and teasing apart the evolutionary significance and the underlying mechanisms is not trivial. Thus, despite our enthusiasm, a systems biology approach to social behaviour may not be appropriate or practical for all questions. Collectively, the chapters in this book suggest two alternative yet immensely fruitful focused approaches that should continue to be productive (Fig. 21.2). On the one hand, many chapters discuss investigations of natural, sexual and social selection acting on social traits, and test how these selective processes influence evolution of brains, neuroendocrine systems and genes (Chapters 1–3, 10 and 11). This top-down approach helps understand how the environment puts pressure on cognitive abilities

and development, and how these selective processes affect genes and genetical evolution.

On the other hand, researchers investigate how specific genes, and gene products (hormones, proteins) in particular parts of the brain or the body, drive behaviour (Fig. 21.2a: bottom-up approach). Initial attempts of the bottom-up approach are illustrated in the fruit fly, honey bee, fire ant and voles (Chapters 1 and 11, profiles by Gene Robinson, Mike Ritchie and Laurent Keller). Again, however, there needs to be integration. Studying genes in social isolation provides limited information, because, if nothing else, social environments are likely to influence gene expression (Toth *et al.* 2007; Wang *et al.* 2008).

Both the bottom-up and top-down approaches to social behaviour, however, face significant challenges. First, rather than gene *or* environment, there are influences from both genes *and* environment, *plus* interactions between genes and environment (Fig. 21.2a; Chapters 1 and 2). Behaviour may well be characterised by an influence of the interaction between genes and environment rather than this being an exception. In addition, an environment is not really only one thing, but rather a host of variables that may interact with each other – and these often change rapidly over both time and space, producing complex density-dependent or density-independent effects (Chapters 10, 11 and 18). Further, virtually unexplored both theoretically and empirically, an association between genes and environment could also influence behaviour. It is expected that organisms sometimes seek out an environment that best matches their genetic make-up: this would generate a genotype-by-environment association (specific genotypes are only found in specific environments) rather than a genotype-by-environment interaction. In addition, traits may be transmitted epigenetically (like bird song: Chapter 3), so a simple genetic approach to social traits can only provide limited information. Finally, studying genetic influences on behaviour allows us to explore the complexity of inheritance in detail. Behaviour may be exactly the sort of trait that will lead to a fuller understanding of how genotypes map onto complex phenotypes.

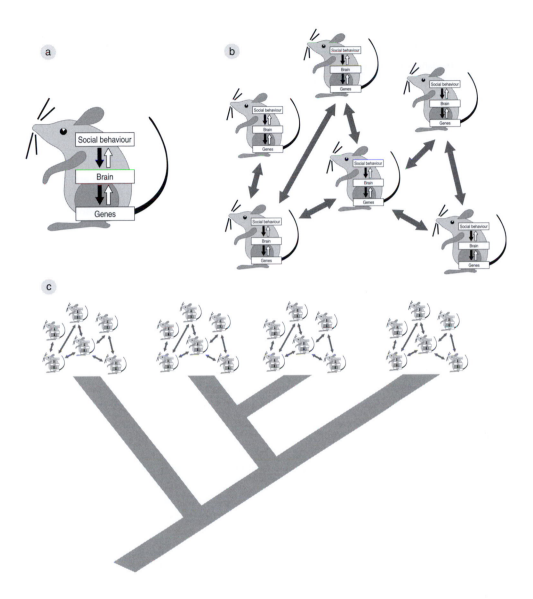

Figure 21.2 Different levels of sociobiological research. (a) The top-down approach (black arrows) and the bottom-up approach (white arrows). (b) Increased complexity occurs when there are interactions between individuals within a population. (c) Including phylogenetic information allows a study of social behaviour over evolutionary time, which we call socio-phylogeography.

Like inheritance, selection can be more complicated when social interactions are involved. The selective advantage (or cost) of a social trait depends not only on the ambient environment (e.g. climate, habitat, etc.) but, importantly, on other individuals that make up the social environment (Chapters 2, 4, 6, 10, 11 and 18), resulting in social selection (Wolf *et al.* 1999). The fluctuating landscape (Fig. 4.1, Chapter 4) is a useful analogy here: by adopting one specific form of behaviour over another, the animals change the fitness implications for their group member, neighbour or mate. Therefore, the locations of the hills and valleys in this fitness landscape constantly change, because an individual's behaviour has implications for the fitness of other individuals and vice versa. It is therefore not surprising that a controversy over group versus individual selection persists (see Chapter 6 and profiles by Edward Wilson and Paul Rainey), as selection in a social contexts does seem to result in special properties. Whether this is better attributed to groups or to individuals is still to be decided.

21.5 Constraints and limitations

Behaviour inherently involves complexity. Therefore it is not surprising that the dichotomous descriptions that have characterised sociobiological research since its conception can stimulate research programmes, but are rarely resolved in favour of one over the other. Generally we end up at a point where both sides have components that best describe the natural world. Thus, while dichotomies serve to generate initial interest and for a focus for research, most have a limited useful lifespan. For example:

- *Nature* versus *nurture*. Chapter 1 makes a convincing case that this debate is futile and unlikely to ever produce a definitive answer. Following the cake analogy used by Dawkins (1981) and others, it is impossible to say what percentage of the cake is recipe and what percentage is ingredients. Clearly, both are needed.

- *Genetic determinism* versus *culture*. This dichotomy is a version of nature versus nurture, usually applied to humans. Humans are clearly unique among animals in many respects, but all animal species are unique in one way or another. They differ in that they have specific adaptations to their environment. Humans, of course, are peculiar in that they have a particularly diverse and sophisticated behavioural repertoire combined with a complex society. Nevertheless, pretending that culture plays no role for any animal other than humans is as untenable as pretending that genes play no role in human behaviour. This is, however, radically different from genetic determinism, as highlighted in

a number of chapters that illustrate how behaviour differs from other traits in its response to environmental influences.

- *Learned* versus *innate*. This is an old argument that just won't seem to go away. In many respects it restates the nature versus nurture argument. A simple thought experiment shows the fallacy of this dichotomy: for learning to have evolved, there must be some genetic basis to the variation in learning ability. If species vary in their ability to learn, and learning is adaptive (experiencing selection), learning is both genetic *and* environmental. It may well be that some species are able to learn better than others, but that is a matter of degree. Furthermore, where researchers have looked for learning, it is often found. This is true for even 'simple' organisms such as invertebrates.

- *Cooperation* versus *conflict*. Both are fundamental ideas that have existed in sociobiological research ever since Darwin (1859, 1871) and Kropotkin (1902). Cooperation is often seen as the defining feature of social behaviour (Tinbergen 1953, West *et al.* 2007). Conflict has also structured investigations of interactions between both related and unrelated individuals (Trivers 1972, 1974, Parker 1979, Arnqvist & Rowe 2005). Recent evolutionary investigations of parent–offspring interactions, mating interactions and sibling interactions are all typically centred on explaining the resolution of conflicts between social partners (Parker *et al.* 2002). There is no question that there is considerable evidence supporting the role of conflict in structuring behaviour. Yet in most of these scenarios cooperation must occur as well. The initial evolution of communication must involve shared interests. Sexual conflict reflected in mating interactions exists only because sexually reproducing species have to cooperate to produce offspring. A complete resolution of conflict by avoiding the opposite sex is evolutionary suicide. It is rarely (if ever) possible to say 'a behaviour is driven by 90% cooperation and 10% conflict.' It may even be that these two are not on a single axis (D. C. Queller, personal communication).

- *Kin selection* versus *group selection*. The theoretical foundation of kin selection and group selection are the same (Chapter 6), and it is hard to imagine an experiment that would unambiguously show that evolution of a given social trait is entirely driven by one of these, but not the other, in a natural system. Nevertheless, it is important that experiments are carefully designed and terminology used with caution (West *et al.* 2007). Adaptive evolution is likely to emerge from diverse forms of selection.

21.6 The unity of sociobiology research

Is there a unifying theory of sociobiology? At the end of this project we have come to two possible answers. On the one hand, yes, of course, we have a theory of adaptive evolution by natural selection, and we see no evidence that social evolution would be distinct (or beyond) Darwin's theory of natural selection (Chapter 6). On the other hand, perhaps our current view of how natural selection operates is not complete, especially with respect to social behaviour. Interacting phenotypes and social selection (Chapter 2), social network theory (Fig. 21.2b, Chapter 9) and evolutionary game theory (Chapter 4) are justified in claiming to be theoretical bases of social behaviour. It will be interesting to watch how these different pieces of theory develop in the future, especially how they coexist and inform each other. Further, combining these microevolutionary details with macroevolutionary information can yield exciting advances (Fig. 21.2c), which we expect will continue to accelerate. Regardless, what is clear is that sociobiology requires a theory of complexity. How do interactions evolve? How do socially contingent traits differ from other traits in their expression? It is these properties and questions that lead us to believe that behaviour serves as a model trait requiring a systems approach that involves an understanding of more than just component parts.

21.7 Conclusions and future directions

Theoretical, experimental and phylogenetic analyses of social traits have produced a wealth of insights and knowledge that are an essential part of science,

culture and societies. In the near future we anticipate progress in nearly all the aspects of social behaviour discussed in this book. We have advocated adopting a systems biology approach to studying social behaviour because we believe a holistic approach is both feasible and likely to yield surprising results. In addition, we identify three avenues of research that we feel are likely to provide important advances:

(1) Better integration of theory with data is needed. The theory of social behaviour is advancing rapidly, and empirical research is needed to uncover the selective value, mechanisms and constraints adopted in a particular theoretical scenario. Empiricists often argue that models are complicated and difficult to grasp, whereas theoreticians often complain that existing data are too simple to test the models adequately. Some of the best theories require a long time to flourish; for instance, Darwin's theory of sexual selection by female choice lay largely dormant for nearly 100 years until it became part of the mainstream research agenda. Yet mate choice is now so widely accepted that we are now seeing calls for attention to be paid to male–male competition (Emlen 2008, Hunt *et al.* 2009)! Such a timeframe, however, is not appealing to a funding agency with a three-year turnover, or to a PhD student with 3–4 years of funding. We believe that the bridge between theory and data needs to be built from both sides. Books such as ours hopefully highlight novel ground for pursuing this desire.

(2) With the development of inexpensive sequencing and the availability of complete genomes for an increasing number of organisms, the bottom-up approach is booming. Indeed, researchers working with non-model organisms benefit from genomic resources produced in model organisms. The gene → brain → behaviour approach should be tested in natural or realistic environments. A sociogenomic approach (see profile by Gene Robinson) is likely to produce fundamentally novel insights.

(3) Behavioural ecologists and comparative biologists have generated a wealth of hypotheses for how selection as a result of the environment

should lead to evolutionary change in a population. The top-down approach (environment → behaviour) should be applied in genetic/neuro-ethological model organisms, where it should be possible to expand it to test the links more fully, generating an environment → genetics → brain → behaviour model. Comparing neuroendocrine systems, genes and genomes across closely related species that exhibit radically different social behaviour in a phylogenetic framework (Chapter 5) would be immensely powerful. Such an integrative approach might best be termed *socio-phylogeography* (Fig. 21.2c).

There is no shortage of fascinating questions, profitable approaches – and surprises – available to students of social behaviour. Researchers in this field have led the way in testing and understanding evolutionary concepts over the past 150 years. However, the ideas and experimental designs penetrate many aspects of biology beyond just evolution. Integrating the study of genes, ecology and evolution into investigations of social behaviour is likely to ensure that biology as a whole will continue to benefit from the creative input of those who examine social behaviour.

Acknowledgements

This chapter greatly benefited from the comments of Martijn Hammers, Gene Robinson, Tamás Székely (Jr) and Jildou van der Woude. Our research and collaboration in this area has been fostered by two EU grants (GEBACO and INCORE).

References

Arnqvist, G. & Rowe, L. (2005) *Sexual Conflict*. Princeton, NJ: Princeton University Press.

Badyaev, A. V., Acevedo Seaman, D., Navara, K. J., Hill, G. E. & Mendonça, M. T. (2006) Evolution of sex-biased maternal effects in birds: III. Adjustment of ovulation order can enable sex-specific allocation of hormones, carotenoids, and vitamins. *Journal of Evolutionary Biology*, **19**, 1044–1057.

Blount, J. D., Metcalfe, N. B., Birkhead, T. R. & Surai, P. F. (2003) Carotenoid modulation of immune function and sexual attractiveness in zebra finches. *Science*, **300**, 125–127.

Clutton-Brock, T. H. (1991). *The Evolution of Parental Care*. Princeton, NJ: Princeton University Press.

Darwin, C. (1859) *On the Origin of Species by Means of Natural Selection*. London: John Murray.

Darwin, C. (1871) *The Descent of Man, and Selection in Relation to Sex*. London: John Murray.

Dawkins, R. (1976) *The Selfish Gene*. Oxford: Oxford University Press.

Dawkins, R. (1981) In defence of selfish genes. *Philosophy*, **56**, 556–573.

Dunlap, J. C. (1999) Molecular basis for circadian clocks. *Cell*, **96**, 271–290.

Eggert, A.-K. & Müller, J. K. (1997) Biparental care and social evolution: lessons from the larder. In: *The Evolution of Social Behavior in Insects and Arachnids*, ed. J. E. Choe & B. J. Crespi. Cambridge: Cambridge University Press, pp. 216–236.

Eggert, A.-K. & Müller, J. K. (2000) Timing of oviposition and reproductive skew in cobreeding female burying beetles (*Nicrophorus vespilloides*). *Behavioral Ecology*, **11**, 357–366.

Elwood, R. W. (1994) A switch in time saves mine. *Behavioural Processes*, **33**, 15–24.

Emlen, D. J. (2008) The evolution of animal weapons. *Annual Review of Ecology, Evolution and Systematics*, **39**, 387–413.

Fewell, J. H. (2003) Social insect networks. *Science*, **301**, 1867–1870.

Fitzpatrick, M. J., Ben-Shahar, Y., Smid, H. M. *et al.* (2005) Candidate genes for behavioural ecology. *Trends in Ecology and Evolution*, **20**, 96–104.

Grafen, A. (1984) Natural selection, kin selection and group selection. In: *Behavioural Ecology: an Evolutionary Approach*, 2nd edn, ed. J. R. Krebs & N. B. Davies. Oxford: Blackwell, pp. 62–89.

Gray, S. M., Dill, L. M. & McKinnon, J. S. (2007) Cuckoldry incites cannibalism: male fish turn to cannibalism when perceived certainty of paternity decreases. *American Naturalist*, **169**, 258–263.

Houston, A. I., Székely T. & McNamara, J. M. (2005) Conflict over parental care. *Trends in Ecology and Evolution* **20**, 33–38.

Hunt J., Breuker, C. J., Sadowski, J. A. & Moore, A. J. (2009) Male–male competition, female mate choice and their interaction: determining total sexual selection. *Journal of Evolutionary Biology*, **22**, 13–26.

Krebs, J. R. & Davies N. B. (1978) *Behavioural Ecology: an Evolutionary Approach*. Oxford: Blackwell.

Krebs, J. R. & Davies N. B. (1984) *Behavioural Ecology: an Evolutionary Approach*, 2nd edn. Oxford: Blackwell.

Krebs, J. R. & Davies N. B. (1991) *Behavioural Ecology: an Evolutionary Approach*, 3rd edn. Oxford: Blackwell.

Krebs, J. R. & Davies N. B. (1997) *Behavioural Ecology: an Evolutionary Approach*, 4th edn. Oxford: Blackwell.

Kropotkin, P. A. (1902) *Mutual Aid: a Factor of Evolution*. New York, NY: McClure Philips.

Looby, P & Loudon, A. S. I. (2005) Gene duplication and complex circadian clocks in mammals. *Trends in Genetics*, **21**, 46–53.

Merrow, M., Spoelstra, K. & Roenneberg, T. (2005) The circadian cycle: daily rhythms from behaviour to genes. *EMBO Reports*, **6**, 930–935.

Müller, J. K. & Eggert. A.-K. (1990) Time-dependent shifts between infanticidal and parental behavior in female burying beetles: a mechanism of indirect mother-offspring recognition. *Behavioral Ecology and Sociobiology*, **27**, 11–16.

Neff, B. D. & Sherman, P. W. (2002) Decision making and recognition mechanisms. *Proceedings of the Royal Society B*, **269**, 1435–1441

Oldekop, J. A., Smiseth, P. T., Piggins, H. D. & Moore, A. J. (2007) Adaptive switch from infanticide to parental care: how do beetles time their behaviour? *Journal of Evolutionary Biology*, **20**, 1998–2004.

Panaitof, S. C., Scott, M. P. & Borst, D. W. (2004) Plasticity in juvenile hormone in male burying beetles during breeding: physiological consequences of the loss of a mate. *Journal of Insect Physiology*, **50**, 715–724.

Panda, S., Hogenesch, J. B. & Kay, S. A. (2002) Circadian rhythms from flies to humans. *Nature*, **417**, 329–335.

Parker, G. A. (1979) Sexual selection and sexual conflict. In: *Sexual Selection and Reproductive Competition in Insects*, ed. M. S. Blum & N. A. Blum. New York, NY: Academic Press, pp. 123–166.

Parker, G. A., Royle, N. J. & Hartley, I. R. (2002) Intrafamilial conflict and parental investment: a synthesis. *Philosophical Transactions of the Royal Society B*, **357**, 295–307.

Perrigo, G., Belvin, L. & Vom Saal, F. S. (1992) Time and sex in the male mouse: temporal regulation of infanticide and parental behavior. *Chronobiology International*, **9**, 421–433.

Rendall, D. & DiFiore, A. (2007) Homoplasy, homology, and the perceived special status of behavior in evolution. *Journal of Human Evolution*, **52**, 504–521.

Robinson, G. E. & Ben-Shahar, Y. (2002) Social behavior and comparative genomics: new genes or new gene regulation? *Genes, Brain and Behavior*, **1**, 197–203.

Robinson, G. E., Grozinger, C. M. & Whitfield, C. (2005) Sociogenomics: social life in molecular terms. *Nature Reviews Genetics*, **6**, 257–270.

Robinson, G. E., Fernald, R. D. & Clayton, D. F. (2008) Genes and social behavior. *Science*, **322**, 896–900.

Scott, M. P. (1998) The ecology and behavior of burying beetles. *Annual Review of Entomology*, **43**, 595–618.

Scott, M. P. & Panaitof, S. C. (2004) Social stimuli affect juvenile hormone during breeding in biparental burying beetles (Silphidae: *Nicrophorus*). *Hormones and Behavior*, **45**, 159–167.

Scott, M. P., Trumbo, S. T., Neese, P. A., Bailey, W. D. & Roe, R. M. (2001) Changes in biosynthesis and degradation of juvenile hormone during breeding by burying beetles: a reproductive or social role? *Journal of Insect Physiology*, **47**, 295–302.

Scott, M. P., Panaitof, S. C. & Carleton, K. L. (2005) Quantification of vitellogenin-mRNA during maturation and breeding of a burying beetle. *Journal of Insect Physiology*, **51**, 323–331.

Smiseth, P. T., Ward, R. J. S. & Moore, A. J. (2006) Asynchronous hatching in *Nicrophorus vespilloides*, an insect in which parents provide food for their offspring. *Functional Ecology*, **20**, 151–156.

Stamps, J. A. (1991) Why evolutionary issues are reviving interest in proximate behavioral mechanisms. *American Zoologist*, **31**, 338–348.

Stanewsky, R. (2003) Genetic analysis of the circadian system in *Drosophila melanogaster* and mammals. *Journal of Neurobiology*, **54**, 111–147.

Takahashi, J. S., Shimomura, K. & Kumar, V. (2008) Searching for genes underlying behavior: lessons from circadian rhythms. *Science*, **322**, 909–914.

Tinbergen, N. (1953) *Social Behaviour in Animals with Special Reference to Vertebrates*. London: Methuen.

Toth, A. L. & Robinson, G. E. (2007) Evo-devo and the evolution of social behavior. *Trends in Genetics*, **23**, 334–341.

Toth, A. L., Varala, K., Newman. T. C. *et al.* (2007) Wasp gene expression supports and evolutionary link between maternal behavior and eusociality. *Science*, **318**, 441–444.

Trivers, R. L. (1972) Parental investment and sexual selection. In: *Sexual Selection and the Descent of Man, 1871–1971*, ed. B. Campbell. Chicago, IL: Aldine, pp. 136–179.

Trivers, R. L. (1974) Parent–offspring conflict. *American Zoologist*, **14**, 249–264.

Trumbo, S. T. (1997) Juvenile hormone-mediated reproduction in burying beetles: from behavior to physiology. *Archives of Insect Biochemistry and Physiology*, **35**, 479–490.

Trumbo, S. T., Borst, D. W & Robinson, G. E. (1995) Rapid elevation of juvenile hormone titer during behavioral assessment of the breeding resource by the burying beetle, *Nicrophorus orbicollis. Journal of Insect Physiology*, **41**, 535–543.

Wang, J., Ross, K. G. & Keller, L. (2008) Genome-wide expression patterns and the genetic architecture of a fundamental social trait. *PLoS Genetics*, **4** (7), e1000127.

West, S. A., Griffin, A. S. & Gardner, A. (2007) Social semantics: altruism, cooperation, mutualism, strong reciprocity and group selection. *Journal of Evolutionary Biology*, **20**, 415–532.

Williams, G. C. (1966) *Adaptation and Natural Selection.* Princeton, NJ: Princeton University Press.

Wilson, E. O. (1971) *The Insect Societies.* Cambridge, MA: Harvard University Press.

Wilson, E. O. (1975) *Sociobiology: the New Synthesis.* Cambridge, MA: Harvard University Press.

Wolf, J. B., Brodie, E. D. & Moore, A. J. (1999) Interacting phenotypes and the evolutionary process II. Selection resulting from social interactions. *American Naturalist*, **153**, 254–266

Wu, Q. & Brown, M. R. (2006) Signaling and function of insulin-like peptides in insects. *Annual Review of Entomology*, **51**, 1–24.

Species index

Subject index